Healthy Sexuality

Third Edition

Richard Blonna
William Paterson University

Lillian Cook Carter
Towson University

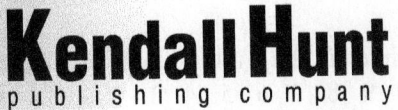

Kendall Hunt
publishing company

Cover design by Will Blonna

Kendall Hunt
publishing company
www.kendallhunt.com
Send all inquiries to:
4050 Westmark Drive
Dubuque, IA 52004-1840

contents in brief

contents

Chapter 3

Male Sexual Anatomy and Physiology   67

Chapter 4

Chapter 5

Chapter 6

Chapter 9

Chapter 10

Chapter 11

Chapter 12

Chapter 13

Human Reproduction   417

Chapter 14

Chapter 15

Chapter 16

Chapter 17

preface

As an introductory text in human sexuality, *Healthy Sexuality* is based on the fundamental information and concepts that have evolved from the body of research in this field. We firmly believe in a biopsychosocial model of human sexuality. In this view, humans become sexual beings and evolve as a result of a continual interaction between biological and psychosocial forces.

We also believe that human sexuality is intimately tied to overall health and wellness. Our overall level of health and wellness plays a big part in our sexuality. *Healthy Sexuality* examines how the components of wellness—physical, intellectual, emotional, social, spiritual, and environmental/occupational—influence our sexual health. Additionally, our sexuality is a key component of our health. The book points out how the healthy expression of our sexuality can improve our overall level of health and wellness.

Essential to being healthy, people have to come to grips with themselves as human beings, to make sound sexual decisions and self-actualize their sexual selves. Although we do cover sexual health concerns and risks (unintended pregnancy, sexually transmitted diseases, date rape, and so on), *Healthy Sexuality* takes a pro-sex rather than a problem-oriented approach to sexual issues. We make no apologies for focusing on the positive, life-enhancing aspects of healthy sexuality instead of presenting sexual topics as a series of problems to overcome.

In the spirit of diversity, we have included information relative to differences between races and ethnic groups, as cited in the most current data generated by the Centers for Disease Control. We use the federally sanctioned language in referring to these groups. We have carefully integrated issues of sexual orientation throughout the book wherever appropriate rather than presenting this as a stand-alone topic in a single chapter. We have incorporated sexual orientation issues into the body of the text, through case studies and in illustrations and photographs. In this way, we hope to project the view of sexual orientation as a healthy part of human sexuality, not a "problem" to be discussed in a separate chapter.

Features of the Text

- The opening page of each chapter begins with a set of **Student Learning Objectives** designed to put the chapter's content into a meaningful framework, to introduce readers to the content of each chapter and personally connect them to the material.
- **Case Studies** throughout each chapter are drawn from the authors' work with students and clients over the years in a number of settings. The case studies cover a diverse cross section of people and are designed to illustrate how the material in the chapter connects to real individuals in everyday situations. You'll meet people like Jorge, a college student who learned the meaning of no the hard way. Although the names have been changed, the cases are authentic.
- **Critical Thinking** questions are inserted next to each case study and bring up questions for readers to answer for themselves. In Chapter 15, for instance, you'll be asked to ponder the issue of discussing one's sexual/medical history with a potential sex partner. You'll be asked to assess the pros and cons of this approach and how a person actually goes about such a task. These questions have no right or wrong answers; they are exercises in critical thinking and represent possible topics for the instructor to consider for group discussion.

- **Personal Exploration Activities** in each chapter allow students to participate in a fun and revealing activity, in which they can explore their feelings and opinions on issues of sexuality. In Chapter 4, for example, students can discover all the things they would never do if of the opposite sex.
- **Healthy Sex Hints** within each chapter are practical, step-by-step suggestions for achieving optimal sexual health and well-being related to the accompanying discussion. Healthy Sex Hints cover a broad range of topics from aphrodisiacs in Chapter 7 to how to perform breast or testicular self-exams in Chapters 2 and 3 respectively.
- **Sex in Society** boxes throughout the text present unusual, interesting, and sometimes controversial material related to the discussion. They add interest and expand upon the basic topic. Sex in Society boxes explore a range of topics such as "Body Image as a Lifelong Concern" in Chapter 4 to the "The HIV Highway" in Chapter 17.
- The text includes an integrated discussion of **Sex and Disability** issues as they relate to healthy sexuality. Our emphasis throughout the text has been that wellness is a continuum and throughout our lives our position on it changes. At any given time in our lives we might have high-level wellness across one or more of the six dimensions of health as we struggle with other dimensions. Disabilities, although they challenge us and sometimes limit some of our options and choices, are presented as just one of many factors that affect our place on our continuum. In Chapter 11, for instance, we examine how living with an ostomy impacts one's sexual response and behavior. In other chapters we introduce people with a host of conditions ranging from being in wheelchairs to having Parkinson's Disease and explore how these challenges affect their sexuality.
- Each chapter integrates **Wellness Syntheses** into key content areas throughout the chapter. These are designed to tie the chapter content to the six dimensions of health and wellness—physical, intellectual, emotional, social, spiritual, and environmental/occupational in a meaningful way. A key facet of our text, this feature demonstrates the linkages between sexuality to health and wellness throughout the text.
- Throughout the text, **Marginal Definitions** identify and highlight key terms that are defined in the margins. These marginal definitions are used to clarify the chapter's content and give the student easy access to the meanings of vocabulary essential to their understanding.
- To further personalize learning, we have added **Personal Assessment** activities at the end of each chapter. These assessment activities are tools for readers to use to apply what they have learned to their own lives—and thereby improve their health and well-being. These assessments range from "Things that Turn Me On" in Chapter 7 to a "Sexual Communication Satisfaction Questionnaire" in Chapter 11.
- The **Thought Questions** and **Test Yourself** quiz at the end of the chapter offer readers an opportunity to assess their mastery of the course material.
- Each chapter contains a list of **References** that includes all of the works cited in the chapter. We have tried to blend the classic works in the field with new material from reputable sources. Besides these features we incorporate data to support the textual presentation through **illustrative tables** and **figures** from the most current sources available, complemented by the classic studies by Kinsey, Masters and Johnson, Laumann and colleagues, and other respected researchers in this field. Finally, the judicious use of **diverse photographs** and **drawings** illustrates important information under the principle that a picture is worth a thousand words.

acknowledgments

First, I acknowledge two people who were early influences in my development as a human sexuality professional. Drs. Richard Cross and Sandra Leiblum of the University of Medicine and Dentistry of New Jersey first opened my eyes to the field and my own sexuality many years ago in one of their intensive sexuality seminars for medical students and invited professionals. Their ease and professionalism in dealing with sexual matters left a lasting impression on me. They provided my first exposure to the scientific, professional study of sexuality and validated sexuality as a scientific discipline worthy of serious study.

I'd also like to thank my mentor and role model, Dr. Marvin Levy of Temple University, for standing out as the epitome of what I consider a "healthy sexuality professional." With his rugged, athletic masculinity, scholarly wisdom, and health background, Marv created an image in my mind of someone able to place sexuality squarely in the framework of health rather than a series of problems to be addressed and feared. I was lucky to come under his influence at a crucial time in my life as a young husband and developing professional. I'm thankful for his guidance in both areas of my life.

I'd like to thank Clifford G. Freund, my mentor with the New Jersey State Department of Health (NJSDH). Cliff nurtured my early career as an STD professional and supported my initial interests in sexuality and education. He had the faith in my work and the wisdom to give me the freedom to explore issues and develop as a sexuality professional.

Lastly, I'd like to thank my co-authors for their contributions to the text. The fact that *Healthy Sexuality* is a balanced, diverse, health-oriented sexuality book is due in great part to the hard work of Jean Levitan and Lillian Cook Carter. Both of these wonderful women have dedicated their professional careers to teaching human sexuality in an honest, open, and supportive way and it shows in their writing and attention to detail. Thanks, Jean and Lillian.

—R.B.

It is not possible to express the thanks I owe to Murray Vincent, an incredible teacher who inspired me to become a health educator. His sexuality class was creative, thought provoking and an amazing growth producing experience. It was because of him that I got my first job teaching sexuality in a college and it was a perfect gift. I also want to thank my students who have taught me probably more than I have taught them. It is because of them that I continue to love working in the area of sexuality. And finally, thanks to Bal, my urologist husband, who is a great resource for confusing issues in the medical aspects of sexuality, and to Rich and Jean who have been wonderful partners in this book.

—L.C.C

Though my graduate school experience was years ago, the training and learning that took place under the mentorship of Deryck Calderwood and the faculty of New York University, along with the incredible work accomplished with classmates, set the foundation for this text. Since then, the professional friendships and constant learning that comes from the Society for the Scientific Study of Sexuality (SSSS) and my network of sexuality educators (ASET) have bolstered my grounding in healthy sexuality.

My gratitude and appreciation extend to Eva Goldfarb, Ernie Green, Konnie McCaffree, Janet Pollack, Donna Ezrol, Arlene Scala, Anthony Nesto, Nancy Begin, Elizabeth Schroeder, Elizabeth Casparian, Emily Joslin-Roher, and my many students whose openness and sharing not only keep me up-to-date but enrich this book. Sue Scott, Dan and Judy Lyons, and Linda Truesdale helped me with the draft manuscript, enabling me to keep to my deadlines. Finally, the incredible understanding, patience, and support of my family throughout the writing process are beyond measure.

—J.L.

We'd like to thank the following people at Kendall/Hunt Publishing: We thank Sue Saad for the opportunity to write this book. Without Sue's belief in the book there would be no second edition of *Healthy Sexuality*. She saw a great book that was about to die and resurrected it. Thanks Sue for your persistence in bringing this book back.

We'd like to thank our Project Manager Stefani DeMoss for framing out the project and keeping us on task. Thanks for helping us with the resources we needed to get the book to press in a record-breaking window of opportunity. We'd also like to thank Elizabeth Roberts for her help with securing the necessary permissions to key material.

Thanks to Will Blonna for a beautiful new cover. The colors are dazzling. Thanks to Jill Martin for her help in researching Richard Blonna's chapters. Jill, you really made updating the chapters easy. Many thanks to Susan Willis for her time and expertise in photographing the various contraceptives methods for Chapter 14.

To our reviewers and class testers—Scott Acrement, Canyon College; Consuelo Bonilla, Kean University; Carol Chenault, Calhoun State; F. Scott Christopher, Arizona State University; Paul Finnicum, Arkansas State; Kay Foland, South Dakota State; Lois Goldblatt, Arizona State University; Elyse Gruttadauria, State University of New York College at Brockport; Lynne Hamelton, West Chester Community College; Edward Hart, Bridgewater State College; Dianna Hurlbut, Irvine Valley College; Eileen Johnston, Glendale Community College; Andrew Kanu, Virginia State University; Richard Larkin, Harper College; Katrina Lubbers, University of Nebraska; Don Matlosz, California State University–Fresno; Susan Molstad, Northwestern State University of Louisiana; Lin Myers, California State University–Stanislaus; Marilyn Myerson, University of South Florida; Bobby Ogletree, Southern University of Illinois at Carbondale; Christine Osgood, Mesa Community College; Dianna Peck, Western Illinois University; Miguel Perez, California State University–Fresno; Valerie Pinhas, Nassau Community College; Catherine Sherwood-Puzzello, Indiana University; Stanley Snegroff, Adelphi University; Sherm Sowboy, California State University–Fresno; Richard Stacy, University of Nebraska; Sonja Swanson, Palm Beach Community College; Tom Tatchell, University of Toledo; Maria Theresa Wessel, James Madison University; William Yurkiewicz, Millersville University—we extend thanks for their time, dedication to thoroughly reviewing the text, and their thoughtful comments that enabled us to improve the manuscript.

Finally, we thank our colleagues in the Department of Community Health at William Paterson University and the Department of Health Sciences at Towson University for providing a supportive work environment.

Richard Blonna   Lillian Cook Carter

about the authors

RICHARD BLONNA, ED.D, CHES, NCC, has been teaching human sexuality for more than 20 years. His initial work in the field was in education and control of sexually transmitted diseases. He served as an STD investigator, counselor, supervisor, and trainer for the New Jersey State Department of Health (NJSDH) STD Control Program. He also worked for the NJSDH as a health education consultant for the AIDS and family planning programs. He has taught human sexuality at Temple University and, most recently, William Paterson University, where he also teaches health counseling, epidemiology, and stress management.

LILLIAN COOK CARTER, PH.D, CHES has been teaching human sexuality at the university level for more than 30 years. She is a health educator at Towson University teaching human sexuality, mental health and stress reduction, and wellness.

chapter

one

Exploring Healthy Sexuality

Student Learning Objectives

After reading this chapter, students will be able to:

- Define *human sexuality*.
- Define *health* and *wellness*.
- Describe the key components of healthy sexuality.
- Explain how the six dimensions of health and wellness impact one's sexuality.
- Compare and contrast behaviors that enhance or inhibit healthy sexuality.
- Describe the key sources of sexual information.
- Evaluate sources of sexuality information.
- Describe the major findings of the key researchers of sexuality over the past 100 years.
- Describe the components of informed decision making.
- Understand some of the health challenges to sexuality.

activity teaser: How "real" are the relationships we see on TV? Find the answer in the Personal Exploration Activity on page 11.

case study 1.1

Maria

Maria, age 25, identifies as Puerto Rican American.

Maria is a full-time, commuter student in her senior year. She is engaged to Nick, a 22-year-old Italian American, also completing his senior year. Maria was finishing up her final project in Dr. Blonna's Human Sexuality class and came in to discuss her paper.

"I'll never forget this conversation," Dr. Blonna recalled, "because it came from such an unlikely source that it was striking. Maria was the quintessential urban woman; tough, street-smart, wise beyond her years, with a cynicism born from years of living in northeastern New Jersey."

I just finished writing my paper and took some time to think through some of the assessments that I took and the work that we did in class this semester. I can't believe how much I've changed in just 16 weeks. I took this class because I was curious about my sexuality and my relationship with Nick.

I was mostly interested in the, you know, the sexual behavior part. I thought that maybe I could learn a few ways to spice up our sex life.

I can't believe how much more I learned about my sexuality and how I never realized how much a part my health played in it. I never even realized what health really was and how things like my spirituality, fitness, and environment influenced it. I took a couple of fitness and body image assessments, and it made me realize that I have never really been comfortable with my body. I guess that is why I have had such a hard time really relaxing with Nick when I am naked and enjoying sex even though he's told me a thousand times he loves my body and likes me just the way I am.

Dr. Blonna asked Maria to tell him about the other parts of her assessment, her spirituality and environmental health.

I rediscovered my spirituality this semester. I guess I had lost touch with it because I'd spent a lot of time over the past few years questioning my faith and the church I grew up in. You helped me realize that it is normal to question our faith and that faith transcends any specific religion. You also made me realize that it was important to not give up my faith as I sorted through my spiritual beliefs and tried to find a connection to something that worked for me. I've kind of started that by doing more things that connect me with nature. I haven't given up on my religion, but I find I am able to think about it differently outdoors than by sitting in church. Nick and I have started getting away from the hustle and bustle of the city on weekends. We've started to drive to the mountains and take long hikes in the woods. We've found some really amazing places within two hours from home that are quiet, peaceful, and beautiful. We really felt that "connection" you talked about in class. We've even gone to the beach in the winter and had the whole place to ourselves. Sometimes we just walk hand-in-hand

Critical Thinking

Maria and Nick are able to escape from the hustle and bustle of their everyday environment and spend time walking in the woods or along the beach. What other strategies could be used to make sure that health needs are met when such escapes are not possible?

for miles without even saying a word to each other. It's like some bond has developed that transcends us. I don't know, it sounds crazy but it's made me appreciate everything a little more.

I guess that I can see the holistic thing you've been talking about in class and in the textbook. I mean, like I am getting in shape by doing all of this walking and nature stuff. My relationship with Nick has never been better. We have this new connection, and I've got to admit we've found that some of these places are great for spontaneous sex. I also think I am beginning to find some kind of rekindling of my spiritual self. Being outside, quietly taking it all in, feeling in touch with my body, feeling sexy toward my man, all of this stuff just seems to make me feel some connection with something bigger than myself.

Maria's case illustrates how one's health plays a crucial role in healthy sexuality. The interplay of the different dimensions of health manifests itself in many ways in our sexuality. As you can see with Maria, often the dimensions of health overlap. Where does our environmental well-being end and our spirituality begin? Where does our physical health stop and our emotional health start? Maria so eloquently describes the interconnections between our health and our sexuality.

Sexuality remains a critical force shaping our lives. It is part of how we see ourselves and impacts our **self-esteem.** It is ever-present as we relate to others on both romantic and platonic levels. Students, as well as the population at large, are constantly confronted with media messages on enhancing sexuality through the use of various products. Sexual themes remain prominent in all forms of entertainment, including books, film, television, and music. As we continue living in the 21st century, students may be struggling to sort out the conflicting messages about "healthy sexuality." Compared to students growing up in the previous century, so much more information is open and accessible. There are choices that are better understood, with the power of the Internet to answer questions that in previous generations may not even have been asked. More and more, individuals are demanding their rights to be who they are in terms of their sexuality.

As health educators, we hold to the position that good decision making is grounded in having accurate information, an opportunity to develop a personal value system, and discussion of possible and probable outcomes of behavior. We advocate the accompanying opportunity to become aware of the variety of sexual lifestyles and concerns of those who are unlike ourselves.

Self-esteem A way of looking at oneself; may be high or low

Our Sexual Climate

To try to figure out how best to make healthy personal decisions in a climate of contrasts is confusing and problematic. Americans talk about sex and sexuality all the time. It is a favorite subject of the media. Some conservative media pundits criticize our culture for its overemphasis on sex. They claim that sexual themes dominate our culture and the media and that the government has gone too far in allowing the free expression of sexuality. Some liberal commentators say exactly the opposite. They claim that our culture is sexually restrictive and downright puritanical.

As examples of a restrictive culture, they cite abstinence-until married sexuality education in the schools, restrictions on reproductive rights, and resistance to the legalization of domestic partnerships/gay marriage. Still others claim that our culture sends mixed messages about sexuality. It is used to market and sell almost everything, yet many schools are not allowed to teach about sexuality in a comprehensive, forthright way.

The reality is that government and society influence our sexuality in many ways, some positive, some negative, and some ambiguous. We are sexual beings from conception to death, and our sexuality evolves and grows regardless of official sanctions or restrictions. We learn about sex whether we do or do not have sexuality education in our schools. It is not a question of *whether* we learn. It's more a matter of the *quality* of what we learn. A key to understanding sexual learning is to realize that we learn about sexuality and what it means to be a man or woman even if no one ever sits us down and has a heart-to-heart talk about the "birds and the bees." And that classic explanation of where we came from is only a small part of understanding ourselves.

Quality sexuality programs result from well-thought-out curricula, with goals and objectives for student learning. Curricula are based on accurate information, in which the pursuit of knowledge is encouraged rather than restricted. Students have a chance to examine their values and the factors that contribute to healthy and appropriate personal decisions. All states do not require sexuality education and in some states certain topics may be prohibited. In our information-rich culture, such censorship further highlights the conflicts students face when attempting to move toward sexual health.

In many ways the sexual learning that takes place outside any classroom is far more influential, as it is constant, both verbal and nonverbal, and often insidious. Students can easily relate the types of misinformation they acquired from friends throughout their childhood and simultaneously often report that their parents didn't talk with them about sexuality issues. In reality, though, parents convey information, impart values, and serve as **role models** whether a formal, face-to-face, serious conversation ever takes place between parent and child. A frown or a raised eyebrow can convey disapproval just as a nod, smile, or laugh indicates support. To be silent on an issue, to omit sexuality from the daily discourse in our lives, to never bring up sexuality as part of the conversation around the dinner table sends a strong message about its being a taboo subject.

Role model A person whose behaviors are imitated by others

Some of what we see and learn, unfortunately, does not present the healthiest picture of sexuality. Sometimes our parents, caregivers, friends, teachers, and media figures do not provide us with the best role models or information for healthy sexuality. The sexual scripts we receive may not promote healthy relationships and in some cases may actually jeopardize our lives. For example, if women are taught that they must be thin to be sexually attractive, what connection might that "lesson" have to eating disorders such as anorexia and bulimia? If men are taught that they are entitled to sex and that women want to be dominated, what connection does that "lesson" have to dating violence and rape? Sometimes the very people and institutions charged with teaching us and nurturing us fail or, worse yet, sexually abuse us.

So what is human sexuality? **Sexuality** is a broad term that refers to all aspects of being sexual. Many people think human sexuality refers to sexual behavior—what people do, how often they do it, and so on. Although sexual behavior is an important part of being sexual, human sexuality encompasses much more than that. Sexuality involves our genetic inheritance, our anatomy and physiology, and the reality of being a sexual creature in a biological sense. It also encompasses our thoughts and feelings about our body and what it means to be a man or a woman. It involves our ethics, values, and the cultural mores we've assimilated through our family, ethnic group, and religious affiliation.

Our sexuality extends beyond the self to encompass our friendships, intimate relationships, and sexual relationships. Lastly, our sexuality does not exist in a vacuum. It is influenced by and influences our environment. Our institutions (schools, governments, and so on), neighborhoods, communities, campuses, states, and countries, and their policies, help shape the person we are and our options as a sexual being.

Sexuality A broad term referring to all aspects of being sexual

Factors That Contribute to Our Sexuality

Our sexuality is influenced by many factors throughout our lives, each impacting our development in similar or unique ways. No researcher or theorist has the widely accepted, definitive explanation for how each of us becomes who we are. Some rely heavily on biology, looking to our genetic inheritance as a prescription for how we will develop. Others hold the culture and the socialization process to be the critical forces that shape our lives. Some believe the psyche processes information as a result of experiences perceived as positive or negative, which in the end cause the individual to become the person he or she is. Finally, some maintain that the person we are is a result of the interaction of heredity/genetics, family socialization, culture, and personal experience.

Without being able to clearly determine which factor is most influential, we do know that we all receive strong and perhaps conflicting messages about sexuality from family, friends, school, media, religion, and the culture. **Sexologists,** those who study sexuality through various rigorous research methodologies, provide input into our knowledge base. Developing a healthy sexuality involves processing that information and, as individuals, internalizing that which is useful.

Sexologists Specialized researchers of sexual subjects from a variety of disciplines including psychology, biology, medicine, nursing, and health

Family

The family has historically been viewed as a critical force in our development. The examination of family influence can focus on both genetic predispositions as well as scripted ways of behaving. Are our ways of being due, therefore, to "nature," "nurture," or combinations of both? From a biological perspective, family represents those to whom one is related "by blood," and, consequently, we may be like our parents and siblings. Complicating that perspective, however, are the various reproductive technologies available today, redefining aspects of the biological connection to parents.

Nuclear family A family made up of the mother, father, and their children

Are we the persons we are because of how we were reared? In a social sense, the term *family* has taken on broader connotations as people's living arrangements take on a variety of forms. Divorce, remarriage, stepfamilies, blended families, and single families introduce new models.

The traditional **nuclear family,** consisting of a married man and woman and their biological children, represents less than half of all households in the United States today. The primary caregiver thus may assume a greater role in a child's development than previously. The challenge comes in trying to evaluate the impact of various family arrangements on a family's members.

The impact of parental influence on sexuality is still open to debate. For example, the societal concern with homosexuality has led courts—almost exclusively, until more recent times—to award children to the heterosexual parent in custody cases resulting from divorce. The concern is that gay or lesbian parents will influence their children to be gay or lesbian. That the heterosexual parents of the gay and lesbian adults were unable to influence their children's orientation is not given the same credibility.

As we will discuss later, good parenting skills, rather than the parents' sexual orientation, are key to raising healthy children. The family influences the development of healthy sexuality in numerous ways. Through family, we learn gender roles and expectations, are taught about love and affection, learn patterns of touch, develop a sense of our physical selves, and assume patterns of social interaction. In each of these areas, our experiences can lead to healthy or unhealthy development.

In some areas of parenting, a number of approaches can lead to healthy sexual development. It is generally accepted that parents should be loving and supportive toward their children. Children who receive physical affection will, in turn, be more likely to be able to give affection to others. Embedded in such general advice, however, are individual patterns that may be criticized. For example, research has shown that boy children stop

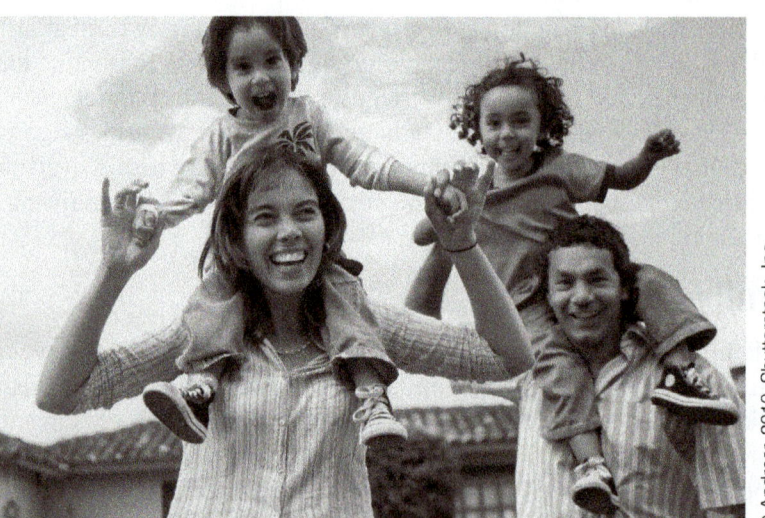

Children learn about sex from their families without it ever being mentioned.

© Andresr, 2010. Shutterstock, Inc.

receiving physical affection earlier than girls, who may continue to be hugged and kissed throughout their lives. Does the change in the type of touch boys receive impact their adult patterns?

In terms of **gender role** expectations, most parents reinforce gender-stereotyped behaviors very early on. Boys are expected to play aggressively and to enjoy trucks, Legos, action figures, and the like. Girls get socialized to plan for motherhood, beauty, and domestic tasks. The women's movement of the late 1960s and early 1970s questioned the impact of gender stereotyping on the healthy development of boys and girls. Years later, television commercials for children's toys reveal little departure from the traditional gender role expectations. Toy manufacturers, in their defense, claim they are marketing to the children who will buy their products. When they have attempted to market toys in a more gender-neutral manner, their efforts have not been successful. Families have different views on what is socially acceptable and what toys they want to purchase, yet children seem to develop their own preferences regardless of their parent's efforts.

Gender role The different behaviors and attitudes that society expects of females and males

Friends

One's peer group has always maintained a powerful role in shaping our attitudes and values about sexuality. Depending on the friends with whom we socialize, we have various experiences at different ages. Teens may refer to others as "being in the fast crowd"—which may mean that more sexual activity and drinking take place. Kids may refer to others as "geeks" or "nerds"—meaning that, though smart, they seem to lack social skills and have interests that are "not cool." Regardless, peer pressure, social judgments, and opportunities all interact to influence healthy development. At the same time, those very influences can leave a negative mark dominated by low self-esteem, depression, and feelings of inadequacy.

Most students report that the bulk of their sexuality education comes from talks with friends. They say that some friends passed along accurate information, and others spoke with authority while dispensing inaccurate information. Students have reported that, as children and teens, they saw sexually explicit pictures, magazines, and videos at a friend's home—all supposedly belonging to "my friend's dad." The sneaking around and the searching through hidden material convey a message about sexuality.

Culture

Anthropologists have defined **culture** as anything and everything that humans learn. Implied within that is a learned set of rules for appropriate behavior. In practice, when addressing issues of culture, what actually may be under study are influences of race, class, religion, and ethnicity. All cultures have established rules to regulate sexual activity (Mindlin, Wallace, & Kapell, 2002). Some are viewed as restrictive, and others are seen as permissive.

Even though Western cultures share certain traditions and values—such as patriarchy, monogamy, having children within marriage—actual behavior varies from one group to another. As the United States becomes

Culture The sum of the learned set of rules governing the behavior of people, often focused on the influences of race, class, religion, and ethnicity

case study 1.2

Karen, with Eyes Wide Open

Karen, age 24, is white.

I remember, as a kid, traveling with the "in crowd" in middle school. There was a group of about 25 of us, and we started having boy-girl parties around the sixth grade. A couple of girls were considered the "pretty ones," and they had the boyfriends. I always got invited to the parties but ended up "watching" rather than participating. There were kissing games, close dancing, and the girls with developed chests invariably let some of the boys "cop a feel." I remember my mother, in particular, being very concerned that certain kids were "bad influences." Despite her reservations about some of my peers, I wasn't being approached, so there were no decisions for me to make. I was watching and learning . . . just not being asked to participate.

I had one friend who my mother worried was a "bad influence." Her parents were divorced, her father was out of the picture, and she was living with her elderly grandparents. One weekend she invited me to join her on a visit to her mother's apartment in the city. My friend confided that her mother had two different boyfriends; in retrospect, I realize that her mom had slept with both of them. I remember feeling uncomfortable watching my friend's mother walk around the apartment in her underwear, sit on her boyfriend's lap, and kiss him. Somehow I knew that my own mother would have been very upset if she knew what type of education I was getting!

an increasingly pluralistic society, it is forced to confront what may seem to be "foreign" practices. For example, female genital mutilation (discussed more fully with female anatomy and physiology in Chapter 2) is a custom practiced primarily in parts of Africa. Today, U.S. health care providers find themselves caring for girls and women who have undergone this mutilating experience.

Newspapers and magazines will report on international cases where punishments are meted out for those individuals whose sexual behavior violates the established culture. One case involved a couple living on the run in England. The woman was afraid that her father or brother was going to kill her because she had defied her culture by choosing her partner. Western ideas of falling in love, being able to decide whom to marry, and the like, were in direct conflict with her Muslim upbringing, which dictated that the bride's father arrange the marriage, with her input having little or no value. In 2003, pressure from outside nations resulted in a Nigerian court saving a woman from being stoned to death. She had given birth to a child as a result of being raped, yet her village court had labeled the crime adultery, requiring her to be punished.

Both these case studies (1.1 & 1.2) confront students with cultural practices different from what is common in the United States. Our cultural beliefs have also been cited as justification for involvement in war, and have made us the target for terrorism abroad and at home. The wars in Iraq and Afghanistan, the terrorist attacks of 9/11, the Boston Marathon attack, and the subsequent vulnerability we have felt on our home soil have changed us all forever.

Loss, grief, and fear brought on by the aforementioned events have changed our collective culture and have many implications for personal wellness and sexuality. They affect our trust, our ability to form intimate loving relationships, and our sexual desire (Davey, 2002; Dettmer, 2001). Studies have shown that blood levels of testosterone, the hormone of sexual desire, diminish in response to such events (Tsigos & Chrousos, 1996). Debra Straw (2001), a professor from Burlington, Vermont, writing in *Community College Week,* describes this so eloquently in the following passage: "One young woman, normally an A student, told me last week that she has been getting B's and that she has been taking depression medication and getting therapy as a direct result of what has been happening in the larger world. These young people now live in fear and uncertainty. Their American Dream seems to have been blown away" (p. 3).

The terrorist attacks of 9/11 threatened the diversity that is so vital to a well-rounded college experience (Garmon, 2001). Terror, fear, anger, and suffering impacted the previous level of acceptance and understanding of students from different cultures, particularly those of the Middle East. Some campuses across the nation reported backlash against Middle Eastern students, professors, and staff, and Islamic studies and culture (Boulard, 2001). This creates a campus climate that is not healthy and safe. We firmly believe that for healthy sexuality to occur, one's environment must be safe and conducive to a free expression of ideas and lifestyles. When tolerance and acceptance are replaced by intolerance and rejection, everyone suffers.

Popular Culture

Terrorism and threats of war, however, do not seem to interrupt popular culture's fascination with sexuality. Television programs in the early 2000s increasingly have brought the viewer into the lives and bedrooms of dating couples.

People meet on television, date in front of a camera, get sexually involved in front of a camera, and even marry, sometimes to someone either picked by their parents or voted on by viewers. While television has become more direct about sexual humor and sexual content, it has also taken greater responsibility in discussing sexual issues in a more forthright manner. Cable television can be credited for leading the way for greater openness; competition for viewers has brought the traditional networks along. For example, the History Channel developed a few multipart series on sexuality, looking at sexuality in the 20th century and another beginning in ancient times. Viewers can also find segments on sexual issues on such news programs as *20/20, Dateline,* and *Primetime,* along with a variety of topics covered by public television stations.

The sexuality of the rich and famous continues to be scrutinized. The years 2002–2003 were witness to Michael Jackson, the pop singer, coming under intense scrutiny for his interest in children, with possible charges of sexual abuse. Catholic priests across the United States were brought to task for the years of sexual abuse covered up by the church hierarchy. Rabbis

personal exploration activity
All That Glitters Is Not Gold

The goal of this activity is to stimulate you to take a critical view of ideas and actions related to sexuality that are presented in the media as normal and healthy. Your task is to determine whether they are healthy or unhealthy for relationships and whether they fit your values. Gather a few of your friends together to watch one of your favorite television shows that deals with romantic relationships. *How I Met Your Mother* and *Modern Family* are the kinds of shows that fit well with this activity. Your task while watching the show is to individually list the relationship behaviors as either healthy/realistic or unhealthy/unrealistic. Examples to watch for are couples talking at the same time and never listening to what the other says, one partner treating the other with respect, and similar behaviors. When the show ends, compare your list with the lists of your friends. Do you all see the behaviors in the same way, or do your friends see something as healthy when you think it is unhealthy? If you find differences, explore with your friends the reasons for your views. Ask your friends what healthy/realistic behaviors they would like to have in a loving relationship. Do they think the behaviors we watch in the media hurt the way we relate to one another?

were arrested for soliciting sex online. As always, the romantic lives of politicians were fair game for media scrutiny.

A cursory examination of popular magazines today will reveal more and more skin, especially that of women's bodies. The *Sports Illustrated* Swimsuit Issue is not that different in appearance from a *Playboy* magazine printed decades earlier. Both have well-written articles of interest, yet the sensual photography of the female models makes the magazines big sellers. The lingerie company Victoria's Secret distributes catalogues and designs store windows displaying female underwear in a seductive manner.

Popular music, particularly that focused on youth, has lyrics about sexuality that are explicit, direct, and often angry. Whereas country singers have long shared the details of dysfunctional relationships, the Dixie Chicks raised some eyebrows when they sang about the murder of a man with a history of beating his wife. Rappers sing and shout about reactions to body parts and sexual activity.

Women get referred to as "bitches," and young kids will sing along to songs focused on oral sex and sexual intercourse. U.S. culture is saturated with sexual messages, yet at the same time political leaders debate whether or not honest, factual information dare be presented to youth.

K–12 Schools

Schools are charged as the institutions primarily responsible for transmitting knowledge and helping children learn about the world. As a logical extension, schools are to play a key role in sexuality education. Even so, the debate has raged for decades regarding the role schools should play, the depth of information they should convey, at what ages children should learn information about sexuality, and how, if at all, schools can teach in a "value-free" way. Programs that have been successful have been conducted by working closely with parents, clergy, and community leaders to develop curricula that are acceptable. The efforts in this regard far exceed those in other subject areas such as English or history. Research shows that most parents support sexuality education in the public schools.

The National Guidelines Task Force, under the auspices of SIECUS (1997), identified six key concepts that should be part of comprehensive sexuality education programs: human development, relationships, personal skills, sexual behavior, sexual health, and society and culture. A broad spectrum of professionals, including the American Medical Association, National Education Association, U.S. Centers for Disease Control, and Planned Parenthood Federation of America published *Guidelines for Comprehensive Sexuality Education,* which expands on the teaching of 36 sexuality-related topics presented from an age-appropriate perspective (SIECUS, 1996).

Since the *Guidelines'* publication in the early 1990s; however, opponents to comprehensive sexuality education have seen their position supported with federal funding for programs that teach abstinence until marriage. There is little doubt that concerns about sexually transmitted disease (STD) and HIV infections among young people have fueled the abstinence education movement. In 1997, the federal government earmarked multimillion-dollar grants to the states for the development of **abstinence-based curricula** (see Table 1.1). Such funding was both continued and

Abstinence-based curricula Are school programs that advocate not having sex before marriage

Table 1.1 Federal Guidelines for Abstinence Education

"Abstinence education" means an educational or motivational program which:
A. Has, as its exclusive purpose, teaching the social, psychological, and health gains to be realized by abstaining from sexual activity.
B. Teaches abstinence from sexual activity outside marriage as the expected standard for school-age children.
C. Teaches that abstinence from sexual activity is the only certain way to avoid out-of-wedlock pregnancy, sexually transmitted diseases, and other associated health problems.
D. Teaches that a mutually faithful monogamous relationship in the context of marriage is the expected standard of human sexual activity.
E. Teaches that sexual activity outside of the context of marriage is likely to have harmful consequences for the child, the child's parents, and society.
F. Teaches young people how to reject sexual advances, and how alcohol and drug use increases vulnerability to sexual advances, and
G. Teaches the importance of attaining self-sufficiency before engaging in sexual activity.

Source: Cited in the *Federal Register, 62* (March 13, 1997), 49.

increased in 2002, with presidential and legislative support. Nonetheless, the Kaiser Family Foundation (2000) conducted a national study finding that the overwhelming majority of parents, teachers, principals, and students want some form of sexuality education taught in secondary school. The majority of parents wanted students to learn about HIV/AIDS and other STDs, the basics of pregnancy and birth control, how to deal with the pressure to have sex, the emotional issues and consequences of being sexually active, how to use and get birth control methods and abortion, and issues related to sexual orientation.

College

Young or old, resident or commuter, full-time or part-time, college students realize that college impacts sexuality in many ways. A college campus is a unique environment. Unlike high school, college is a place of limitless intellectual and personal freedom, where ideas and the pursuit of knowledge reign supreme. It is a place where knowledge, attitudes, and behavior are supposed to be examined and challenged. It is also a place of great personal and intellectual diversity, where people of all walks of life come together to learn and grow. For many of us it is the first time we have ever experienced such freedom and diversity.

The freedom and diversity of college extend into our sexuality. Away from home and in a new environment, we are exposed to people, ideas, experiences, and situations that challenge us and help shape us as sexual beings. The combination of personal freedom and the opportunity to try out new ideas, behaviors, and lifestyles is exciting. Our college years are a time of great personal growth. Many of us develop intimate, loving, sexual relationships in our college years that remain with us for a lifetime. College life also is a time for making choices. The decisions we make also can remain with us for a lifetime. Our decision-making ability is put to the test on a regular basis. Sexual choices are among the most important decisions we have to make. Decisions about who we are and what it means to be men and women, who we are attracted to, how we want to live and express our sexuality, what our sexual needs and wants are and how we will fulfill them are but a few of the decisions we will make during our college years.

Evaluating Sexuality Research
Research Methods and Sources of Information

As we strive toward a personally healthy sexuality, a critical task for all of us is to evaluate the information we receive. **Sexology,** the discipline that scientifically studies sexuality, is often conducted by researchers, some of whom refer to themselves as *sexologists*. Because the field of sexuality is truly interdisciplinary, researchers may primarily identify themselves as biologists, psychologists, sociologists, anthropologists, health educators, nurses, historians, physicians, and so on. Wiederman (2001) identifies 19 professional journals whose primary focus is publishing research on human sexuality. In addition, professional organizations in the field also publish newsletters and reports, which add to the knowledge base.

Sexology is the discipline that scientifically studies sexuality

Table 1.2 Contributions of Experts on Sexuality

Researcher(s)	Research	Years	Comments
Richard von Krafft-Ebing	*Psychopathia Sexualis*	1886	Viennese psychiatrist who introduced Victorian public to fetishism, sadomasochism, transvestism, homosexuality
Havelock Ellis	*Psychology of Sex*	1897–1910	Challenged negative views toward masturbation and narrow definitions of normal behavior
Alfred Kinsey and associates	*Sexual Behavior in the Human Male* *Sexual Behavior in the Human Female*	1948 1953	A pioneer undertaking involving thousands of males and females interviewed about their sexual behavior
William Masters and Virginia Johnson	*Human Sexual Response* *Human Sexual Inadequacy*	1966 1970	The first research efforts to photograph and physiologically record thousands of instances of sexual arousal, orgasm, masturbation, and coitus. Followed by brief effective treatment for sexual problems.
Morton Hunt	*Sexual Behavior in the 1970s*	1974	Showed consistencies and changes in sexual behavior a generation after the Kinsey findings
Philip Blumstein and Pepper Schwartz	*American Couples*	1983	Study of sexual and affectional behavior of couples
Shere Hite	*The Hite Report on Female Sexuality* *The Hite Report on Male Sexuality* *Women and Love* *Good Guys, Bad Guys*	1976 1981 1987 1991	Although statistically unrepresentative an early attempt at qualitative research yielding valuable insights to behavior
Popular culture	Magazine surveys: *Redbook, Cosmopolitan, Playboy*	1980	Surveyed more than 100,000 readers; findings often apply more to magazine's readers than to all adults
Richard Green	*The "Sissy Boy" Syndrome*	1987	Controversial study on the origins of homosexuality

(continued)

Table 1.2 Contributions of Experts on Sexuality *(continued)*

Researcher(s)	Research	Years	Comments
Edward Brecher	*Love, Sex, and Aging*	1984	One of the first large-scale scientific studies of sexuality in older people
John Money Anke Erhardt	*Man and Woman, Boy and Girl* *Gay, Straight and In-between*	1972 1988	Now-controversial study of gender anatomy, and identity. Attempted definitions of the biological and psychological determinants of sex, sexuality, and gender.
Edward Laumann, John Gagnon, Robert Michael, and Stuart Michaels	*The Social Organization of Sexuality: Sexual Practices in the United States*	1994	Comprehensive examination of practices within social settings and their meanings
Vern and Bonnie Bullough	*Sin, Sickness, and Sanity; Women and Prostitution: A Social History; Cross Dressing, Sex, and Gender*	1957– present	Review of extensive historical data on a variety of subjects
Michel Foucault	*The History of Sexuality*	1980	Argues that sexuality is socially constructed, including orientation
Centers for Disease Control	Youth Risk Behavior Surveillance System (YRBSS)	1999 2009	Federally sponsored ongoing research conducted in collaboration with federal, state, local, and private sector agencies to examine health risk behaviors of youth to develop better health programs. Specific attention paid to tobacco and drug use, diet and exercise, violence and injury, and sexual behaviors connected to STD/ HIV and unintended pregnancies.

It has often been difficult for researchers to secure adequate funding for sexuality research. Government funding has been most available if the research agenda can be closely demonstrated to impact public health. To some, however, the very study of human sexuality is suspect; others can appreciate the need to know and how much there is to learn. Table 1.2 profiles some of the more prominent research and researchers. The studies were conducted in different ways—some through questionnaires, some through interviews, some by observation, and so forth—although it would be fair to argue that better funding may have yielded broader samples and more comprehensive information.

As mentioned, a growing number of professional journals are focused on sexuality research. At the same time, there are limitations on the types of research conducted. Although a wide variety of questionnaires have been designed and administered, most sexuality research involves surveying selected populations. Often, university academics rely on the input of students, groups who are at the very least better educated and literate. In contrast, it would be far more difficult to assess information from populations who may not speak English, trust researchers, or even communicate about sexuality issues.

Ethical and practical considerations also impact what kinds of research are conducted. Observing and surveying children may be problematic, as parental permission must be secured; determining when an issue may be most related to the developmental stage of the child can become political and contentious. Some research is best conducted as a longitudinal study, where a population can be examined over time; the costs associated with such a design, however, can be prohibitive. In other cases, topics such as understanding sexual functioning related to a particular disease may pose challenges in securing an adequate sample size.

Because disciplines have their own established perspectives, the research presented may have other limitations or biases. Key criteria separate good research from poor research. Issues such as bias, sampling issues, honesty, and access, all contribute to the quality of sexuality research findings.

When applying research findings to one's personal life, practical questions to consider include the following: Are you like most people? If not, how aren't you? If you are part of a sexual minority—identifying, for example, as bisexual—how does this affect your lifestyle? If some expert claims that a sexual behavior is problematic and you engage in it, will your behavior change? Should it? Who *is* this expert when it comes to helping you make decisions about your sexuality?

Sexuality Researchers

Because of the interdisciplinary nature of the field of sexology, individuals and teams of researchers have conducted research exploring various aspects of sexuality. Some of the prominent names in the field have examined human sexual response and subsequently developed strategies to help people respond more fully and positively. Others have focused their work on patterns of behavior, differentiating for gender, race, culture, and ethnicity, where possible. Theorists have worked on questions of gender, orientation, and identity. Others have looked at relationship patterns. Almost all traditional styles of research have been utilized over the years to help provide a fuller understanding of human sexuality. Descriptive research formats have been widely used to survey a myriad of attitudes, values, and experiences. Experimental designs have yielded better understanding of sexual functioning and dysfunction. Qualitative research, in which individuals have been interviewed in depth, has provided the richness and contexts that statistical reports omit.

sex in society 1.1

Criteria Associated with Good Research

We are bombarded with sexual information every day. Countless studies and reports are released and presented by the media. "Experts" report new findings that challenge our notions about sexual issues. Here are some guidelines for evaluating sources of sexual information and research:

1. **Evaluate the researchers.** Reputable researchers are well known in their fields, have some kind of university or agency affiliation, and are members in good standing in professional organizations, and their research is not connected to or funded by for-profit businesses.
   - Who did the research?
   - Was the study done by reputable researchers?
2. **Evaluate the researchers' track record.**
   - Have they conducted scientific studies before?
   - Is their previous research respected and accepted in the field?
3. **Evaluate the sample.** Two issues related to the population studied will tell you the most about the quality of the study: sample size and randomness.
   - How large is the sample? (In general, the larger the sample, the better the study.)
   - Were the samples chosen randomly (subjects chosen at random from a larger pool of eligible), or were the subjects taken from a convenience sample (an intact group; students in a certain class—prison population, army recruits, subscribers to a certain magazine, and so on)?
4. **Evaluate the methods.** In general, first-person observable reports (person-to-person interview or direct observation) are better than other ways of gathering data (such as mailed questionnaires and telephone interviews). Sexuality research is unique, though. Anonymity protections in many situations will help guarantee better results. Unfortunately, when facing a questioner, respondents may be sensitive to reactions to their answers and consequently give desired answers rather than honest ones.
   - How was information about the subjects obtained?
5. **Evaluate replication.** Studies that are replicated with different samples and come up with similar findings are more likely to stand the test of time. Research linking smoking to lung cancer, for example, has been replicated with samples from different countries over the past decade and yielded similar results.
   - Has the study been replicated with a different population resulting in the same findings?
6. **Examine the impact.** Read reviews and reports of the study in reputable journals.
   - Have other researchers in the field received the study well?

A Wellness Approach to Understanding Sexuality

One way to explain and understand our sexuality is to look at it from a more holistic approach. Think of how Maria from Case Study 1.1 described how the dimensions of health affected her sexuality. A person cannot study something such as body image, for example, without looking at issues related to individual personality, family and peer influences, and societal expectations. The focus of this textbook is on healthy sexuality and strategies for maximizing our sexual potential.

Healthy sexuality enables a person to develop to the fullest potential. It requires being knowledgeable. It involves personalizing information and

Healthy sexuality is the safe and open exploration and development of our potential as human beings

using it to make informed decisions about your life and the world around you. Making good decisions about yourself and others is an essential part of healthy sexuality.

It involves our personal level of well-being, the health of our relationships with others, and the nature of the environment in which everything occurs. The best way to conceptualize this approach to understanding human sexuality is to use a health and wellness model to describe it.

Health and Wellness Defined

In 1947 the World Health Organization (WHO) defined **health** as "the state of complete mental, physical, and social well-being, not merely the absence of disease" (p. 35). WHO's definition was the first globally accepted conceptualization of health and stood the test of time for more than a decade.

Although multifaceted, this definition of health was flawed, according to members of a new movement called **holistic health**. The holistic health movement came into being in the 1960s as an attempt to expand the view of health that WHO had promulgated.

One of the early pioneers in the field, Halbert Dunn (1962), believed that the WHO vision of health characterized it as a static state. Rather than call health a state of well-being, Dunn preferred to view it as a continuum. Developing and maintaining a high level of health means moving toward optimal functioning. Health is a conscious and deliberate approach to life and being, rather than something to be abrogated to doctors and the health care system. Like your health in general, your sexual health is viewed as moving along a continuum, reaching optimal states as a result of your decisions and behavior (see Figure 1.1).

In addition, Dunn recast the notion of well-being to revolve around functioning. How well does the organism function? Dunn viewed functioning as evidence of well-being. Although people will have setbacks in their quest for optimal functioning, the direction in which their lives are moving becomes an important criterion for evaluating their well-being. In this movement, daily habits and behaviors, and overall lifestyle, assumed primary importance.

Originally, the scope of well-being was limited to three dimensions: physical, social, and mental. Adherents of holistic health argued that the mental dimension has two components: the intellectual (rational thought processes) and the emotional (feelings and emotions). Each of these domains

Health Total mental, physical, and social wellbeing, not merely the absence of disease

Holistic health The process of moving toward optimal functioning across the physical, social, spiritual, emotional, and intellectual dimensions

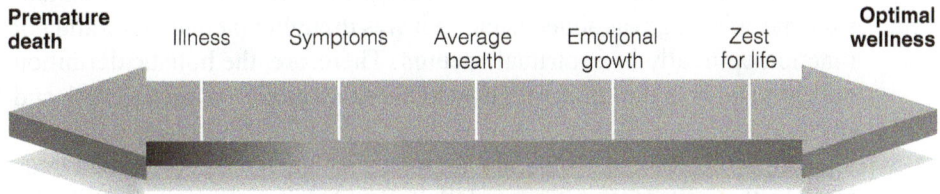

Figure 1.1 *Health and Wellness Continuum* Health can be viewed as a continuum. Where we are on the continuum at any given time is strongly influenced by our lifestyle.

sex in society 1.2

Diversity in Sex Research

One of the long-standing criticisms of many human sexuality studies is the lack of diversity in their subjects. Most of the classic studies in the field have focused on white, heterosexual, middle-class subjects. The two best-known sexuality works—Kinsey's studies of male and female sexual behavior and Masters and Johnson's work on sexual response—are both based on such a sample. Both were conducted decades ago, when diversity received much less attention. The lack of diversity seems to affect three distinct minority subgroups: lower socioeconomic status populations, racial minorities (blacks, Asians, and Hispanics/Latinos), and gays, lesbians, and bisexuals.

To complicate matters, although these three categories of populations are underrepresented in major studies of sexual response and behavior, they are overrepresented in other types of sex research, such as those focusing on STDs and teen pregnancy.

The problem may represent a lack of aggressive recruitment of nonwhite, non-middle-class, nonheterosexual subjects in major sexuality research (particularly studies that are privately funded) and an overreliance on sampling from public clinic populations (people with STDs, family planning), which tend to have higher minority representation.

Studies of gay, lesbian, and bisexual populations also have been clouded by methodological problems associated with sampling. Studies of gay men draw heavily from men who frequent gay bars, subscribe to gay publications, are incarcerated, or attend gay public events. Less is known about lesbian women. A true cross-sectional sample of gay men and lesbians representing various socioeconomic and racial/ethnic lines is needed.

Methodological issues related to sampling and sample size have been cited as the primary problems related to obtaining more diverse samples. It is harder to target recruitment efforts for lower socioeconomic status, minority, and gay/lesbian populations. Targeting narrow segments of these populations (for example, gay men attending gay bars) is easier and has a higher-yield recruitment than mainstream sources such as newspapers, random-digit telephoning, and the like. Narrowing the scope of recruitment, however, means that sampling may miss a true cross-section of the population targeted for study.

Can these studies accurately reflect human sexual behavior and response if they omit large segments of the population? Are there differences between and among various racial and ethnic groups, socioeconomic segments, and different sexual orientations, that might lend greater insight into the true nature of human sexuality?

Finally, newer research has attempted to draw conclusions and examine differences in attitudes, values, and behaviors of groups drawn from a broader range of backgrounds. Students must remember, however, that the United States has increasingly drawn immigrants into our midst who do not answer surveys, may not speak English, or may even feel that sexuality is not a topic to be discussed with anyone outside the immediate family circle.

---

deals with a different aspect of psychological well-being. A final dimension, the spiritual, was added because it was thought that humans could not function optimally in a spiritual vacuum. Therefore, the holistic definition of health has five dimensions: physical, social, emotional, intellectual, and spiritual.

In the 1970s and 1980s, the definition of health was expanded once again by the wellness movement (Ardell, 1985). Adherents defined wellness as "an active process of becoming aware of and making choices toward a more successful existence" (National Wellness Institute, 2002). Added to the previous dimensions was that of environmental health. Currently, some

Wellness The state of optimal health and wellbeing

The components of wellness

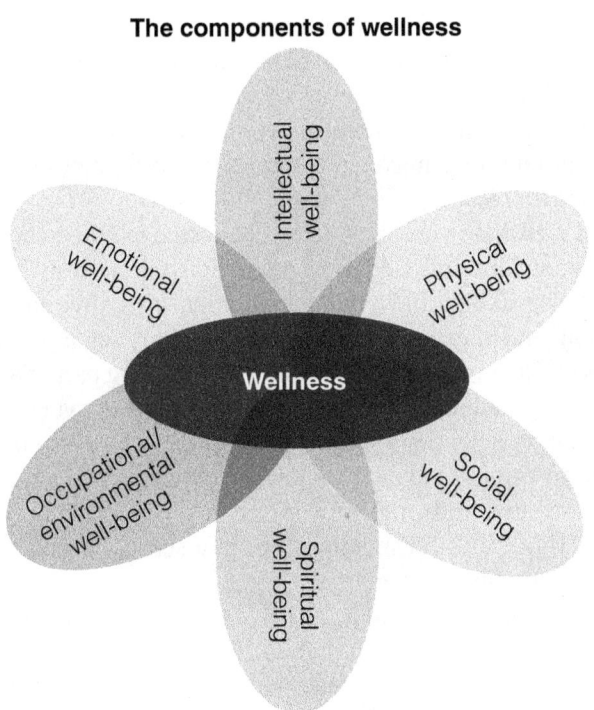

Figure 1.2 *Six-Dimensional Wellness Model* Wellness is a multifaceted phenomenon. Source: Adapted from Bill Hettler, M.D., 1979; http://hettler.com, 2003.

authors are adding vocational/occupational health to the definition, arguing that one's environment includes the work site and accompanying health issues related to job and career.

What is critical to wellness is to understand that it is a process of becoming healthier. The journey (becoming the best one can be) is more important than the ending. The process of wellness involves becoming increasingly more aware of health and making healthy choices. Success is individually determined and is based on the ability to live life to its fullest. A key element of the wellness model is striving for balance. When all of the six dimensions are at high levels and in balance, we have optimal health and well-being. When the dimensions are out of balance or one is severely lacking, we have lower levels of health and well-being. Figure 1.2 illustrates this concept.

The Six Dimensions of Wellness

The first dimension, **physical well-being,** is reflected in how well the body performs its intended functions. Absence of disease—although an important influence—is not the sole criterion for health. The physical domain is influenced by one's genetic inheritance, nutritional status, fitness level, **body composition,** and immune status, to name just a few.

Intellectual well-being is the ability to process information effectively. It involves the capability to use information in a rational way to solve problems and grow. It includes issues such as creativity, spontaneity, and openness to new ways of viewing situations. To maintain a high level of intellectual well-being, one must seek knowledge and learn from one's experiences.

Physical well-being A component of wellness reflected in how well the body performs its intended functions

Body composition The fat and nonfat components of the human body; important in assessing recommended body weight

Intellectual well-being A component of wellness referring to the ability to process information effectively and rationally

Emotional well-being A component of wellness that refers to being in touch with one's feelings, having the ability to express them, and being able to control them when necessary.

Social well-being A component of wellness that involves connection to others through various types of relationships

Environmental well-being A component of wellness that reflects our ability to function in our immediate environment, such as home, school, and work, as well as being able to deal with the world at large

Micro-environment The part of one's environment that is immediate and includes living situation, campus, neighborhood, home, and work site and family, friends, and associates who populate these places

Macro-environment The environment that extends beyond the micro and includes one's city, state, country, and the world at large

Spiritual well-being A component of wellness that involves feeling connected to something beyond oneself

Occupational/vocational well-being A component of wellness that reflects our ability to use our unique skills/talents to work that is meaningful and rewarding

Emotional well-being means being in touch with one's feelings, having the ability to express them, and being able to control them when necessary. Optimal functioning involves the understanding that emotions are the mirror to the soul. Emotions help us get in touch with what is important in our lives. Our emotions make us feel alive and provide us with a richness of experience that is uniquely human.

Social well-being involves being connected to others through various types of relationships. Individuals who function optimally in this domain are able to form friendships, have intimate relationships, give and receive love and affection, and accept others unconditionally. They are able to give of themselves and share in the joys and sorrows of being part of a community. This community includes both formal and informal networks. Formal networks include organizations such as churches, professional organizations, fraternities, sororities, and campus groups requiring official membership, dues, and standards. Informal networks such as an intramural sports team do not have rigid rules for membership. In a sense, your social networks are a big part of your environment.

Environmental well-being involves high-level functioning on two levels. The most immediate environment, the **micro-environment,** consists of school, home, neighborhood, and work site. The people with whom we interact in those places link the environment to the social aspects of our health. This environment greatly affects our health and personal safety by influencing whether we are at risk for and fear issues such as theft, crime, and violence. The quality of our air and water, noise pollution, crowding, and other issues that impact our stress levels are also affected. Our social support system is also part of this environment.

The **macro-environment,** the level of well-being at a larger level— state, country, and the world at large—also affects our wellness. The impact of things discussed earlier in the chapter—the wars in Iraq and Afghanistan, the terrorist attacks of 9/11, and other things such as violence, international disputes, racism, sexism, heterosexism, ageism, and so on—all influence us daily to some extent. Decisions that our political leaders make, such as engaging in wars or determining where we store radioactive wastes, affect the way we think and live our lives. Our ability to stay focused and whole is constantly challenged by the media, which bring the entire world and its problems into our living rooms each night. We need to learn to think globally, act locally, and be happy despite the myriad of problems in the world.

Spiritual well-being involves feeling connected to something beyond oneself. One way to express spirituality is by participating in organized religious activities. This usually means believing in a supreme being or higher supernatural force and subscribing to a formalized code of conduct to live by. In a secular sense, spirituality could manifest itself through connection to something greater than oneself. Whether it is being part of a community, working to save the environment, helping feed the needy, or being committed to world peace, the underlying feeling is a perception of life as having meaning beyond the self.

Finally, **occupational/vocational well-being** involves issues related to job wellness. Occupational/vocational well-being encompasses everything from the safety of our particular work site to the nature of your career. Work site wellbeing includes physical (air, water, physical plant, machinery, and

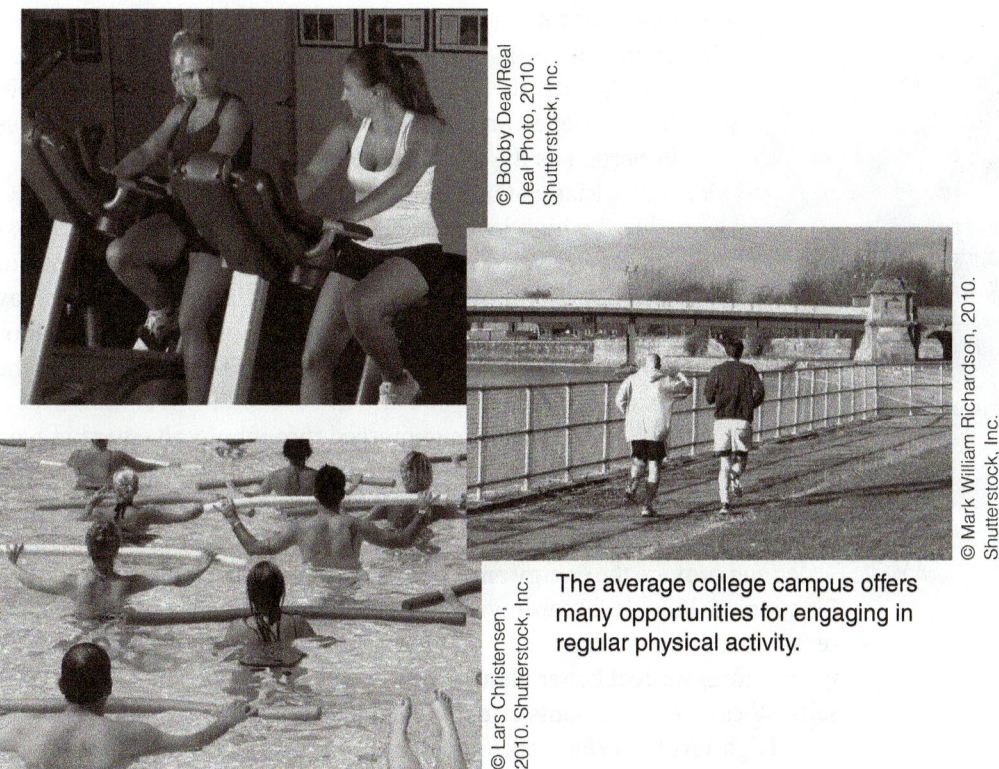

The average college campus offers many opportunities for engaging in regular physical activity.

so on) and social (relationships with coworkers, management, health and wellness facilities and activities) factors. Our personal wellness is affected by the health of our work site. Employers and work sites vary tremendously in relation to health. Some strive for optimal levels, encouraging employees to take advantage of a myriad of health-enhancing programs and services, whereas others meet the minimum acceptable standards for health and safety set by the government.

Besides the specific health of the workplace, different jobs/careers pose varying threats to our well-being as a result of the nature of the work. Some jobs such as police and military service are risky because of possible exposure to hostile combatants. Other occupations such as firefighters, emergency medical service workers, coal miners, and oil rig operators are risky because they place employees in dangerous environments. Other occupations entail high stress due to deadlines, competition, or other factors.

Wellness and Human Sexuality

Our sexuality both contributes to overall health and well-being and is affected by it. High-level sexual health can be a positive force in our lives. It contributes to the full functioning of our body, mind, spirit, and social relationships. When we are engaged in healthy sexual activity and have a healthy outlook concerning our sexuality, we can maximize our potential as men and women. Conversely, our sexuality is affected by our overall level of health and well-being. Sexual response (from desire to arousal and orgasm) is greatly influenced by our overall level of well-being. We simply are less interested in sex and perform poorly when we have low-level health and wellness.

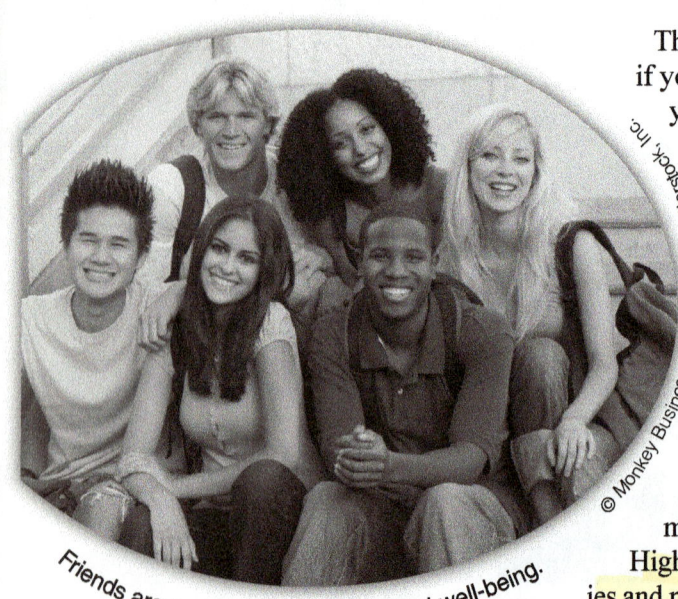

Friends are an important part of social well-being.

© Monkey Business Images, 2010. Shutterstock, Inc.

The important thing is to be moving toward optimal health, even if you never achieve it. If your current level of health is lower than you would like, the main thing is to take steps to improve it. The experience and process of improving, the journey, is as important as the current level of functioning.

Many of us have limitations that keep us from achieving the high levels of health that others enjoy. A wellness perspective of health and sexuality helps us accept our limitations and maximize the potential within us. You may never have the body of the man or woman of your dreams, but you can enjoy healthy sexuality if you strive to be the best you can be.

Our values are expressed through involvement in paid and nonpaid activities that are personally rewarding for us and make a contribution to the well-being of the community at large. High-level *physical well-being* can make us feel better about our bodies and provide the energy and capacity to maximize sexual pleasure and functioning. High level cardiovascular fitness and muscle tone can enhance sexual functioning and pleasure. When our bodies are healthy and optimally functioning, we feel better about how we look and move, and have higher self-esteem—two elements critical to healthy sexuality.

High-level *emotional well-being* can help us understand and cope with the myriad of feelings that being sexual creates. It helps us cope with the emotional roller coaster that most of us face when confronted with issues such as gender identity, sexual orientation, puberty, dating, and preventing unintended pregnancy. A high level of emotional well-being helps us understand and accept our emotions related to these and other sexual issues.

High-level *intellectual well-being* helps us process sexual information, think critically, and make sound decisions regarding our sexual health. The ability to sort through the often-conflicting barrage of sexual information and advice requires an ability to seek out information, evaluate facts, seek clarification of unanswered questions, solve problems, and relate this information to our own needs, wants, and values.

High-level *social well-being* enhances our sexuality and provides a safe forum to explore it and share it with others. Having solid friendships, intimate relationships, and sexual partnerships with people we care about, love, and trust allows us to explore our developing sexuality in a safe way.

Our sexual health is based in our ability to form healthy relationships with others. *Intimacy* is the ability to be open and honest and to feel close with another person. It enhances relationships but is not part of all the relationships we form. For example, you may be open and honest with a college roommate with whom you live day to day. In contrast, you may not find it appropriate or feel comfortable discussing personal concerns with colleagues at work. Relationships that involve an obvious power dynamic—such as boss and employee—often dictate that we are prudent in what we disclose and how intimate we become.

The expression "blood is thicker than water" has been used to explain the support we often expect from family. Friends may come and go, but your family is always your family. In truth, some people have wonderfully inti-

case study 1.3

Donna's Journey to Sexual Health

Donna, 40, is white.

I'm 40 years old, and I like myself. I accept myself. I can be who I am. But it wasn't always like that. As I look back, I realize that my sexuality has played a very significant role in my life.

Sexuality is a significant part of everyone's life, yet if you stray from the center, the average, the expected, then the journey at the very least has more bumps in it than for most.

We can get into a whole list of identities—woman, daughter, lover, student. I see labels as political designations. You try them on to see which ones fit. Can you find "one" that encompasses a total human being? I don't think so. In the last 5 years I've taken "transgendered" as one of my primary identities, yet I am also a mother of two boys. I am committed to a woman as a partner. I am a recent college graduate with a full-time job that isn't what I've always hoped to be doing with my degree, but it pays the bills. And when I clear out some of my debts, I hope to pursue graduate school at some point.

I've always been "inappropriate." My mother was always into dressing me to be the pretty little girl, and in 6 seconds I would destroy her efforts. I wanted to climb trees, play in the dirt, and have fun—all sorts of things you couldn't do in a dress. My hair was always very long to please my mother. My way to manage that was to always keep it in pigtails. Once on my own, I started dressing in drag, with short hair and men's clothing. I came out to my family when I was 16, but to my painful surprise found the reception in the lesbian community most unwelcome. Being butch and dressing like a man back in the 1970s was not "politically correct." I remedied my sense of not fitting in and trying to sort everything out by marrying a man and trying to live as a heterosexual woman. I was very successful at that game for close to 20 years, being the dutiful wife and mother.

Today it's a 50–50 shot as to whether people think I'm a man or a woman. It used to bother me a lot when people were confused. Now, I find it amusing and really don't care. I have a job where I can be free to be who I am, sharing the ups and downs of my life with people who are friends. I don't fit neatly into the transgendered community, nor do I have "gender dysphoria." My body is my body, and I accept it. I wear men's clothing primarily because they fit better, both body and psyche. I build muscle in "male-patterned" ways, my voice has gotten deeper over time, and my neck is thick. The blood tests I've had in the past all indicate "normal hormone parameters" for a woman.

I feel that I've experimented a lot to find out what is most comfortable and to learn who I am as a sexual person. Not that my journey has ended, but I better understand the road to healthy sexuality. And self-acceptance is a great place to start.

Critical Thinking

How does Donna illustrate some of the problems associated with trying to attach a label to someone's sexuality?

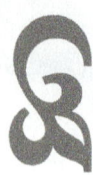

healthy sex hints 1.1

Making Informed Decisions

The following is a simple decision-making model that may help you make better decisions about your sexuality.

1. *Establish your goal.* Try to put in a broader context the decision you are making about an issue. ("How will this decision affect my goal?")
2. *List the pros and cons.* In two columns on a sheet of paper, list the consequences of saying either yes or no to the question you are trying to make a decision about. Don't scrimp. Put down all of them, no matter how trivial they might seem.
3. *Prioritize the pros and cons.* Rank the pros and cons from most important to least important.
4. *Weigh the pros and cons.* Although one column might be greater than the other (many more pros than cons, for instance), the top one or two items on the shorter list might carry much more weight.
5. *Ponder the results.* Examine the lists, and discuss them with one or two people whose opinions you value.
6. *Listen to your instincts.* Sometimes something may seem to be right for the average person but may not feel like the best thing for you. Your rational/intellectual evaluation of your lists, and your significant other's advice, provide you with two pieces of information; your gut-level intuition provides you with another.
7. *Decide.* Action is important. You must make a decision and move on with your life.
8. *Give it time.* Once you make a decision, give yourself time to experience the effects of that decision. At first it may seem that you made the wrong decision. Only time will tell.
9. *Reevaluate.* Go through this model again to reevaluate your decision once a sufficient amount of time has passed.
10. *Don't beat yourself up!* You are human! Sometimes you will make the wrong decisions. Learn from your mistakes, and try not to make the same ones twice. Persecuting yourself and putting yourself down are not productive and will not help you make better decisions.

mate relationships with family, whereas others have disengaged from their family or contact them only in times of need. When one's sexual lifestyle is perceived at odds with family expectations, family ties may be strained or severed, with friendships providing the intimacy and support needed.

Someone once noted that if heterosexual women could relate to their male partners and hold them to the same expectations they have for their female friends, romantic relationships would be in a better state. This observation points to the subtle ways by which we change the script when we look toward developing healthy romantic relationships. Identifying what is unhealthy in someone else's relationship is often easier than seeing the weaknesses in one's own relationships.

High-level *environmental well-being* extends from our personal living space, to our school and work space, to the world beyond. As such, it

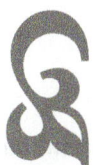

healthy sex hints 1.2

Creating Healthy Environments

- *Help create a healthy sexual environment within your community.* Be a role model for healthy sexuality. Lead by example, whether through words or actions.
- *Get involved in organizations that actively champion sexual rights.* If you can't or don't want to get publicly involved with them, support organizations financially. Make a contribution to acknowledge and support their work.
- *Be an advocate within any organization in which you are involved, such as youth sports, church or temple, fraternity/ sorority, and the like.* If you see or hear things that work against creating or maintaining a healthy sexual environment, speak out.

is often the one area of our health where there is the least personal control. As we age and become independent, our environment extends beyond the family into the immediate community. Community standards for safety and support vary from place to place. Official government, police, and school policies on diverse issues such as treatment of known sexual offenders, sexual harassment in the community, gay rights, sexual abuse, prostitution, prevention and treatment of sexually transmitted diseases, and so on, all influence one's sexual health. Unofficial community standards interact with official policies to create a climate within a community that either supports sexual development and expression or sets up barriers to it.

A primary environment for college students is the campus. Campus policies, especially for residential students, have a great impact on issues related to sexual health. Colleges are becoming increasingly aware of the necessity of formalizing policies on issues such as the prevention of, and treatment of students with, HIV/AIDS, sexual harassment and assault, sexual health services, and so on.

The focus on *occupational/vocational well-being* can be subsumed within a broad definition of *environment*. The jobs and careers we choose reflect who we are as people. They also set the stage for meeting partners and developing relationships that give our lives meaning. As a nation, we are spending increasing amounts of time related to work, both on the job and in commutation. Some individuals find themselves with two or more hours needed to "get to and from work," followed by a full work day, then the advisable seven hours of sleep, needs for exercise, quality time with family, and more; as a result, stress overload becomes "mathematically" apparent. Chemical and radiation exposure at work, along with overall safety of the workspace, affects health in general and aspects of sexual health in particular. Fertility can be affected. Pain and injury can certainly impact sexual functioning.

High-level *spiritual health* connects us with a higher power. It puts our sexuality in a broader context, providing a different perspective from which to view ourselves and our behavior. It also links our lives with a broader purpose and historical continuity that reaches beyond the self and mere personal fulfillment. We feel as though we are part of something that transcends our present place and time.

Health Challenges

As we've pointed out in this chapter, wellness functions along a continuum, with various dimensions impacting our sexual health throughout our lives. Ideally, college students and young adults are not confronted with serious health challenges. In reality, some already have or will find themselves managing chronic, sometimes debilitating illnesses and/or disabilities. Some of those illnesses and disabilities directly affect sexuality, whereas others may do so indirectly. Students have reported problems with substance abuse, eating disorders, and gambling. Others break bones, injure backs, and have accidents that may leave them in a wheelchair. Managing bouts of depression, having panic attacks, or being diagnosed with an obsessive-compulsive disorder all take their toll on socializing and getting close to others. For those who contract an STD such as genital warts, which is viral and long-term, the issue of how and what to tell a future partner adds to the regular issues related to dating.

We take the position that sexual health requires understanding ourselves and others—the people intimately in our lives and those in our communities. Toward that end, when an individual is confronted with health challenges, the specific condition can become a limitation. Although we all have limitations of one kind or another, health challenges become most limiting when they *define* us rather than when being viewed as a *part* of who we are. Optimal sexual health requires that we be able to identify available resources and strategies to enable the highest levels of functioning possible. Table 1.4 provides some of the resources available. Increasingly, the Internet has provided the much-needed link for those who previously may have felt isolated from information and support.

Table 1.4 Resources Available to Support Health Challenges

Professional Journals

Journal of Sexuality and Disability

Sexuality and Disabilities

Selected Web Sites and Phone Numbers

Sexuality and Disability Webliography: www.bccpd.bc.ca
A Web site of suggested readings compiled by the Wellness and Disability Initiative.

Spinal Cord Injury: www.sexualhealth.com
A Web site with information and resources on sex and disability.

Mental Health: http://Ulifeline.org
A Web site designed for college students. Sponsored by the Jed Foundation, named for a college student who committed suicide. The site has linkages to resources related to mental health, suicide prevention, drug abuse, and more.

Depression and Bipolar Support Alliance: www.dbsalliance.org
Web site support for those living with mood disorders.

STDs

American Social Health Association: www.ashastd.org
Provides information and resources about sexually transmitted diseases.

National AIDS hotline: (800) 342-2437

Gay Men's Health Crisis line: (212) 807-6664; www.gmhc.org
These two resources focus primarily on HIV/AIDS.

Chronic Illness/Cancer

Chronic Fatigue: www.chronicfatiguesupport.com
A Web site sponsored by ProHealth, Inc., with an expert medical advisory board.

Testicular Cancer Resource Center: http://tcrc.acor.org
Provides information for patients, caregivers, and physicians.

Susan G. Komen Breast Cancer Foundation: www.komen.org
Provides breast cancer research funds as well as educational and support services.

Drug Use

Bacchus & Gamma Peer Education Network: www.bacchusgamma.org
This is an association of college and university peer education groups focused on alcohol and other safety issues for students.

Alcohol hotline: (800) ALCOHOL

Alcoholics Anonymous: http://alcoholics-anonymous.org
The white pages of phone books list local chapters.

Cocaine hotline: (800) COCAINE

Narcotics Anonymous: http://www.na.org/
The white pages of phone books list local chapters.

Eating Disorders

National Eating Disorders Association: www.NationalEatingDisorders.org
Provides educational and treatment information on eating disorders.

National Association of Anorexia Nervosa and Associated Disorders (ANAD): www.anad.org
Provides hotline counseling, education, and referrals.

Personal Assessment

The purpose of this personal assessment is to increase your awareness of areas in your life that increase risk of disease, injury, and possibly premature death. A key point to remember is that you have control over each of the lifestyle areas discussed.

Awareness is the first step in making change. After identifying the areas that require modification, you will be able to use the behavior modification techniques presented in Chapter 10 to bring about positive lifestyle changes.

Directions

Put a check by each statement that applies to you. You may select more than one choice per category.

A. Physical Fitness

_____ I exercise for a minimum of twenty to thirty minutes at least three days per week.

_____ I play sports routinely (two to three times per week).

_____ I walk for fifteen to thirty minutes (three to seven days per week).

B. Body Fat

_____ There is no place on my body where I can pinch more than one inch of fat.

_____ I am satisfied with the way my body appears.

C. Stress Level

_____ I find it easy to relax.

_____ I rarely feel tense or anxious.

_____ I am able to cope with daily stresses without undue emotional stress.

D. Car Safety

_____ I have not had an auto accident in the past four years.

_____ I always use a seat belt when I drive.

_____ I rarely drive above the speed limit.

E. Sleep

_____ I always get seven to nine hours of sleep.

_____ I do not have trouble going to sleep.

_____ I generally do not wake up during the night.

F. Relationships

_____ I have a happy and satisfying relationship with my spouse or boy/girlfriend.

_____ I have a lot of close friends.

_____ I get a great deal of love and support from my family.

G. Diet

_____ I generally eat three balanced meals per day.

_____ I rarely overeat.

_____ I rarely eat large quantities of fatty foods and sweets.

H. Alcohol Use

_____ I consume fewer than two drinks per day.

_____ I never get intoxicated.

_____ I never drink and drive.

I. Tobacco Use

_____ I never smoke (cigarettes, pipe, cigars, etc.).

_____ I am not exposed to second-hand smoke on a regular basis.

_____ I do not use smokeless tobacco.

J. Drug Use

_____ I never use illicit drugs.

_____ I never abuse legal drugs such as diet or sleeping pills.

K. Sexual Practices

_____ I always practice safe sex (e.g., always using condoms or being involved in a monogamous relationship).

Scoring

1. **Individual areas:** If there are any unchecked areas in categories A through K, you can improve those aspects of your lifestyle.
2. **Overall lifestyle:** Add up your total number of checks. Scoring can be interpreted as follows:
   23–29 Very healthy lifestyle
   17–22 Average healthy lifestyle
   ≤ 16 Unhealthy lifestyle (needs improvement)

From *Health and Fitness: A Guide to a Healthy Lifestyle*, 3rd Edition by Laura Bounds et al. Copyright © 2006 by Kendall Hunt Publishing Company. Reprinted by permission.

Thought Questions

1. What is human sexuality? What are its components?

2. What is the definition of *health*, according to the World Health Organization?

3. What complaints did the wellness movement have with the WHO conceptualization of health?

4. What is the definition of *wellness*? What are its six components?

5. Define healthy sexuality, incorporating the elements of wellness.

Test Yourself

1. Which generalization about sexuality in our culture is most accurate?
   a. Our culture is clearly becoming more sexually permissive, as reflected in the content of our television programming.
   b. Our culture is clearly becoming more sexually restrictive, as evidenced by growing financial support for abstinence-until-marriage education.
   c. Our cultural climate has not changed significantly for decades.
   d. Sexual messages in our culture are contradictory and diverse.

2. Guidelines developed for comprehensive sexuality education programs highlight the importance of teaching about all but which of the following:
   a. Abstinence-until-marriage strategies
   b. Human development
   c. Relationship skills
   d. Society and culture

3. In evaluating sexuality research, which among the following is least important?
   a. The size of the sample responding
   b. The gender of the researcher
   c. The professional affiliation of the researcher
   d. How the information was gathered

4. The criticism that there has been a lack of diversity in research subjects is highlighted by the fact that:
   a. most subjects are white, heterosexual, and middle class.
   b. most research is conducted on the East and West coasts of the United States.
   c. more research has been conducted on women than men.
   d. few subjects are over 35 years of age.
5. According to Dunn, personal well-being is connected to:
   a. regular visits to physicians and other health practitioners.
   b. personal habits and lifestyle.
   c. the health of your parents and other relatives.
   d. age and ethnic background.
6. John feels depressed a lot and is told about a Web site where college students can get information about mental health, along with a referral. By checking the site out, he will be attending to which aspects of his well-being?
   a. Physical and spiritual
   b. Emotional and intellectual
   c. Emotional and physical
   d. Intellectual and environmental
7. Sarah has decided to move into a campus apartment with friends. Her decision should improve which components of her well-being?
   a. Physical and social
   b. Environmental and emotional
   c. Social and environmental
   d. Emotional and physical
8. Students who exercise regularly are more likely to
   a. feel better about their bodies.
   b. get better grades.
   c. have more friends.
   d. gain weight over time.
9. Increasingly, college campuses have policies focused on sexuality-related issues. Policies related to all but which of the following should be expected?
   a. HIV/AIDS
   b. Sexual assault and date rape
   c. Sexual harassment
   d. Premarital sex
10. The model for making informed decisions recommends all but which of the following strategies?
   a. Identify the pros and cons.
   b. Weigh the pros and cons.
   c. Rate what is most important to least important.
   d. Think about what is right, not what your gut instincts tell you to do.

Web Resources

American Association of Sex Educators, Counselors, and Therapists
www.aasect.org/

Professional organization devoted to the promotion of sexual health by the development and advancement of the fields of sex therapy, counseling, and education. There is a selection of associated Web links and the "contemporary sexuality" section providing general items of interest on sexuality.

Answer
http://answer.rutgers.edu/

Answer is a national organization with resources to help young people and adults find reliable information about sexuality and sexuality education.

Go Ask Alice
www.goaskalice.columbia.edu/

Columbia University's Health Education Program, offering information and e-mail advice on sexual health, sexuality, communication, and relationships. The primary goal is to make health and wellness a life priority for students, staff, and professors.

Sexuality Information and Education Council of the U.S.
(SIECUS)
www.siecus.org

National nonprofit organization that promotes comprehensive education about sexuality and advocates the right of individuals to make responsible sexual choices. This site details information on sexuality, contraception, and sexual abuse and assault.

The Society for the Scientific Study of Sexuality (SSSS)
www.SexScience.org

The Society for the Scientific Study of Sexuality is dedicated to advancing knowledge of sexuality. It believes in the importance of both the production of quality research and the application of sexual knowledge in educational, clinical, and other settings. The site provides links to professional meetings, journals in the field, other SSSS publications, professional contacts, and more.

Discovery Health
http://health.discovery.com/

This the Discovery Channel's health Web page. It has excellent sexual health information (click on sexual health icon on the left side). It also offers an array of online health assessments through the following link: http://health.discovery.com/tools/assessments.html.

National Wellness Institute (NWI)
http://www.nationalwellness.org/

Founded in 1977, the National Wellness Institute has steadfastly provided health promotion and wellness, professionals' unparalleled resources, and services that promote both professional and personal growth. Besides a membership division, NWI hosts the National Wellness Conference. Held annually in Stevens Point, Wisconsin, at the University of Wisconsin for over 25 years, it is the most highly acclaimed conference for wellness and health promotion professionals.

The Sexual Health Network
www.sexualhealth.com

The Sexual Health Network is dedicated to providing easy access to sexuality information, education, mutual support, counseling, therapy, health care, products and other resources for people with disabilities, illness, or natural changes throughout the life cycle and those who love them or care for them.

Online Health Assessments
http://health.discovery.com/tools/assessments.html

Take as many of the additional assessments as you wish. Make sure to explore all of the available assessments under all three menus (general health, personality, nutrition).

References

American College Health Association. (1996). *Policy guidelines for HIV/AIDS on campus.* Washington, DC: Author.

Ardell, D. (1985). *The history and future of wellness.* Dubuque, IA: Kendall/Hunt.

Boulard, G. (2001, December 24). After September 11th students find themselves under a magnifying glass. *Community College Week, 14*(10), 2–4.

Davey, J. (2002, September 30). One day in September. *Community College Week, 15*(4), 4.

Dettmer, J. (2001, October 29). New York shows strength in adversity. *Insight on the News, 17*(40), 13.

Dunn, H. (1962). High-level wellness in the world of today. *Journal of the American Osteopathic Association, 61,* 9.

Garmon, J. (2001, December 24). Making sense, not war. *Community College Week, 14*(10), 4–6.

Henry J. Kaiser Family Foundation. (2000). *Sex education in America: A view from inside the nation's classrooms.* Chart pack. Menlo Park, CA: Author.

Kirgiss, K. (2002, February). Taylor-made service: After the terrorist attacks, 99 students from Indiana's Taylor University drove to New York to help however they could. *Campus Life, 60*(7), 62–64.

Lane, K. (2002, January 21). After the fall: Against the ruined backdrop of Ground Zero, the wounded Borough of Manhattan community college is struggling to rebuild. *Community College Week, 14*(12), 6–11.

Manisses Communication Group. (2002, September 16). Survey finds impact of September 11th stretches across the country. *Mental Health Weekly, 12*(35), 1–3.

Mindlin, A. C., Wallace, E. E., & Kapell, M. (2002). Cultural and religious determinants of sexual behaviors: A crosscultural analysis of the available literature. *Michigan Academician, 34*(1), 6–8.

National Abortion and Reproductive Rights Action League Foundation. (2001). *Who decides? A state-by-state review of abortion and reproductive rights.* Washington, DC: NARAL and the NARAL Foundation.

National Wellness Institute. (2002). Definition of wellness [Online]. Available: www.nationalwellnessinstitute.home.

Office of the Surgeon General. (2001). *The surgeon general's call to action to promote sexual health and responsible sexual behavior.* Washington, DC: U.S. Government Printing Office.

Seong-Ngoo. (2002, May). Psychological burden after September 11th tragedy. *Student British Medical Journal, 138.*

Sexuality Information and Education Council of the U.S. (1996). *Guidelines for comprehensive sexuality education* (2nd ed.). New York: Author.

Sexuality Information and Education Council of the U.S. (1997). Guidelines for comprehensive sexuality education fact sheet [Online]. Available: www.siecus.org/pubs/fact/fact0003.html.

Sexuality Information and Education Council of the U.S. (2001, August–September). Issues and answers: Fact sheet on sexuality education. *SIECUS Report, 29*(6) [Online]. Available: www.siecus.org/pubs/fact/fact0007.html.

Straw, D. (2001, December 24). A separate peace in a wartime classroom. *Community College Week, 14*(10), 4–6.

Tsigos, C., & Chrousos, G. P. (1996). Stress, endocrine manifestations and disease. In C. L. Cooper (Ed.), *Handbook of stress, medicine, and health.* New York: CRC.

Weis, D. (2002, May). Another stab at sexual theory [a review of *The Role of Theory in Sex Research,* edited by J Bancroft]. *Journal of Sex Research, 39*(2), 158–160.

Wiederman, M. (2001). Why understanding research? In *Understanding sexuality research.* Belmont, CA: Wadsworth.

World Health Organization. (1947). Constitution of the World Health Organization. *Chronicles of the World Health Organization, 1,* 29–43.

chapter
two

Female Sexual Anatomy *and* Physiology

Student Learning Objectives

After reading this chapter, students will be able to:

- Identify and locate the key structures of the female sexual anatomy;
- Describe the main functions of the key female sexual structures;
- Identify and describe the functions of the key female sex hormones;
- Explain the erogenous potential of the female sexual structures;
- Perform a breast self-exam;
- Identify the signs, symptoms, and treatment for common female sexual disorders;
- Describe a variety of screening tests used to diagnose common female sexual disorders.

activity teaser: How much do you know about female anatomy? Find the answer in the Personal Exploration Activity on page 35.

case study 2.1

"The Vagina Workshop" from *The Vagina Monologues* by Eve Ensler

The subject of this piece is an anonymous woman in her late 30s to 40s.

Ensler prefaces this piece as belonging to one of the women she interviewed from a group in their late 30s and early 40s. The woman had learned about her body and orgasm at one of the body workshops taught by Betty Dodson.

. . . I found it quite unsettling at first, my vagina. Like the first time you see a fish cut open and you discover this other complex world inside, right under the skin. It was so raw, so red, so fresh. And the thing that surprised me most was all the layers. Layers inside layers, opening into more layers. My vagina, like some mystical event that keeps unfolding another aspect of itself, which is really an event in itself, but you only know it after the event.

. . . It was better than the Grand Canyon, ancient and full of grace. It had the innocence and freshness of a proper English garden. It was funny, very funny. It made me laugh. It could hide and seek, open and close. It was a mouth. It was a morning. And then it momentarily occurred to me that it was me, my vagina: it was who I was. It was not an entity. It was inside of me.

> ### Critical Thinking
>
> It is important for women to love and accept their genitals. We take better care of that which we love. We may then choose to share our genitals only with those who deserve us.
>
> Is it comfortable for you to examine your genitalia?
>
> Why is it important for women to look and understand how they are built?

Many of the structures and functions of sexual anatomy are really quite similar when comparing females and males. Indeed, an underlying theme in this book is the emphasis on how women and men are more similar than different. That being said, however, women's unique role in reproduction and the experiences associated with monthly menstruation across much of a woman's life require women to be aware of their bodies in a way different from men. Those experiences also make it challenging to separate the sexual from the reproductive function of the anatomy.

External Female Sexual Structures

Vulva The external female genitalia

The formal term used to describe all of the external female genital structures collectively is the vulva. The **vulva** includes the mons pubis (also known as mons veneris), labia majora and minora, clitoris, hymen, introitus, and vestibule. These are shown in Figure 2.1.

Mons Veneris

The mons veneris is named after the Greek goddess of love. In Latin, mons veneris means "the mound of Venus." The mons veneris, commonly called the pubic area, is the softly protruding cushion of fat, skin, and pubic hair that covers the pubis symphysis, the juncture of the pubic bones of the pelvis. Although it serves no reproductive function, the mons is sensitive to stimulation during sexual arousal. Its pad of fatty tissue provides a soft cushion to maximize pleasure during sexual activities, particularly those involving grinding circular movements.

personal exploration activity

What Do You Know?

After drawing and labeling the female sexual anatomy, you will be able to identify what is accurate and inaccurate about your knowledge of the female anatomy.

Before reading this chapter on female anatomy, take a few minutes to see how much you know or don't know about the female sexual anatomy. Take a sheet of paper and draw from memory the internal and external female sexual anatomy. If possible, get one of your friends of the opposite sex to team up with you to do this drawing. This will be more fun and will show which sex has the most knowledge of the female anatomy. Once you have drawn the anatomy, label the following parts: clitoris, ovaries, uterus, vagina, cervix, labia majora, labia minora, mons pubis, urethra, ureter, fimbria, and bladder.

When you have finished, compare your drawing to the one in this chapter. Are you surprised by how little or how much you know? How comfortable were you drawing this sexual anatomy? Ask one of your friends to do this activity. Does your friend's drawing indicate that they have good knowledge of the female anatomy? How comfortable were they drawing the sexual anatomy?

Labia Majora

The two **labia majora** form the outermost vaginal lips. The labia are folds of skin covering fatty tissue and are covered with hair on the outside. The inner portion of the labia majora is covered with numerous sweat and oil glands.

In the unaroused state, the labia majora remain closed, providing protection for the vaginal opening and clitoris. The skin of the labia, like that of the male scrotum, is normally darker in color than the rest of a woman's body. During sexual arousal, underlying erectile tissue engorges with blood,

Labia majora The larger, outer vaginal lips

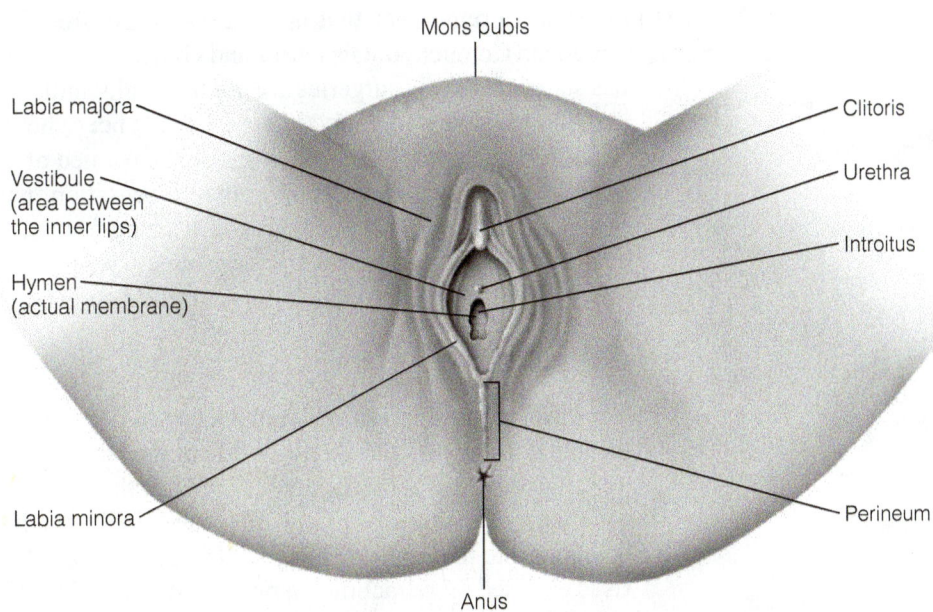

Figure 2.1 *The External Genitalia*

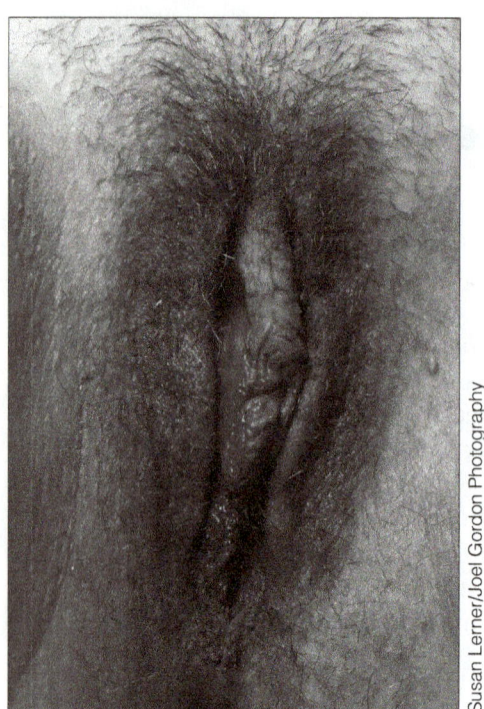

The appearance of the vulva varies woman to woman.

Susan Lerner/Joel Gordon Photography

Labia minora The smaller, inner vaginal lips

Bartholin's glands Small glands adjacent to the vaginal opening that secrete a small amount of lubricant during arousal

Clitoris A small, highly sensitive, organ located at the top of the labia minora

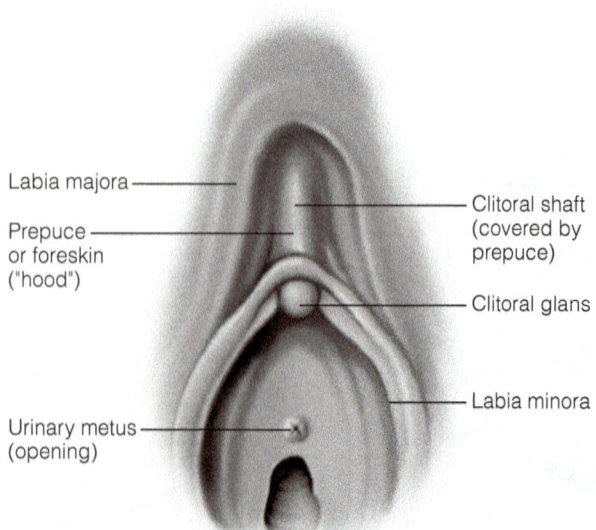

Labia majora

Prepuce or foreskin ("hood")

Clitoral shaft (covered by prepuce)

Clitoral glans

Labia minora

Urinary metus (opening)

Figure 2.2 *The Clitoris*

causing the labia to swell, deepen in color, and open like "the petals of a flower" (see "Betty Dodson's Art"- Sex in society 2.1), exposing the vaginal opening and clitoris.

The sweat and oil secretions of the labia majora are capable of producing a cheesy substance called *smegma, which can collect under the clitoral hood causing irritation.* Routine washing with soap and water around the labia and after pulling back the clitoral hood helps ensure cleanliness and prevents the accumulation of smegma under the clitoral hood.

Labia Minora

The **labia minora** are a second set of vaginal lips located within the larger labia majora. Thinner than the labia majora, the labia minora have spongy tissue containing oil and sweat glands and are richly endowed with blood vessels and nerve endings. The top portion of the labia majora fuse to form the clitoral hood, or *prepuce.* Unlike the labia majora, the minora are hairless. In the unaroused state they, too, remain closed, providing a second line of protection for the vaginal opening and clitoris.

The labia minora are highly sensitive to sexual stimulation and engorge with blood during sexual stimulation, opening up and exposing the vaginal opening and clitoris. Within the labia minora are **Bartholin's glands**, which secrete a small amount of lubricating fluid during sexual arousal. Once thought to provide the major portion of lubrication during arousal, it is now understood that vaginal lubrication comes from the walls of the vagina, rather than any significant amount of secretion from these glands. Bartholin's glands are homologous in structure and function to the bulbourethral (Cowper's) glands in males.

The media has convinced some women that their labia minora hang down too far or are the wrong shape and so they need labia plasty- surgery to reduce size and reshape the labia. The procedure is often described as minor but it is important to remember that no surgery is risk free. The American Congress of Obstetrics and Gynecology (2007) has stated that these surgeries are not medically indicated and that the safety and effectiveness has not been shown. In addition, they believe women should be warned of the complications such as infection, altered sensation, pain during intercourse and adhesions and scarring from these procedures. Labia come in various shapes, size and color making us all very individual, not in need of surgery.

Clitoris

The **clitoris** is a small structure made up of erectile tissue located at the top of the vestibule where the labia majora join. It is made up of three parts—the glans, the shaft, and the root, or *crura,* and evolves from the same tissue that develops into the penis on the male. The glans of the clitoris is exposed by retracting the prepuce or clitoral hood.

The clitoris is a structure solely designed for sexual pleasure; it has no urinary or reproductive function. It is not

sex in society 2.1

Betty Dodson's Art

The vulva has long been the subject of artistic expression. The vulva has often been portrayed as a flower, with the labia representing its petals, moist with the dew of sexual arousal, unfolding to reveal the secrets of love and lust contained within.

For more than 30 years, author, artist, and lecturer Betty Dodson has been celebrating female form and function. She has had over 100 exhibitions, and her artwork has adorned countless galleries throughout the world. Her sketches of the vulva capture the variety and uniqueness of female external genitalia. She combines artistic expression with sexual health activism.

Her book *Sex for One: The Joy of Self Loving* is a celebration of female sexuality. In the book, Dodson chronicles her own personal journey from a woman who questioned her own sexual response and ability to enjoy orgasm to a champion of women's sexual health. For decades, Dodson has run workshops devoted to helping women become orgasmic by using masturbation to liberate their sexual energy. Her artwork adorns her book, illustrating the sensual nature of female sexuality.

Source: From *Sex for One: The Joy of Self Loving* by Betty Dodson, copyright © 1974, 1983, 1987 by Betty Dodson.

involved in the passing of any body fluid, in contrast to the penis, which has a role in sexual response, reproduction, and urination. Because of this, many females don't discover their clitoris until preadolescence or older. Figure 2.2 depicts the clitoris.

The clitoris is richly endowed with nerve endings. Although it appears externally as much smaller than the male penis, the clitoral glans has 8000 sensory nerve endings, more than any other body part (Cornforth, 2009). Because of its dense concentration of nerve endings, the clitoris is sensitive to over stimulation, and the prepuce will move forward to cover and protect it from excessive stimulation. The glans is exposed during sexual arousal but the underlying structures of the clitoris are not. New research suggests that these underlying structures may play a larger role in sexual arousal than previously believed. Johnson (2004) uses an iceberg analogy to explain how the glans of the clitoris is similar to the tip of an iceberg. Most of the mass of the clitoris continues under pelvic bone, turns down and surrounds the vagina from above and both sides.

In the unaroused state, the clitoris is hidden by the prepuce. During sexual arousal, the spongy tissue of the clitoris engorges with blood, causing the clitoris to grow, become erect, and protrude from the prepuce, which retracts as the labia minora unfold. The clitoris is highly sensitive to sexual stimulation. Because of this high sensitivity, females often find it more arousing and comfortable when the clitoris is stimulated gently on either side instead of being directly stimulated. Adequate clitoral stimulation plays a key role in female sexual response and orgasm.

Methods effective for arousal include manual, oral, and mechanical stimulation of the clitoris. During intercourse, if there is no pressure on the clitoris, manual stimulation can be used to enhance arousal. Discussion of the clitoris has often been missing from the education of young women. The clitoris is the center of sexual arousal, and U.S. culture has historically been reticent to discuss sexual pleasure with young girls. See chapter 7, sex in society 7.3, Rethinking the Role of the Clitoris in Sexual Arousal, for a more detailed description of the role of the clitoris during sexual arousal.

Vestibule

Vestibule The area within the labia minora that includes the hymen, introitus, and urethral opening

The **vestibule** is the area between the labia minora that is covered with the hymen and contains the openings to the vagina and urethra. In a sense, the vestibule represents the entrance to the vagina. During sexual arousal, the vestibule is sensitive to stimulation of all kinds. Like the labia and clitoris, it is richly endowed with nerve endings.

Urethral Opening

Urethral opening The opening to the urethra, lying behind the clitoris and in front of the vaginal opening

The **urethral opening** in the female lies behind the clitoris and in front of the vaginal opening. Because it is difficult for a female to see and locate, some people have mistakenly thought that a female urinates out the vagina. The urethra itself is an internal structure.

Hymen and Introitus

Hymen The membrane that lines the introitus

Introitus The vaginal opening

The **hymen**, named for the Greek god of marriage, is a thin mucous membrane that partially covers the opening to the vagina, the **introitus**. There is no biological function for the hymen. The hymen is intact at birth but typically becomes perforated by the time a young woman reaches puberty, allowing the passage of menstrual flow. Various activities ranging from sports and exercise to inserting fingers or other objects into the vagina during masturbation are capable of perforating the hymen.

Although the hymen is durable, its opening is capable of being stretched or enlarged through intercourse, masturbation, or insertion of a tampon. Many people believe that the presence of a hymen is proof of a woman's virginity. This belief also is not true.

Figure 2.3 illustrates the three main types of hymens. The most common is the *annular*, in which the tissue surrounds the entire opening of the vagina and is open in the middle. The *cribiform* hymen has a web of tissue over the introitus and several small openings. The *septate* has a single band of tissue that divides the introitus into two parts. In rare occurrences, girls

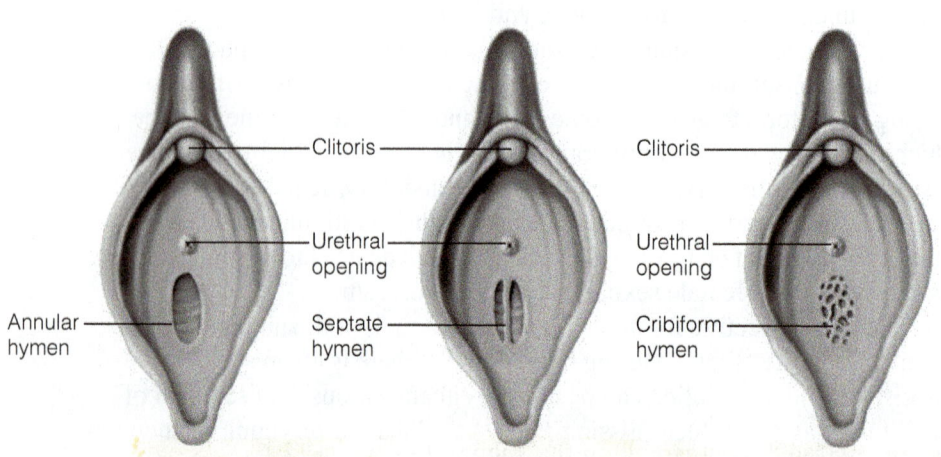

Figure 2.3 *Types of Hymens*

are born with the hymen completely covering the opening of the vagina, which is not discovered until she starts menstruating. This causes the fluid to build up in the vagina. When this happens, a physician must make a small opening to allow the menstrual flow.

If the hymen is still present at the time of first intercourse, penetration by the penis can produce some discomfort or even bleeding if the hymen is torn. Prior to first intercourse, a female can stretch her hymen by inserting 1 to 2 finger(s) into the vagina and pushing toward the front , sides and back of the vagina. If necessary, a physician may also cut the hymen or stretch the hymen with dilators. However, there is usually little trouble inserting the penis through the hymen if the male is gentle and has taken enough time in foreplay to allow the female to become adequately lubricated.

Perineum

The female **perineum** is the area between the thighs bounded in the front by the pelvis joint (the *symphysis pubis*) and in the rear by the coccyx (tailbone). The muscular tissue is covered by a layer of skin. Although it is not normally considered part of the female sexual anatomy, the perineum plays a part in sexual response because the entire area is endowed with nerve endings and is highly responsive to sexual stimulation. As with men, the nature and intensity of stimulation desired in this area varies from woman to woman and encounter to encounter.

Perineum The area of muscle and skin between vagina and anus

The major difference between the perineum in women and men is its role in childbearing. The perineum of pregnant women is subject to tearing of the skin and muscle tissue during childbirth. This is usually the time when they first become aware of this region. During delivery, pressure from the emerging fetus can exert a tremendous force on the perineum, first stretching, then tearing, the muscle and skin. The muscles and skin will heal, although some women report less sensitivity, as nerve endings can be injured and require additional time to recover. Women are encouraged to massage the perineum with vitamin e oil during pregnancy to minimize the risk of tearing.

Anus

The anus in women is exactly the same as in men and, as such, is capable of similar responsiveness during sexual activity. Sexual stimulation can be enjoyed manually, orally (**anilingus**), and through anal intercourse. Some women use anal intercourse as an alternative to vaginal coitus because they think that by doing this, they can "preserve their virginity" and still enjoy sex. (See Healthy Sex tips 8.5)

Anilingus Oral stimulation of the anus

Underlying Structures

Although only the vulva is visible, there are underlying structures that are important to sexual arousal (see Figure 2.4). The area is rich in erectile tissue, with a network of nerves and blood vessels that become engorged, comparable to the spongy tissue of the penis. The vestibular bulbs run along the

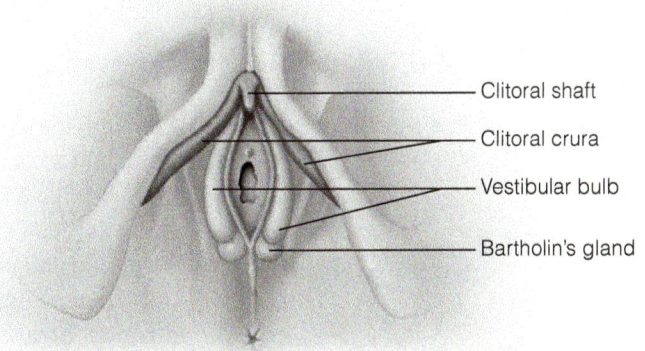

Clitoral shaft
Clitoral crura
Vestibular bulb
Bartholin's gland

Figure 2.4 *Underlying Structures*

sex in society 2.2

Female Genital Mutilation

The practice of female genital mutilation (FGM) is a centuries old tradition in some cultures, primarily in western, eastern and north-eastern Africa, and in some countries in Asia and the Middle East (World Health Organization, 2013).

It is estimated that 140 million girls and women worldwide are living with the consequences of female genital mutilation. (World Health Organization, 2013). The procedure ranges from removal of the clitoris, removal of the clitoris and labia minora, or removal of the clitoris and entire labia with the area stitched closed. Other harmful procedures include piercing, scraping and cauterizing the genital area. Although the procedure is most commonly performed between the ages of 2 and 15, some girls have had it done within the first week of life (Rising Daughters Aware, 1999; WHO, 2013). This cultural and religious custom has been done to reduce females' ability to experience sexual pleasure and ensure marital fidelity. The cultures that practice FGM do not believe a woman should derive pleasure from sex. The physical health risks of the procedure are many with immediate consequences including shock, bleeding, sepsis, urinary retention, open sores in the genital area, and damage to nearby genital tissues. Long term consequences include infertility, recurrent bladder infections, the need for more surgery, childbirth complications and the deaths of newborns (WHO, 2013).

Female genital mutilation is recognized internationally as a violation of human rights of girls and women. In 1012 the United Nations General Assembly accepted a resolution on the elimination of female genital mutilation. In recent years many organized groups, most prominently the World Health Organization and the United Nations Children's Fund, have condemned this treatment of females and are continuing to pressure the countries and cultures that still practice genital mutilation to end it. U.S. representatives to the World Bank and other financial institutions oppose loans to countries that widely practice genital cutting and have no anti-FGM educational programs. In 24 African countries there are laws prohibiting FGM. In most countries, there is a decline in female genital mutilations and most women and men in these practicing countries support the elimination of the practice (WHO, 2013).

In the United States, the Federal Prohibition of Female Genital Mutilation Act of 1995 passed in September 1996, provides for prison sentences for anyone who performs this procedure on a female under 18 years of age. That law does permit the surgery if it is "necessary to the health of the person on whom it is performed." Other countries that outlaw the procedure include England, Canada, France, Sweden, and Switzerland.

vagina, with the crura of the clitoris extending up toward the pelvic bone. The structures engorge with blood during sexual arousal, causing the labia, clitoris, and vagina to enlarge, swell, and deepen in color.

The muscles in the area also play a significant role in arousal. As discussed in Healthy Sex Hints 2.1, strengthening the pelvic floor muscles through Kegel exercises has clear health and sexual benefits.

Breasts

Lactation The process of producing and secreting milk from the breasts

Although the main function of the female breast is **lactation**, it has taken on erotic and sexual significance in American and other cultures. Breast size and shape have become markers for attractiveness, sexiness, femininity, and motherhood. The breasts are composed of mammary glands, fatty tissue, the nipple and areola, and underlying muscle and ligaments.

Increasingly, women—even teen girls—are choosing to surgically alter their breasts. Large-breasted females may choose reduction surgery for appearance and comfort while small breasted women may want to increase the size of their breast.

Mammary Glands

The **mammary glands** are divided into 15 to 20 lobes or compartments separated by fatty tissue. Each lobe is made up of several smaller components called lobules.

Imbedded in the lobules are milk-secreting cells called alveoli. Following childbirth, special hormones trigger the production and secretion of milk from the alveoli. Milk secreted from the alveoli is stored in chambers called mammary ducts and are drained through nursing.

Swelling of glandular tissue and storage of milk typically cause the breasts of nursing women to enlarge significantly. Breast size returns to normal after nursing ceases. (We will discuss lactation and nursing more fully in Chapter 13.)

Breast swelling, and in some cases painful tenderness, often precedes menstruation, as the breasts (like the uterus) prepare for potential pregnancy.

Mammary glands Glands within the breasts that produce milk for lactation

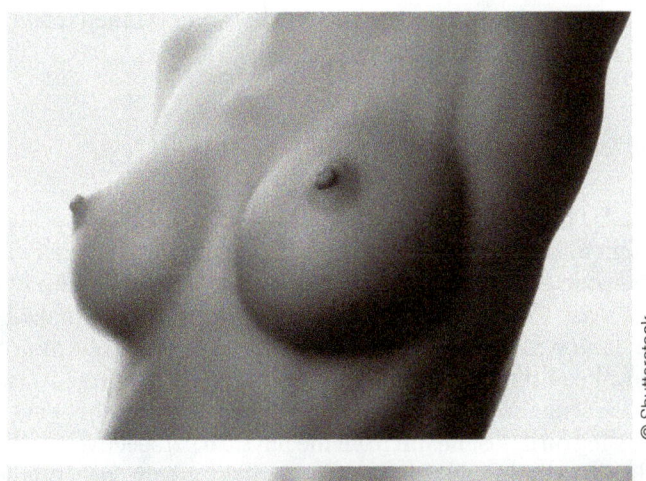

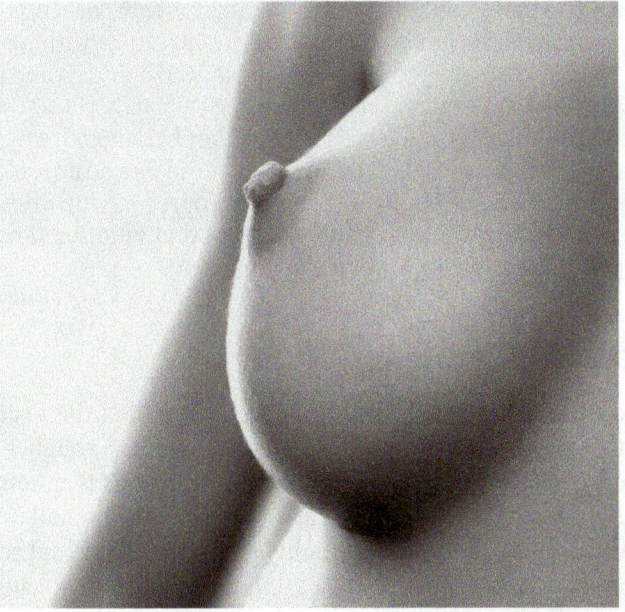

The female breast comes in a variety of shapes and sizes.

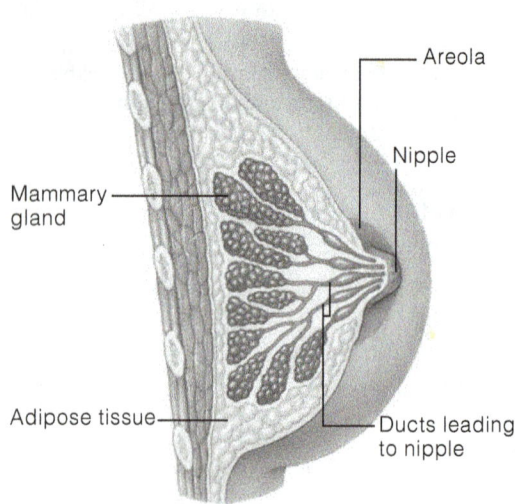

Figure 2.5 *Structures of the Female Breast*

Fatty Tissue

Breast size and shape in a woman who is not nursing are determined primarily by heredity and the amount of adipose or fatty tissue present in the breast. Figure 2.5 highlights the different structures of the breast.

Because of the cultural emphasis on breast size, surgical breast augmentation (enlargement) and reduction procedures have become much more common. In 2012, breast augmentation was the number one plastic surgery performed with approximately 286,000 women having breast augmentation surgery. In addition, 89,000 women had breast lifts and 42,000 had breast reduction surgery (American Society of Plastic Surgeons, 2012). The number of augmentation procedures had been as low as 32,000 in 1992. A 2008 study of women who had had breast augmentation, lift, or reduction found the women reported improved self esteem and quality of life. Of these women, 99 percent were so satisfied that they would have the surgery again (American Society of Plastic Surgeons, 2008). As with any surgery, breast augmentation and reduction procedures are not without risks. Some women report problems with breast feeding that are related to implants.

❧ *Physical and Emotional Wellness* ❧

Concern for the appearance of one's breasts highlights how the emotional dimension of health interfaces with the physical dimension. Many females spend money to increase the size of their breasts with implants or to decrease the size. Plastic surgeons are available to make breasts smaller, larger, more even, or higher and/or to replace one or both that may have been removed due to disease. Because breasts in American culture are sexualized and significant to women's sense of being attractive, focusing on breast health from the physical perspective may become secondary to a woman's concern that her breasts are "acceptable."

The physical dimensions of breast health can change with menstruation, pregnancy, breastfeeding, menopause, and aging. Some females are prone to breast cysts related to their menstrual cycles. Some are amazed at the changes in the breast when they breastfeed, whereas for others concerns over breast changes can stand as an impediment to their desire to breastfeed. Breast health requires paying attention to the breasts and their changes and ensuring that emotional concerns do not get in the way of proper care.

Areola and Nipple

Areola The brownish or pink ring of tissue surrounding the nipple of the breast

At the end of the breast is a ring of darker skin called the **areola**. In the center of the areola is the nipple. The areola is slightly rougher in texture than the rest of the breast because it contains oil glands that help lubricate the nipples during breastfeeding. The areola also contains small muscles and many nerve endings. This makes it highly responsive to sexual stimulation. Nursing mothers also report that suckling their babies can cause sensual feelings that can be a source of confusion.

case study 2.2

Pubic Hair

When I was younger, I could not wait for my body to change and become a 'grown up' body. My first pubic hair was greeted with great excitement and pride. I grew the most wonderful bushy pubic hair and looked forward to showing it off to the future love of my life. The time finally came when I thought I had found the perfect guy with whom to share my body. I was so proud when I first undressed only to find that he thought my pubic hair was ugly and disgusting. He pressured me until I agreed to remove it to please him. What a disaster! I shaved, only to find that it grew back in a few days and itched like crazy. So then I went to a salon to have a bikini wax. That took longer to grow back but was it was pretty uncomfortable when they pulled the wax and hair off and it really seemed expensive on my budget. For my grand finale, I tried tweezing since that would be cheap but it almost killed me. After all that, I decided my pubic hair was just fine as it was. I liked it and if he did not, then maybe he wasn't truly the right one for me. This experience really made me look at what I am willing to do to my body to please someone. I am now with this amazing guy who loves all parts of my body, just as they are. His attitude makes our physical intimacy so relaxing and this relaxation makes the physical pleasure incredibly intense.

Critical Thinking

Do sexual partners have the right to persuade a partner to make physical changes? How far are you willing to go to change for your partner?

The nipple is located within the areola and contains smooth muscle fibers, milk ducts, and many nerve endings. The nipples and areola are highly sensitive, and their smooth muscle fibers can contract upon stimulation, causing them to stiffen and become erect. Nipples also can stiffen and become erect in response to cold and nonsexual tactile stimulation.

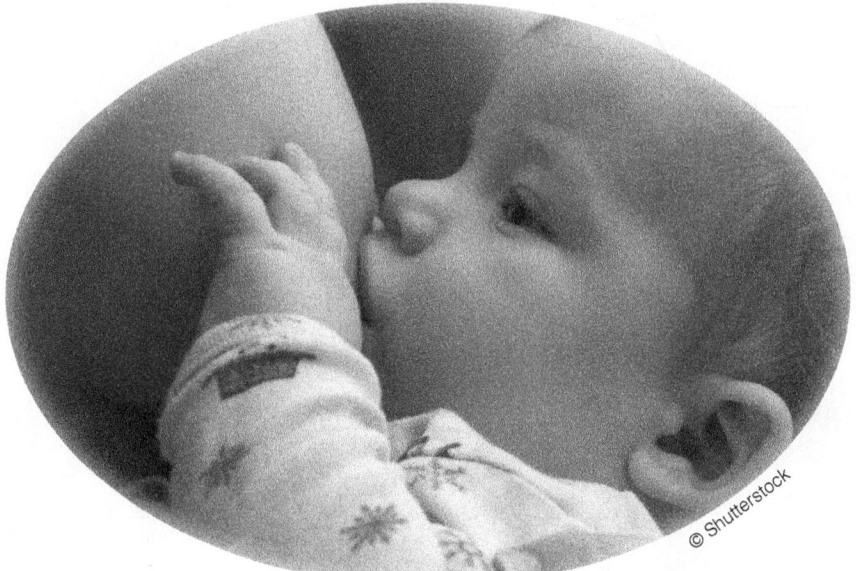

Breastfeeding is strongly encouraged as a healthy and economical way to nourish a baby.

Breast health was once thought to include monthly breast self exams by all women. The philosophy and thinking about this action has changed however. The US Preventative Services Task Force (2009) and the Canadian Preventative Services Task Force both recommend against women doing monthly breast self exam (BSE). There is no data to support that breast self exams decrease breast cancer deaths. However, these exams are likely to decrease the chances of her going for a clinical assessment and biopsy. Therefore both groups recommend against doing breast self exam. Mammograms are recommended every two years for women age 50-74 for early detection of breast cancer to help protect breast health. Deciding to screen women under 50 should be on an individual basis (USPSTF, 2009).

Internal Female Sexual Structures

The internal structures of the female anatomy include the vagina, uterus, cervix, fallopian tubes, and ovaries (Figure 2.6). The urethra in the female lies outside the reproductive system, yet, along with the bladder, it is affected by pregnancy, menstruation, and sexual behavior.

Urethra and Bladder

The urethra in the female runs from the bladder to the vestibule, and it is much shorter than that of the male (1 inch compared to 9 inches in the male) making her more vulnerable to infections. It is relatively easy for bacteria from outside the body to enter the urethra and lead to bladder infections known as **urinary tract infections (UTIs).** *Escherichia coli* bacteria from the rectum and irritation from sexual intercourse can lead to bacterial bladder infections , necessitating antibiotic treatment. Using the diaphragm as birth control can also increase a woman's risk of bacterial UTI's. An inflammation of the bladder, called **cystitis**, can occur due to irritants such as feminine hygiene sprays or spermicidal jellies(Mayo Clinic, 2012). Drinking plenty

Urinary Tract Infections (UTI) Bacterial infection of the bladder

Cystitis Bladder inflammation

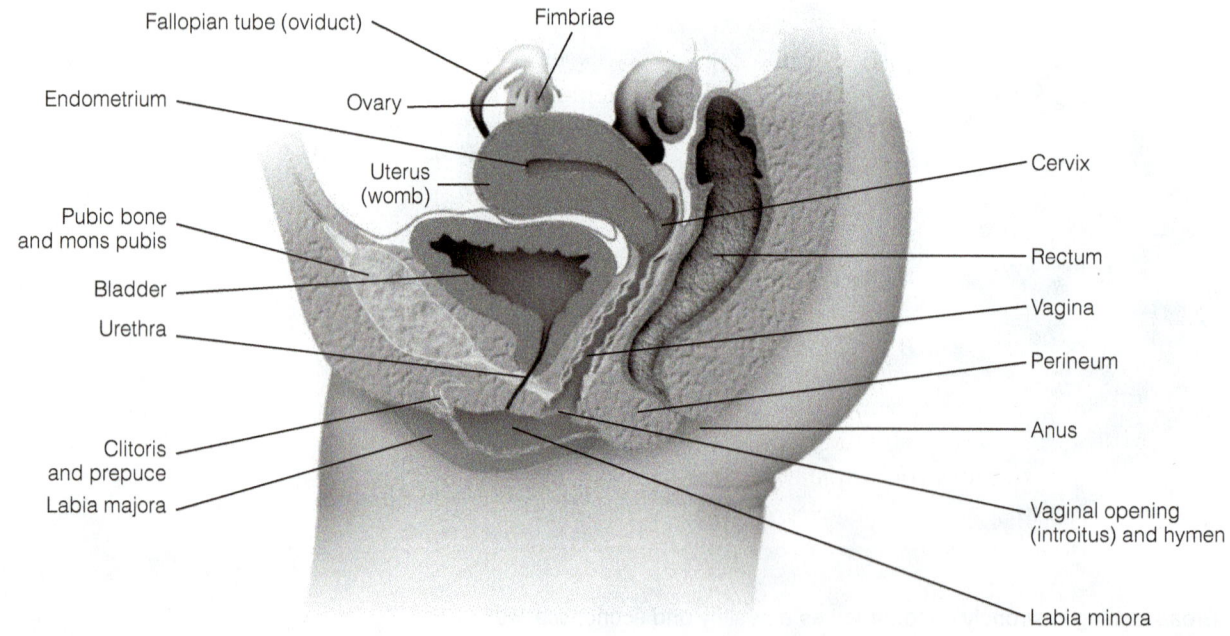

Figure 2.6 *Internal Sexual Structures*

of fluids, urinating frequently, washing gently around vagina or anus with mild (not harsh) soaps, urinating after intercourse and wiping from the front to back when you use the bathroom can enhance urinary health. The bladder in the female lies next to the anterior wall of the vagina and in close proximity to the uterus. The role of the bladder is to hold urine and when this stretchy pouch is full, the female feels the need to urinate. Because of its location, women's sense of needing to urinate can be affected by menstruation, pregnancy, lovemaking activities, and pelvic exams.

Vagina

The **vagina** is a thin-walled muscular tube, about 3 to 4 inches long, lying between the bladder and the rectum, which connects to the cervix at one end and opens up to the outside of the body at the other. The vagina is tilted upward at a 45-degree angle extending toward the small of the back.

The walls of the vagina contain an outer layer of muscular tissue and an inner layer of mucous membrane. The mucous membrane tissue produces a thin, clear, moderately acidic (pH 3.5–4) discharge that provides an efficient self-cleaning mechanism. During sexual arousal, these same tissues engorge with blood, producing a thin, slippery lubrication that reduces friction and facilitates intercourse.

The outer third of the vagina contains the most muscle tissue and nerve endings. The interior and rear part, which connects with the cervix,

Vagina A tubular organ connecting to the uterus, which serves both reproductive and erotic functions

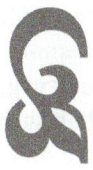

healthy sex hints 2.1

Pelvic Floor (Kegel) Exercises

You can practice contracting your pelvic floor muscles to prevent or reduce sagging of the organs and urinary incontinence (losing urine when you cough, sneeze, or laugh), to strengthen your orgasms, and to prepare for childbirth. Before you begin your exercises make sure your bladder is empty. A good way to locate these muscles is to spread your legs apart while urinating and to then start and stop the flow of urine. Your ability to do this is one indication of how strong your muscles are. If you are not sure if you have found the correct muscle, insert your finger into the vagina and tighten the muscles as if you are stopping the flow of urine, then release, You should feel the muscle tighten on your finger.

When you have correctly identified the muscles, begin exercising these muscles by squeezing, and holding for 6-8 seconds, then relax for 10 seconds. It is essential to isolate the pelvic floor muscles. If you contract your buttocks or abdomen while doing the exercises, you are doing them incorrectly. Repeat these contractions 10 times in a row. to make up one set of exercises. Repeat the set of 10 contractions 3 times every day. The exercises are only effective when done regularly and the more you do them, the more they will help. You can do them at any time—sitting in a car or bus, talking on the telephone, or even as a "wake-up" exercise. After just 6 weeks, many report better muscle tone, increased sexual pleasure during intercourse, and stronger orgasms.

Source: *Mannheim, J. (2012). Kegel exercises-self care. Online:http://www.nlm/nih.gov*

is relatively devoid of nerve endings. In the unaroused state, the vagina resembles a collapsed space similar to a balloon without air in it. Because the vagina is a muscle, it can expand to accommodate objects of varying sizes ranging from a tampon, penis, or sex toy to a newborn's head. Myths and stories exist, nonetheless, alluding to male or female partners being incompatible: "He's too big for me," "She's too loose for him," and so on. Being sexually active or having a baby will not make the woman's vagina "too big" since the vagina is a muscle. However, all females need to perform Kegel exercises three times a day to maintain and strengthen the muscle tone of the vagina and pelvic floor. (Mannheim, 2012). The technique guidelines are explained in healthy sex hints 2.1.

G-spot An area on the front wall of the vagina

On the front wall of the vagina, midway between the introitus and cervix, is an area known as the **G-spot**, or Grafenberg spot, named for the physician who first identified that portion of the vagina as having erotic potential. Research conducted in the 1980s focused on whether all women had such a spot, if all women found stimulation to the area arousing, and what exactly was the chemical makeup of the fluid propelled from the urethra in some women at the time of orgasm. Deep manual stimulation or penile stimulation can cause the area to swell, leading to an orgasm that has a strong, vaginal component. Overall, research on the G-spot has been related to discussions of female ejaculation, tissue referred to as a female prostate gland, and a redefining of the components of female orgasm (Zaviacic & Whipple, 1993).

The vagina is also known as the birth canal because of its function as the exit point for the newborn during childbirth. The vagina has both reproductive and sexual pleasuring functions. Unlike the penis, the vagina is not involved during urination. Urine is excreted through the urethra, whose opening is located above the vaginal opening in the introitus.

The vagina is actually a self-cleansing structure. To ensure vaginal health, the average, healthy woman needs to do nothing more than shower or bathe daily (making sure to wash the vulva). She has no need to douche, wear minipads (if not menstruating), or use feminine hygiene sprays to perfume the vaginal area. Douching and/or using feminine hygiene sprays can change the pH of the vagina and cause a vaginal infection.

The walls of a normal, healthy vagina produce a thin, clear to yellow colored, slippery discharge that cleanses the vaginal lining and does not indicate any problem. The discharge and the vagina in general have a characteristic musky odor that sex partners often consider erotic.

Changes in the amount, consistency, color, and odor can be used to assess whether you have a vaginal infection. If the amount of discharge increases, changes in color (from clear to bright yellow, green, or white), consistency (from thin and slippery to thick and curdish), or odor (becomes foul smelling), it could indicate a vaginal infection.

Vaginal health can be enhanced by taking steps to increase overall health and vaginal health. Using condoms when sexually active and being in a monogamous relationship will help protect the vagina from STDs. All females should be vaccinated for human papillomavirus that can cause warts and vaginal cancer. In addition, they should also be vaccinated for hepatitis A and B, which are spread through sexual contact, The vaginal tissues are very sensitive so avoid douching, perfumed soaps, feminine sprays and scented tampons. If sex toys are used, be sure to clean them after each use. Antibiotics can cause vaginal yeast infection and should be taken only when really needed. Some antihistamines used for allergies can cause vaginal dryness which can be irritating during intercourse. She may need to change to a medication that does not have this side effect. Spermicides and the NuvaRing can cause vaginal irritation so finding a different and effective contraceptive will protect vaginal health. Anxiety and stress can decrease sexual arousal and vaginal lubrication so relaxing before intercourse will decrease vaginal dryness and irritation (Mayo Clinic, 2012). Marijuana use before and during intercourse may contribute to vaginal dryness so she may want to avoid using. She may also want to use a water based lubricant to protect against irritation during intercourse. The couple could make using the lubricant an erotic, fun part of foreplay.

Uterus

The **uterus** is an organ that is sized and shaped like a pear. It is connected to the vagina at its narrow end. The end, or cervix, of the uterus is attached to the vagina and protrudes into the end of the vaginal canal. The wider end (the fundus) extends backward and is held in place by a broad uterine ligament. The uterus is tipped slightly forward.

The uterus is composed of three layers of tissue. The innermost layer, called the **endometrium**, undergoes a cycle of transformation each menstrual period as it prepares for implantation of a fertilized egg. The endometrium is where a fertilized egg implants and grows during pregnancy. If fertilization does not occur, the endometrium breaks down and is shed during menstruation.

The next layer of tissue, the **myometrium**, makes up the bulk of the uterus. This is thick muscular tissue capable of providing the powerful contractions necessary to dislodge endometrial tissue during menstruation or deliver a developed fetus during childbirth. This layer is capable of expanding the size of the uterus from that of a pear, pre-pregnancy, to a small watermelon during pregnancy, and then returning to near its original size within 2 months after birth.

The myometrial contractions associated with menstruation can cause severe cramping and pain which is called dysmenorrhea. At the end of this chapter, we will discuss self-help strategies to reduce these and other symptoms associated with menstrual discomfort. The third and outermost layer of uterine tissue is called the **perimetrium**.

Cervix

The **cervix**, located at the lower end of the uterus, is described as the neck of the uterus and is about one inch long. It resembles a small ring or button, the center portion tightly contracted and blocked with a plug of mucus. The cervix feels similar to the way the tip of your nose feels. Running through the cervix is the cervical canal, a small passageway connecting the vagina to the uterus. It is filled with irregularly shaped spaces called *crypts*. The cervical opening, or *cervical os,* remains closed and blocked with mucus during most of a woman's menstrual cycle. As a woman's fertile time approaches, the mucous plug thins, allowing a passageway through the cervix into the uterus. Figure 2.7 shows the cervix and related structures.

Uterus Also called the womb, a fist-sized muscular structure that houses the developing fetus during gestation

Endometrium The inner blood lining of the uterus

Myometrium The muscular, middle layer of the uterus

Perimetrium The outer lining of the uterus

Cervix The neck of the uterus, which extends into the inner end of the vagina

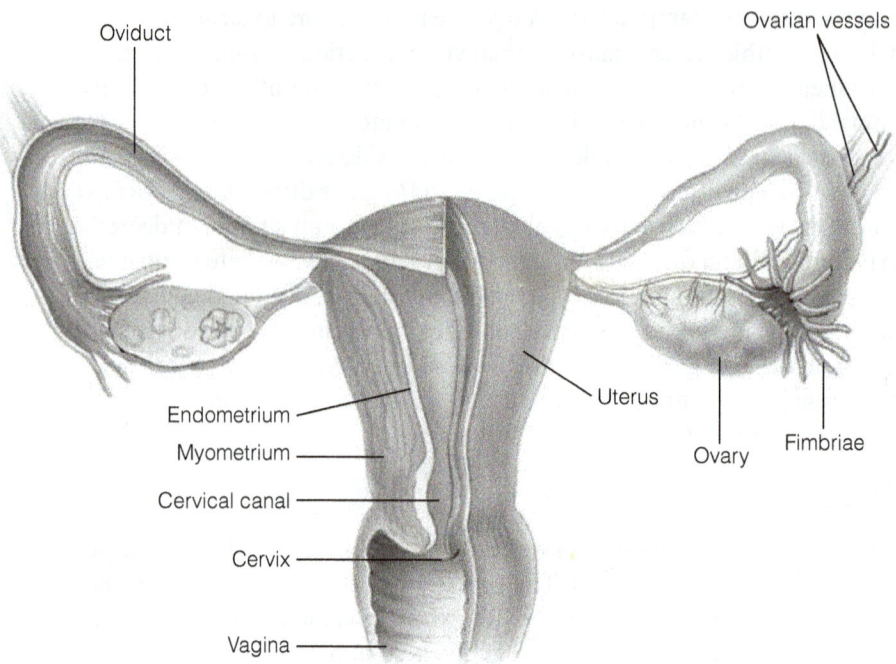

Figure 2.7 *The Cervix and Related Structures*

T-zone Transformation zone of the cervix, where columnar epithelial tissue of the uterus meets with squamous tissue of the vagina

During adolescence, the tissue of the cervix changes or transforms. This transformation zone is referred to as the **T-zone**. Cervical tissue (columnar epithelial tissue) is different from vaginal tissue (squamous mucous membrane tissue). During childhood, a young girl's cervix is covered with more columnar epithelial tissue than squamous tissue. As she matures, the amount of exposed columnar epithelial tissue decreases. The T-zone becomes smaller, encompassing the cervix and cervical canal. The T-zone is the area most commonly infected by gonorrhea, chlamydia, and other STDs during unprotected vaginal sexual intercourse. Because columnar epithelial tissue seems much more susceptible than squamous tissue to STD infection, all women (particularly young women) who are having vaginal intercourse should protect this area with barrier contraceptives such as a condom or diaphram.

The cervix is also a common site for the development of cancer in women. STD infection of the T-zone in young women can be a precursor of cervical cancer in later life. This is particularly true of infection with viral organisms (human papillomavirus, herpes simplex virus) introduced into the cervix during adolescence. It literally lays the seeds for the development of cervical cancer that appears a decade or more later. Each year 19,000 cancers caused by HPV are diagnosed in women and cervical cancer is the most common of these. About 8000 cancers caused by HPV occur in men each year and oral cancer is the most common (American Cancer Society, 2013). The Human papillomavirus vaccine protects both males and females from these unnecessary cancers,

To protect the health of the cervix, the Human papillomavirus vaccine is recommended for routine use in females and males ages 11-12 to help prevent cervical cancer caused by HPV. The vaccine is also recommended for 13- 26 year olds who have not yet been vaccinated. All three shots should be given before the first sexual contact, ensuring the greatest protection from the virus. Human papillomavirus is spread by skin to skin contact during any type of sexual activity with another person (Center for Disease Control, 2013). Currently only one third of teen girls and only one percent of teen males receives all three shots (CDC, 2012). Starting at age 21, cervical cancer screening (a pap smear), is recommended every three years. It is recommended that women not be screened before age 21 (US Preventive Services Task Force, 2012). Women, who begin having intercourse after age 20, have a lower risk of cervical cancer. Waiting to have intercourse, using condoms to protect the cervix and reducing the number of sexual partners is a great combination of actions to best protect the cervix.

Fallopian Tubes

The two **fallopian tubes**, also known as *oviducts* and *uterine tubes,* approximately 4 inches long, stretch from either side of the fundus of the uterus to the ovaries. Unlike the male vas deferens, which connects to the epididymis, the fallopian tubes do not actually connect with the ovary. Each fallopian tube stops just short of the ovary and is held in place with ligaments that attach it to the peritoneal cavity. The open end of the fallopian tube is funnel shaped, with fingerlike projections called *fimbriae,* which shadow but do not connect with the ovaries. The fallopian tubes are made up of smooth muscle tissue and are lined with hair like projections called *cilia.*

During ovulation, an egg released from the ovary is drawn into the fallopian tube by the fimbriae. No one knows for sure how this happens, but once inside the tube, the egg is moved along by a combination of smooth-muscle contractions and the wavelike action of the cilia. For the egg to be fertilized and implanted within the uterus, a viable sperm must be waiting in the fallopian tube or reach the egg within 24 hours. Figure 2.8 shows how the female egg develops and moves.

Fallopian tube cilia are highly susceptible to destruction from infection. Destruction of these cilia is a common byproduct of infection with gonorrhea or chlamydia. Once the cilia are destroyed, they do not grow back. In addition, infections can cause scarring of the fallopian tubes. Either of these can result in infertility or **ectopic pregnancy**. The term ectopic refers to the process in which the fertilized egg implants in a part of the body other than the uterus, most often in the fallopian tubes. Fertilized eggs can also implant in the abdominal area or cervical canal. Ectopic pregnancies cannot go to term and, if not treated promptly, can be life-threatening. The most common early symptoms of an ectopic pregnancy include abdominal or pelvic pain and light bleeding (Mayo Clinic, 2012).

It is estimated that 1 in 15 sexually active adolescents has Chlamydia. Therefore, to protect the health of the fallopian tubes sexually active women must make sure they do not have Chlamydia. The American Congress of Obstetrics and Gynecology recommends yearly Chlamydia screening for all sexually active women age 25 and under. A urine test is all that is needed and allows non invasive screening. Chlamydia is a silent infection and if left untreated it may cause pelvic inflammatory disease (PID) and if this is not treated it may cause infertility, ectopic pregnancy or chronic pelvic pain. Annual screening of sexually active women is also recommended for gonorrhea since it has the same destructive effects on the fallopian tubes (Burstein, Jacobs, Kissin, & Workowski, 2013)

Fallopian tubes Also called oviducts, extending from the fundus of the uterus to the ovaries; serve as the passageway for the ova

Ectopic pregnancy Implantation of an egg outside the womb

Follicle development

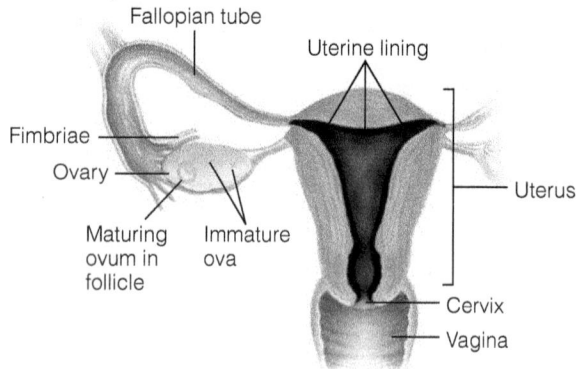

Ovulation

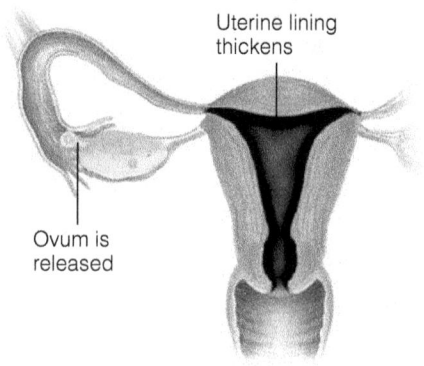

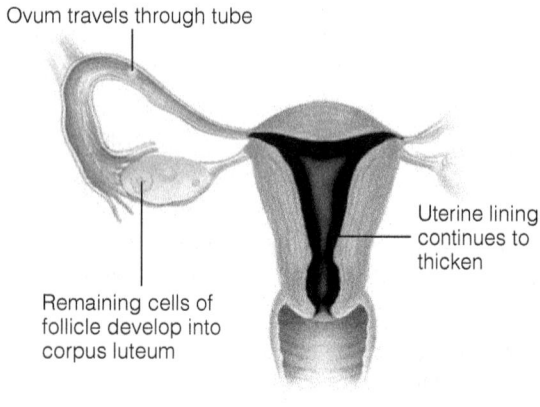

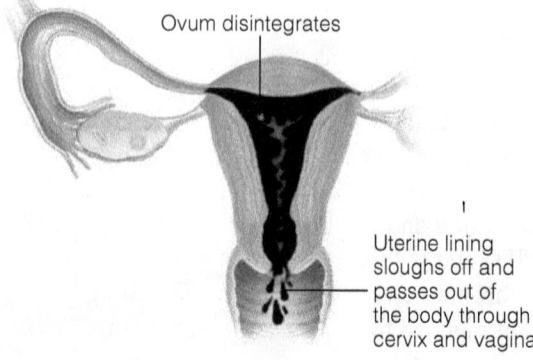

Figure 2.8 *Movement of the Egg*

Ovaries

The **ovaries** are the size and shape of almonds. Each is located adjacent to a fallopian tube and is held in place in the peritoneum by connective tissue that anchors them to the broad uterine ligament. Like the male testes, the ovaries have two primary functions: fertility and hormone production. The ovaries produce ova (eggs) and the two important female sex hormones, estrogen and progesterone.

Reproductive Physiology

Two distinct cycles—the menstrual (also known as *uterine*) and ovarian—work in concert to control reproduction. Each cycle is regulated by hormones secreted by various endocrine glands. These cycles and their respective hormones are introduced here and described in greater detail in Chapter 13, "Human Reproduction."

Menarche is the term to define the onset of the menstrual cycle in girls. The age of menarche is similar to what it was in 1973 with only ten percent of girls experiencing menarche before 11 and ninety percent of girls reaching menarche by age 14 (Chumlea, Schubert, Roche, Kulin, Lee, Himes, & Sun, 2003).

Menopause has become a term somewhat harder to define, yet the traditional definition is 12 consecutive months of amenorrhea, meaning the absence of a period, without a woman having had surgery or any medical treatment that stops menstruation. The average age for menopause is 51 (Mayo Clinic, 2013). Overall, females menstruate approximately 13 times a calendar year, over a 40-year time frame, minus pregnancy. Consequently, menstruating is a fundamental part of being female, occupying a significant part of a woman's life.

Ovarian Cycle

Unlike male sperm, which are freshly produced in unlimited numbers, women are born with approximately 400,000 immature ova. The health and viability of the ova are affected by age and various environmental factors. Exposure to radiation, toxic chemicals, and other hazards can impair the health of the ova. In general, the viability of ova declines with age.

In a normal cycle, one immature egg matures, is released, and either is fertilized or dies and is discarded with the menstrual flow. This three-phased process is called the **ovarian cycle** (see Figure 2.9). Each cycle has a follicular, ovulatory, and luteal phase. For purposes of illustration, a typical 28-day cycle is used here.

Women's cycles can vary significantly; hormonal changes, stress, weight loss, exercise, and other factors can all impact cycle length. A woman who is monitoring her body to determine ovulation needs to understand that ovulation occurs 14 days from the end of the cycle. While the follicular phase can vary in length, the luteal phase tends to be consistently 2 weeks in length.

1. The *follicular phase* consists of the first 10 days. During this time, a **follicle** grows, preparing to release a mature egg.
2. The *ovulatory phase,* days 11 to 14, consists of final preparation for and release of a mature egg.
3. The *luteal phase,* days 14 to 28, revolves around the activity of the **corpus luteum.** The corpus luteum's role of secreting progesterone to sustain the rich endometrial lining necessary for implantation varies depending on whether fertilization occurs.

Ovaries Two almond shaped structures that contain and release ova and secrete the hormones estrogen and progesterone

Menarche The onset of the menstrual cycle in girls

Menopause The absence of a period for 12 consecutive months, without surgery or medical treatment

Ovarian cycle A three phased period of time covering maturation of a follicle, release of ovum, and secreting role of corpus luteum

Follicle An egg sac in the ovary

Corpus luteum The follicle after it has released its ovum and begins to produce progesterone

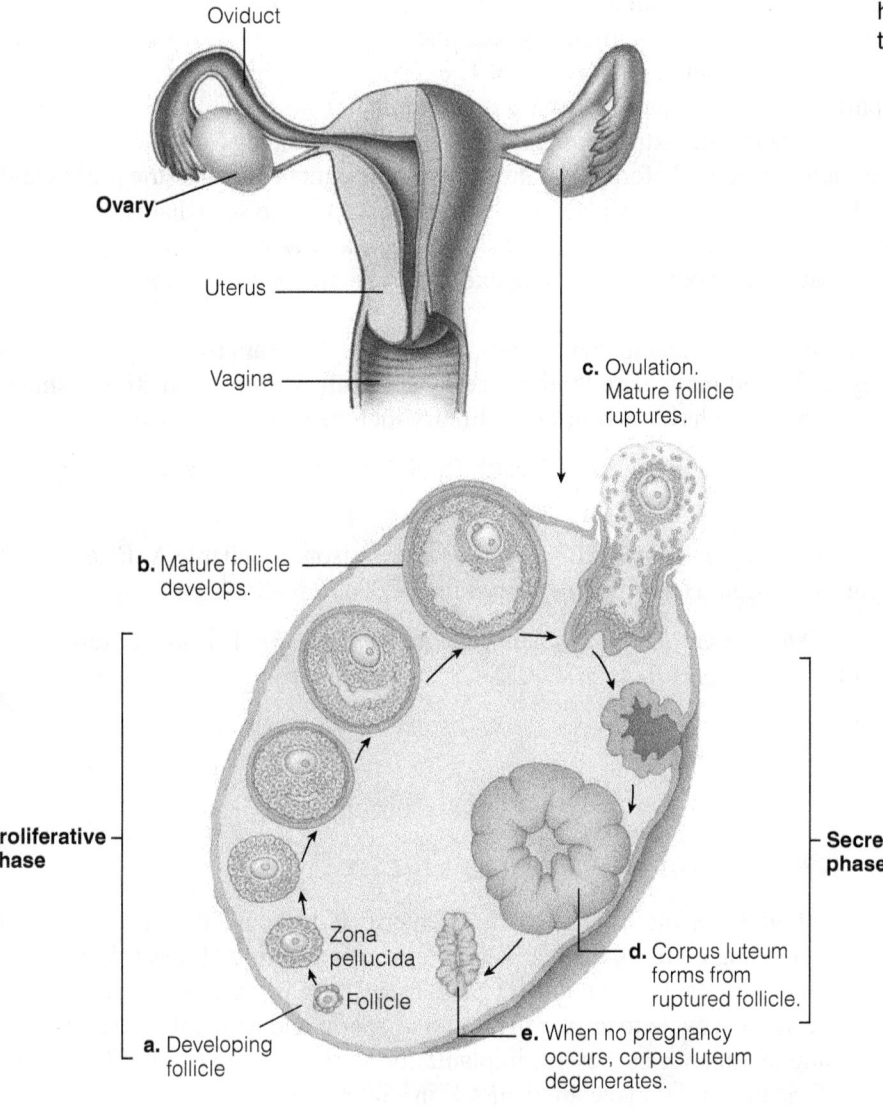

Oviduct

Ovary

Uterus

Vagina

c. Ovulation. Mature follicle ruptures.

b. Mature follicle develops.

Proliferative phase

Secretory phase

Zona pellucida

Follicle

a. Developing follicle

d. Corpus luteum forms from ruptured follicle.

e. When no pregnancy occurs, corpus luteum degenerates.

Figure 2.9 *The Ovarian Cycle*

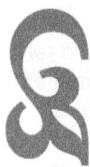

healthy sex hints 2.2

Taking Care of Your Reproductive Health

For many women, going to the gynecologist or other reproductive health care provider is a visit they don't look forward to. In particular, the pelvic exam tends to arouse the most anxiety and discomfort. Draped from the waist down, lying on their back on the exam table with their feet in stirrups, legs spread wide apart, vulva completely exposed, they wait, feeling vulnerable.

Even when performed by the most sensitive of clinicians, the pelvic examination can be stressful. The examination is designed to allow the clinician to examine visually and manually a woman's internal and external sexual anatomy. To facilitate this examination, a speculum is used to spread the walls of the vagina, and a light is used to illuminate the vaginal walls and cervix.

The examination consists of looking at the vulva and internal structures for any abnormalities—unusual growths, erosions, lumps, rashes, or discharges. After visually examining the area, the clinician manually probes the various structures, feeling for any changes in size or shape. A *bimanual examination* means using two hands to palpate structures such as the cervix, uterus, fallopian tubes, and ovaries. During this procedure, the clinician places one hand on the patient's abdomen and inserts two fingers from the other hand into the vagina. The clinician then feels for any abnormalities. Often these palpations will cause pain if disease is present.

Patient-centered clinicians take extra time and care to prepare patients for what is about to happen. They explain each procedure before it is done, helping the patient adjust to the probes and prods that are part of the examination. They also offer patients the option to see what is happening through the use of floor and handheld mirrors. Little things such as warming a speculum before inserting it and helping patients relax with breathing exercises can go a long way toward making the examination less offensive.

Women are encouraged to understand their bodies, prepare for the exam by thinking through the questions that they have, and make sure their concerns are dealt with in a sensitive manner. Three excellent reference books to have in your home library include these:

> *Our Bodies, Ourselves,* Boston Women's Health Book Collective (New York: Simon & Schuster, 2011)

> *The New Harvard Guide for Women's Health,* Karen J. Carlson, Stephanie A. Eisenstat, and Terra Ziporyn (Boston: Harvard University Press, 2004)

> *The V Book: The Doctor's Guide to Complete Vulvovaginal Health,* Elizabeth Stewart and Paula Spencer (New York: Bantam, 2002)

Menstrual or Uterine Cycle

Although the main function of the uterus is to house the implanted and developing embryo, the cyclic nature of reproduction allows this for only a few short days each month. The menstrual cycle coincides perfectly with the ovarian cycle to ensure the union of sperm and egg at the best possible time to enhance successful implantation in the endometrium. The phases of the menstrual cycle are depicted in Figure 2.10.

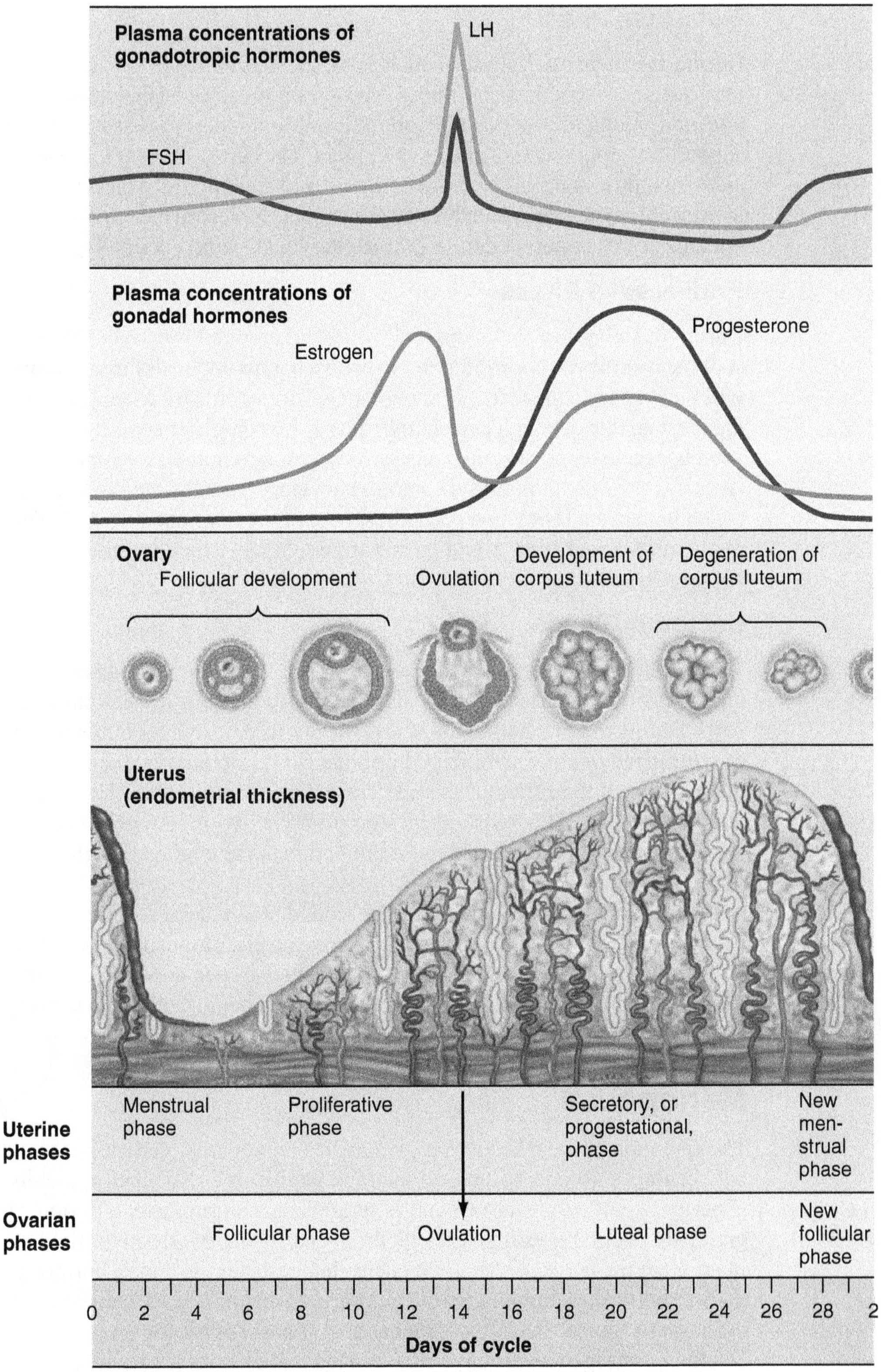

Plasma concentrations of
gonadotropic hormones

LH

FSH

Plasma concentrations of
gonadal hormones

Estrogen

Progesterone

Ovary

Follicular development

Ovulation

Development of
corpus luteum

Degeneration of
corpus luteum

Uterus
(endometrial thickness)

| Uterine phases | Menstrual phase | Proliferative phase | | Secretory, or progestational, phase | New menstrual phase |
| Ovarian phases | Follicular phase | | Ovulation | Luteal phase | New follicular phase |

0   2   4   6   8   10   12   14   16   18   20   22   24   26   28   2

Days of cycle

Figure 2.10 *The Menstrual (Uterine) Cycle*

Menstrual Phase

During the menstrual phase, which lasts approximately 3 to 5 days, the uterus sheds its endometrial lining. The strong muscles of the uterus contract and slough off the rich network of tissue and blood vessels built up to support fetal implantation and development. The cervix dilates to allow the menstrual fluid, a mixture of blood. mucus and endometrial tissue, to work its way out of the uterus and through the vagina. To absorb menstrual fluids, females can use internal tampons or sanitary pads worn externally.

Proliferative Phase

During this phase of the menstrual cycle, the uterine lining rebuilds. The endometrium literally proliferates with a rich network of tissue and blood vessels, preparing the uterus for pregnancy. To support a pregnancy, the lining must be thick enough and endowed with the complex network of blood vessels necessary to sustain successful implantation and development of an embryo for the 9 months of prenatal development. During the buildup, the endometrium relies on a constant source of the hormone estrogen. This phase takes about 9 days and ends with ovulation which occurs 14 days before menstruation starts.

Secretory Phase

The secretory phase begins with ovulation and lasts about 14 days or until the onset of the menstrual phase. The secretory phase is divided into two parts. During the first half of the phase, the uterus prepares for implantation of a fertilized ovum. Luteinizing hormone (LH), secreted by the pituitary gland, triggers the ruptured ovarian corpus luteum to secrete high levels of progesterone. This extra progesterone mixes with estrogen, causing the endometrium to thicken even more and become engorged with blood vessels.

If fertilization does not occur, the second phase of the secretory cycle begins with a decline in LH, and progesterone levels. This causes the corpus luteum to degenerate and causes a decrease in estrogen and progesterone. This loss of hormones causes the endometrium to begin sloughing, starting the menstrual phase again.

Menopause

Perimenopause A period of gradually declining estrogen levels produced by the ovaries

The cessation of the menstrual period, called menopause, generally occurs between ages 40 and 55 and on average begins at 51. Women typically experience 5 to 10 years of what is termed **perimenopause**, a period of gradually declining estrogen levels produced by the ovaries, culminating in no more menstrual periods. Physical changes from declining hormones include hotflashes, thinning of the genital area that may lead to discomfort during intercourse, sleep disturbances and increased risk for osteoporosis. Declining estrogen levels have been related to higher rates of osteoporosis and heart disease in postmenopausal women. Some women may be prescribed either estrogen replacement therapy (ERT) or hormone replacement therapy (HRT), which is a combination of estrogen and progesterone to decrease menopausal symptoms. In addition, some hormone protocols include testosterone replacement therapy, which can help improve sex drive.

There is some controversy surrounding the use of hormones for menopause so women should educate themselves and discuss it with their health care provider.

Vaginal dryness can affect sexual enjoyment but can be improved with estrogen applied directly on the vaginal tissues with a tablet, ring or cream. Low dose antidepressants or the drug Gabapentin can help reduce hot flashes. There are several drug choices that will help women avoid osteoporosis (Mayo Clinic, 2013).

Many women want to avoid using drugs or may want to do more in addition to the above ideas. Taking control of one's health during menopause is an important step in this life transition. Some women gain weight during this period due to the slowing of metabolism. Regular daily exercise will increase metabolism and help her regulate her weight. Weight bearing exercises, running/weight lifting, are also effective in preventing osteoporosis. Exercise reduces anxiety; an issue brought on by changing hormones. Menopause is a perfect time in life to focus on eating in a healthy way and decreasing the empty calorie foods that increase body weight. Getting plenty of sleep by avoiding too much caffeine and alcohol are effective in improving health and managing menopause. Yoga, tai chi and qi gong are also helpful in reducing hot flashes. If she is experiencing vaginal dryness, water based vaginal moisturizers and lubricants will help. Staying sexually active will increase blood flow to the vagina resulting in improved vaginal health (Mayo Clinic, 2013.) All of the healthy changes listed can be practiced early in life to help females achieve a healthy body and mind long before the change of menopause.

❧ *Emotional and Social Wellness* ❧

Because the menstrual cycle is such a fundamental part of being female, it is important that women learn to manage this part of their health. For some, menstruation means little more than remembering to carry the necessary hygiene products. To others, however, each cycle can be fraught with intense pain, mood swings, irritability, and an overall desire to be left alone.

The cessation of menstruation can bring relief and joy to some women. No more cramps. No more hassles. No fear of pregnancy. Others, however, feel a loss when they no longer experience the menstrual cycles that have been a part of their lives for so long.

Interacting with Health Care Practitioners

For optimum health a woman must take care of her total body. The medical specialty focused on women's reproductive health is called **gynecology**. In practice, many physicians who specialize in gynecology also complete a residency in **obstetrics**, a specialization focused on pregnancy and childbirth. **Family practitioners** offer comprehensive health care, including monitoring pregnancies and delivering babies. Women's reproductive health can also be monitored by nurse midwives and nurse practitioners.

Gynecology The medical specialty focused on women's reproductive health

Obstetrics A specialization focused on pregnancy and childbirth

Family practitioners Physicians who offer comprehensive health care, including monitoring pregnancies and delivering babies

sex in society 2.3
Disparities in Reproductive Health Care

Both national and international concerns about HIV/AIDS have generated attention to an overall lack in reproductive health care for women of color. Groups at both levels have sought to frame women's health as a women's rights issue. As such, women need to be treated fairly by the health care system, with adequate information, services, and treatments being available.

In the United States, the Sister Song Women of Color Reproductive Health Project was founded in 1998 to address how racial, gender, and economic discrimination impact the reproductive rights of women of color. The four primary ethnic populations represented are Black/African American, Latina/Hispanic, American/Indigenous, and Asian/Pacific Islander. Within the project are a number of women-of-color organizations that conduct research, provide direct services, and/or work to develop and implement advocacy strategies.

It is estimated that of 36 million women of color living in the United States, almost one-fourth are uninsured. Native American women have the lowest screening rates for cervical cancer among all ethnic groups. Asian/Pacific Islanders living in the United States often confront language barriers that impede adequate health care delivery. Their cultural values also put them at odds with ideas that they should feel in control of their bodies. Latina women traditionally seek advice from family members before turning to professionals, a practice which has contributed to delayed utilization of health care services. They have higher rates of cervical cancer, Caesarian deliveries and sterilization abuse. African American women have high rates of cervical and breast cancer, yet they typically have not been adequately screened by Pap smears and mammograms (Ross, Brownlee, Diallo, Rodriguez, & the Latina Roundtable, 2001). Attempts to provide adequate health care must incorporate the sometimes-unique concerns that race, gender, sexual orientation, and poverty create.

Source: Adapted from L. J. Ross, S. L. Brownlee, D. D. Diallo, L. Rodriguez, and the Latina Roundtable, "The SisterSong Collective: Women of Color, Reproductive Health and Human Rights," *American Journal of Health Studies, 17*(2) (Spring 2001), 79–89.

Physicians who offer comprehensive health care, including monitoring pregnancies and delivering babies

❧ *Physical and Intellectual Wellness* ❧

To ensure optimal physical well-being, girls should be taught about their body and learn to love, respect and care for their genitalia. As girls approach puberty, they need to be aware of the changes that will take place in their body and their sexual anatomy and physiology. The new information females will learn include the changes associated with menstruation and fertility, increasing sexual desire, hygiene, prevention of sexually transmitted disease and unintended pregnancy, and breast self-examination.

As women age, fitness, proper nutrition, and weight management all become increasingly important for optimal sexual health. Throughout adulthood, proper functioning of female sexual anatomy, positive body image, and other sexual health issues are affected by the level of physical well-being. So much information is available through publications targeted at women as well as the tremendous resources of the Internet that becoming an informed consumer is both easy and expected. As good consumers, all women should carefully evaluate the reliability and validity of this easily accessed information.

Health Issues

Although most women can expect to stay healthy, various health issues/disorders can affect female sexual anatomy and physiology. For many of these health issues, making healthy behavior choices can decrease the likelihood of experiencing the disorder.

Endometriosis

Endometriosis, one of the most common gynecological diseases, is a disorder of the endometrium resulting from migration of the byproducts of menstruation into the fallopian tubes, ovaries, and abdominal cavity. The shed endometrial tissue, called *implants,* adheres to these structures and continues to respond to the effects of hormones during the menstrual cycle. The most common symptoms of endometriosis are sharp pain, cramps, and heavy bleeding during menstruation. The first choice of treatment for endometriosis is oral contraceptives.

Endometriosis A condition in which pieces of the endometrium migrate to the fallopian tubes, ovaries, or abdominal cavity

Uterine Fibroids

Uterine fibroids are noncancerous tumors located throughout the uterine muscle wall (myometrium) that affect 20-40 percent of premenopausal women (MD Consult, 2013). Symptoms of fibroids include heavy bleeding, difficulty urinating, and pelvic pain. Small tumors usually do not produce noticeable symptoms. Treatments include drug therapy and surgery.

Uterine fibroid Noncancerous tumors located throughout the muscle wall of the uterus

Fibrocystic Breast Disease

Fibrocystic breast disease is a disorder involving the swelling, and resulting "lumpy" configuration, of breast tissue. The breasts, like the uterus, change as ovulation and menstruation approach. The secretory cells surrounding the mammary ducts secrete fluids that seep into the fibrous connective tissue in the lower parts of the breast, and breast tissue swells. This fluid sometimes creates pockets of fluid that appear to be cysts.

Breast Cancer

Breast cancer develops when cancerous cells proliferate, causing one or more tumors.

These tumors may metastasize, with malignant cells spreading throughout the body in lymph fluid and the bloodstream. Excluding skin cancer, breast cancer is the most common cancer of American women and is the second leading cause of deaths from cancer in women, surpassed only by lung cancer. The often quoted, "1 in 8 chances of getting breast cancer", is scary for most women. It is also a misleading quote since it is more accurate to examine the chances of getting breast cancer by age group as shown below.

A 40 year old has a 1 in 14 chance of getting breast cancer by age 70

A 60 year old has a 1 in 28 chance of getting breast cancer by age 70

A 70 year old has a 1 in 14 chance of ever developing breast cancer (Sohal, Baustian, Rao, Choy, Sweet, & Jones, 2010)

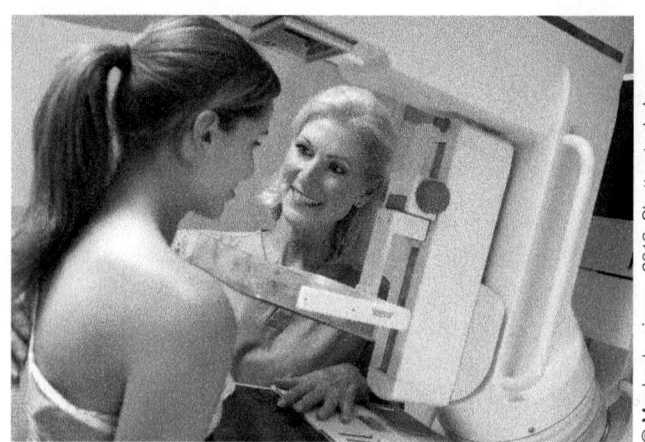

A mammogram can detect lumps too small to feel during breast self-exam.

There is increasing concern that women are being scared into early mammograms and that we are over treating breast cancer. It is estimated that in 2008 breast cancer was over diagnosed in more than 70,000 women and that screening is having only a small effect on the rate of death from breast cancer (Bleyer & Welch, 2012). "According to a survey of randomized clinical trials involving 600,000 women around the world, for every 2,000 women screened annually over 10 years, one life is prolonged but 10 healthy women are given the diagnosis of breast cancer and unnecessarily treated, often with therapies that have life-threatening side effects"(Orenstein, 2013, pg 39). Because mammography has both benefits and harms, the recommendation is to have a mammogram every other year if you are between 50-74. If you are outside of that age group it should be a personal decision after being fully informed of the risks (USPSTF, 2012). All breast cancers are not alike; there are at least four genetically distinct breast cancers. The most likely treatment for early stage breast cancer will be surgery (either a mastectomy or lumpectomy) with either chemotherapy or hormonal therapy (Sohal et al, 2010).

Gender (being female), age and a having a parent, sibling or child with breast cancer are the strongest predicting factors for having breast cancer. These factors cannot be controlled but there are ways a woman can reduce her risk for developing breast cancer. Moderate risk factors include smoking, alcohol consumption and obesity. A woman can take control and avoid smoking, drink only in moderation and either maintain a healthy weight or lose weight if needed.

Exercise and eating fruits and vegetables have been shown to protect against breast cancer so women should incorporated daily exercise and a variety of fruits and vegetable into their lives. Additional risks under a woman's control include late childbearing (after 30), never having children, and never breast feeding a baby. If a woman is planning to have children she may wish to consider doing so before age 30 and breast feeding her baby (Sohal et al, 2010).

Vaginitis

Vaginitis Inflammation and irritation of the vagina

In **vaginitis**, the vagina becomes inflamed, resulting in one or more of the following symptoms: discharge, dryness, burning upon urination (if the inflammation spreads into the urethral opening), and pain during intercourse. The discharge associated with vaginitis is often overlooked or mistaken for a woman's normal vaginal fluid. Three characteristics of vaginal discharge—quantity, color, and odor—can vary in response to vaginitis. The discharge associated with vaginitis is usually profuse (quantity), ranging from frothy white to greenish yellow (color), and changes from a woman's normal scent to a foul, even fishy-smelling odor. Sometimes vaginitis causes vaginal dryness instead of discharge. This unusual dryness results in pain.

The urethra can become inflamed as a result of either the discharge or unusual dryness. When the urethra is inflamed, urination is painful. Painful intercourse is another common symptom of vaginitis.

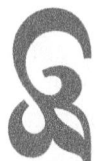

healthy sex hints 2.3

Promoting Optimal Vulvovaginal Health

1. Do not make your private parts private to you. Examine yourself.
2. Get involved in your health care. Go on the Internet. Get information. Ask questions.
3. Wash the vulva daily with warm, soapy water.
4. Avoid douching. The vagina is a self-cleansing organ. Douching does not prevent pregnancy or infection and can destroy healthy bacteria present in the vagina.
5. Avoid scented products such as vaginal hygiene sprays and perfumed soaps. Do not use talcum powder on the vulva.
6. Be careful about what you insert into your vagina (make sure all sex toys and other objects are safe and clean before inserting them).
7. Do not progress from anal intercourse to vaginal intercourse (a common way to transfer germs from the rectum to the vagina) without first washing your partner's penis.
8. Never force vaginal penetration (make sure your vagina is well lubricated before inserting anything into it).
9. Become familiar with the amount, consistency, color, and odor of your normal daily discharge.
10. If the discharge changes, see a health care provider.

Source: Elizabeth G. Stewart and Paula Spencer, *The V Book: A Doctor's Guide to Complete Vulvovaginal Health* (New York: Bantam, 2002).

Vaginitis is diagnosed through a combination of clinical examination and laboratory tests. Various forms of vaginitis have different combinations of symptoms. An experienced clinician often can make the diagnosis based on the symptoms and will most likely treat with prescription or over the counter drug therapy. Self-treatment of vaginitis (especially involving douching) is not recommended without an accurate diagnosis of the condition.

Cervical Cancer

Cervical infection with HPV is the primary risk factor for cervical cancer. Cervical cancer is the end stage of cervical dysplasia. *Cervical dysplasia* refers to the presence of abnormal or precancerous cells at the cervix. Also known as cervical *intraepithelial neoplasia* (CIN), it is more common than both breast and uterine cancers. The good news is that it is almost 100 percent curable if detected early and there is now an FDA approved HPV vaccine that protects against 70% of cervical cancers. As discussed earlier, The American Cancer Society recommends that all females ages 11-12 be routinely vaccinated for HPV. The vaccine is also recommended for females ages 13-26 who have not yet been vaccinated (American Cancer Society, 2013). Early detection of cervical cancer also can prevent its spread into the uterus. Early changes in the cells lining the cervix can be detected through a procedure called the Pap test. It is recommended that women not get a pap test prior to age 21 and then to get a pap test every other year from

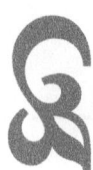

healthy sex hints 2.4

Reducing the Risks for Cervical Cancer

The major risk factors for cervical cancer are:
- early onset of intercourse (beginning in early adolescence);
- lifetime number of sexual partners (risks increase as numbers increase);
- history of STD infection (particularly viral STDs such as HPV and HSV);
- not using barrier contraception (condoms, diaphragm).

To lessen your risk:

1. *Be vaccinated for HPV, ideally prior to first sexual contact.*
2. Delay onset of intercourse (women who begin having intercourse after age 20 have a lower risk).
3. Reduce your number of total sexual partners (having one, uninfected sex partner is lowest risk).
4. Use barrier contraceptives (male and female condoms work best) to protect the T-zone.
5. Women should have their first cervical screening at age 21 and can be screened every 2 years between 21 and 30. Women 30 and older who have had three consecutive test may be screened every 3 years. (American Congress of Obstetricians and Gynecologist, November 2009).

age 21-30. After 30, if they have 3 normal tests then they can wait 3 years between tests (US Preventive Services Task Force, 2010).

Uterine Cancer and Ovarian Cancer

Uterine cancer, rare in women under age 45, usually affects the endometrial lining. Early symptoms include abnormal bleeding or spotting. Women can decrease their risk of uterine cancer by using hormonal contraceptives, being physically active and maintaining a healthy weight (CDC, 2012).

The majority of women (90%) who get ovarian cancer are over age 40. It accounts for only 3 percent of all cancers among women. Symptoms include vaginal bleeding, pelvic and/or back pain, and bloating. Factors that protect women from ovarian cancer are using the hormonal birth control pill for 5 years or longer and giving birth to a child (CDC, 2012).

Premenstrual Syndrome (PMS)

Premenstrual syndrome (PMS) A condition preceding menstruation, characterized by a myriad of physical and psychological symptoms

Premenstrual syndrome (PMS) is characterized by a myriad of physical and psychological symptoms that appear anywhere within 2 weeks of the onset of menstruation and end after menstruation begins. Up to 40% of women report having one or more of a variety of physical and psychological symptoms. Some common symptoms include bloating, weight gain, breast swelling and tenderness, fatigue, difficulty in sleeping, headache, appetite change or food cravings- especially sugary foods, chocolate and carbo-hydrates, joint or muscle pain, tension, irritability, mood swings, anxiety,

healthy sex hints 2.5

Self-Help for PMS

Various treatments are available to help women who have PMS. For years, stress management and dietary changes have been advocated as part of a comprehensive PMS treatment program. Recently, prostaglandin inhibitors have been recommended. The following are some strategies that might work for you:

1. Have a daily exercise program.
2. Eat a well-balanced diet high in complex carbohydrates, low in fat, and containing moderate protein.Eat at least three meals a day (it may be preferable to eat many smaller meals). This will provide the best fuel and an even release of energy throughout the day.
3. Avoid excess sugar and snacks high in sugar and fat. This step, coupled with tip 2, will help avoid the extreme high and low blood sugar levels associated with mood swings.
4. Avoid excess sodium intake (table salt and salt in food), which will help reduce bloating related to fluid retention.
5. Have an orgasm. This activity can help release pent-up vaginal and uterine muscle tension.
6. Try relaxation activities such as diaphragmatic breathing, imagery, meditation, and systematic muscle relaxation.These activities can help reduce stress and induce relaxation.
7. Have your partner (or a professional) give you a lower-back massage. It will help relieve muscle tension and induce relaxation.
8. Soak in a warm bath, Jacuzzi, or hot tub, or apply heat to the abdominal area with a heating pad or water bottle.The warmth will help you relieve muscle tension and induce relaxation.
9. Try antiprostaglandin medications. Prostaglandin inhibitors reduce the intensity and duration of cramps. Mild prostaglandin inhibitors include ibuprofen (marketed as Motrin). Stronger prescription medications include naproxen (Naprosyn), naproxen sodium (Anaprox), and mefenamic acid (Ponstel).

depression and difficulty concentrating. The cause is not yet determined but may be linked to sensitivity to changing hormone levels during the menstrual cycle. Stress is not thought to be a cause but can make it worse. The symptoms of PMS are so varied that women often attribute to the menstrual cycle symptoms that are not related. Women may find it helpful to note on a calendar the dates they experience certain symptoms and the dates they have their menstrual cycle. After a few months it will be easy to identify the symptoms that are consistently related to the menstrual cycle and those that are simply "life symptoms." This information can be helpful in planning around problem days if there are any.

Dysmenorrhea

Often, the myometrial contractions associated with menstruation cause dysmenorrhea, resulting in cramping and pain that can be severe. As you might recall from our discussion earlier in this chapter, the myometrium is a thick layer of muscular tissue capable of providing the powerful contractions necessary to dislodge endometrial tissue during menstruation or expel a developed fetus during childbirth. Myometrial contractions are triggered

Dysmenorrhea Painful menstruation

Prostaglandins Hormones that can cause muscle contractions and have been associated with menstrual pain

by the release of powerful hormones called **prostaglandins**. Dysmenorrhea is often caused by excessively high levels of prostaglandins. This can cause more intense contractions that last longer than usual.

Toxic Shock Syndrome

Toxic shock syndrome (TSS) is caused by infection with the *Staphylococcus aureus bacterium,* an organism that can live in the vagina without threatening a woman's health. Overgrowth of the bacteria, however, can result in TSS, which is life-threatening. Toxins produced from TSS infection produce initial symptoms including a sudden high fever (102 degrees Fahrenheit or higher), headache, dizziness, confusion, diarrhea, vomiting, muscle aches, and a sunburnlike rash. If untreated, TSS can cause kidney or liver failure, resulting in death in about 5 percent of all cases. If diagnosed early, TSS is easily treated with antibiotics (Jones, Ferri, Baustian, Danakas, Murray, Jain, & Linger, 2010).

Initial research found that TSS was associated with tampons, especially the superabsorbent type. This finding led to the removal of Rely brand tampons from the market. Subsequent studies found that cervical caps, diaphragms, and contraceptive sponges also pose a risk for developing TSS if they are used during menstruation. Since first being reported in 1980, the incidence of toxic shock syndrome has continued to decline.

To reduce the risk of TSS, it is recommended that women not use superabsorbent tampons, frequently change the ones they do use (at least three times per day), use a sanitary pad at least once in a 24-hour period, and when menstruating do not use a cervical cap, diaphragm, or the contraceptive sponge.

Personal Assessment

Body Image: Female

Body image refers to our evaluation and perception of our body, specific body parts, and their functioning. It includes the messages (positive and negative) that we tell ourselves about our bodies, our self-esteem, and the behaviors and choices we make as a result. The following inventory will help females assess their body image.

Rate each body part listed here using the following scale: extremely satisfied = 5; satisfied = 4; neutral = 3; dissatisfied = 2; extremely dissatisfied = 1.

1. eyes _____ 2. ears _____ 3. nose _____

4. hair _____ 5. teeth _____ 6. mouth _____

7. weight _____ 8. face _____ 9. shoulders _____

10. breasts _____ 11. arms _____ 12. calves _____

13. hands _____ 14. height _____ 15. stomach _____

16. buttocks _____ 17. hips _____ 18. thighs _____

19. feet _____ 20. sex organs _____ 21. overall body _____

Scoring:

105–80 Very positive body image
 20–40 Negative body image
 60–80 Positive body image
  0–20 Very negative body image
 40–60 Ambivalent about your body

Rate each item below, using the following scale: very comfortable = 5; comfortable = 4; neutral = 3; uncomfortable = 2; very uncomfortable = 1.

_____ 22. Looking at my nude body in the mirror.

_____ 23. Performing self-examinations of my nude body.

_____ 24. Being nude when I am alone.

_____ 25. Being nude when I am with my lover.

_____ 26. Being nude when I am around my kids.

_____ 27. Sunbathing in the nude.

_____ 28. Swimming in the nude.

_____ 29. Walking around the house nude.

Scoring:

32–40 Very comfortable with nudity
12–16 Uncomfortable with nudity
21–32 Comfortable with nudity
 0–12 Very uncomfortable with nudity
16–21 Ambivalent about nudity

Complete the following sentences:

30. The thing I like best about my body is _____

31. The thing I dislike most about my body is _____

Thought Questions

1. What is the best way to ensure good vaginal health?

2. (a) What are the cervical crypts and the transformation zone?

   (b) Describe their significance in the transmission of STDs.

3. How are the ovaries and testes alike and different?

4. What are the phases of the menstrual cycle?

5. What is the role of female sex hormones in female sexuality?

Test Yourself

1. Females are born with approximately how many immature ovarian follicles?
   a. 40,000
   b. 40 million
   c. 400,000
   d. 400

2. Which term refers to the cessation of menstruation?
   a. Menarche
   b. Dysmenorrhea
   c. Endometriosis
   d. Menopause

3. Young women are advised to have a pelvic exam
   a. only if having vaginal sexual contact.
   b. every other year starting at age 21.
   c. only if heterosexual.
   d. once they get married.

4. The Pap test is designed to detect cancer of the
   a. cervix.
   b. vagina.
   c. breast.
   d. colon.

5. Female deaths associated with reproductive cancers are highest when cancer is found in the
   a. cervix.
   b. uterus.
   c. fallopian tubes.
   d. ovaries.

6. Which part of female anatomy is not considered part of the vulva?
   a. Labia majora
   b. Vagina
   c. Mons pubis
   d. Clitoris

7. The structure most critical for female sexual arousal is the
   a. uterus.
   b. vagina.
   c. clitoris.
   d. mons pubis.

8. Female genital mutilation is a practice
   a. widely found among immigrants to the United States.
   b. designed to enhance female fertility.
   c. supported by the United Nations.
   d. rooted in religious and cultural customs.

9. All but which are true regarding the size of a woman's breasts?
   a. Size is correlated with sexual pleasure.
   b. Size is related to heredity and body fat.
   c. Size can be temporarily affected by pregnancy and lactation.
   d. Cosmetic surgery can be used to increase or decrease breast size.

10. A woman's menstrual blood includes tissue from which part of the uterus?
    a. Cervix
    b. Endometrium
    c. Myometrium
    d. Os

Thought Questions

1. What is the proper term for the external female genitalia?

2. What are the components of the external female genitalia?

3. What is the nature of the hymen?

4. What are the internal structures of the female sexual anatomy?

5. What are the characteristics of the vagina in the normal and aroused states?

Web Resources

National Women's Health Information Center
www.4woman.gov

Developed by the U.S. Department of Health and Human Services, this site provides up-to-date research and information related to a wide variety of women's health concerns.

National Women's Health Network
www.Nwhn.org

A clearinghouse for a variety of women's health topics. It produces a bimonthly newsletter, *The Network News,* and works as a major advocacy group for women's health issues.

Harvard Women's Health Watch
www.health.harvard.edu

This group interprets medical information for the general reader. A monthly newsletter is also available.

OBGYN.net Women's Health
www.obgyn.net

Valuable information concerning all areas of women's health with links to many sites. Information covered in this site includes diseases and conditions, interactive tools, health information resources, forums, directories, organizations, publications, and international resources.

Food and Drug Administration
www.fda.gov/cdrh/mammography/certified .html

Federal Drug Administration–certified mammography facilities by region in the United States.

Susan G. Komen Foundation
www.Komen.org

An interactive Web site providing breast cancer screening and treatment information. It includes conversations with survivors, searchable A–Z guide, after-treatment care, insurance issues, and more.

References

American Cancer Society. (2008). American Cancer Society Recommendations for Human Papillomavirus (HPV) Vaccine Use To Prevent Cervical Cancer and Pre-Cancers [Online]. Available: www.cancer.org.

American College of Obstetricians and Gynecologists. (2007). Vaginal rejuvenation and Cosmetic Vaginal Procedures. Available: www.acog.org-Resources-And-Publications/ Committee

American Society of Plastic Surgeons. (2008). "Fantastic Four" of Breast Procedures Leave Women Extremely Satisfied. [Online] Available: www.plasticsurgery.org/ media/ press releases.

American Society of Plastic Surgery (2013). Plastic Surgery Statistics. Available: www.plasticsurgery.org

Bleyer, A. & Welch, G. (2012). Effects of three decades of screening mammography on breast cancer incidence. The New England Journal of Medicine. 367, pp 1998–2005

Boston Women's Book Collective. (1998). *The new our bodies, ourselves.* New York: Simon & Schuster.

Burnstein, G., Jacobs, A., Kissin, D., & Workowski, K., (2013). Changes in 2010 STD Treatment Guidelines. Available: www.acog.org

Center for Disease Control and Prevention (2012,August). Ovarian Cancer. Available:www.cdc.gov

Center for Disease Control and Prevention (2012,August). Uterine Cancer. Available:www.cdc.gov

Center for Disease Control and Prevention (2013, February). HPV vaccine for preteens and teens.. Available:www.cdc.gov

Chumlea, W., Schubert, C., Roche, A., Kulin, H., Lee, P., Himes.J,. & Sun, S. (2003). Age and menstruation and racial comparison in girls. Pediatrics. 111(1) pp 110–113.

Comforth, T, (2009, July 17). The Clitoral Truth. Womens Health About .com. Available: http://womenshealth.about.com/cs/sexuality/a/clitoraltruthin_31

Dodson, B. (1996). Sex for One. New York: Three Rivers Press.

Ensler, E. (1998). The vagina workshop. In The vagina monologues. New York: Villard.

Ferri, F., Baustian, G., Murray, J., Danakas, G., Jain, T., & DeMarco, B.(2011). Dysmenorrhea. First Consult. Available: www.mdconsult.com

Ferri, F., Baustian, G., Murray, J., Danakas, G., Jain, T., & DeMarco, B.(2007). PMS. First Consult. Available: www.mdconsult.com

Johnson, J (2004). Exposed at last; the truth about your clitoris. pp 387–389. In Worcester N,

Mannheim, J. (2012). Kegel exercises-self care. MedlinePlus. Available: http://www.nlm.nih.gov

Mayo Clinic (2012, February). Ectopic Pregnancy. Available:www.mayoclinic.com

Mayo Clinic (2012, February).Vagina: What's normal and what's not. Available: www.mayoclinic.com/health/vagina/MY01913

Mayo Clinic (2012,April).Cystitis. Available: www.mayoclinic.com/health/cystitis /DS00285

Mayo Clinic (2013, January).Menopause. Available: www.mayoclinic.com/health/menopause /DS001199

Mayo Clinic (2013, January).Menopause. Available: www.mayoclinic.com/health/menopause /DS001199

MD Consult (2013). Fibroids. Available; www.mdconsult.com

Orenstein, P. (2013, April 30). The problem with pink. New York Times Magazine.

PLANetWIRE. (2002). Saving women's lives [Online]. Available: www.planetwire.org.

Ross, L. J., Brownlee, S. L., Diallo, D. D., Rodriguez, L., & the Latina Roundtable. (2001, Spring). The Sister Song Collective: Women of color, reproductive health and human rights. American Journal of Health Studies, 17(2), 79–89.

Smith, R. A., Cokkinides, V., & Eyre, H. J. (2003). American Cancer Society Guidelines for the early detection of cancer, 2003. CA: A Cancer Journal for Clinicians, 53, 27–43.

Sohal, D., Baustian, G., Rao, D., Choy, C., Sweet, E., & Jones, R.(2010). Breast Cancer. First Consult. Available: www.mdconsult.com

Stewart, E. G., & Spencer, P. (2002). The V book: A doctor's guide to complete vulvovaginal health. New York: Bantam.

US Department of Health and Human Services (2010, May) Cervical Cancer Fact Sheet. Available: womenshealth.gov/publications/our-publications/fact- US Preventative Services Task Force (2012). Cervical Cancer Screening. Available: uspreventativeservicestaskforce.org

US Preventative Services Task Force (2013). Screening for breast cancer appendix F. Available: uspreventativeservicestaskforce.org

WebMd (2007, April 3). Normal menstrual cycle: Menarch and the teenage menstrual cycle. [online] Available: www.Webmd.com

WebMd (2009, August 12) Kegel exercises: an overview. Available: www.webmd.com

WebMd (2012,) What to know about ectopic pregnancy.Available: www.webmd.com

Whipple, B., Gerdes, C., & Komisaruk, B. (1996). Sexual response to self-stimulation in women with complete spinal cord injury. Journal of Sex Research, 33(3), 231–240.

World Health Organization (2013, February). Female Genital Mutilation

Available: www.who int/en/

Writing Group for the Women's Health Initiative Investigators.

(2002, July 17). Risks and benefits of estrogen plus progestin in healthy postmenopausal women. Journal of the American Medical Association, 288(3).

Zaviacic, M., & Whipple, B. (1993). Update on the female prostate and the phenomenon of female ejaculation. Journal of Sex Research, 30, 148–151.

chapter
three

Male Sexual Anatomy *and* Physiology

Student Learning Objectives

After reading this chapter, students will be able to:

- Identify and locate key structures of the male sexual anatomy;
- Describe the main functions of the male sexual structures;
- Identify and describe the functions of the key male sex glands;
- Explain the erogenous potential of the key male sexual structures;
- Perform a testicular self-exam;
- Identify the signs and symptoms of, and treatment for, eight common male sexual disorders;
- Describe a variety of screening tests used to diagnose common male sexual disorders;
- Describe a variety of disabilities and their effects on male sexuality.

activity teaser: How much do you know about male anatomy? Find out in the Personal Exploration Activity on page 89.

case study 3.1

Penis Size and Self-Esteem

Jordan, 19, gay, identifies as African American.

Jordan, a sophomore, attends a large urban northeastern university.

For the longest time I can remember being hung up on the size of my penis. I remember, as a kid, getting my mom's tape measure and measuring the length and circumference of my penis. I never talked to my friends about size because I was convinced mine was smaller than theirs. My dad used to kid me about how small mine was when he'd see me in the shower. I'd get intimidated by his because it seemed so big. I probably should have talked to him about it, but I couldn't. He wasn't so approachable, and, like I said, he always seemed to be making fun of mine. Maybe this was his way of trying to break the ice and get a conversation going. I don't know. I doubt it.

Anyway, I guess I just kind of felt that mine was small, and if I tried to bring it up with my friends, they'd laugh at me or, worse yet, I'd find out that theirs were really bigger than mine. I sent away for this stuff from the back of a magazine that was "guaranteed" to make your penis grow. The only thing it did was make my penis burn. It must have been some kind of liniment or something. I decided from that point on that I'd have to be satisfied with what I have. My current lover thinks my penis is big enough to satisfy him and that has really put me at ease.

Critical Thinking

How far would you go to change a feature of your body that you currently are dissatisfied with?

One of the more interesting things about healthy sexuality is the great diversity we are capable of bringing to our sexual response. Whether we are straight or gay, male or female, our bodies are capable of responding in a myriad of pleasurable ways if we take the time to understand them and explore their potential. After our discussion of female anatomy in Chapter 2, we will now focus on male anatomy and physiology as an additional step in understanding our bodies.

Much of male sexual anatomy is external. Most men touch their genitals frequently during urination, and because of this, men tend to be familiar with the external parts. Even though men tend to be comfortable with their external sexual anatomy and physiology, sexual health extends to understanding the proper functioning of the internal structures also. Many of the internal and external sexual structures of both men and women are capable of responding sexually. Proper stimulation can provide intense sexual pleasure. We vary tremendously in how we like to stimulate (and have our partners stimulate) these structures. We will discuss this further at various points in this and other chapters.

External Male Sexual Structures

The external structures of the male sexual anatomy (see Figure 3.1) include the penis and scrotum, as well as the perineum, anus, and breasts. The last three, although not traditionally considered parts of sexual anatomy, are included here because of their potential as **erogenous** structures.

Erogenous Capable of producing sexual excitement

68

Penis

Like many structures in the human body, the penis has more than one function. Both sperm and urine pass through the penis on their way out of a man's body. The same organ used to pass liquid waste is capable of providing exquisite sexual pleasure. This duality of function is often cited as a reason for feeling squeamish about engaging in **fellatio.**

Structure of the Penis

The penis (Figure 3.2) consists of two main parts: the shaft and the glans. The shaft of the penis consists of two cylinders of spongy tissue—the larger cavernous body (*corpora cavernosa*) and one smaller spongy body (*corpus spongiosum*)—wrapped in thick membrane sheaths. Similar to a common household sponge, this cylindrical tissue has many pockets of open space or cavities that are richly endowed with blood vessels, allowing them to fill with blood during sexual arousal. This is how a penis becomes erect during sexual arousal.

A key to understanding this is to visualize how a sponge expands as its cavities fill with water. Contrary to popular belief, the penis has no bone or cartilage and very little muscle tissue. Slang terms such as *boner* and *hard-on* derive their origin from the firm, protruding nature of the spongiosum during erection. The spongy cylinders are held together by **connective tissue** attached to a loose wrapping of skin. The penis is capable of great expansion and changes in size because of its spongy tissue and loose covering of skin.

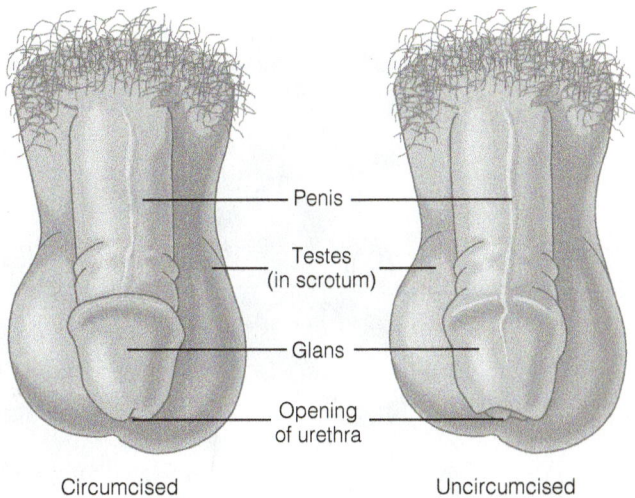

Figure 3.1 *Male External Genitalia* The male external genitalia includes the penis, scrotum, and perineum.

Fellatio Oral stimulation of the penis

Connective tissue Tissue that supports or binds other tissue

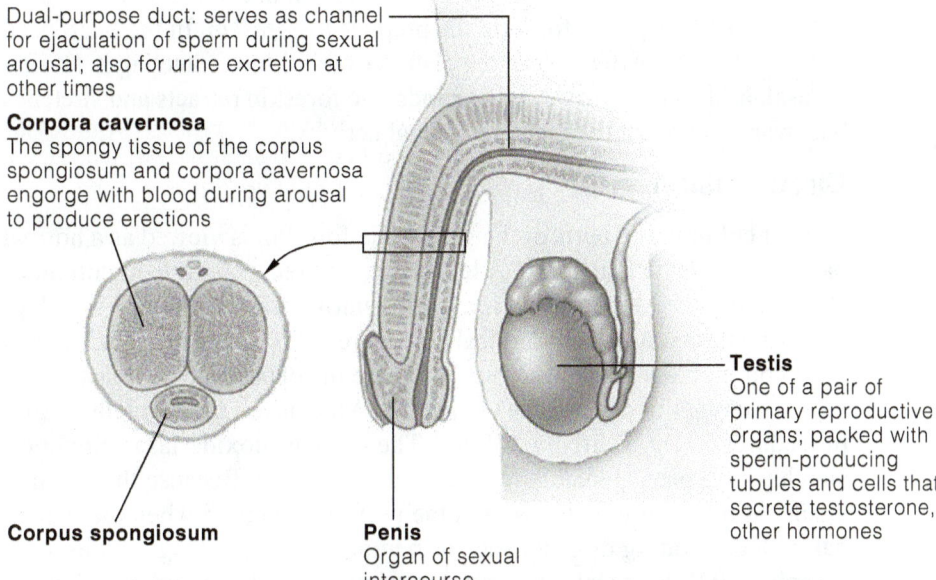

Urethra
Dual-purpose duct: serves as channel for ejaculation of sperm during sexual arousal; also for urine excretion at other times

Corpora cavernosa
The spongy tissue of the corpus spongiosum and corpora cavernosa engorge with blood during arousal to produce erections

Corpus spongiosum

Penis
Organ of sexual intercourse

Testis
One of a pair of primary reproductive organs; packed with sperm-producing tubules and cells that secrete testosterone, other hormones

Figure 3.2 *The Structure of the Penis* The penis consists of three cylinders of spongy tissue wrapped in a muscular sheath.

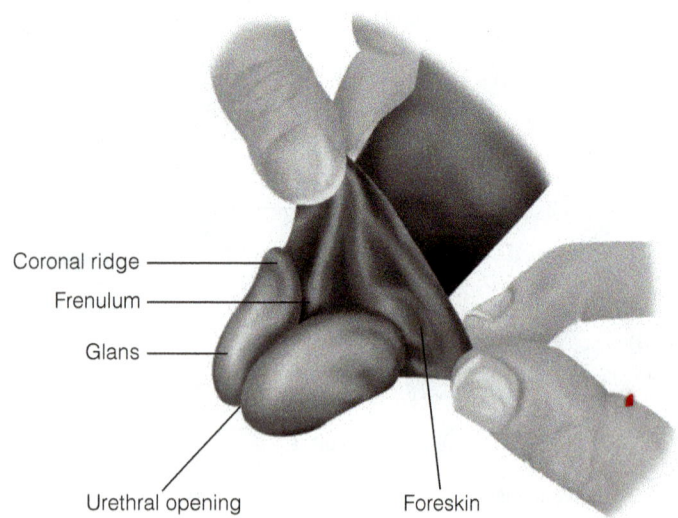

Coronal ridge ——————
Frenulum ——————
Glans ——————

Urethral opening   Foreskin

Figure 3.3 *Glans and Foreskin* The frenulum, located on the underside of the glans, is the most sensitive part of the penis.

Glans penis The end of corpus spongiosum, which is composed of the head of the penis and the urethral opening

Urethra Dual-purpose duct: serves as channel for ejaculation of sperm during sexual arousal; also for urine excretion at other times

Circumcision Surgical removal of foreskin of penis

The corpora cavernosa run side by side along the entire length of the penis, attaching to the abdominal cavity by their roots, the crura. The cavernous body lies above the corpus spongiosum and wraps around it, appearing to create two cylinder-like structures on either side. The corpus spongiosum also runs the entire length of the shaft, forming the head or **glans penis.** When the penis is erect, the corpus spongiosum is what gets hard and protrudes, forming a pronounced ridge along the underside of the penis. The **urethra** runs through the corpus spongiosum.

The entire penis is responsive to touch. The amount and type of touch that men like vary from man to man and sexual encounter to encounter. Even though the entire penis is responsive to touch, the greatest concentration of nerves is on the glans penis, illustrated in Figure 3.3. Two regions of the glans in particular—the coronal ridge and the frenulum—are the most richly endowed with nerve endings and capable of providing the greatest pleasure.

The *coronal ridge* forms the mushroom-like cap of the penis, separating it from the shaft. The *frenulum* is the triangular patch of tissue on the underside of the penis where the ridge pinches in to give the glans its distinctive shape. Both the corona and the frenulum are involved during arousal but are stimulated more precisely through oral sex and manual stimulation. The latter two forms of stimulation allow more individual control over the type and amount of pressure and stimulation than through intercourse.

The loose layer of skin that covers the shaft of the penis attaches at one end to the base of the penis near the abdomen and at the other end just behind the coronal ridge of the glans. The skin continues forward, extending beyond the glans penis, forming the prepuce or *foreskin.* In the unaroused state, the foreskin extends over the glans, covering and protecting it. During arousal, as the penis grows and expands, the foreskin retracts and stretches backward, exposing the glans for sexual activity.

Circumcision

In most cultures and parts of the world, the foreskin is viewed as a normal part of male sexual anatomy, is left intact, and receives little attention. In the United States, the foreskin is usually removed during the first few days following birth through the surgical procedure called **circumcision.** The two most common methods of circumcision are the clamp and the plastibell.

Two types of clamps, the Gomco and Mogen, are used with the clamp procedure (Peleg & Steiner, 1998). The carbon dioxide laser circumcision has also been available for use since the 1980s. Because this method results in minimal blood loss, it is the preferred method when the patient has a blood-clotting disorder such as hemophilia (How, Ong, Jacobsen, & Joseph, 2003). Surgical outcomes associated with laser circumcision are comparable to the traditional methods (How et al., 2003). Removal of the foreskin leaves the glans penis exposed. Most circumcisions done today are for religious, cultural, or aesthetic reasons. Circumcision is an important, required ritual in Judaic and Islamic religious practice.

❧   *Social and Spiritual Wellness*   ❧

The issue of circumcision clearly illustrates how the social and spiritual dimensions of wellness impact men's sexual health. Our parents or caregivers, the core of our social network when we are infants, are our initial resource and primary sex educators. They make the initial decisions regarding our sexual health, and provide us with guidance in developing healthy lifestyles that optimize sexual functioning. Parents are charged with the responsibility of making decisions about issues like circumcision. After the decision is made, they are responsible for teaching their sons about the proper hygiene and care of their circumcised penises. Our parents are influenced by their social milieu. They are products of a culture (and subculture), and their decisions regarding our health are influenced by this fact.

Their social well-being is also affected by their socioeconomic status and religious/spiritual beliefs. Spirituality and religiosity influence sexual health and anatomy and physiology. Circumcision often is part of a religious tradition. Most circumcisions are performed for religious and cultural beliefs and not because of purely intellectual decisions.

As men age, their parents' influence is supplanted by that of friends, peers, teachers, coaches, and intimate partners. These people in their social environment often give advice, share information, and in a direct or indirect way help put sexual health issues into a broader perspective. For instance, an uncircumcised boy may begin to have doubts about his penis if most of his peers are circumcised. This might make him uncomfortable in social settings such as a locker room. Later in his sexual development, the preferences of his intimate sex partner(s) may impact his happiness at being circumcised or uncircumcised.

Prior to 1971, the American Academy of Pediatrics (AAP), the nation's foremost pediatric professional organization, had recommended circumcision of newborn males for health concerns associated with smegma and its supposed links to cervical cancer in women and penile cancer in men. *Smegma* is a mixture of oily secretions from sebaceous glands on the skin of the penis, dead epithelial cells, dirt, bacteria, and sweat. Smegma buildup is prevented through simple washing with soap and water and pulling the foreskin back to cleanse this area of the penis. It can be compared to other routine procedures such as washing behind the ears regularly.

Beginning with the 1971 edition of its procedures manual, and reiterated in subsequent revisions in 1975 and 1983, the American Academy of Pediatrics Task Force on Neonatal Circumcision found no absolute indication for routine circumcision. In 1999, the task force reexamined the issue in light of new research on circumcision status and urinary tract infections and sexually transmitted diseases. It concluded at the time that newborn male circumcision had potential medical benefits and advantages as well as disadvantages and risks.

The most recent report and recommendations of the American Medical Association (AMA) support those of the AAP Task Force on Neonatal Circumcision released on March 1, 1999. The Council on Scientific Affairs of the AMA reports that although circumcision decreases the incidence of urinary tract infection in the first year of life, the low incidence of this condition minimizes its potential benefits compared to the risks inherent in circumcision (AMA, 2003).

case study 3.2

A Tough Decision

Jeno, 54, Jaana, 52, married to each other, both identify as Polish American.

Jeno and Jaana emigrated to the United States in 1973 and attended medical school together. They chose not to circumcise their son Jon (age 20) when he was born, but he has since been circumcised.

JAANA: Jon was born in a hospital birthing center within a major metropolitan hospital where Jeno and I had done our residency. After reading the literature on circumcision, doing rotations through labor and delivery, and discussing it with the other residents, we decided against having the procedure done.

JENO: I was raised a Roman Catholic, and Jaana and I are very religious, but our religious beliefs really had nothing to do with our decision. Being born in Poland and living in several Eastern and Western European countries growing up [his father was a diplomat], most of my friends were uncircumcised. I was concerned about my son's experiences in America where circumcision was the norm. Many of the things I had read in the 1970s and 1980s projected that the rate of circumcision would drop dramatically in the coming decades. We figured that by the time our son was in school most of his friends would be uncircumcised.

JAANA: Unfortunately, it didn't work out that way. In fact, it was just the opposite. Jon was usually the only boy in his class who was uncircumcised. None of his friends were uncircumcised, and he felt very self-conscious about it. He started to develop anxiety about going to gym class and participating in sports that required him to shower and change among his peers.

JENO: After much soul searching, Jaana and I decided to have Jon circumcised at age 12. We didn't want him to go through puberty and then have the procedure done. Fortunately, everything went smoothly, and his recovery was uneventful.

I thought that not having him go through the procedure at birth would save him from unnecessary surgery, but as it turned out, he had the procedure done anyway. He is glad he had it done and says he understands why we decided what we did.

Critical Thinking

How would your culture, social relationships, and spirituality influence your sexual health decision-making regarding having your son circumcised?

This report reinforces the Academy of Pediatrics' position, based on two years of study of the most recent data available concerning neonatal male circumcision. The AAP (1999) report states that existing scientific evidence demonstrates potential medical benefits of routine newborn male circumcision; however, these data are not sufficient to recommend routine neonatal circumcision. Parents should determine what is in the best interests of their child (Buie, 2005).

There is an association between circumcision and HIV risk. Studies have shown that uncircumcised men have a two- to eightfold increased risk of HIV infection compared to circumcised men (*AIDS Weekly* Staff, 2002).

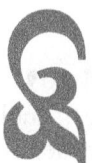

healthy sex hints 3.1

Deciding on Circumcision

Male circumcision is a common procedure, generally performed during the newborn period in the United States. Parents of newborn males must decide whether to have the infant circumcised.

In 2007, the American Academy of Pediatrics (AAP) formed a multidisciplinary task force of AAP members and other stakeholders to evaluate the recent evidence on male circumcision and update the Academy's 1999 recommendations in this area.

In 2012, after an exhaustive review of all available evidence related to the advantages and disadvantages of newborn circumcision, the American Academy of Pediatrics (AAP) reversed its previous policy of not recommending that male babies be routinely circumcised.

In the most recent policy statement the AAP wrote that the health benefits of newborn male circumcision outweigh the risks and that the procedure's benefits justify access to this procedure for families who choose it.

The following facts are intended to help you make an informed choice about circumcision for your child.

1. Specific benefits identified by the AAP included the prevention of urinary tract infections, penile cancer, and transmission of some sexually transmitted infections, including HIV.
2. The American College of Obstetricians and Gynecologists has endorsed this statement.
3. As with any surgical procedure, circumcision involves a small risk for the newborn.
4. Research indicates that uncircumcised boys have a slightly higher rate of urethral infection than circumcised boys.
5. Many fathers prefer that their son's penis look like theirs.
6. No evidence is available that uncircumcised sons of circumcised fathers suffer any psychological distress over this difference.
7. If you opt to have the procedure done, you have the right to indicate who will perform your son's circumcision.

Based on this information, if you had a newborn son, would you have him circumcised?

Source: The American Academy of Pediatrics (2012). *Circumcision Policy Statement. Pediatrics Vol. 130 No. 3 September 1,* 2012. pp. 585 -586

The increased risk is attributed to the nature of the cells in the mucosal lining of the foreskin. When exposed to HIV in laboratory settings, this tissue was infiltrated at a much greater intensity than other tissue. The increased sensitivity of foreskin tissue to HIV is the suspected link to the increased risk. This link is currently being explored by Dr. Robert Bailey, from the University of Illinois, in a prospective study of 1,400 African American men (*AIDS Weekly* Staff, 2002).

Another way to study this risk is to examine the rate of HIV among sample of circumcised and uncircumcised men from the same population. In a another study of over 3,000 men from a township near Johannesburg, Cohen (2005) reports that researchers found that circumcision can offer 65 percent protection from acquiring HIV infection. This lower rate of infection was found in the circumcised men despite the fact that they reported 18 percent more sexual contacts that the uncircumcized men. Researchers caution that the results from one region of South Africa may be difficult to generalize to all circumcised and uncircumcised men.

Erection Filling of the penile spongy tissue with blood during vasocongestion, resulting in a hard, erect, penis

Penis Size

The average penis is approximately 3 to 4 inches when flaccid (soft). In a recent study of penis size, when erect, the average length among subjects was found to be 6.02 inches, with a variation from 3.4 to 9.44 inches. Average penis girth (circumference) at erection was found to be 4.96 inches with a variation from 2.24 to 7.4 inches (Harding & Golombok, 2002). Most of the variation in penis size occurs during erection. Erection has been called "the great equalizer" because smaller penises seem to grow more during erection than larger ones, so the extremes tend to equalize when erect.

Obsession with penis size has a long history. Most young boys are curious about their penis size, and use rulers and tape measures to actually measure their penises. They are concerned that their penises are smaller than their peers'. By late adolescence, most boys grow out of their fears and obsessions about the size of their penises.

Much of the adult male concern about penis size stems from the perception promoted through inaccurate media coverage suggesting that size equates to virility and sexual performance. Penis size is a central theme in both straight and gay erotica and pornography. Male pornographic actors are recruited as much for the size of their penises as their ability to act.

Researchers Masters, Johnson, and Kolodny (1996) found that penis size had little physiological effect on women's sexual response. The vagina, they point out, is capable of adjusting to penises of varying sizes from small to large. The inner depth of the vagina can be reached by a man with an average-size penis by using intercourse positions (such as rear entry) that facilitate deeper penetration. An unusually long penis can extend beyond the depth of the vagina. A slightly shortened vagina also can be the byproduct of a hysterectomy. Partners can accommodate for any discomfort by adjusting intercourse positions and avoiding those that facilitate deeper penetration.

The inner depths of the vagina, the area stimulated by the probing of a larger penis, is relatively devoid of nerve endings. Most of the nerve endings in the vagina are located in the outer third, thereby accessible to all sizes of penises. The most sensitive area for sexual stimulation is actually the clitoris, not the vagina. Female arousal is related to adequate clitoral stimulation; clitoral stimulation is not contingent on penis size (or even the presence of a penis) at all.

The relationship of penis size to anal sexual intercourse is similar to that of vaginal sex. The length of the rectum and bowel is longer than the vagina, allowing for either deeper penetration or a longer penis. Unlike the vagina, the rectum does not produce lubrication. Men and women who engage in anal intercourse should use water-based lubricant to facilitate ease of penetration and thrusting. In Chapter 7 (sexual behavior), we offer a full range of health hints associated with anal sexual activity.

Although penis size has little physiological relationship to sexual response, it can play a big part in one's psychological functioning. Men, whether straight, gay, or bisexual, who are overly concerned with or anxious about the size of their penis seem to be more likely to develop sexual disorders than men who don't share this concern (Masters et al., 1996). Men who are overly concerned about their penis size can become anxious about sexual relations and develop sexual arousal disorders and even inhibited sexual desire.

sex in society 3.1

Penis Size Throughout History

People have been preoccupied with penises and penis size throughout time. Penis artifacts, ranging from pottery to temple decorations to statues with grinning characters possessing huge penises, have been recovered across the globe. Nearly 2,000 years ago, the Romans worshipped Priapus, the god of fertility. Priapus symbolized both passion and fertility. Although small in stature, Priapus had a huge penis. Every bride of the Roman aristocracy was supposed to lose her virginity by sacrificing it on the altar of Priapus.

In Greece, giant penises adorned the classic columns used to support its massive structures. In India, the temple of Kama Sutra is decorated with characters having oversized penises. The erotic pen-and-ink art of Japan has, as its focal point, couples lost in their passion, their elaborate silk robes parted, capturing their

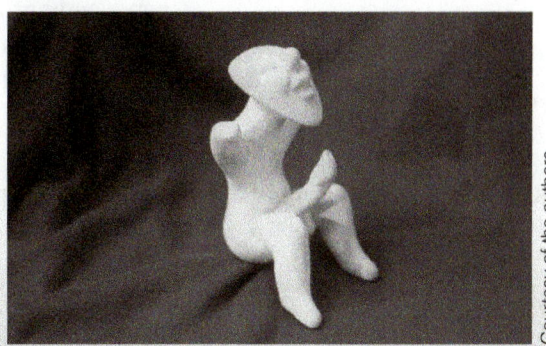

Priapus was always portrayed with an unusually large penis.

genitalia. The men all possess oversized penises that they are thrusting into their enraptured lovers.

No wonder that men are convinced that the size of their penises determines their masculinity.

Scrotum

The **scrotum** is a sac or pouch with two chambers that house the testes. Each testicle is cradled in its own scrotal pouch, suspended by a *spermatic cord* and *cremaster muscle.* A midline, or *raphe,* divides the scrotum into left and right halves. The scrotum has a sparse covering of hair and is usually darker in pigmentation than skin elsewhere on the body.

The scrotum normally hangs loosely, away from the body. This provides an optimal temperature of about 93 degrees Fahrenheit for the testicles. In a sense, the scrotum acts like a thermostat, regulating temperature by pulling the testicles closer to the abdominal cavity in colder temperatures and letting them hang loosely and away from the body under warmer circumstances.

The scrotum is composed of a thin layer of muscle tissue called the *tunica dartos* covered by skin. The skin attaches to the body at the base of the penis. During sexual arousal, exposure to cold, or threat of physical harm, the tunica dartos contracts and works together with the cremaster muscle to pull the testicles closer to the abdominal cavity for warmth and protection. In doing this, the scrotal sac shrinks and becomes taut.

Like the penis, the scrotum is responsive sexually to various forms of stimulation and pressure. When stimulating the scrotum, care must be taken, since each man varies in sensitivity to stimulation.

Scrotum A double-chambered pouch of tissue that hangs loosely from the base of the penis, containing the testicles

Perineum

The **perineum** is an area between the thighs, bounded in the front by the pelvis joint (symphysis pubis) and in the rear by the coccyx (tail bone). The perineum can be divided into two triangles of muscle tissue, the first

Perineum The erogenous area of skin extending from the base of testicles to the anal opening

containing the base of the penis and the scrotum and the second containing the anal opening. The muscular tissue is covered by a layer of skin. Although not normally considered part of male sexual anatomy, the perineum plays a part in the male sexual response because the entire area is endowed with nerve endings and is responsive to stimulation.

Again, the nature and intensity of stimulation to this area vary from man to man, and encounter to encounter.

Anus

Anus The opening of the bowel, through which fecal matter is eliminated from the body

The **anus,** or opening of the bowel, is another body part with multiple functions. Although the primary function of the anus is to eliminate solid waste from the body, it also serves as a part of male sexual anatomy.

The anal canal is about 11.5 inches long and is composed of two sets of sphincter muscles. The internal anal sphincter muscle is made up of smooth muscle tissue, and the external anal sphincter is composed of skeletal muscle. The anal sphincters act like the strings of a purse to open and close the anus. The anus is normally closed, except during defecation and sexual stimulation. Anal tissue is slightly elastic. The bowel or anus produces no natural lubrication.

The anus is richly endowed with nerve endings, can be stimulated manually or orally, and is enjoyed sexually by gay and straight men alike.

As a result of the AIDS epidemic, this behavior is being talked about more openly. Gay and straight couples have discovered that sex toys can be inserted into the anus to provide sexual pleasure that entails less risk than anal intercourse. We will discuss this in greater detail in Chapters 7 and 15.

Breasts

The breast is not usually discussed as a part of the male sexual anatomy. Although men's breasts are not typically thought of as erogenous, heterosexual women and gay men find the sight and feel of men's breasts to be sexually appealing. In addition, many men enjoy having their breasts stimulated manually or orally during sexual contact.

Structurally, men's breasts have the same components as women's: nipple, areola, fat, and glandular tissue. Men's breasts, however, have much less underlying fatty and glandular tissue than women's do, and men do not lactate. Men's breasts normally do not enlarge during puberty. A small percentage of men develop a condition known as *gynecomastia,* which will be discussed in greater detail later in the chapter.

Breast size and concerns about other external sexual anatomy and body shape in general are a source of stress for many men. A "manly" torso, with well-developed pectoral (chest) muscles, broad shoulders, and a tapered waist, is the ideal that the media and society present to us. Many men become obsessed with trying to achieve the perfect body and, toward that end, try everything from binging and purging to taking steroids. Separating good health from physical perfection is something we have to learn (see Case Study 3.3 Charlie: All Bulked Up and Nowhere to Go).

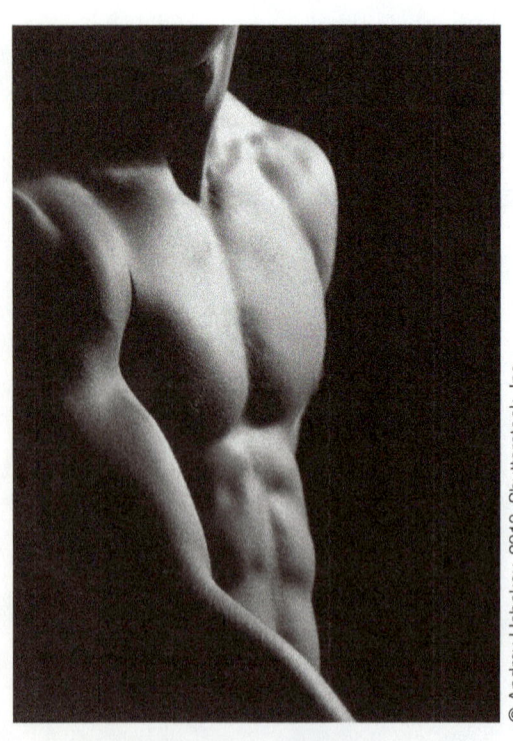

© Andrey Ushakov, 2010. Shutterstock, Inc.

The standards for male perfection promoted by media images are often unattainable for the vast majority of men.

case study 3.3

Charlie: All Bulked Up and Nowhere to Go

Charlie, 22, a student-athlete, identifies as Irish-American.

Charlie is a friend of Dr. Blonna's son who recently quit his small, NCAA Division 3 college football team after 2 1/2 seasons. He quit for a combination of reasons but mostly because of his coach's insistence on his bulking up. Here is his story.

"I'm 5'10" and in high school I made All-County as a defensive lineman. I weighed about 210 pounds and I was solid as a rock. I'm not sure what my body fat percentage was but I had a 34" waist and like a 44" chest. My grades and board scores were not too good and since I'm only 5'10" I didn't get any scholarship offers from any Division 1 teams. A few Division 3 coaches told me they could get me in if I played football.

I decided to go to XXXX State because they had a decent Communications major and I've always wanted to be a sportscaster. The coach told me that I had to come to summer football camp at 225lbs, so I started eating like a maniac and hitting the weight room even more. I knew I could have done it if I used steroids like a lot of the other linemen, but I didn't want to go that route. Boy, was my mom glad to get rid of me in August. I was eating everything she and my dad brought into the house.

I came into summer camp for my freshman season at 226, but felt heavy and slow. Most of the weight was muscle but my waist increased to 36" and I just felt too heavy. As it turned out I hurt my back during the first week and didn't play at all that year. The coach redshirted me and told me to come back next year, but to put more weight on.

I worked out all year, ate everything in sight, and came into camp for my Sophomore year at 230. I was huge. My waist was now pushing 38" and I looked like the hulk. I had never weighed so much, and I swear. When girls saw me coming, they walked the other way because I was so big. I hated it. I felt like a freak and couldn't find any clothes to wear. I made the team but had a sub-par year. I didn't start and mostly played on special teams. I only had a couple of minor injuries but I just felt too heavy and slow. My coach told me I just needed to do more speed work and he knew I could carry 240 pounds if I just accepted it and worked harder. He said I'd start next year if I came into camp at 240 lbs.

Once again I hit the weight room big time and continued to eat everything, take a host of different supplements, and spent a fortune on protein powder and creatine. I came into camp at 240 lbs., but felt miserable. All winter and spring I was anxious and felt very self-conscious. I had to fight to keep my waist at 38", even though I was working out like a madman. I had to eat a lot to hold onto the weight. I couldn't find any clothes that fit and didn't date at all. I drank a lot of beer and really was angry at the world.

I reported to summer camp in my Junior year only to find that my starting spot on the defensive line was taken by some kid who transferred in

(continued)

77

from a Division 1 school in the Midwest. The coach gave me some bullshit about toughing it out for the team and I just lost it. I told him to take his team and shove it. I quit on the spot and never looked back. I was a little more than a year away from graduating and had an opportunity to take an internship at a major TV station in a big city near the campus during the Spring semester.

I managed to drop about 20 pounds during the fall by just eating a normal amount of food, cutting out the supplements, and doing more cardio work. I got my waist down to a 36 and I'm still working to get it back to 34 inches and to get my weight down to between 200-210 pounds. I'm back to being pretty solid and feel great. I even started dating again and the internship is working out great. I doubt if I'd have even interviewed for it if I were still playing. I'd be too self-conscious of the way I looked.

Did the ends justify the means in Charlie's quest to get bigger, faster, and stronger in order to make the football team? What physical consequences could he have faced had he not changed his mind and reversed his course?

❧ *Physical Wellness* ❧

Physical wellness affects men's sexual health from conception until death. A mother's physical health and lifestyle affect the normal development of her baby. Factors such as prenatal nutrition, drug and alcohol use, and weight management can influence fetal structural development. To ensure optimal physical well-being, boys must be taught about their bodies and understand issues such as proper hygiene and protection of their genitals during sports and other activities.

To protect the genitals against injury from trauma, all male athletes participating in contact sports should use a plastic protective cup within their athletic supporters.

As boys approach puberty, they need to be aware of the changes that will take place in their bodies and their sexual anatomy and physiology. They need to understand issues such as nocturnal emissions and ejaculation, increasing sexual desire, hygiene, prevention of sexually transmitted disease and unintended pregnancy, and testicular self-exam. Fitness, proper nutrition, weight management, not smoking or abusing drugs and alcohol—all become increasingly important in sexual health as males age.

Often, physical and other disabilities impact on physical well-being. Rather than respond to all disabilities in a stereotypical way, we need to understand the extent of any limitations the disability imposes, and strive to maximize all remaining functions.

Internal Male Sexual Structures

The internal male sexual structures are illustrated in Figure 3.4.

Testes

The **testes** are oval-shaped male **gonads** housed in the scrotum. During the third trimester of fetal development, the testes form inside the abdominal cavity, and descend into the scrotum. The testes are held in place within the scrotal sac by the spermatic cord, which passes through the inguinal canal attaching to the wall of the abdomen and the cremaster muscle, which connects with the lower part of the internal oblique abdominal muscle (see Figure 3.5).

When one or both testicles have not descended by birth, the infant is diagnosed with **cryptorchidism.** In most cases the testicles will descend by the end of 5 years. If they do not descend by this time, surgical or hormonal treatment may be necessary to get them to fall into place. Undescended testicles are a risk factor for infertility, inguinal hernia, and testicular cancer.

The testes have two primary functions: sperm production and hormone production. Each oval-shaped (1.5 inches long by 1 inch in diameter) testis is divided into 300 to 400 cone-shaped lobules. Each lobule contains two to three tightly coiled *seminiferous tubules* and endocrine cells called *interstitial* or *Leydig cells.* **Spermatogenesis** occurs within the seminiferous tubules. The Leydig cells produce the male sex hormone testosterone. If

Testes Two almond-shaped male gonads responsible for sperm and hormone production

Gonads The primary endocrine glands in men (testes) and women (ovaries) that influence sexuality

Cryptorchidism Undescended testicle(s)

Spermatogenesis Sperm production

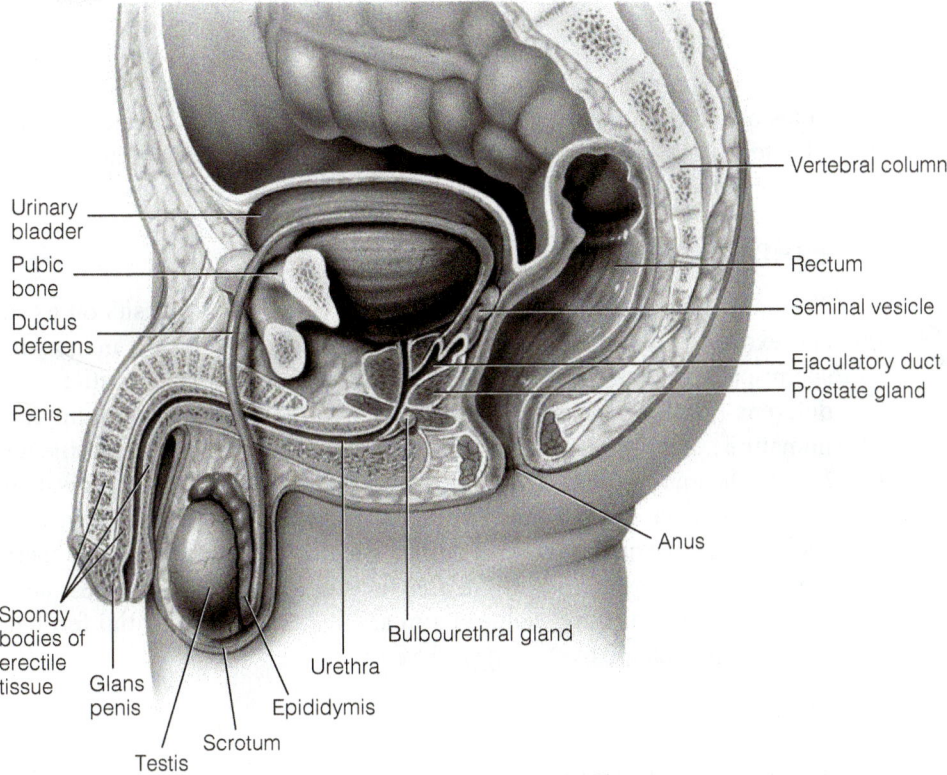

Urinary bladder
Pubic bone
Ductus deferens
Penis
Spongy bodies of erectile tissue
Glans penis
Testis
Scrotum
Epididymis
Urethra
Bulbourethral gland
Anus
Vertebral column
Rectum
Seminal vesicle
Ejaculatory duct
Prostate gland

Figure 3.4 *Male Internal Sexual Structures* The male internal sexual structures have reproductive and sexual arousal functions that are similar to female internal structures.

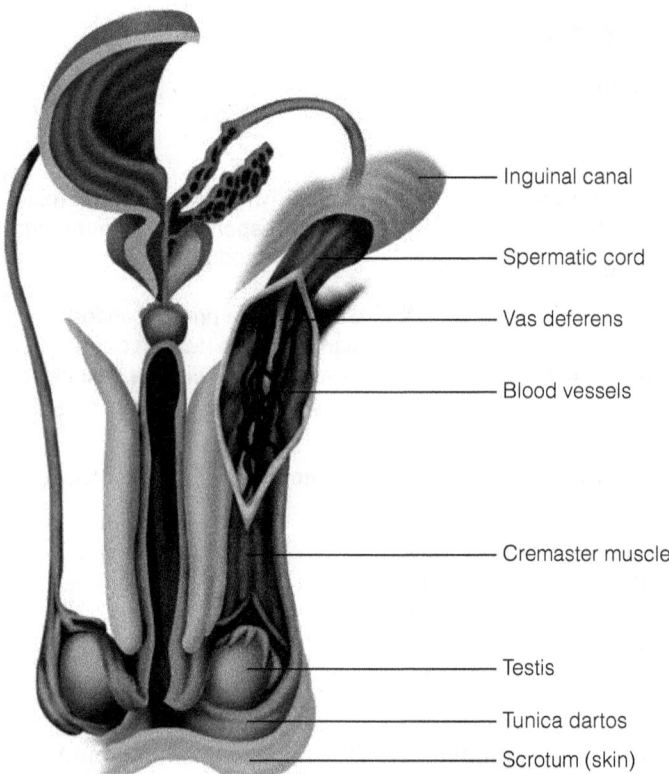

Inguinal canal

Spermatic cord

Vas deferens

Blood vessels

Cremaster muscle

Testis

Tunica dartos

Scrotum (skin)

Figure 3.5 *Testes and Spermatic Cord* The testes are anchored to the abdominal wall by muscles in the spermatic cord.

Testosterone the main hormone associated with sexual desire

Epididymis A C- or comma-shaped structure that sits along top of each testicle and serves as storage chamber for immature sperm

Vas deferens A tube extending from testicles to prostate gland, where it converts into urethra; responsible for transporting sperm and other ejaculatory fluid

laid end to end, the seminiferous tubules (each between 1 and 3 feet long) from both testicles combined would stretch almost 0.5 miles.

Sperm production begins at puberty and can continue until death, although the rate of production does diminish with aging. Some men fear "running out" of sperm. In fact, sperm are produced on an ongoing basis. Many things can interfere with sperm production, resulting in a low sperm count. Examples of the range of conditions that can lower sperm production as a result of damage to the testicles are injuries incurred during participation in sports and other circumstances, tight clothing, and exposure to toxic chemicals. **Testosterone,** the main hormone associated with sexual desire, also is produced first during puberty, and its production ends with death.

No evidence shows that sperm have anything to do with energy production and loss. Many men (including athletic coaches, trainers, and associated personnel) erroneously believe that depletion of sperm (through sexual activity) will weaken athletes and hamper their performance.

Because of this, coaches sometimes sequester their teams before games or matches to prevent these athletes from having sex. We will discuss the influence of testosterone and other hormones on sexual response in greater detail in Chapter 7. Sex in Society 3.2, provides an interesting view of how castration, eunuchs and sexual desire among other things.

Epididymis

The **epididymis** is a *C-* or comma-shaped, coiled duct that sits on top of and extends along the back of each testis. Each of its heads merges the sperm-producing seminiferous tubules, and each tail connects with the vas deferens (*ductus deferens*). Within the coiled, 20-foot-long epididymis, immature sperm produced in the seminiferous tubules become motile and fertile. The journey of the sperm from head to tail takes about 20 days. During this time, the sperm receive nutrients and mature fully, and the inactive sperm undergo a quality-control procedure. Defective and immature sperm are "weeded out" before they are able to be ejaculated. This process helps ensure that only healthy, viable sperm are available for potential fertilization of a ripe female ovum (egg).

Vas Deferens

The **vas deferens** are two long, thin ducts that originate in the base of the testis and extend up and around the bladder and into the prostate gland. There, they merge with the urethra. Each vas deferens is responsible for transporting mature sperm from the epididymis to the urethra. Each vas

sex in society 3.2

Castration, Eunuchs and Erection-Obsessed Societies

In a fascinating review of the historical literature, Richard Wasserburg (2004) describes the role of eunuchs throughout history. Wasserburg feels that eunuchs are very misunderstood in most Western cultures. He claims that "erection-obsessed societies" equate penile potency with power and effectiveness. In contrast, penile impotency is viewed as a sign of weakness and ineffectiveness. In a sense, Wasserburg notes, to refer to someone a eunuch *is* to label him an ineffectual wimp.

In fact, this is far from the truth. Wasserburg cites how, for most of the last 4,000 years, all of the reigning imperial Asian regimes have had eunuchs play a major role in the administration and management of their governments. He illustrates how members of this "castrated caste" have served as key officials and advisors to the administrations of Assyria, Babylon, Persia, China, Byzantium, various early Islamic societies, and the Ottoman Empire. Contrary to the image of eunuchs as impotent, powerless, and marginalized members of society, Wasserburg documents their power as diplomats, chamberlains, and ambassadors, wielding significant political influence and power.

Wasserburg discusses how the modern stereotype of eunuchs presents them as pathetic, penis-less, mutilated creatures, whose sole function was to protect women from the sexual pursuits of powerful men. Wasserburg claims that this was a small role played by eunuchs in history and is linked primarily to the early part of the 16th century and the Ottoman Empire. Even this role, however, has been distorted by cultures that don't understand the service and loyalty of eunuch guards who sacrificed their sexual desire to serve their rulers.

Eunuchs played a unique role in the history of Christianity, according to Wasserburg. Freed from lust and sexual desires, eunuchs rose through the ranks of the church to become bishops and archbishops. In a sense, their purity and freedom from sexual desire were viewed as a sign of greater spiritual purity. Some eunuchs, such as Saint Ignatius, even attained sainthood.

Another common misconception regarding eunuchs is that castration makes men incapable of fighting. Wasserburg cites how eunuchs played various roles in the military throughout history, some even rising to the rank of general.

The modern image of eunuchs as sexless creatures guarding the harem creates a very asexual image of eunuchs, which is also misleading. Although removing the testicles does remove the major source of testosterone, the hormone associated with sexual desire, it does not preclude erections and the ability to have intercourse. As Wasserburg notes, low levels of sexual desire does not mean that a man is incapable of having sex. Although a eunuch may not feel compelled to have sex out of need or desire, he can still satisfy the desire of others. In fact, as Wasserburg notes, serving others is what eunuchs do best.

This last observation is interesting in light of the over 40,000 men in North America each year who are, in Wasserburg's words, " castrated either chemically or surgically" to slow the progress of prostate cancer (p. 18). While most people might disagree with this description Wasserburg (2004) that this is really what they are. Perhaps if we were less "erection-obsessed" as a culture we could help these men view this loss as an opportunity to re-examine their sexuality and their ability to please their partners. Maybe this would help them reassess what sexual desire and gratification were all about.

Source: Wasserburg, R (2004). Eunuch Power in Old Byzantium. *Gay & Lesbian Review*, (11) # 3, pp18–20. May/June, 2004.

deferens joins the ejaculatory duct of the seminal vesicles just prior to entering the prostate gland.

The smooth muscle tissue of the vas deferens contracts during ejaculation, moving sperm as it does so. The sperm mix with secretions of the seminal vesicles, prostate gland, and Cowper's glands to form the milky-white fluid released through ejaculation. Each ejaculate contains about 1 teaspoon of fluid.

Vasectomy A male contraceptive method resulting in sterilization by cutting the vas deferens Inguinal canal

During a **vasectomy,** the vas deferens are located, a piece is cut out of each, and the end is tied or burned off. This prevents sperm from mixing in the ejaculate. We will discuss this method of male sterilization more fully in Chapter 14.

Seminal Vesicles

Seminal vesicles Small structures connected to the vas deferens which release fluids that nourish and buffer sperm as they are ejaculated

The **seminal vesicles** are two saclike glandular structures located behind the urinary bladder. Each gland is about 2 inches long, and tapers into a short duct that joins with the vas deferens to form the ejaculatory duct. The seminal vesicles produce an alkaline fluid that is high in the sugar fructose. The alkalinity helps neutralize the acidity of the urethra, protecting sperm as they pass through it. The fructose provides energy the sperm need to reach their ultimate destination, a mature female egg, or ova. Seminal vesicle fluid contributes 60 to 70 percent of the total amount of fluid ejaculated.

Prostate Gland

Prostate gland A chestnut-sized gland connected to the neck of the bladder and vas deferens, which secretes alkaline fluid and enzymes that are part of ejaculatory fluid

The **prostate gland** is about the size and shape of a chestnut. The prostate produces several enzymes that play a role in activating sperm. These enzymes are released in a milky-white alkaline fluid that mixes with seminal vesicle fluid and sperm to make up about 30 percent of the total fluid ejaculated.

The prostate is located immediately in front of the rectum, enabling digital (by finger) examination to detect any changes in shape and size. A routine prostate examination is recommended for all men over 40 years of age as part of their preventive health checkups. Some men find stimulation of the prostate (through digital penetration or receptive anal intercourse) sexually arousing. Others find any contact with the prostate uncomfortable.

Cowper's Glands

Cowper's glands Bulbouretheral glands, located below seminal vesicles, which produce pre-ejaculatory fluid that lubricates the vas deferens and urethra and protect sperm that are being ejaculated

The **Cowper's glands,** also known as the *bulbourethral glands,* are ducts that secrete a thick, clear mucus during the plateau stage of sexual arousal, prior to ejaculation. This alkaline, preejaculatory fluid provides an additional buffer for sperm against the acidic environment of the urethra as the sperm make their way out of the body.

Advocates of birth control have long speculated that enough live sperm can be present in preejaculatory fluid to cause an unintended pregnancy. This has not been proven, however, in scientific studies of preejaculatory fluid. Two studies intended to determine the ability of preejaculatory fluid to transmit HIV found that the preejaculate was free of spermatozoa (Ilaria et al., 1992; Pudney, Oneta, Mayer, Seage, & Anderson, 1992). Some sperm may remain in the urethra following ejaculation.

The two variables that contribute to the presence or absence of live sperm within the urethra are *time* (sperm live 3 to 5 days) and *urination* (urination flushes the urethra and the acidity kills sperm). If live sperm are present in the urethra before a man urinates, they possibly could get mixed into the preejaculatory fluid secreted by the Cowper's glands and thus increase the risk of pregnancy.

personal exploration activity

What Do You Know?

After drawing and labeling the male sexual anatomy, you will be able to identify what is accurate and inaccurate about your knowledge of the male anatomy.

Before completing this chapter on male anatomy, take a few minutes to see how much you know or don't know about the male sexual anatomy. Take a sheet of paper and draw from memory the internal and external male sexual anatomy. If possible, get a friend of the opposite sex to team up with you to do the drawing. This will be more fun and will show which sex has the most knowledge of the male anatomy. Once you have drawn the anatomy, label the following parts: penis, bladder, testicles, Cowper's glands, ureter, scrotum, urethra, vas deferens, seminal vesicles, epididymis, ampulla, corona, glans penis, and prostate gland.

When you have finished, compare your drawing with the one in this chapter. Are you surprised by how little or how much you know? How comfortable were you drawing this sexual anatomy? Ask one of your friends to do this activity. Does your friend's drawing indicate that he or she has good knowledge of the male anatomy? How comfortable was your friend drawing the sexual anatomy?

Diseases and Disabilities Related to Male Sexual Anatomy

The most common disorders of the male sexual anatomy are benign prostatic enlargement BPH), prostatitis, prostate cancer, urethritis, urethral strictures and trauma, phimosis and balanitis, hydrocele, Peyronie's disease, testicular cancer, gynecomastia, and male breast cancer.

Benign Prostatic Enlargement (BPH)

BPH is a noncancerous enlargement of the prostate gland. Because the prostate gland surrounds the urethra, any prostatic swelling, irritation, or infection can obstruct the flow of urine. Men with BPH usually have problems with urination, such as a weak, hesitant, or interrupted stream of urine or an urgency to urinate, more frequent urination (especially at night), and leaking or dripping. In extreme cases, urination is impossible.

The risk for BPH increases with age. BPH occurs in about 10 percent of men by the age of 40, more than 50 percent of men by age 60, and close to 90 percent of men in their 70s and 80s (American Cancer Society [ACS], 2003a; Coley, Barry, Fleming, & Mulley, 1997). The cause of BPH is unknown. Diagnosis is usually made by a rectal exam or measurement of urine flow using a flow meter. In some cases **cystoscopy** is used to diagnose BPH. The urethra is anesthetized, and a cystoscope is inserted into the urethra. The instrument has a light and camera lens that allow the physician to observe the inside of the urethra and the bladder.

Treatment of BPH depends on the size of the enlargement and the extent of complications. Up to one-third of all cases clear up spontaneously. Drugs can be used to help shrink a mildly enlarged prostate gland.

Cystoscopy Direct visual examination of interior of urethra, urinary bladder, and kidneys by inserting a cystoscope (optical viewing tube) into the urethra

Balloon dilation—a new treatment similar to what is used to open clogged coronary arteries—stretches the urethra and facilitates the passage of urine, alleviating the condition until the prostate can shrink. If no spontaneous shrinkage occurs, surgery is performed to remove the enlarged part of the prostate pressing against the urethra.

Prostatitis

Prostatitis Inflammation and irritation of the prostrate gland

Prostatitis is an inflammation of the prostate gland. The symptoms of prostatitis are lower back and pelvic pain, a sensation of heat and tenderness in the area, a thin discharge from the penis, and swelling in the genital area. The two types of prostatitis are infectious and congestive.

- *Infectious prostatitis* is caused by bacterial or viral infection. Treatment usually involves taking antibiotics.
- *Congestive prostatitis* is associated with failure to ejaculate prostatic fluid.

Prostate secretions are produced in response to a man's sexual behavior patterns. Reducing the frequency of sexual activity disrupts the pattern of production and removal of prostatic fluid. If prostatic fluid is not ejaculated, it begins to decompose and build up, causing congestion. Congestive prostatitis usually responds to warm baths and prostate massage (ACS, 2003d).

Prostate Cancer

Prostate cancer has become the most common type of cancer among men, and it is the second leading cause of cancer deaths in males (lung cancer is number one) (ACS, 2003c, 2003e). In 2003, it was estimated that in that year approximately 220,900 men in the United States would develop prostate cancer, and approximately 28,900 would die from the disease (ACS, 2003c). The lifetime risk for clinical prostate cancer among men in the United States is approximately 10 percent; approximately 3 percent die of this disease. Prostate cancer mortality increased an average of 1 percent per year between 1973 and 1990. Since 1990, the prostate cancer death rate in the United States has fallen an average of 1.1 percent annually, the decrease totaling 6.7 percent from 1991 to 1995 (ACS, 2003d; Dennis & Resnick, 2000).

These changes in incidence are consistent with the introduction of a successful screening test that detects slower-growing tumors and with an effect of lead time bias due to the early detection of prostate cancer beginning in the late 1980s and early 1990s (Hankey, Feuer, Clegg, Fever, Midthune, & Fay, 1999). Prostate cancer is a very slow-growing cancer. The early warning signs of prostate cancer are frequent or difficult urination, blood in the urine, painful ejaculation, and lower back pain. Risk Factors: Major risk factors are age, family history, race, and possibly dietary fat.

Age

The risk of acquiring prostate cancer increases after age 50, and greater than 70 percent of all prostate cancers are diagnosed in men over the age of 65. Prostate cancer is rare in men under 50 years of age (ACS, 2003d).

Race

Between 1995 and 1999, the rate of prostate cancer in African American men was 60 percent higher than that of white men. Much of this disparity is attributed to an increase in early diagnosis through stepped-up screening using the PSA blood test among African American men (ACS, 2003b). Despite this increase in early diagnosis, African American men are still more likely to be diagnosed at an advanced stage, and are twice as likely to die of prostate cancer than white men (ACS, 2003d). Late-stage diagnosis of cancer is usually attributed to lack of access to health care and preventive health services.

Diet

Men who eat a lot of red meat and diary products have a lot of fat in their diet and appear to have a greater chance of developing prostate cancer. No one is sure which of these factors is responsible for increasing risk, but men with diets high in meat and dairy products tend also to consume less fruits and vegetables. Nutrients such as lycopenes (found in high levels in some fruits and vegetables, such as tomatoes, grapefruit, and watermelon), vitamin E, and the mineral selenium may lower prostate cancer risk (ACS, 2003d; Herbert, Hurley, Olendzki, Teas, Ma, & Hampl, 1998).

Family History

Having a father or brother with prostate cancer doubles a man's risk of developing this disease. The risk is even higher for men with several affected relatives, particularly if their relatives were young at the time of diagnosis. These data imply a genetically inherited risk for prostate cancer. Research has linked the BRCA1 or BRCA2 genes with breast, ovarian, and a small percentage of prostate cancers (ACS, 2003d).

Early Detection and Diagnosis of Prostate Cancer

The prostate gland, as previously described in this chapter, is a chestnut-sized gland located immediately in front of the rectum. Although several other cell types are found in the prostate, over 99 percent of prostate cancers develop from the glandular cells. Glandular cells make the seminal fluid that is secreted by the prostate. Because of its location, the prostate gland can be reached through digital examination.

Early detection is potentially important because the survival rate of patients diagnosed in early-stage disease is much higher than that of patients diagnosed with late-stage disease (Mettlin, Jones, & Murphy, 1993; ACS, 2003d). The main screening tests in use today for the early detection of prostate cancer are digital rectal examination (DRE), measurement of the serum concentration of prostate specific antigen (PSA), and transrectal ultrasound (ACS, 2003d; Catalona, Richie, Ahmann, Angier, & Holman, 1994; Coley et al., 1997).

Digital Rectal Examination (DRE)

DRE involves the insertion of a gloved, lubricated finger into the rectum and the palpation of the prostate gland (see Figure 3.6). DRE is used to identify any abnormalities, including nodules or changes in size and shape

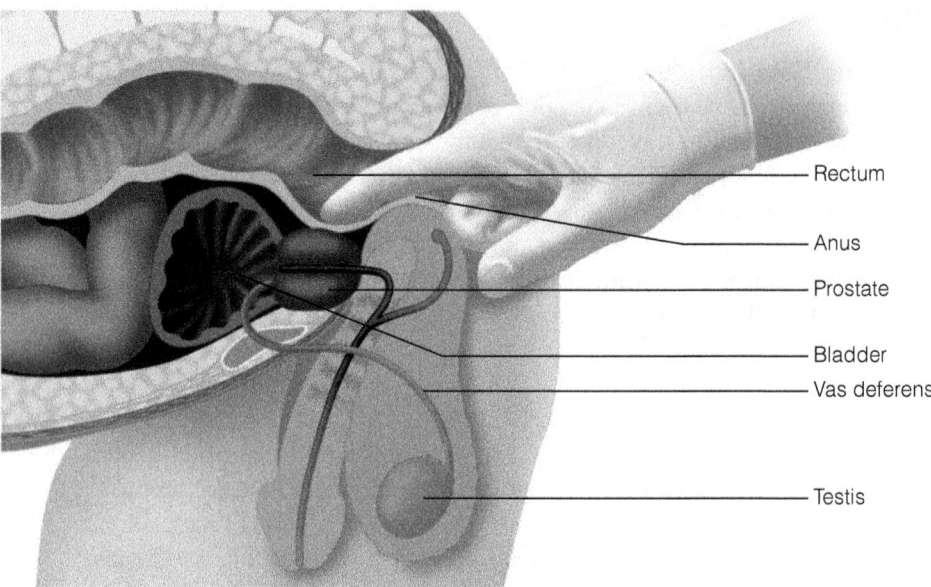

Figure 3.6 *Digital Rectal Examination* A digital rectal examination is a routine examination performed in a clinician's office.

that may indicate the presence of cancer. The use of DRE as a screening tool for early detection is limited because it can't always pick up the presence of small tumors and those deep within the prostate gland (ACS, 2003d; Catalona et al., 1994).

Prostate-Specific Antigen (PSA)

PSA is an antigen normally produced by the prostate gland. Healthy men have levels of PSA of 4 nanograms per milliliter of blood. Men with prostate cancer usually have PSA levels above 4 (ACS, 2003d; Catalona et al., 1994). If a man's level is above 4 but less than 10, he has about a 25 percent chance of having prostate cancer. If it goes above 10, his chance of having prostate cancer is over 67 percent and increases further as the PSA level rises (ACS, 2003d).

Many factors other than prostate cancer can influence PSA levels. It increases with enlargement of the prostate (called *benign prostatic hyperplasia,* or BPH), a common condition in older men. It can also increase with prostatitis. Because PSA elevations are not specific for prostate cancer, the PSA test has a high false-positive rate when used as a screening tool. On initial screening, 8 to 15 percent of men will have a PSA greater than 4 nanograms/milliliter, and only 1.5 to 4.1 percent will have a positive biopsy (ACS, 2003d; Mettlin, Murphy, Babaian, Natarajan, Nemeto, & Nemeto, 1997).

The combined use of DRE and PSA can yield higher results than either test alone. The PSA assay detects about one-third of diagnosed cancers in asymptomatic men that are missed by DRE, whereas DRE detects about 20 percent of those missed with PSA. In studies employing both DRE and PSA, about 25 percent of screened men require further assessment, but no more than 4 percent will be diagnosed with cancer (ACS, 2003d; Catalona et al., 1994).

Transrectal Ultrasound (TRUS)

TRUS uses sound waves to make an image of the prostate on a video screen. When performing TRUS, the health care provider inserts a small probe into the rectum, and sound waves enter the prostate. This creates sound echoes that are picked up by the probe and turned into a picture on a computer monitor. TRUS is not recommended as an initial screening test because of its expense and intrusive nature, but it can be employed to confirm results detected by the PAS or DRE examinations (ACS, 2003d).

The Prostate Biopsy

After a man has a positive PSA, DRE, and/or positive TRUS screening test, a core needle biopsy is the main method used to diagnose prostate cancer. A *biopsy* is a procedure in which a sample of tissue is removed and then examined under a microscope. During a core needle biopsy, the physician inserts a narrow needle through the wall of the rectum into several areas of the prostate gland and removes cylinders of tissue about 1/2 inch long and 1/16 inch across. These samples are examined in the laboratory for cancerous changes. Anywhere from 6 to 13 samples are taken to get a representative sample of the gland that will show how much of the gland is affected by the cancer (ACS, 2003d).

Prostate Cancer Stages

Prostate cancer, like other forms of the disease, is reported by stage. Treatment options vary according to the stage of the disease.

> *Stage I:* The cancer has not spread to lymph nodes or elsewhere in your body. Less than 5 percent of the tissue was cancerous.
>
> *Stage II:* The cancer has not spread to the lymph nodes or elsewhere in any of these cases, and more than 5 percent of the tissue contained cancer.
>
> *Stage III:* The cancer has begun to spread outside the prostate and may have spread to the seminal vesicles, but it has not spread to the lymph nodes or elsewhere in the body.
>
> *Stage IV:* The cancer has spread to tissues next to the prostate (other than the seminal vesicles), such as the bladder's external sphincter (muscles that help control urination), the rectum, and/or the wall of the pelvis, and/or it has spread to the lymph nodes or to other, more distant sites in the body (ACS, 2003d).

Treatment

Prostate cancer treatment varies according to several factors:

- The man's age and expected life span;
- The man's feelings about the side effects associated with each treatment;
- Any other serious health conditions;
- The stage and grade of the cancer;
- The likelihood that each type of treatment will be curative.

Treatment options include surgical removal of the prostate, radiation, radiation "seed" implantation, hormone therapy, chemotherapy, and cryotherapy.

Each has its own pros and cons and needs to be evaluated in relation to the factors discussed earlier. Some of the treatments can result in urinary incontinence and impotence, and therefore may be unacceptable (ACS, 2003e).

Urethritis

Urethritis Inflammation and irritation of urethra

Dysuria Burning upon urination

Discharge Draining of pus from the urethra

Urethritis is the inflammation and irritation of the urethra. The two most common symptoms of urethritis are **dysuria** and **discharge.** Urethritis can be caused by a variety of things, including mild injury, exposure to irritants, and infection.

The urethra can incur mild injury from too vigorous masturbation or other sexual activity. The tissue is temporarily damaged and becomes sensitive to the passage of urine. The urethra also can become irritated from exposure to harsh soaps or other personal hygiene products. Mild injury and irritation usually resolve within a day or two without any special treatment.

Urethral infections can be sexually transmitted or non-sexually transmitted. (We cover sexually transmitted infections in great detail in Chapter 15.) Non-sexually transmitted urethritis is usually associated with poor personal hygiene and infection with micro-organisms. Daily washing or bathing of the genitals will remove most micro-organisms capable of causing urethritis. Uncircumcised men who do not practice normal daily hygiene have a slightly higher risk for infectious urethritis. Infectious urethritis is treated with antibiotics, and responds rapidly to treatment.

Urethral Strictures

A *urethral stricture* is a scar anywhere along the urethra. The scar can be congenital (present at birth) or the result of an injury, untreated urethral infection, or multiple cases of urethritis (Swanson & Forrest, 1984). The scar can cause urinary hesitancy, decreased force and caliber of urine stream, postvoid dribbling, and excessive nighttime urination. Strictures are treated surgically either by dilating the urethra or surgically removing the stricture (Swanson & Forrest, 1984).

Urethral Trauma

Trauma to the urethra can cause damage to the urethral walls or, in extreme cases, severing of the urethra. In milder trauma, ice and rest can reduce swelling and prevent further trauma. In more severe trauma, a catheter is often inserted and left in place until surgical repair and antibiotic treatment is completed (Swanson & Forrest, 1984).

Phimosis and Balanitis

Phimosis A tight foreskin that cannot be retracted fully

Balanitis Inflammation of the glans penis

Phimosis is a condition of uncircumcised men who have a tight foreskin that is not fully retractable. **Balanitis** is an inflammation of the glans penis. By adolescence, more than 95 percent of all uncircumcised males have fully retractable foreskins. Although it was once thought that all newborn males had fully retractable foreskins, studies in the 1960s and 1970s showed that fewer than half of newborn males had fully retractable foreskins.

Newborns and young, uncircumcised boys often have some degree of tightness in their foreskins. A tight foreskin usually is not a problem in prepubescent boys. As long as the urethral opening and urine flow remain unobstructed, this condition has no negative health risks. Phimosis that occurs in a young man who has gone through the physiological changes and growth of puberty can be corrected with a variety of treatments, ranging from topical steroids to surgery designed to loosen the foreskin and separate it from the glans.

Phimosis also can be caused by infection as a possible complication of urethritis. The discharge associated with urethritis can get trapped under the foreskin, causing balanitis and inflammation of the foreskin, which results in increased tightness and difficulty retracting the skin. Because both conditions are associated with the infectious urethritis, antibiotic treatment of this infection usually reduces swelling and alleviates balanitis and phimosis. In rare instances, emergency circumcision is done to relieve the swelling and pain associated with infectious phimosis (AAP, 1999).

Hydrocele

A **hydrocele** is an accumulation of fluid in any saclike cavity or duct. Hydroceles are commonly found in the scrotum. Fluid accumulates in the *tunica vaginalis,* a small, closed sac that covers most of the testes. The condition is caused by an inflammation of the testis or epididymis or obstruction in blood or lymphatic fluid within the spermatic cord.

A hydrocele can develop as a result of congenital malformation or from injury during any period in a man's life. Hydroceles usually require surgical repair. In some cases the sac may be aspirated and the fluid removed. This usually is considered a temporary treatment because in most cases the sac will refill with fluid. A hydrocele is distinguished from the small, solid lump associated with testicular cancer; hydroceles are larger, fluid-filled sacs.

Hydrocele Accumulation of fluid in any sac, cavity, or duct

Peyronie's Disease

Peyronie's disease is similar to Dupuytren's contracture, a deformity of the hand in which there is a contracture of fingers toward the palm, often resulting in functional disability. Peyronie's disease is a condition in which collagen plaques form on the shaft of the penis and interfere with erection and sexual intercourse. The condition usually manifests itself through a

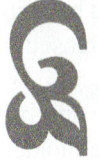

healthy sex hints 3.2

Preventing Urethral Trauma

Many cases of urethral trauma can be prevented by using risk-reducing protective devices. Protective plastic cups that fit securely in athletic supporters provide excellent protection against most sports-related trauma. Newer bicycle seats are designed with a protective groove or gap along the middle of the surface that comes in contact with the urethra.

Other ways to avoid trauma are to always read user manuals and understand safe ways to operate equipment and machinery that can cause blunt force to the lower body.

Do you routinely use these strategies?

curve in the penis. The curve can range from a slight bend to an angle severe enough to make intercourse impossible. Treatment involves collagenase injections and/or surgery.

❧ *Emotional Wellness* ❧

Issues related to men's sexual health can provoke strong emotions. A diagnosis of testicular cancer, for example, can conjure images ranging from deformity to death. High-level emotional well-being can make the difference between facing the challenge of cancer and working with health care providers to ensure that everything possible is done, or turning your back to the problem and hoping it will go away by itself. High-level emotional wellness involves recognizing, accepting, and working with our emotions. It involves asking for help when needed, and taking responsibility for your feelings.

Testicular Cancer

Testicular cancer is a relatively rare form of cancer (representing less than 2 percent of all cancers). Although fairly uncommon, it is the leading cancer killer of men under 35 years of age. Most cases of testicular cancer affect men between the ages of 15 and 40 years (ACS, 2003c; Landis, Murray, Boldon, & Wingo, 1999).

Risk Factors

The major risk factor for testicular cancer is cryptorchidism (undescended testicle). About 14 percent of the cases of testicular cancer are attributed to cryptorchidism (ACS, 2003d). Most of these cases occur in the undescended testicle, but 25 percent occur in the normally descended testicle. Some experts believe that performing surgery to lower the testicle prior to the onset of puberty can reduce the risk of developing some tumors in the testicle (ACS, 2003d).

Family history can also increase risk. Research indicates that a history of testicular cancer in one brother can increase risk in other male siblings. Cancer in one testicle slightly increases the risk for cancer in the other testicle. Certain occupations (mining, oil and gas workers, food- and beverage-processing workers, janitors, and utility workers) have an increased risk for testicular cancer.

The rate of testicular cancer has increased for both white and black men although the rate of increase is greater for white men. The incidence among white American men is five times that of African American men and double that of Asian American men. The reason for this difference is unknown. Worldwide, the risk of developing this disease is highest among men living in the United States and Europe, and lowest among men living in Africa or Asia (ACS, 2005).

Symptoms

Ninety percent of all men with testicular cancer have a painless or uncomfortable lump in the testicle or testicular enlargement or swelling. The remaining 10 percent notice no specific problem in their testicles but often report a sensation of heaviness or aching in the lower abdomen or scrotum. In rare cases, men with certain testicular tumors notice breast tenderness or swelling caused by an overproduction and release of the hormone human chorionic gonadotropin (HCG).

Many conditions can mimic the signs and symptoms of testicular cancer. The most common are injury and orchitis, both of which often cause pain and swelling that can be mistaken for testicular cancer symptoms. These can easily be ruled out by a physician, through examination and testing.

Testicular Cancer Stages

There are three stages of testicular cancer:

Stage 0: Preinvasive cancer of the testicular germ cells is present.

Stage 1: No cancer has spread to the lymph nodes or distant organs.

Stage 2: The cancer has spread to regional lymph nodes.

Stage 3: The cancer has spread to nonregional lymph nodes.

Diagnosis and Treatment

Most cases of testicular cancer are diagnosed through a combination of medical history (to rule out injury, preexistent medical conditions, and so forth), blood tests (to look for proteins and enzymes associated with the disease), ultrasound (to rule out fluid buildup and other conditions), and biopsy (to detect the presence of cancer growth) (Schmidt, Mettlin, Natarajan, Mench, McGinnis, & Piver, 1986; ACS, 2003d).

Treatment of early-stage testicular cancer typically consists of removing the cancerous tumor and administering chemotherapy. The chemotherapy is usually a prophylactic treatment to reduce the likelihood that the cancer has spread beyond the local lymph nodes. More rigorous combinations of surgery, chemotherapy, and radiation treatment might be indicated for later-stage testicular cancer. The long-term survival rates for early-stage testicular cancer treatment are excellent. Most men treated for testicular cancer have no loss of fertility, sexual desire, or sexual response (ACS, 2003e).

Gynecomastia

Gynecomastia, the abnormal swelling or enlargement of one or both of a man's breasts, is usually temporary and benign. If it occurs around the time of puberty, it usually is the result of a temporary hormonal imbalance. If it occurs later in life, it may be attributable to a tumor of the testis or pituitary, taking medications that contain estrogen or other steroids, or liver failure associated with cirrhosis or other causes. In cases where gynecomastia does not resolve spontaneously, corrective surgery may be necessary, especially if it is contributing to psychological stress and illness.

Gynecomastia Enlargement of one or both breasts in men

Male Breast Cancer

Breast cancer is primarily a disease occurring in women; however, men can have it, too. Male breast cancer accounts for less than 1 percent of the overall incidence and mortality of breast cancer. Even though men are at low risk of developing breast cancer, they should be aware of risk factors, especially family history, and report any changes in their breasts to a physician. Early detection improves the chances for successful treatment (Lawson, 2003).

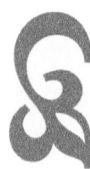

healthy sex hints 3.3

Testicular Self-Exam

Why It's Done

Testicular self-exams help you learn the normal feel and appearance of your testicles. That may make it more likely that you'll notice subtle changes, should they occur. Changes in your testicles could be a sign of a common benign condition, such as an infection or a cyst, or a less common condition, such as testicular cancer.

Who should consider regular testicular exams?

It's not clear which men should consider regular testicular exams. Though often promoted as a way to detect testicular cancer, testicular exams aren't proven to reduce the risk of dying of the disease. Testicular cancer is a relatively uncommon type of cancer. It's also highly treatable at all stages, so finding testicular cancer early doesn't make a cure more likely.

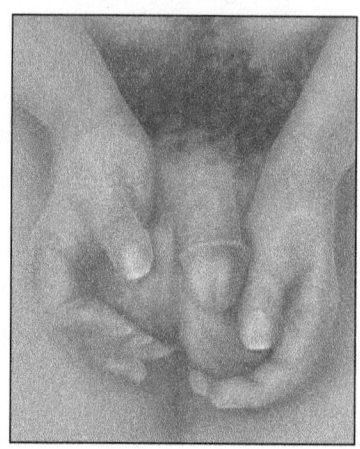

Testicular self-exam should be performed monthly while in the shower.

Doctors and medical organizations differ on their recommendations for testicular exams. The U.S. Preventive Services Task Force doesn't recommend testicular exams because a benefit has never been proven. The American Cancer Society recommends discussing cancer-related health issues, such as testicular self-exams, with your doctor during routine checkups. If you're concerned about your risk of testicular cancer, discuss the issue with your doctor. Together you can decide whether regular testicular self-exams are right for you.

The Mayo Clinic (2013) recommends that you do this at least once a month.

Source: Reprinted from the MayoClinic.com article "Testicular Exam" (http://www.mayoclinic.com/health/testicular-exam/MY00776/DSECTION=why-its-done)

Personal Assessment

Body Image: Males

Body image refers to our evaluation and perception of our body, specific body parts, and their functioning. It includes the messages (positive and negative) that we tell ourselves about our bodies, our self-esteem, and our behaviors and choices as a result. The following inventory will help males assess their body image.

Rate each body part listed below using the following scale: extremely satisfied = 5; satisfied = 4; neutral = 3; dissatisfied = 2; extremely dissatisfied = 1.

1. eyes _____   2. ears _____   3. nose _____

4. hair _____   5. teeth _____   6. mouth _____

7. weight _____   8. face _____   9. shoulders _____

10. chest _____   11. arms _____   12. calves _____

13. hands _____   14. height _____   15. stomach _____

16. buttocks _____ 17. hips _____   18. thighs _____

19. feet _____   20. sex organs _____ 21. overall body _____

Scoring:

105–80 Very positive body image
 60–80 Positive body image
 40–60 Ambivalent about your body
 20–40 Negative body image
  0–20 Very negative body image

Rate each item below, using the following scale: very comfortable = 5; comfortable = 4; neutral = 3; uncomfortable = 2; very uncomfortable = 1.

_____ 22. looking at my nude body in the mirror

_____ 23. performing self-examinations of my nude body

_____ 24. being nude when I am alone

_____ 25. being nude when I am with my lover

_____ 26. being nude when I am around my kids

_____ 27. sunbathing in the nude

_____ 28. swimming in the nude

_____ 29. walking around the house nude

Scoring:

32–40 Very comfortable with nudity
21–32 Comfortable with nudity
16–21 Ambivalent about nudity
12–16 Uncomfortable with nudity
 0–12 Very uncomfortable with nudity

Complete the following sentences:

30. The thing I like best about my body is _____

31. The thing I dislike most about my body is _____

Thought Questions

1. Describe the nature of penile erectile tissue. How does it facilitate erection?

2. Discuss the pros and cons of circumcision.

3. What are the major functions of the scrotum?

4. What two major processes occur within the testicles? Where do they occur in the testicles?

5. Describe the route of the ejaculate from the testes to expulsion from the end of the penis.

6. What is the role of testosterone in male sexuality?

7. Describe how you can reduce your risks for all of the sexual disorders discussed in the chapter.

Test Yourself

1. The shaft of the penis consists of two cylinders of _____ tissue.
   a. spongy
   b. mucous
   c. muscle
   d. connective

2. Erection of the penis is caused by
   a. bony tissue within the penis.
   b. cartilage that moves into place during sexual arousal.
   c. engorgement of spongy tissue.
   d. muscle tension in the penis.

3. The most recent recommendations regarding circumcision of newborn males is
   a. circumcision should be performed on all males for health reasons.
   b. circumcision is not recommended under any circumstances.
   c. circumcision should only be performed to save the life of the child.
   d. circumcision is considered elective surgery.

4. Which of the following is *not* a part of male sexual anatomy?
   a. Seminal vesicles
   b. Cervix
   c. Urethra
   d. Prostate gland

5. The two primary functions of the testes are
   a. hormone and sperm production.
   b. sperm and egg production.
   c. hormone and lubricant production.
   d. sperm and pheromone production.

6. The vas deferens and urethra
   a. meet at the cervix.
   b. merge at the prostate gland.
   c. are shared by male and female sexual anatomy.
   d. contain miles of tiny passageways.

7. Which of the following best describes the significance of prostate cancer?
   a. It is relatively uncommon in men.
   b. It is the number one cause of death in men.
   c. It is the second leading cause of cancer death in men.
   d. It is the most common cause of cancer in men but is rarely fatal.

8. Which of the following best describes the significance of testicular cancer?
   a. It accounts for about 2 percent of cancers in men.
   b. It is the number one type of cancer in men.
   c. It is the second leading cause of cancer death in men.
   d. It is the leading cause of cancer in men but is rarely fatal.

9. The American Cancer Society recommends that a digital rectal exam (DRE) be performed
   a. annually for men over 40.
   b. every 5 years for men over 50.
   c. only when symptoms are present.
   d. every 5 years for men over 21.

10. Testicular self-exam (TSE) should be performed
    a. every year by a qualified physician.
    b. monthly by all men.
    c. every 5 years after the age or 50.
    d. annually for men over 40.

Web Resources

Male Health Center
www.malehealthcenter.com

The first center in the United States specializing in male health. The center takes a holistic approach to health and covers impotence, prostate disorders, sexually transmitted diseases, vasectomy, cancer screening, and wellness.

Men's Health Network
www.menshealthnetwork.org

An information and educational organization that recognizes men's health as a specific societal concern and is committed to promoting issues affecting men's health. See "Library" and "Men's Links" for 54 pages of links to magazines and journals, books, organizations, miscellaneous resources, and men's health resources.

Men's Web Health Page
WebMD Men's Health Center hppt://men.webmd.com

This web site provides the latest information on a variety of men's health concerns.

American Cancer Society
www.cancer.org

The home page for the definitive source of information about cancer for men.

American Medical Association's Patient Education Page
www.ama-assn.org/ama/pub/category/3158.html

This is the home page for the AMA's patient education section. In it you will find information on a variety of health issues. The following address is a link to their report on circumcision: www.ama-assn.org/ama/pub/article/2036-2382.html.

Discovery Health Channel Prostate Cancer Assessment
http://health.discovery.com/centers/cancer/cancermain/prostate/prostate.html

This link is a questionnaire, provided by the online Discovery Channel, to help give you an idea about your individual risk for prostate cancer based on proven medical and scientific evidence. It will provide you with an overall summary of your risk factors and how they compare to those for the general population. It is an approximation of your risk; the results should not be interpreted as an absolute risk value.

Rather, you should use your individualized results to assess those factors that you can modify to minimize your risk of developing prostate cancer.

References

AIDS Weekly Staff. (2002, September 30). *AIDS Weekly*, pp. 4–6.

American Academy of Pediatrics (2012). Circumcision Policy Statement. *Pediatrics Vol. 130 No. 3 September 1*, 2012. pp. 585–586

American Cancer Society (2005a). Cancer Reference Information. Detailed Guide to Testicular Cancer. Revised: 07/01/2005 http://www.cancer.org/docroot/CRI/content/CRI_2_4_3X_Can_Testicular_Cancer_Be_Found_Early_41.asp

American Cancer Society. (2003a). Can prostate cancer be found early? [Online]. Available: www.cancer.org/ docroot/CRI/content/CRI_2_4_3X_Can_prostate_ cancer_be_found_early_36.asp.

American Cancer Society. (2003b). Cancer facts and figures for African Americans 2003 [Online]. Available: www.cancer.org/downloads/STT/861403.pdf.

American Cancer Society. (2003c). Cancer facts and figures 2003 [Online]. Available: www.cancer.org/downloads/ STT/CAFF2003PWSecured.pdf.

American Medical Association. (2003). *Neonatal circumcision* [Online]. Council on Scientific Affairs Report #10. Available: www.ama-assn.org/ama/pub/article/2036-2382.html.

Buie, MF (2005). Circumcision: The Good, the Bad, and American values. American Journal of Health Education, 36 (2) (March/April, 2005). Pp102–108.

Catalona, W. J., Richie, J. P., Ahmann, F. R., Angier, N., & Holman, J. R. (1994). Comparison of digital rectal examination and serum prostate specific antigen in the early detection of prostate cancer: Results of a multicenter clinical trial of 6,630 men. *Journal of Urology, 151,* 1283–1290.

Cohen, J. Male Circumcision Thwarts HIV Infection. Science v. 309 (August 5, 2005) p. 860.

Coley, C. M., Barry, M. J., Fleming, C., & Mulley, A. G. (1997). Early detection of prostate cancer. I. Prior probability and effectiveness of tests. *Annuals of Internal Medicine, 126,* 394–406.

Dennis, L. K., & Resnick, M. I. (2000). Analysis of recent trends in prostate cancer incidence and mortality. *Prostate, 42,* 247–252.

Hankey, B. F., Feuer, E. J., Clegg, L. X., Fever, E. J., Midthune, D. N., & Fay, M. P. 1999). Cancer surveillance series: Interpreting trends in prostate cancer—part I: Evidence of the effects of screening in recent prostate cancer incidence, mortality, and survival rates. *Journal of the National Cancer Institute, 91,* 1017–1024.

Harding, R., & Golombok, S. E. (2002, August). Test–retest reliability of penile dimensions in a sample of men. *Archives of Sexual Behavior, 31* (4), 351–358.

Herbert, J. R., Hurley, T. G., Olendzki, B. C., Teas, J., Ma, Y., & Hampl, J. S. (1998). Nutritional and socioeconomic factors in relation to prostate cancer mortality: A crossnational study. *Journal of the National Cancer Institute, 90* (21), 1631–1647.

How, A. C. S. W., Ong, C. C. P., Jacobsen, A., & Joseph, V. T. (2003). Carbon dioxide laser circumcisions for children [Online]. Available: http://link.springer-nv.com/ link/service/journals/00383/contents/02/00894/s00894/s00383-002-089.

Ilaria, G., Jacobs, J. L., Plosky, B., Koll, B., MacLow, C., Armstrong, D., & Schlegal, P. N. (1992). Detection of HIV-1DNA sequences in pre-ejaculatory fluid. *Lancet, 340* (8833), 1469.

Landis, S. H., Murray, T., Boldon, S., & Wingo, P. A. (1999). Cancer statistics, 1999. *CA: A Cancer Journal for Clinicians, 49,* 8–31.

Lawson, W (2003). Mammograms for Men? Breast Cancer is not just a Woman's Disease. Psychology Today. 36 (5) September/October, 2003, p 28.

Mayo (2013). *Testicular Self-Examination. Mayo Foundation for Medical Education and Research.* Available online at: http://www.mayoclinic.com/health/testicular-exam/MY00776/DSECTION=why-its-done.

Masters, M. H., Johnson, V. E., & Kolodny, R. (1996). *Human sexuality* (6th ed.). New York: HarperCollins.

Mettlin, C., Jones, G. W., & Murphy, G. P. (1993). Trends in prostate cancer care in the United States, 1974-1990: Observations from the patients care evaluation studies of the American College of Surgeons Commission on Cancer. *CA: A Cancer Journal for Clinicians, 43,* 83–91.

Mettlin, C. J., Murphy, G. P., Babaian, R. J., Natarajan, N., Nemeto, D., & Nemeto, L. (1997). Observations on the early detection of prostate cancer from the American Cancer Society National Prostate Cancer Detection Project. *Cancer, 80,* 1814–1817.

Peleg, D., & Steiner, A. (1998, September 15). The Gomco circumcision: Common problems and solutions. *American Family Physician, 58* (4), 891–899.

Pudney, J., Oneta, M., Mayer, K., Seage, G., & Anderson, D. (1992). Pre-ejaculatory fluid as a potential vector for the transmission of HIV-1. *Lancet, 340* (8833), 1470.

Schmidt, J. D., Mettlin, C. J., Natarajan, N., Mench, H. R., McGinnis, L. S., & Piver, S. (1986). Trends in patterns of care for prostate cancer, 1974–1983: Results of surveys by the American College of Surgeons. *Journal of Urology, 136,* 416–421.

Swanson, J. M., & Forrest, K. A. (1984). *Men's reproductive health.* New York: Springer.

Wasserburg, R (2004). Eunuch Power in Old Byzantium. Gay & Lesbian Review, (11) # 3, pp18–20. May/June, 2004.

chapter *four*

Sexual Identity

Student Learning Objectives

After reading this chapter, students will be able to

- Identify the components of sexual identity and appreciate its complexity.
- Describe the components of gender development.
- Evaluate the impact of biological, psychological, sociological, and cultural factors on gender development.
- Evaluate the impact of biological, psychological, sociological, and cultural factors on sexual orientation.
- Analyze the similarities and differences in the development of a variety of sexual orientations.
- Understand the challenges of "coming out."
- Discuss the more common forms of gender incongruities.

activity teaser: What would it be like to change sexes for a day? See the Personal Exploration Activity on page 119.

case study 4.1

Emily

Emily, 23, is white.

In these past 6 years, I haven't hooked up with a man, but I still feel uneasy about identifying as either lesbian or bisexual. "Lesbian" speaks to the fact that I date women, but naming myself as a lesbian does not mean that I am closed off to the potential of being with a man. "Bisexual," although allowing for fluidity, isn't really me. I pursue sexual and romantic relationships with women, not men. Queer—that's the word that says me best. "Queer" is like the antilabel label for me, a way to say "I'm here and I'm different" but at the same time not demand that I make any promises about what choices I might make in the future. "Queer" connects me to a political community that is inclusive of many different expressions of gender and sexuality. I identify as a queer femme, and what attracts me the most are alternative forms of masculinity, butch women, and female-to-male transgendered people.

Of course, many LGBT (lesbian, gay, bisexual, transgendered) people find the term queer offensive because the term has been derogatory. For this reason, I am deliberate about which label I use depending on whom I'm talking to. When I talk to someone who does not have much experience or knowledge of the LGBT community, I usually identify as a lesbian because that label is easier for them to understand. Because I am a queer femme, most people assume that I am straight. I identify as queer or femme with other queers and with straights who are both supportive of and sophisticated in their understanding of queer identity. Being queer celebrates my gender and sexuality in all its fabulousness and lets me feel comfortable being myself.

Critical Thinking

How do you feel about the use of the word queer? In what ways does our sexual identity become a political issue?

A basic philosophical question about sexuality is, Why are we the sexual beings we are? Some find a spiritual or religious answer to the question, looking toward their Supreme Being for the answer. Others turn to science and claim factual answers. Some question why, after decades of argument and research, scientists and theorists in the 21st century are still embroiled in the "nature versus nurture" controversy. Still others do not even appreciate why the question is being asked in the first place.

We are using the term *sexual identity* in a comprehensive way, to include the various factors that affect how we see ourselves. Individual sexual health requires that we appreciate the impact biology has on our being. The experiences one has in life, occurring in varied social and cultural contexts, help frame how we see ourselves. Sexual identity becomes a part of who we are as whole people: we have physical bodies, we show them to the world in a variety of ways, and we form romantic attachments with others. Ideally, our healthy sexual identities leave us comfortable with our bodies, expressing ourselves in ways that are true to who we "are." Our sexual identities develop from the interaction of several variables:

1. **Biological/anatomical sex** focuses on the anatomical parts associated most closely with reproductive capabilities and sexual arousal, specifically internal and external reproductive organs. The term *natal sex* has been used to describe that part of identity connected to what is visible at birth (Bockting, 1999). Included as well are the influences of the endocrine system hormones, as reflected in **secondary sex characteristics** and the process of sexual differentiation in the brain.

2. **Gender identity,** the private sense of maleness or femaleness, and **gender role,** the exhibited and shared behaviors that reinforce gender, bring sexual identity beyond the physical domain. In the scheme of things, how we see and express ourselves is expected to correlate with our anatomy. Therapists who provide services to those with sexual identity concerns have preferred the term *social sex role,* which goes beyond *gender role*—the outward presentation of gender—to include culturally defined sexual stereotypes and what the individual adopts from a spectrum of masculinity to femininity (Bockting, 1999; Kleigman, 2011)

3. **Sexual orientation** defines romantic and erotic attachments in choice of partners. One can be drawn to male partners, or to female partners, or be receptive to both men and women.

The question of why we are the sexual beings we are has no simple answer. Sexuality is complex, and our understanding of it continually grows. A number of questions have been, and are continuing to be, researched:

- What factors contribute to the individuals we are? Can those factors be controlled? Altered?
- At what point, if any, is our sexual identity fixed? Is this locked in our genes?
- Are parents and other caregivers the principal forces in shaping our sexuality?
- How powerful are the actual experiences we have in determining how we see ourselves, and how we make decisions?

In this chapter, we will explore the various dimensions of sexual identity, keeping in mind the following principles:

1. The research that has been conducted to date is not conclusive or definitive. Ongoing research from biologists, psychologists, sociologists, anthropologists, sexologists, the medical community, and others supports a variety of positions. Most likely, the persons we are result from an interaction among a variety of forces.

2. The culture has forced a dichotomous view of sexual identity. A person is supposed to be either male or female, heterosexual or homosexual, masculine or feminine. In working toward a healthy sexual identity, we might, instead, think of issues along various continua.

3. The premise that sexuality "just is" and that by some magical age one has evolved into a healthy, self-accepting, sexual being is false. The culture has defined rather narrowly what is deemed "acceptable," with an obvious preference for people to be heterosexual, attractive, able-bodied, and young. When we fall outside that norm—which for

Biological/anatomical sex Categorizing individuals based primarily on their reproductive organs, chromosome makeup, and hormone levels; traditionally, one sex is labeled male and the other female

Secondary sex characteristics Physical traits that develop during puberty and signal sexual maturity; examples are developed breasts, armpit and pubic hair, and coarse facial hair

Gender identity One's personal perception and sense of being male, female, or blended

Gender role The ways we express our gender identity—including appearance, clothing, movement, and life choices

Sexual orientation The predominant erotic thoughts one has for members of one's own sex, a different sex, or both sexes. *Heterosexuality* refers to attaching to a partner with different anatomy; *homosexuality* refers to a same-sex partner; *isexuality* refers to attaching to both men and women.

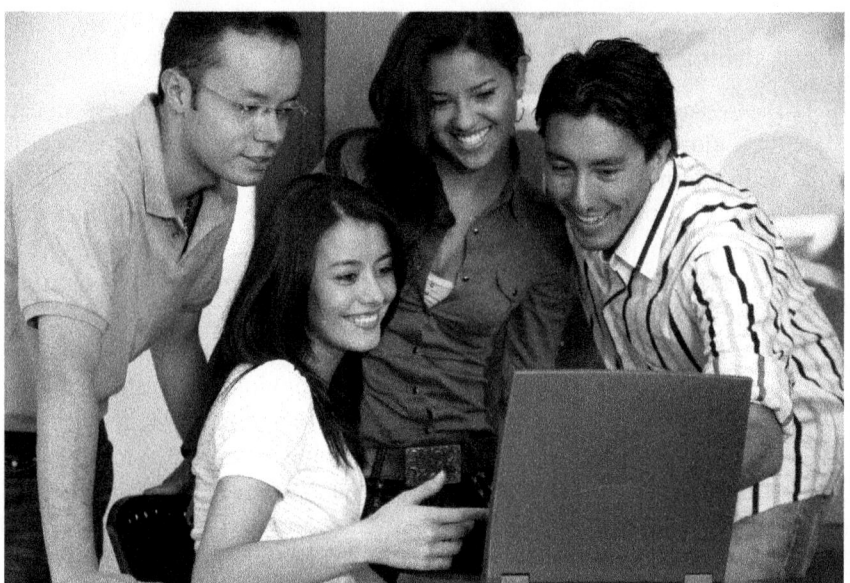

Being better educated and respectful of people with diverse sexual identities promotes greater sexual health.

many is the reality—self-acceptance and acceptance or tolerance from others may be difficult to attain.

To be sexually healthy, we have to become introspective, examine our past, look for explanations and answers, and work through aspects of our sexual identity that are uncomfortable for us. To promote greater sexual health, society, too, has to become better educated and respectful of people with diverse sexual identities.

❧   *Intellectual Wellness*   ❧

It is often said that "knowledge is power." In the area of sexual identity, it is helpful to know that theorists do not agree on why we are who we are. Parents should recognize where they can and cannot influence the sexual development of their children.

Also, the individual should know where to turn for more information. The Internet offers myriad opportunities to click on to useful information. Prior to personal computers, however, groups still found ways to connect. Support groups are available for gay and lesbian youth. Boutiques provide clothing to transgendered men and women. Some hospitals conduct sex reassignment surgery. And most large bookstores today have sexuality sections where individuals can learn more about themselves and people they hold dear and care about.

Continua of Sexuality

Sandra Bem (1995), Charlene Muehlenhard (2000), and others have challenged the approach to sexuality that limits the individual to dichotomous choices about his or her sexuality. You are either "male" or "female." You are either "masculine" or "feminine." You are either "heterosexual" or "homosexual." Needless to say, the culture at large seems to have mandated the dichotomy while simultaneously confusing issues of physical

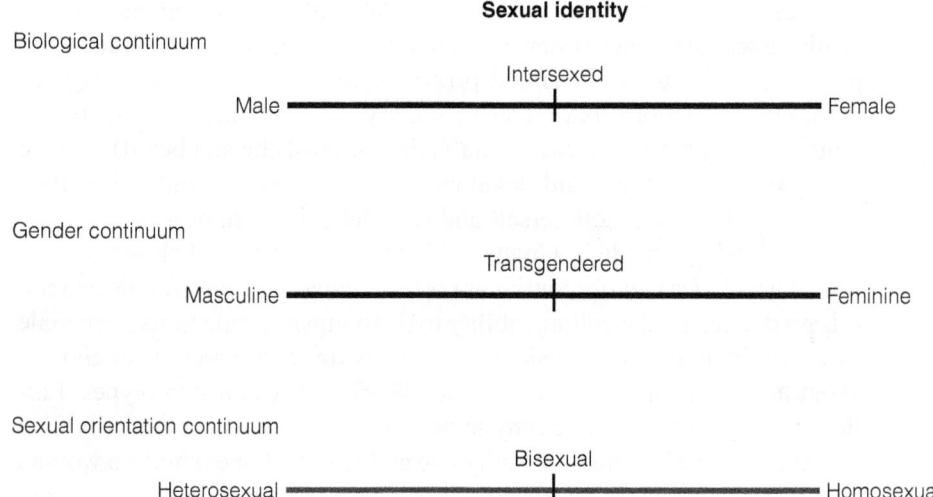

Figure 4.1 *Conceptualization of Sexual Identity* Identities can be fluid and form at various intersections.

sexuality, gender identity, and sexual orientation. Greater sexual health and freedom may come from viewing identity along the continua described in this chapter.

Self-acceptance, as well as a more sophisticated and accurate assessment of others' sexuality, benefits from the recognition that three continua influence our sexual identity (see Figure 4.1). For each variable, the individual can place him or herself at any point along the continuum. Permutations of the intersections are many. As a result, the tremendous diversity within sexuality becomes apparent.

For example, in the traditional model of female sexuality, the female has female reproductive organs—clitoris, vagina, uterus, and so on—and female secondary sex characteristics such as developed breasts, broader hips, and narrow waist. To be viewed as an attractive female, the culture further prescribes an acceptable presentation of those characteristics. The female identifies herself as female, adopts the prescribed female role, enjoys feminine things, and behaves in feminine ways. She sees herself as heterosexual, making herself available to males in the culture. This person assumes positions at the extremes of the three continua.

Above and beyond fundamental questions regarding "feminine things and feminine ways" is the basic reality that this description defines only certain females in the culture. Relying on a broader model of sexual identity, someone who is female can possess female reproductive structures but appear more "masculine" to others. A female could enjoy male clothing and be attracted to women. She could have both male and female reproductive structures and enjoy relating to both men and women sexually. The possibilities and realities are numerous.

The *biological continuum* of identity is often thought to be separated clearly into "male and female," yet some individuals have reproductive structures from both. The term *hermaphrodite* has been used when the gonads of both sexes are present and *pseudohermaprodite* when gestational hormone imbalances have caused the external genitalia to be ambiguous and different from the internal structures (Sherwood, 2004). Today, such

Intersexual An individual possessing some degree of both male and female internal or external reproductive structures; the preferred term, replacing earlier labels of *hermaphrodite* and *pseudohermaphrodite*

Androgynous Expressing characteristics and traits considered stereotypically male and female

Transgendered The preferred term to describe individuals whose gender identity and gender role encompass both masculine and feminine qualities

Heterosexuality Forming sexual relationships with members of the other sex

Homosexuality Forming sexual relationships with members of the same sex

Bisexuality Forming sexual relationships with both men and women

individuals have embraced the preferred label of **intersexual** and, as will be discussed later, have become vocal in their concerns about medical and psychological interventions and practices. Some individuals experience hormone fluctuations that affect secondary sex characteristics, such as a female having male patterned facial hair (a moustache and beard). A male may have soft features and developed breasts. How the individual then goes on to define himself/herself and what label is taken or what cosmetic "corrections" get made is a matter of increasingly personal choice.

The *gender identity* continuum offers numerous points for placement. It is predicated on the cultural ability to distinguish female traits from male traits. Individuals who consider themselves **androgynous** make choices about how they look and act without adhering to sexual stereotypes. Earlier literature defined androgyny in positive terms, in which the individual adopted the healthier traits of both male and female. For example, a woman would not be afraid to voice her opinions, and a man would not hesitate to express his emotions. Clothing, and more significantly one's occupation, would be chosen without gender restrictions. In essence, each would freely choose characteristics and behaviors that best suit his or her personality, not the cultural stereotypes.

Woodhill and Samuels (2003) propose that individuals may be "positively androgynous" or "negatively androgynous" by incorporating desirable or undesirable characteristics. Gender-based characteristics can be positive or negative. The positively androgynous person may demonstrate high levels of compassion, a positive female quality, along with high levels of independence, a positive male quality. In contrast, the negatively androgynous person would demonstrate high levels of submissiveness, a negative female quality, and selfishness, a negative male quality. Their research findings identify positive androgyny as the developmental ideal, associated with higher scores on indicators of mental health and well-being; such individuals have the potential to live a more fulfilled life.

As discussed later in this chapter, those identifying as **transgendered** also place themselves at varying points on the gender identity continuum. For some, their physical appearance is of primary concern. For others the core gender identity is under question, and at some point hormonal and surgical interventions may be sought to become more authentic.

Placement along the *sexual orientation* continuum allows for erotic connections to males, females, or both. Exclusive **heterosexuality** involves erotic relationships with members of the other sex; males would connect with females and females with males. Exclusive **homosexuality** involves erotic relationships between members of the same sex—that is, males with males and females with females. **Bisexuality** is reflected by erotic connections in which the individual relates to both males and females.

Figure 4.1 is intended to provide a visual model for understanding sexual identity. Individuals may place themselves at different points along each continuum, and those points may vary at different times in their lives. The continua can also intersect at various points, resulting in a great diversity of sexual identities.

Biological Sex

Some researchers perceive that "biology is destiny"; biological influences are the strongest influences over our sexuality. At issue are not only one's anatomical parts but also the need to examine influences of hormones on the brain, particularly during gestation and puberty. For many years, the prevailing wisdom held that "nurturing could override nature" (Money & Ehrhardt, 1972).

In 1972, John Money and Anke Ehrhardt wrote of the case of identical twin boys, in which, because of damage to one infant's penis during a circumcision repair, the child received sex reassignment surgery and was reared as a girl. Through strict feminine gender role experiences, the girl was thought to have a secure gender identity. For many years, sexologists relied on this case to highlight that biology was *not* destiny—nurturing behaviors and socialization could override biological beginnings.

Milton Diamond and H. Keith Sigmundson reported that this boy whose identity was changed in early childhood was not well adjusted, as had been previously described in academic circles (Diamond, 1982; Diamond & Sigmundson, 1997). The child struggled with identity issues, rejected playing with dolls, and attempted to urinate in a standing position. A suicide attempt in adolescence led to learning the truth, a cessation of female hormone treatments, and later extensive surgery to restore his masculinity. John Colapinto (2000) published *As Nature Made Him: The Boy Who Was Raised as a Girl,* bringing the story of David Reimer to the public at large. Reimer today is happily married yet understandably quite bitter about the professional treatment that led to an emotionally troubled childhood (Diamond, Sigmundson, & Reimer, 2002). Diamond and Sigmundson have publicly argued for great restraint in treating intersexed children as well as conducting sex-changing surgery in early childhood. Although they recognize that a child must be raised as either a boy or girl, they recommend limiting that nurturing to hair length, clothing, and name and strongly advise against any irreversible surgical intervention (Diamond et al., 2002). Reimer's case gives support to those who argue that the brain has a fixed sexual identity resulting from genetic and gestational influences.

The biological dimension of sexuality leads toward a more dichotomous approach, yet in reality—like the other dimensions to be reviewed—one can evolve in varying ways. The process of **sexual differentiation** embraces the term *different.* Males are different from females. If this is true, in what ways and how significant are the differences?

Sexual differentiation Sexual differentiation The processes by which the embryo/fetus develops into a male or a female; internal and external genitalia develop in distinct ways, as does the brain

Sexual Differentiation

The moment of conception marks our beginning. The union of a sperm and an ovum represents the chromosomal level of development.

Chromosomal Level

Sperm and ova are known as **gametes,** each of which carries 23 individual chromosomes. Together they become the 23 chromosome pairs carrying the complex array of genes that define us. One of those pairs, the sex

Gametes The reproductive cells—sperm and ova

chromosomes, determine our biological sex. If a Y-bearing sperm fertilizes the ovum, the species presumably develops as a male, with the gender chromosomes designated as XY; if the X-bearing sperm fertilizes the ovum, the species develops as female, with the gender chromosomes designated as XX (Figure 4.2). The genetic material within the gender chromosomes then acts to shape the organism in a way that is consistent with that differentiation.

Many factors influence identity. Chromosomes represent the beginning of a process that unfolds over many years, hopefully leading toward a clear identity.

In Utero Development

Gonads The primary endocrine glands in men (testes) and women (ovaries) that influence sexuality

Homologous structures Body parts that develop from the same embryonic tissue (for example, the female clitoris and the male penis)

During the second and third months of pregnancy, the **gonads,** the primary reproductive organs, develop. We refer to the two testicles as male reproductive organs and two ovaries as female. Because these structures evolve from the same embryonic tissue, they are called **homologous structures.** If the embryo follows a male pattern of development, the Y chromosome causes the testicles to produce testosterone, helping shape the structures that will develop. Specifically, the presence of the TDF gene—testis-determining factor—allows for male sexual differentiation. Without it, the fetus develops along female lines, regardless of chromosomes.

Estrogen and testosterone continue to play important roles in sexual development in utero as well as appearance and sexuality after birth. During development, the ratio of the two hormones will produce a child who is anatomically matched to the chromosomes and gonads. If the embryo is chromosomally XX, the ovaries will produce estrogen, which in turn will cause tissue to evolve into the internal and external reproductive organs associated with the female. If the embryo is chromosomally XY, testosterone will direct the tissue to developing into the internal and external reproductive structures of the male. Figure 4.3 shows the sexual differentiation of internal and external structures.

Hormones circulate throughout the developing fetus, affecting the brain, too, through a process referred to as *neural encoding.* Questions arise as to how the male brain may be different from the female brain. Researchers continue to debate whether the brain becomes encoded to later respond to the environment in a biologically predetermined way or whether the

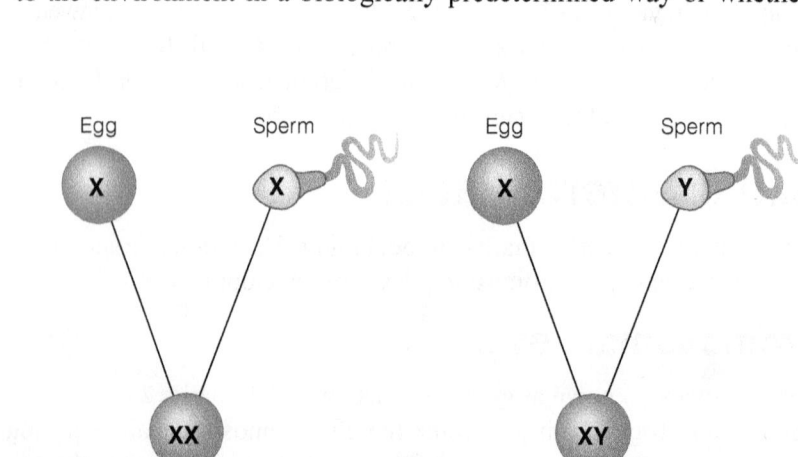

Figure 4.2 *Genetic Sex*

forces of socialization cannot be separated from identity. Although it has been reported that gonadal steroid hormones affect sexual differentiation of the brain in laboratory animals, the same case cannot be made for humans (Coleman, Gooren, & Ross, 1989; Hines & Collaer, 1993). Researchers continue to examine the role of hormones on the brain during both gestation and puberty, working toward a better understanding of differences in male and female brains.

Questions continue, however, as development progresses in the areas of gender identity, gender role expression, and sexual orientation. The pituitary gland in the brain and the hypothalamus interact to regulate the sex hormones estrogen and testosterone. One might ask whether the brain is set up to respond to the environment in a particular way, so that perhaps gender identity and sexual orientation evolve in a predetermined fashion.

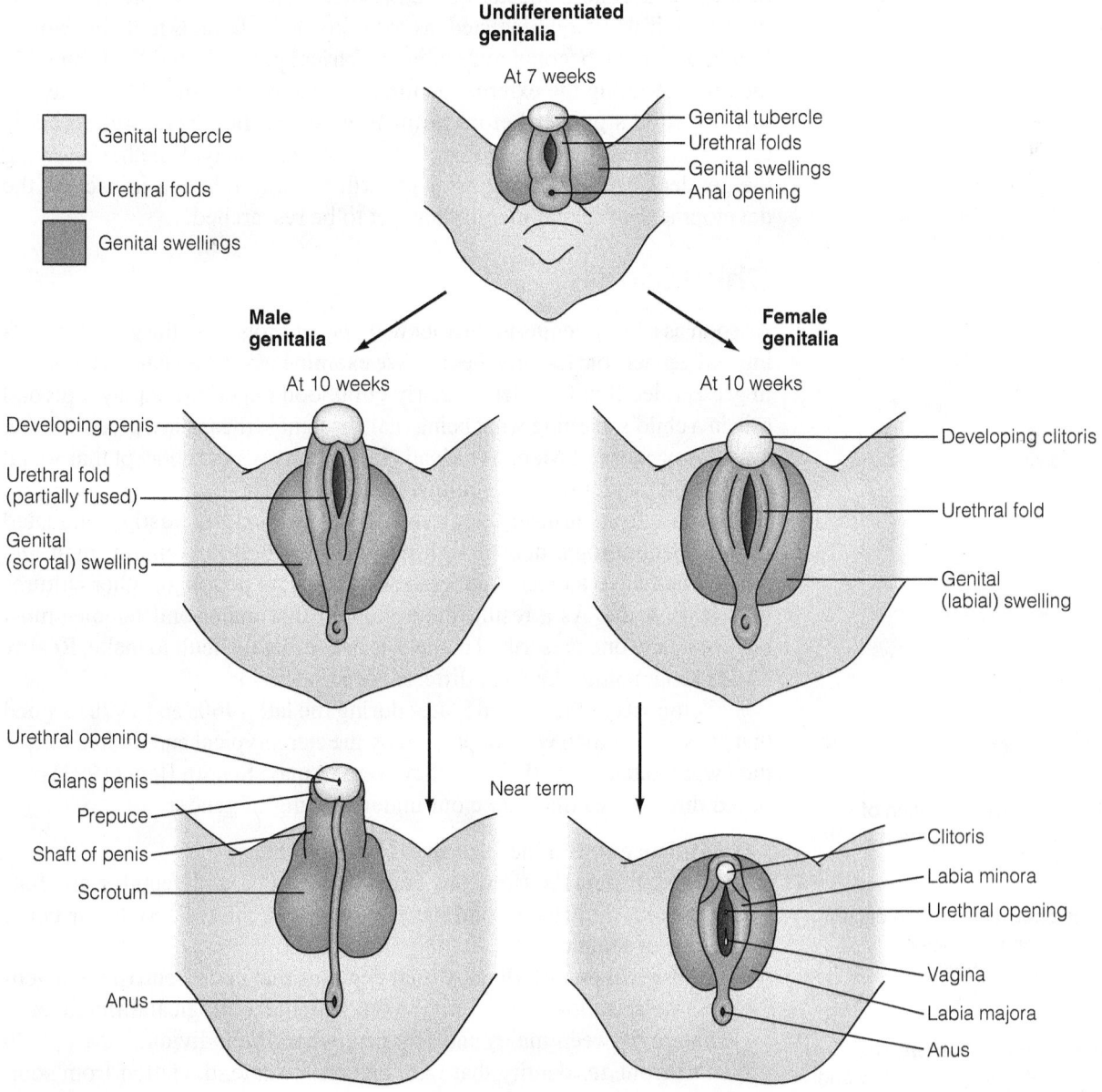

Figure 4.3 *Differentiation of Internal and External Reproductive Structures*

Anthropologists, however, argue that gender identity, gender role, and sexual expression are not strictly a function of biology. Their studies of non-Western cultures challenge commonly held assumptions about the universality of sexual impulses, the importance of sexuality in human life, the private status of behavior, or its assumed reproductive nature (Vance, 1988).

Birth

Traditionally, the next level of differentiation—gender assignment—is thought to occur at birth. Physicians, nurse midwives, and parents look at the external genitals of the baby and proclaim, "It's a girl!" or "It's a boy!" In today's high-tech world of prenatal screening, many couples know the sex of the offspring months before the baby is born. Chorionic villus sampling and amniocentesis—two prenatal screening techniques discussed in greater detail in Chapter 13—provide data about chromosomal abnormalities. In the second trimester of the pregnancy, prospective parents can be informed, if they are interested, as to whether the fetus is male or female. Sonograms have become routine in obstetrical practice, and they can yield pictures revealing the external genitalia. Thus, parents may be well aware of their child's gender before birth. In essence, they have time to begin gender socialization earlier than they could previously. Whether knowing the gender of the offspring prior to birth has any relevant impact on the development of sexual identity has yet to be researched.

Childhood

As soon as a baby begins to interact with the environment, the gender scripting and gender role learning begin. (We examine psychosexual development in greater detail in Chapter 5.) Early childhood experiences play a pivotal role in a child's learning what being male or female means in a given culture. The classic work of Margaret Mead (1935) conveys the concept that social scripts and gender roles are culture-specific.

Apart from primitive cultures, today's world is vastly connected through technology, and though cultural distinctions remain, men and women can have a clearer understanding of how people in other cultures may learn to be. As a result, the argument that males and females must behave in any one prescribed manner is becoming difficult to make. Reality stands testament to the wide differences in behavior.

Feminists in the United States during the late 1960s and 1970s argued that girls and women were oppressed by the stereotypical and limited scripts they were to learn and the roles they were to play. Sandra Bem (1993) proposed three lenses that frame our understanding of gender:

1. **Androcentrism,** defined as male centeredness
2. **Gender polarization,** the belief that males and females are fundamentally different and have mutually exclusive scripts for being male or female
3. **Biological essentialism,** which explains that androcentrism and gender polarization result from the fundamental biological differences in nature between males and females; when the individual attempts to carve out an identity that may be comfortable, deviation from society's script becomes problematic.

Androcentrism A position of viewing the world with the male at its center

Gender polarization The belief that males and females are fundamentally different, with mutually exclusive gender scripts

Biological essentialism The position that biology is destiny and our biology explains our nature

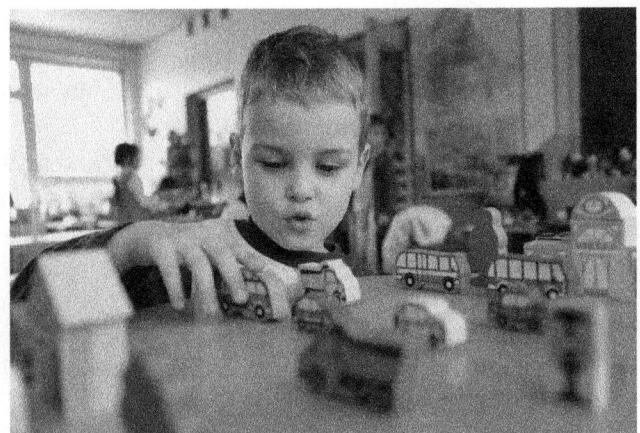

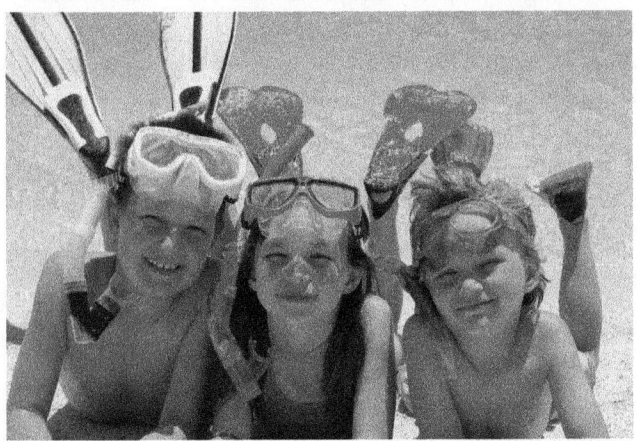

Toys, games, and ideas of fun all affect our sexual development.

Sex role stereotyping—in which girls were to be pretty, nurturing, and domestic to the exclusion of being independent and earning a meaningful wage—is now thought to be damaging to women's overall health and survival. The rigid expectations for males to be strong, financially successful and "in control" are probably equally damaging to male health and survival. Furthermore, it has been argued that stereotypes, by the mere fact that they are exaggerated, are inaccurate and ignore the cultural context in which people live (Brody, 1997).

Dressing children and teaching them about life are roles of the parents and the culture; television, schools, and other institutions play a big part in how children learn about themselves. By 24 months of age, a child is usually able to distinguish between males and females, and by 3 years of age, he or she has developed a gender identity, a clear understanding of being male or female.

Children today do not experience the rigidity in gender role learning that those of previous generations did. It could be argued that the culture has changed somewhat in its tradition of "color-coding" babies—that is, boys wear blue, and girls wear pink. Girls now wear blue, but can boys wear pink? The answer is still no. This may reflect the unspoken parental fear that putting a boy baby in pink clothes will feminize him. The color pink is purported to "sissify" boys, yet girls seem to have the ability to develop normally in spite of wearing blue clothes.

Boys and girls today can make freer choices for play and toys. Boys and girls can play with kitchen sets. Both can play with blocks and Legos. Broader questions remain as to why children are drawn to certain types of toys and what kinds of play are fun versus what kinds of play are needed to reinforce established gender roles. The women's movement in the early 1970s called into question stereotyped gender roles and forced gender play. The prevailing wisdom was that both boys and girls would benefit from broader choices based on interest and skill. Even though children in schools, for example, are no longer pushed to play in the "boys' corner" or the "girls' corner," evidence of gender preferences remains. Activities such as jumping rope, playing with dolls, and dressing up are more stereotypically female, whereas playing with toy guns, pretending to be a soldier, climbing trees, and so forth, are more stereotypically male.

Regardless, examining play activity patterns in children remains only one piece of a complicated puzzle for identity development. A persistent preference for "gender-inappropriate" play or dress may be connected to various states of **gender dysphoria,** whereas greater gender role flexibility may be considered a sign of health.

Gender dysphoria Condition in which there is a distinct difference between a person's biological sex and their gender identity. This may cause confusion or distress for the individual.

Dress-up dolls remain very popular with girls, with Barbie clearly dominating the market. Increasingly, the doll has been criticized for negatively impacting the self-perception of young girls. Barbie seems obsessed with clothes and has features that distort the female form. Yet, Barbie, who celebrated her 50th birthday March 9, 2009, continues to be popular, with numerous versions available. In 1998, the manufacturer announced its plans to make Barbie's proportions more realistic; Barbie added a few pounds yet remained quite thin.

Childhood also is the time when affectional patterns develop, and the basis for whom we find sexually attractive, what behaviors interest us, and with whom we want to romantically attach become set. Our sexual orientation defines whether the object of our attachment is male or female, or whether one becomes receptive to both males and females. In reflecting on their early childhoods, adults may remember being attracted to others in a particular pattern ("I always knew I was attracted to men"). Still, the concept of sexual orientation doesn't really take hold until adolescence and later.

John Money, internationally renowned researcher and clinician, coined the term lovemaps to refer to

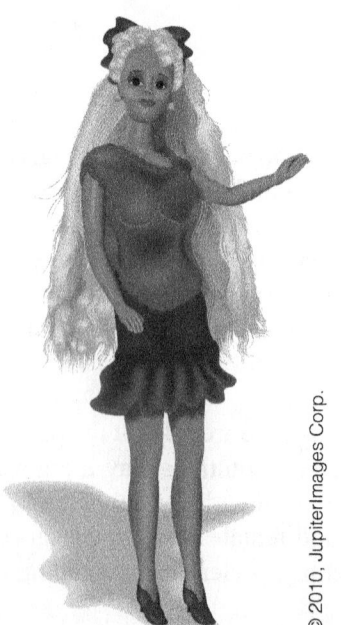

© 2010, JupiterImages Corp.

Picture Barbie has remained very popular despite criticisms about the unrealistic standard she sets.

case study 4.2

The Flower Boy

The flower boy is white and was 4 at the time.

When my sister was planning her wedding, she asked us if our 4-year-old son could be the flower boy. He would walk down the aisle just before the bride and throw rose petals along the path as he went. Though neither of us had ever seen or heard of a flower "boy," we thought that it was a wonderful idea. When we asked our son, he was excited about his important job. It never occurred to us that there would be a problem until we started mentioning, in casual discussions, that our son was going to be the flower boy at the upcoming wedding. Reactions we got from family members and friends (not all, luckily) ranged from astonishment to disgust: "Boys don't throw flowers." "That is a girl's job." "How can you do that to your son? You will humiliate him." "You'll confuse him," and so on. Frankly, we could not believe the reactions people had. After all, we argued, we weren't planning to put him in a dress, and since when were flowers the sole purview of girls? Remember, we are talking about a 4-year-old—a boy who happens to love picking flowers for his mommy and daddy.

In the face of scandal, we became even more committed to seeing this through. The day came, and our son, along with everyone else in the wedding party, was very excited and very nervous.

As he came down the aisle, dressed in his tuxedo, a basket of rose petals in his hand, spontaneous "oohs" and "aahs" could be heard from those assembled. People saw not a radical, genderbending experiment but an adorable 4-year-old spreading beauty and love. We were so proud of him!

Critical Thinking

If and when you have children, how far will you be willing to go to encourage their role flexibility? What will you do that your parents' did or did not do? How will you respond to those who have strong, negative reactions to you encouraging role flexibility in your children?

---

the patterns that develop in the brain, dictating what sexual behaviors will become arousing and pleasurable. His research highlights that lovemaps are formed in early childhood, underlying the power of this phase of development (Money, 1999).

Adolescence

Puberty, marked by surges in estrogen and testosterone, represents another passage in gender development. Secondary sex characteristics develop in both males and females, and sexuality becomes eroticized. For boys, the surge in testosterone prompts an increase in body hair, specifically armpit and pubic hair. The pitch of the voice lowers, the male reaches adult height, muscles develop, and the genitals, both penis and testicles, increase to their adult size. For females, the hips broaden, breasts develop, hair grows on the mons pubis and in the armpits, and the uterus and ovaries begin to function to allow for menstruation and ovulation. For some adolescents, hormones also have the undesirable impact of producing acne.

Heredity also plays a key role in how we end up. To some extent, our adult physical selves reflect the genetic material passed down. If members of your family tend to be hairy, your hairy chest is more likely to reflect your heritage than to make a comment on your masculinity. If you descend from large-breasted women, your large chest reflects that heritage rather than an unusually high estrogen level.

This phase of development is extremely powerful in its impact on self-esteem. Because of the many changes happening to the body, adolescents explore and play with appearance. A sense that we are acceptable as potential partners arises at this time: "Am I pretty?" "Am I thin enough?" "Are my breasts big enough?" "Are my muscles big?" "Is my penis big enough?" "Am I too tall?" "Am I too short?" "Am I OK?"

❧ Pysical Wellness ❧

As we age, particularly at puberty, our physical selves become a statement of gender. Heredity and hormones play a significant role in size, structure, and, to some extent, shape. Once we've matured, we make decisions about appearance—what clothes to wear, how to cut our hair, what we accentuate, what we hide.

In the past several years, males and females alike have been using steroids as a way to increase muscle mass. The evidence is clear that steroids used in this way can be dangerous. Women bodybuilders, for example, may have the desired large muscles but will notice diminished breast size, changes in the menstrual cycle, and more masculine contours to the face, not to mention increased facial hair. Males who use steroids may be excited by the size and strength of their muscles but unprepared for what is commonly called "roid rage," a pronounced and intense level of anger, and decrease in testicle size.

Changes to our health, such as depression or having a serious accident can influence the physical aspects of our identitiy. Having or developing a disability may affect movement, which in turn may affect how we see ourselves and how others react to us. Our view of our body is very closely tied to how we feel about our sexuality.

Our physical body is the machine through which we express our sexuality, therefore taking care of it, in whatever condition it is, and learning to love and accept it is essential for healthy sexuality.

Adolescence is the time when sexual experimentation takes place for many teens. Social norms support the development of a heterosexual orientation— choosing a partner of the opposite sex. Males choose females, and vice versa. For teens who begin to struggle with confusing feelings, the social supports are less obvious. Gay and lesbian youth may find groups that help them clarify their orientation. On the other hand, in reflection, many gay and lesbian adults report "playing the game" during their junior high and high school years. They feigned crushes and dated opposite-sex partners to fit in with their peers.

Developing a clear sexual orientation may not happen during adolescence. For those who know that they are lesbian, gay, or bisexual, being able to be open with others may or may not occur during adolescence. In an ideal world, individuals would be free to explore what makes them comfortable and happy. In reality, those who do not fit the norm, in whatever way, may find themselves lying, keeping secrets, and avoiding expressing who they really are.

Adulthood

In the past, theorists would argue that, by the end of adolescence, one would be moving on to adulthood and therefore should embrace the tasks of adulthood. One's initial adult sexual identity should be complete. In reality, though, we all continue to struggle with questions of who we are, how we want to present ourselves, and what types of partners are most attractive to us. A key piece in adult happiness is having a clear sense of one's sexual orientation. As shown in Figure 4.4, the process of "arriving" at one's sexual identity is a journey that involves many sources of input.

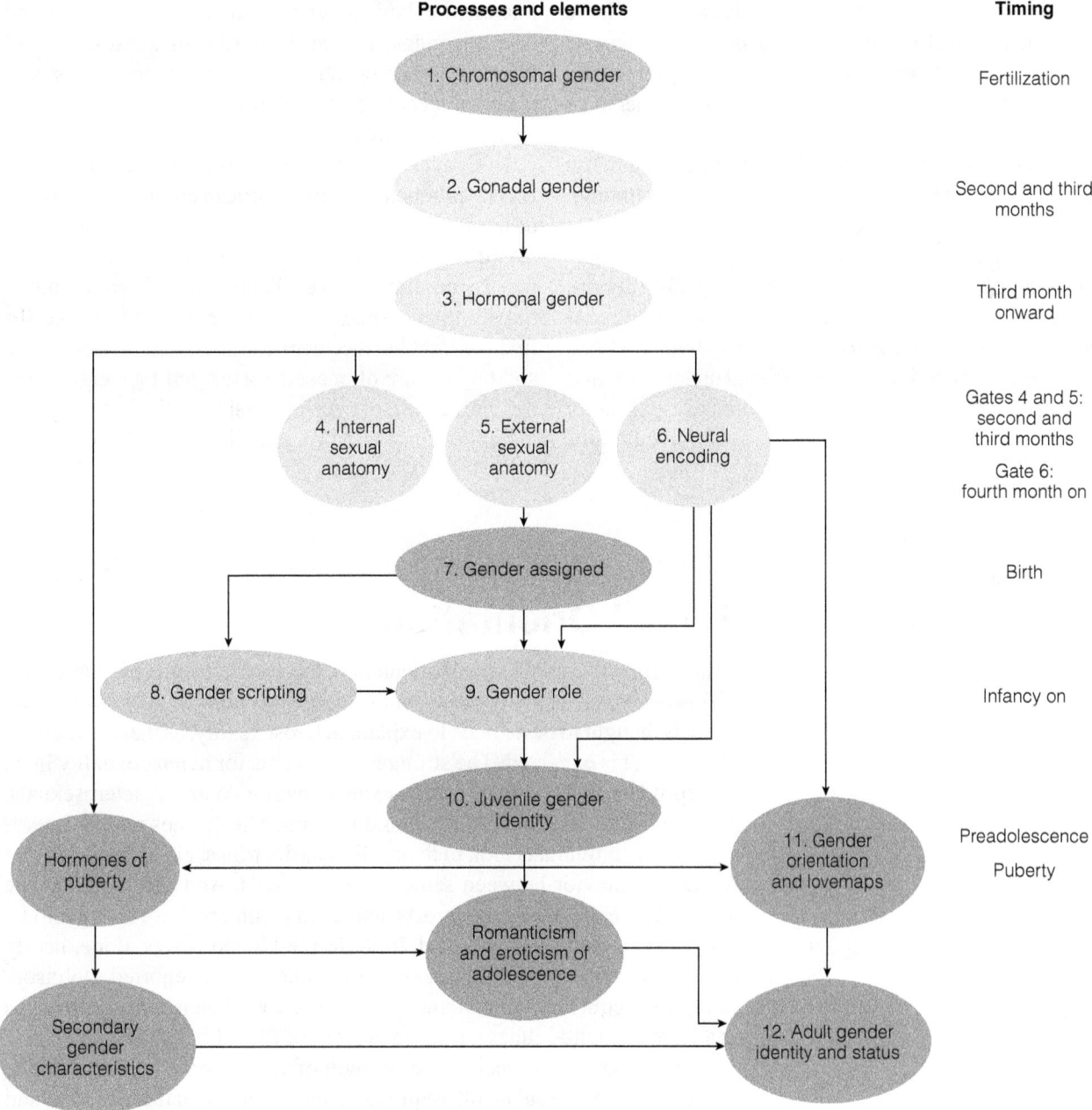

Figure 4.4 *Paths for the Development of Sexual Identity*

Source: *Becoming a Sexual Person,* 2nd Edition, by Robert T. Francouer (Boston: Allyn & Bacon, 1991) p. 74. Based on the work of John Money. Reprinted with permission.

sex in society 4.1

Body Image as a Lifelong Concern

The concept of "body image" refers to how one views one's body. It is a matter of self-perception, formed over years of looking in the mirror, receiving comments both critical and complimentary from others, comparing oneself to friends and models in magazines, and experimenting with looks. Who hasn't looked back at old photographs and wondered " How could I have thought I looked so good?" What is fashionable one year can be passé in the next. Changes in what is seen as desirable can certainly have an impact on a person's health, in all its dimensions.

It has been documented that a desire to be thin has led to elementary-aged girls going on diets. Although the research on eating disorders indicates greater rates among white, middle- and upper-class women, clinicians and researchers are seeing eating disorders in both males and females, regardless of race and ethnicity (Woodside et al., 2001). A person can have a "bad hair day," want to hide his or her head under a hat, and generally feel self-conscious. Individuals with body dysmorphic disorder (BDD), however, have a clinical diagnosis, and they see themselves as ugly, often becoming obsessive about one particular part of their body. Their disordered thinking about appearance can disrupt all aspects of their everyday lives, with some becoming housebound.

Increasingly, high school and college students seem interested in body adornment in the form of tattoos and body piercings. The need to make sure that tattoo and piercing parlors operate under sanitary conditions is of paramount concern for the prevention of infection, both bacterial and viral (for example, HIV).

Concern for appearance and positive body image is very entrenched in the American culture. The process of aging does not cause our desire to be attractive to disappear. Some choose to approach aging in a positive way by continuing to exercise daily and eating nutritiously to maximize their appearance as they age. To find the right balance between attending to appearance and taking care of oneself versus getting caught up in the momentum of ever-increasing options for improving appearance remains a challenge.

Sexual Orientation

In attempting to explain sexual orientation, theorists have often focused their efforts on explaining why some people identify as homosexual or bisexual. There is thought to be no need to explain heterosexuality, as that is the norm. That is what is expected. The strongest arguments for heterosexuality lie in the reproductive aspects of heterosexual behavior. Without heterosexuals, the argument goes, no children would be born. The species would die.

Some individuals look to their religious doctrines, citing passages that condemn behavior between same-sex individuals. And history is replete with violence, gay bashing, arrests, and even death for those thought to be homosexual. Between 2005 and 2008, in the United States alone, nearly 6,000 hate crimes involving sexual orientation were reported (Johnson, 2008). Consequently, some homosexuals have found their sexuality viewed as a form of mental illness, a sin, or a form of illegal behavior.

Although we appreciate the strength of various convictions, we take the position that sexual health requires accepting our sexual orientation and that individuals who are comfortable with themselves are less likely to feel threatened by people who have orientations that are different from their own. The gay and lesbian rights movement has often pointed out, "We are everywhere. We are your children, your brothers and sisters, your parents,

personal exploration activity

All the Things I Would Never Do If I Were the Opposite Sex

The goal of this activity is to inspire you not only to look at behaviors of the opposite sex that annoy you but to identify your own behaviors that hinder your relationships with the opposite sex.

Imagine that you have the ability to change what really irritates you about the opposite sex. All you have to do is make your wish list, and everything you wanted would be granted.

Take a minute and make a list of all the things that the opposite sex does that you really wish they would never do again. After you have finished making your list, show your list to your best same-sex friend and see whether he or she has the same wishes or can add to your list. Then be very brave and show it to your best opposite-sex friend. How does he or she react to your list? Ask this best opposite-sex friend if he or she could make any changes in the behavior of your sex, what would they be? Notice all the behaviors on your friend's list that you presently do. Are you willing to make those changes?

For example: If I were a female I would never
- lead a guy on sexually.
- wear so much makeup.
- always expect the guy to pay for everything.

If I were a male, I would never
- scratch my genitals in public.
- expect sex because I pay for dinner.
- talk with the guys about my sexual experiences.

your friends." The issue is whether an individual can be open about his or her sexuality, and whether you are willing to know that aspect of those with whom you are close.

Theories of Sexual Orientation

Theories on sexual orientation abound, following different tracks. Biological theorists have looked toward genetic, hormonal, and structural differences in the brain to explain homosexuality. Social theorists emphasize learning as a key factor in determining orientation. Wiederman (2001), in his critique of research on orientation, elaborates on the difficulties inherent in studying orientation. While the question of causality may be the primary focus, the experimental research that would be needed to systematically identify key factors cannot be conducted.

It is unethical, for example, to manipulate genetic material in an attempt to identify difference. It would be just as unethical and impossible to manipulate the behavior of parents, or experiment with childhood experiences, in order to assess the impact on later interpersonal attachments. Consequently, much of the research on orientation ends up being speculative and correlational; for example, researchers will survey and interview adults about their past to identify related variables (Wiederman, 2001).

Biological Theories

Studies of sexual orientation among identical twins and fraternal twins show varying rates of being gay or lesbian, yet the rates are not 100 percent. In one study of gay men, with an admittedly small sample, 52 percent of the twins had a gay twin; among lesbians, the rate was 48 percent (Bailey & Pillard, 1991; Bailey, Pillard, Neal, & Agyei, 1993). In studies examining the family connection, both male and female homo- sexuals are more likely to have a family member who is gay than are heterosexuals (Pillard, & Weinrich, 1986; Bailey, & Benishay, 1993). These and other research suggest some genetic component to a homo- sexual orientation.

Research on hormonal influences during gestation has been conducted more carefully with rats than humans. Theorists look to the period of time when sexual differentiation occurs in the brain and the hypothalamus devel- ops, arguing that hormonal imbalances may cause homosexuality as well as gender dysphoria (Ellis & Ames, 1987; Ellis, Ames, Peckham, & Burke, 1988). The hormonal imbalances may be a result of medications, steroid use, or high stress levels. A problem with the research in this area is the basic difficulty of carefully monitoring hormone levels in a large enough sample of pregnant women throughout their pregnancies and then being able to follow, in a longitudinal study, the development of their offspring. That kind of research has not been conducted.

Theorists also have looked to hormonal differences after birth, par- ticularly from a "deficiency" perspective. This approach—which holds that gay men lack adequate testosterone and lesbian women lack adequate estrogen—reflects the old stereotypes that gay men are effeminate and les- bian women are mannish. Most of the research in the area has been done on males, which also becomes a problem. The work conducted on males has not found any differences based on orientation (Banks & Gartrell, 1995). At one time, treatment for male homosexuality involved testosterone therapy. Rather than changing orientation, that therapy just made patients "hornier and hairier." The most publicized research on anatomical brain differences came from the work of Simon LeVay (1991), who dissected the brains of a small sample of gay men and compared them to the brains of straight men and women. He found structural differences in a section of the hypothalamus of the gay men. The research has been roundly criticized for sample size, absence of lesbian women in the sample, and the complicating factor that the gay men had died of AIDS. The research sparked a lot of discussion but offered limited findings.

Psychological and Learning Theories

In looking to psychological theories, particularly psychoanalytic and learn- ing theories, explanations of sexual orientation again have limited uses or reliability. In his *Three Essays on the Theory of Sexuality,* published in the early part of the 20th century, Freud spoke of the child as having an undifferentiated sexuality and having to learn appropriate responses as he or she ages. Part of that learning would be to identify with the par- ent of the same sex, and to seek out a partner of the opposite sex. To be homosexual then could be construed as inappropriate identification. The female child, for example, would identify with her father and seek out women as partners.

For years, the field of mental health, led by psychiatrists, psychoanalysts, and psychologists, considered homosexuality a form of mental illness. Not until 1973 did the American Psychiatric Association remove homosexuality from its *Diagnostic and Statistical Manual of Mental Disorders* (DSM). It is now understood that homosexuality does not cause mental illness. However, society's reaction to homosexuality and treatment of homosexuals can certainly contribute to depression and other mental health issues for some gays.

Very popular for years was the notion that homosexuality in males resulted from a weak or absent father and a strong, domineering, overly intimate mother. In short, parental ways of interacting with their children and between themselves were responsible for the homosexuality of their children. In cases where such a relationship between the parents was found, however, the household also had heterosexual children. It becomes quizzical, to say the least, that the nature of the parental relationship would explain only homosexuality and not heterosexuality. Research has not supported this theory of parents being responsible for their child's sexual orientation thus parents do not need to wonder what they did to influence their child's sexual orientation.

Another false notion has been that homosexuals were seduced into their lifestyle by an older adult. This myth is particularly destructive, for it sets up gay and lesbian adults as seducers, likely to seek out children and adolescents for their personal pleasure. As a result, professions where adults have contact with children (teacher, coach, and so on) become particularly risky places to "come out."

One study extensively interviewed and compared responses from close to 1,000 gay and lesbian adults with those from a sample group of approximately 500 heterosexual males and females (Bell, Weinberg, & Hammersmith, 1981). The interviewees were asked about their child and adolescent years. The results showed no patterns of family dysfunction, no prevalence of positive or negative sexual experiences to explain orientation, and, most important, no predetermination of orientation before adolescence.

Researchers have also had difficulty obtaining samples of adults to study. A common practice has been to seek out volunteers for convenience samples, advertising in publications targeted to the gay, lesbian, and bisexual community. Individuals are asked to recall childhood and adolescent experiences, which are then used to frame a developmental picture. The costs and sample size involved in following very young children over time become prohibitive. The results of such research, however, may be tainted by selective memories and inaccuracies (Wiederman, 2001).

There is much uncertainty about why some have a homosexual orientation but what we do know is that there are no differences in the family and social backgrounds of heterosexuals and homosexuals nor is there any evidence for orientation being related to parenting, sexual abuse or other trauma (Kleigman, 2011).

At the risk of oversimplification in describing various theories, it should become obvious that no one theory of sexual orientation explains it all.(Savin-Williams and Cohen (2004) conclude that sexual orientation is present at conception if caused by genetic factors; begins in prenatal life if caused by biologic and environmental factors that act on the fetus during prenatal development; and is present from early childhood if caused by psychogenic or social factors. Although the genesis of sexual orientation is different for individuals, orientation is thought to be stable and not under our conscious control. "What we have learned over the last 30 years is that you apparently cannot change a person's sexual orientation, though you can change others views about sexual orientation" (Dreger, 2009). Homosexual, bisexual, and heterosexual children can and do have the same biological parents, grow up in the same households, and end up differently along the continuum of sexual orientation.

Labels and Categories

Alfred Kinsey's work on male and female sexuality continues to provide a reference point for work on sexual orientation (Kinsey, Pomeroy, & Martin, 1948; Kinsey, Pomeroy, Martin, & Gebhard, 1953). Along with his colleagues, he developed a 7-point scale that categorized sexual experience, shown in Figure 4.5.

After interviewing more than 10,000 people, Kinsey found it useful to categorize behaviors on a continuum based on sexual experience with same-sex and other-sex partners. If one's behavior was exclusively with a member of the other sex, that person was referred to as a "Kinsey 0." A person whose behavior was exclusively with members of his or her own sex was labeled a "Kinsey 6." All other positions between 1 and 5 represented interest in both men and women. Those in this part of the continuum are the ones most likely to fluctuate in their attraction and commitment to one particular sex (Savin-Williams & Cohen, 2004).

Because the culture often seems to want to classify or label people regarding orientation, only Kinsey 0's would fit the definition of heterosexual. Individuals categorized as Kinsey 6's would be homosexual, and those falling within categories 1 through 5 would be bisexual or ambisexual. The mean age for self labeling as a non heterosexual is middle adolescence. However, many choose not to share this with others causing the mean age for coming out to be after high school, or young adulthood (Savin-Williams & Cohen, 2004).

Later researchers and theorists, as well as groups holding to one or more political positions, have objected to classifying individuals based only

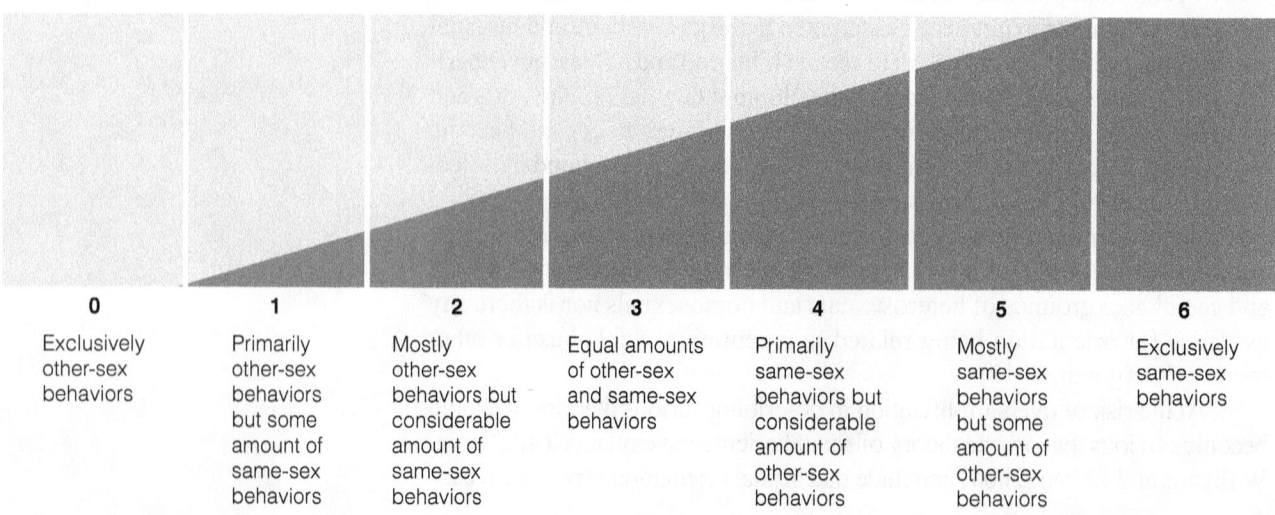

Figure 4.5 *The Kinsey Scale*

on their behavior, as well as questioning the need to classify and label at all. Fred Klein pointed out the limitations of using behavior as the sole variable for labeling. Common sense dictates that *what we do* is only a part of *who we are* and what identity we have. Klein proposed that orientation be assessed on seven factors (Klein, 1978; Klein, Sepekoff, & Wolf, 1985):

1. *Sexual attraction:* To whom do we find ourselves attracted? Who turns us on? Do we respond only to women? Only to men? To both?
2. *Sexual behavior:* When you've engaged in sexual behavior, who have been your partners?
3. *Sexual fantasies:* When you fantasize or masturbate, what sex/gender is your partner?
4. *Emotional or affectional preference:* To whom do you connect on an emotional level? With whom do you "fall in love"?
5. *Social preference:* With whom do you prefer to socialize? With whom do you "go out"?
6. *Lifestyle:* In your community, with whom do you spend most of your time? Are your friends primarily lesbian or gay? Bisexual? Heterosexual?
7. *Self-identification:* How do *you* label yourself? Where do you place yourself on the Kinsey grid?

Awareness of attraction to the same sex often occurs before children reach the age of 10. This sexual attraction may be the earliest and strongest predictor of a person's sexual orientation (Kliegman, 2011). This reality lead The American Academy of Pediatrics to describe the four stages of identity formation for gays and lesbians (Ryan & Futterman, 2001). First, there is "Sensitization," where a feeling of being different is experienced by prepubertal children and adolescents. The second stage, "Sexual Identity Confusion," is marked by a self-awareness of same-gender attraction yet confusion reconciling oneself with what are negative societal stereotypes. The third stage, "Sexual Identity Assumption," is the process of acknowledgment and social and sexual exploration of one's identity. Delving into the gay and lesbian community is more common in late adolescence. Finally, the fourth stage, "Integration and Commitment," represents the individual's ability to incorporate being gay or lesbian into positive self-acceptance, and sharing that part of oneself with others. This stage, if and when reached, typically occurs in adulthood. However, in the face of society's lack of acceptance of gays, some gay people marry and have children before finally admitting to themselves that they are gay. This can take a tremendous toll not only on the gay person, but on the spouse and especially the children. With greater societal acceptance of all orientations, each person would be free to explore and accept his or her orientation early in life. Since this orientation is established early in life, it seems a great loss for so many to struggle even into late adulthood to accept this essential aspect of personhood.

It seems safe to say that society at large presumes people are heterosexual until proven otherwise. And then, if someone's gay or lesbian orientation becomes known, it is not unusual to hear someone remark, "Oh, I didn't know that person was gay." At one time in history, gays and lesbians were called "the invisible minority." The 1969 Stonewall Uprising in New York City, during which a police raid of a gay bar was met with resistance, has been credited as the event that began the gay and lesbian rights movement. That movement has led to more individuals feeling free to be open about

case study 4.3

Marcus's Story

Marcus, 32, identifies as African American.

Growing up the son of a professional football player, I was pretty sure that being attracted to other guys wasn't something I was ever going to talk about to anyone. For as long as I could remember, there was something there that I couldn't define. When I was a kid, there were no gay characters on sitcoms—no Ellen DeGeneres coming out on television. No show like Will and Grace, no Queer Eye for the Straight Guy. No one ever said that being attracted to guys was an OK thing for a guy. The only talking I ever heard about homosexuality was the constant tossing around of the word fag that was just used as a general, all-purpose term for anyone you were mad at. My older brother used to call me a fag all the time, not because I was unlike other guys in any way—that whole sissy-boy thing is pretty much a myth—but because he was my older brother and that's what older brothers do—torment their younger brothers.

Going off to college, I admitted to myself that I was gay and that I would always be attracted to men. But, as a second-semester freshman, I swore that I would never act on it. I wouldn't think about guys. I wouldn't fantasize about guys. I wouldn't date guys. I would search out the perfect best friend, and the two of us would embark on a completely chaste relationship that would be mutually satisfying. Of course, no such guy existed, and several attempts to pin my flagging hopes on various friends of mine ended up in disaster. I had told myself that I would never do anything for which I would be ashamed.

After almost a full year of repressing all feelings of attraction for anyone, I came to realize that perhaps I could be happy and sexually active, and not end up living alone for the rest of my life. My feelings of self-hatred and shame, however, had run far too deep, and I started having anxiety attacks.

Over the next two and a half years, I saw a therapist whose office was about a block off campus.

I went not because I was sick but because I wanted to feel better about myself. Over those two and a half years, I talked to the therapist about how I felt and who I was.

Coming out is a long and hard process for many people, and my story is probably not all that unusual. Many of us still hear and see messages of hatred and spend some time hating ourselves. I'd hope that the positive images seen these days and supportive statements from various celebrities, magazines, books, and movies might make it much easier for gay people who are younger than I am. Some friends—whom I thought would never understand or accept me—have. Now, instead of admitting that I'm gay—as if it were something to be ashamed of—I can say with comfort and confidence that I'm a gay man. And when people get to know me, they'll learn other things about me as well.

Critical Thinking

Do you think that the images presented in the media today make it easier for students to be open about their sexual orientation? Can you think of any changes you could make in what you say and do that would help gays feel more accepted?

sex in society 4.2

Dealing with the Categories

Audre Lorde, a feminist writer, highlighted our culture's need to categorize and stigmatize individuals around issues of race, sex, class, and sexual orientation. "As a fortynine-year-old Black lesbian feminist socialist mother of two, including one boy, and a member of an interracial couple, I usually find myself a part of some group defined as other, deviant, inferior, or just plain wrong" (Lorde, 2001, p. 588). She speaks to the constant drain of energy it takes to respond to a world that oppresses individuals for a variety of qualities—sex, race, social class, ethnicity, and sexual orientation—and challenges the culture to redefine the way it deals with difference.

For sexual health, it is necessary to realize that issues of race and ethnicity cannot be separated from the ways the individual functions in his or her community. The Families of Color Network is a coalition of Asian–Pacific Islanders, Latinos, African Americans, Arab Americans, Native Americans, Caucasians, and biracial individuals who come together as an activist and advocacy group around LGBT issues.

Nila Marrone (2001), in an article for *The SIECUS Report,* identifies issues in the Latino culture, for example, that make dealing with LGBT concerns more difficult:

- Very strong family ties are more common and all family problems must be solved internally by its members.
- The family name and image must be protected.
- Traditions are highly valued, and change is generally not welcome.
- Respect for elders is highly prized.
- There is no tradition for forming or joining support groups.
- Privacy is highly prized.
- Limited economic resources are a serious obstacle to joining civic or support groups.
- Most Latinos are Catholic.

Other racial and cultural groups may share some of these values and characteristics, adding others that are unique to them. Overall, the LGBT community must address its diversity on race, class, ethnicity, religion, politics, and other issues as it works to build the connections stemming from sexuality.

Source: Adapted from N. Marron (April/May 2001), "Advice to Latino Parents of GLBT Children," *SIECUS Report,* 29 (4).

their sexual orientation, although many still report that to "come out" would leave them vulnerable to harassment, violence, and loss of jobs, housing, friendships, and family members. Some states (such as Maryland and New Jersey) have included sexual orientation, along with race, creed, gender, ethnicity, military and veteran's status, and disability, as a basis for which one's civil rights must be protected. In states that do not offer this protection, one can be fired from a job, not allowed to rent an apartment, nor adopt children. The United States military has historically dismissed any soldier who admitted to being gay. However, one of the signs of change in attitudes toward homosexuality is the 2012 decision by the US military to allow openly gay soldiers to serve. The US military joins the Israeli, Canadian and British military in a policy of acceptance and support for homosexual soldiers.

How Many?

The subject of sexual orientation has often led to a need to document "how many." How many people are heterosexual? How many are lesbian and gay? How many are bisexual? As researchers attempt to count, a number of problems arise. What criterion will be used? How easily assessed is a sample, and can it be determined to be generalizable to the population at large?

Kinsey reported that 37 percent of males and 13 percent of females had engaged in adult same-sex behavior to the point of orgasm. He estimated that 2 percent of males and 1 percent of females could be categorized as Kinsey 6's (Kinsey et al., 1948, 1953). A limitation of Kinsey's work, particularly as it pertains to the Heterosexual-Homosexual Rating Scale, is that behavior is emphasized without attending to the other factors that Klein identified.

When the National Health and Social Life Survey (NHSLS) results were reported (Laumann, Gagnon, Michael, & Michaels, 1994), the researchers addressed the difficulty they, or others, have in "counting" homosexuals. A primary problem lies with the definition of *homosexual*. They point out that people change their behavior during their lifetime, that patterns of sexual desire and identification vary, and that, because of oppression, it can be difficult to get respondents both to identify themselves and honestly respond to questions. What they were able to determine was that those who admit to having a same sex attraction (8%) were significantly higher than those who identify as gay, lesbian or bisexual (2%) and those who engage in same sex behavior (7%) (Michael, Gagnon, Laumann, & Kolata, 1994). In comparison, in a different study of college students, 12 % of women and 10% of men admitted to having same sex attraction (Lippa, 2000). As you can see, these research problems and differences make it difficult to paint a definitive picture of homosexuality in the United States.

The NHSLS examined issues of attraction by asking respondents, "In general, are you sexually attracted to . . . only women, mostly women, both men and women, mostly men, only men?" Appeal was measured by "How would you rate this activity: having sex with someone of the same sex . . . very appealing, somewhat appealing, not appealing, not at all appealing?" For self-identification, they asked, "Do you think of yourself as heterosexual, homosexual, bisexual, something else?"

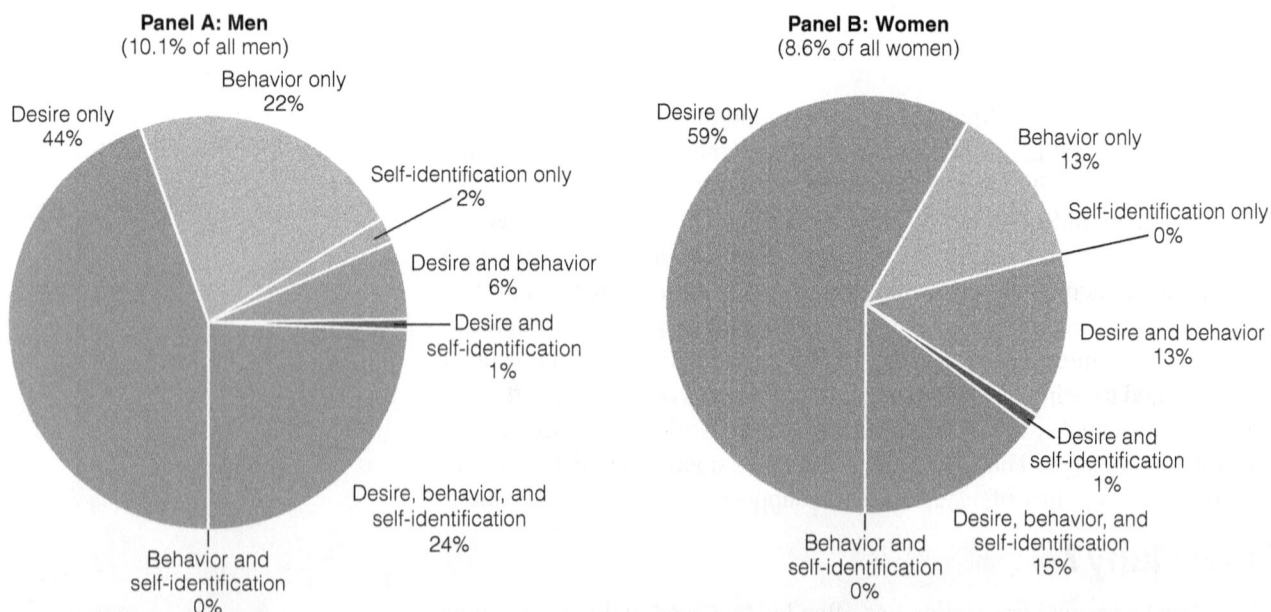

Figure 4.6 *Interrelationship of Three Aspects of Same-Gender Sexuality: Desire, Behavior, and Self*

From *Sex in America* by John Gagnon. Copyright © 1994 by CSG Enterprises, Inc., Edward O. Laumann, Robert T. Michael, and Gina Kolata. By permission of Little, Brown & Company.

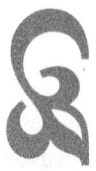

healthy sex hints 4.1

Advice on Coming Out

The decision to be open about one's homosexuality is a personal one, one that heterosexuals don't have to confront. It is almost as if lesbian and gay individuals have to explain to the world that they are not heterosexual, rather than "the world" having considered that possibility.

The risks a person takes for being open about sexual orientation depend on a variety of factors including age, geography, employment, and financial solvency, among others. Although civil rights protections are gradually being extended to people at the local and state levels, no constitutional amendment guarantees civil rights protection regardless of sexual orientation.

The following guidelines are adapted from the brochure *Be Yourself* * (Sauerman, 1998):

1. *Are you sure about your sexual orientation?* Don't raise the issue unless you're able to respond with confidence to the question "Are you sure?" Confusion on your part will increase your parents' confusion and decrease their confidence in your judgment.

2. *Are you comfortable with your gay sexuality?* If you're wrestling with guilt and periods of depression, you'll be better off waiting to tell your parents. Coming out to them may require tremendous energy on your part; it will require a reserve of positive self-image.

3. *Do you have support?* In the event your parents' reaction devastates you, there should be someone or a group that you can confidently turn to for emotional support and strength. Maintaining your sense of selfworth is critical.

4. *Are you knowledgeable about homosexuality?* Your parents will probably respond based on a lifetime of information from a homophobic society. If you've done some serious reading on the subject, you'll be able to assist them by sharing reliable information and research.

5. *What's the emotional climate at home?* If you have the choice of when to tell, consider the timing. Choose a time when they're not dealing with such matters as the death of a close friend, pending surgery, or the loss of a job.

6. *Can you be patient?* Your parents will require time to deal with this information if they haven't considered it prior to your sharing. The process may last from six months to two years.

7. *What's your motive for coming out now?* Hopefully, it is because you love them and are uncomfortable with the distance you feel. Never come out in anger or during an argument, using your sexuality as a weapon.

8. *Do you have available resources?* Homosexuality is a subject most non-gay people know little about. Have available at least one of the following: a book addressed to parents, a contact for the local or national Parents and Friends of Lesbians and Gays, the name of a non-gay counselor who can deal fairly with the issue.

9. *Are you financially dependent on your parents?* If you suspect they are capable of withdrawing college finances or forcing you out of the house, you may choose to wait until they do not have this weapon to hold over you.

10. *What is your general relationship with your parents?* If you've gotten along well and have always known their love—and shared your love for them in return—chances are they'll be able to deal with the issue in a positive way.

11. *What is their moral societal view?* If they tend to see social issues in clear terms of good/bad or holy/sinful, you may anticipate that they will have serious problems dealing with your sexuality. If, however, they've evidenced a degree of flexibility when dealing with other changing societal matters, you may be able to anticipate a willingness to work this through with you.

12. *Is this your decision?* Not everyone should come out to their parents. Don't be pressured into it if you're not sure you'll be better off by doing so—no matter what their response.

Be Yourself highlights the process that most parents go through when told that their child is gay. The stages include shock, denial, guilt, expression of feelings, personal decision-making, and true acceptance. It highlights that each family is unique, and offers suggestions of resources and support.

Source: *Read This Before Coming Out to Your Parents* by T. H. Sauerman, PFLAG Philadelphia, 1998. For ordering information: PFLAG Philadelphia, P.O. Box 176, Titusville, NJ 08560-0176; vrb@pupgg.princeton.edu.

The NHSLS researchers have claimed that their research represented a scientifically accurate survey of sex in the United States, representing nearly all adult U.S. men and women (Michael et al., 1994). Although the researchers are not above criticism, they were able to interview and survey a wider range of people than other studies to date. For what it's worth "toward the count," they found that more people find others of the same gender sexually attractive than have homosexual sex.

Approximately 5.5 percent of women found the idea of having sex with another woman very appealing or appealing, with 4 percent reporting that they were sexually attracted to women. Less than 2 percent had had sex with a woman during the past year, yet slightly more than 4 percent reported having sex with a woman at some time in their lives.

About 6 percent of the men in the NHSLS study reported being attracted to other men, with 2 percent saying they had had sex with a man in the past year. By comparison to females, 9 percent reported having had sex with a man at least once since puberty. When respondents were asked to label themselves, only 1.4 percent of women thought of themselves as homosexual or bisexual, and 2.8 percent of men identified themselves as homosexual or bisexual.

❧   Social and Environmental/Occupational Wellness   ❧

Social health depends on making connections with others. We learn to do that by first making connections with our families, and then making friends and expanding our social groups. Once children interact in schools, turn on a television set, or take a trip to a shopping mall, they become exposed to the various ways that males and females appear and act. Comments of approval and disapproval shape our behaviors; they also can be the basis for whether we feel good or bad about ourselves.

The process to a clear and comfortable sexual identity is not always easy. For those who are gay, lesbian, bisexual, or transgendered, relationships with others may add risk in a way that heterosexuals don't experience: being thrown out of one's home, losing a job, or losing friends. Although people do not segregate themselves socially based on sexuality, at times the ability to join a community of others like you becomes critical to one's health. That community may be on the Internet, at a conference or gathering, in a therapeutic support group, and in the home. Urban areas offer more social opportunities than small towns regarding sexual identity, with such cities as New York City and San Francisco, in particular, being known for their tolerance.

On an individual basis, we all must find a place to call home—a place that feels safe and secure and where we can be ourselves. The homes we grew up in may or may not have been places like this. Health and positive growth require that children be loved and nurtured and allowed to develop in their own unique way.

Some children live in environments that are threatening to their sexual development. Taunts and abuse from schoolmates, threats of, and real, violence from strangers, and, for some, self-abuse and suicide can result from identity issues. No longer should a child who is transgendered be mistaken as schizophrenic. No longer should a child be institutionalized in a mental hospital where shock treatments or other forms of aversive therapy are used to change sexual orientation.

The medical community is better informed—though not necessarily better prepared—to deal with these issues. Laws at the federal, state, and local levels have been slow to protect the civil rights of gay, lesbian, and transgendered individuals.

Creating environments where people can be who they are helps reduce the power of sexual difference and allows society to be enriched with citizens who can safely develop to their full potential. People learn that sexual identity is only one piece of a person's being and that a person can form working relationships and even friendships that allow for differences. Tolerant, respectful, and safe environments improve the opportunities for everyone.

Atypical Paths of Development

As the influences affecting sexual identity come into play, the question persists as to whether one is developing "normally." Regardless of one's definition of *normal,* what, if anything, is to be "done" when development varies? After birth, questions such as "Is the child happy with him- or herself?" "and "Are the parents happy with the child?" may be secondary to concerns expressed from family, physicians, and other outside observers.

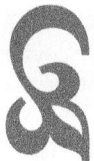

healthy sex hints 4.2

Support in Faith Communities

Spiritual health needs get met in many ways, and having a sense of community is one of them. One of the challenges of considering yourself "religious" and part of the LGBT community is to be able to reconcile religious teachings with your lifestyle. The Internet has enabled groups within various religious communities to provide support and resources. Here is a sample of sites organized by Lambda Families (E. Schroeder, personal communication, September 3, 2002):

Source: Activism to Stop Spiritual Violence: **www.soulforce.org**

Baptist: Association of Welcoming and Affirming Baptists: **www.wabaptists.org**

Catholic: Dignity: **www.dignityusa.org**

Episcopalian: Integrity: **www.integrityusa.org**

Evangelical: Evangelicals Concerned: **www.ecinc.org**

Jewish: The World Congress of GLBT Jews: **www.glbtjews.org**

Lutheran: Lutherans Concerned: **www.lcna.org**

Methodist: Reconciling Ministries Network: **www.rmnetwork.org**

Metropolitan Community Churches: **www.ufmcc.com**

Mormon: Affirmation: **www.affirmation.org**

Presbyterian: More Light: **www.mlp.org**

Quaker: Friends for Lesbian, Gay, Bisexual, Transgender, and Queer Concerns: **www.quaker.org/flgbtqc**

Seventh-Day Adventists: Kinship International: **www.sdakinship.org**

Unitarian Universalist: Interweave: **www.interweave.uua.org**

United Church of Christ: Coalition for LGBT Concerns: **www.ucccoalition.org**

Table 4.1 Atypical Chromosomal and Hormonal Patterns in Prenatal Development

Syndrome	Chromosomal Sex	Gonad	Internal Reproductive	External Reproductive	Secondary Sex Characteristics	Gender Identity
Klinefelter syndrome	Male, XXY	Testes	Normal male	Small penis and testes	Female secondary sex characteristics develop at puberty	Male
Turner syndrome	Female, XO	Nonfunctioning or absent ovaries	Normal female except for ovaries	Underdeveloped genitals	No breast development or menstruation at puberty	Female
Androgen insensitivity syndrome	Male, XY	Testes, but body unable to utilize testosterone	Shallow vagina, lacking normal male structures	Labia	Female secondary sex characteristics develop at puberty; no menstruation	Female
Congenital adrenal hyperplasia	Female, XX	Ovaries	Normal female	Ambiguous, tending toward male appearance; enlarged clitoris may be mistaken for penis	Female secondary sex characteristics develop at puberty	Usually male
DHT deficiency	Male, XY	Undescended testes	Partially formed, but no prostate	Ambiguous until puberty when penis enlarges and testes descend	Male secondary sex characteristics develop at puberty	Female until puberty when male identity taken

Every year children are born who are not genetically, anatomically, or hormonally consistent with one sex or the other. Some situations are immediately apparent, as in ambiguous external genitalia. In other situations the chromosomal makeup may be abnormal, yet the impact of the genetic mosaic may not be obvious until childhood or adolescence. Table 4.1 charts the more common of variations.

U.S. culture traditionally has looked at atypical patterns as problems, and the medical community has become involved where possible to "fix" the child. The terms used to describe ambiguities are clinical. *Pseudohermaphrodism* describes the conditions in which the child is genetically one sex, with mixed external and internal structures. Genetic females whose genitals are masculinized because of an accumulation of androgens from the adrenal glands are referred to as having *congenital adrenal hyperplasia* (CAH), also called *adrenogenital syndrome*. A condition with parallel outcomes—*androgen insensitivity syndrome*—is found in a genetic male whose body does not respond to the testosterone it produces, leading to female external genitalia. Adult individuals with these conditions have recently become more visible and political. They are asking to be referred to as intersexuals and demanding their civil rights.

The Intersex Society of North America (ISNA) is a support, education, and advocacy group founded by and for individuals who are intersexual. The organization opposes the predominant model of treatment that recommends emergency sex reassignment for infants, followed by hormonal treatments and gender role learning that reinforces that assignment. As a result of sharing their experiences, the intersexuals involved with ISNA (1995) claim that these early interventions, considered a form of genital mutilation, have impaired them in many ways.

The ISNA (2013) has recommended a new model of treatment that avoids harmful or unnecessary surgery, requires family therapy by well-trained mental health professionals, and asks that intersexual individuals be empowered to decide on treatment after fully understanding their status. For the overall health of the individual, the organization argues against genital surgery that is primarily rooted in cosmetic concerns.

Other atypical patterns of development that fall along the gender identity continuum may not receive attention or any intervention until the child is older. Broad questions remain as to how strongly a child must identify with gender appropriate appearance and roles and, indeed, what the list of "appropriateness" contains. **Gender variance** and **gender role** non conformity in children can make some adults uncomfortable. Gender variance in childhood describes behaviors that do not conform to the expected behaviors for that child's sex in the culture in which he or she lives. A young boy who wears skirts because his beloved sister wears them and a little girl who will only play with guns and trucks are examples of gender variance or gender non conformity. Gender variance reflecting the exploration of gender identity and gender role is part of normal development. These behaviors may or may not continue after childhood and into adulthood (Kleigman, 2011).

Gender variant gender identity or role that varies from what is typical for the person's biological sex

Gender role a person's role in society typically a male or female

Children with transgender or gender variant identity differ not just in behaviors but in their core gender identity. The transgendered group includes a diverse population that does not fit into the culturally defined description of gender. Transsexuals and cross dressers are some of those included in the transgender category. There are two major sources of stress for the transgendered person. One stressor is the confusion and discomfort with the difference in the sex assigned at birth and gender identity. This discomfort is often referred to as gender dysphoria. The other source of distress is the feeling of not fitting in, of being different than expected by society and not accepted by friends and family (Kleigman, 2011).

Children with transgender or gender variant identity exhibit some characteristic behaviors. Boys prefer typical girl toys such as dolls and enjoy playing house. They avoid rough play and prefer to dress like girls. These boys may wish they were a girl or wish to grow up to be a woman. Girls with gender variant identity avoid the traditional girl activities and seek tomboy play and boys as friends. They may dress as a boy, may refuse to urinate sitting down, and believe they will grow a penis. Only a minority of children's identity concerns last into adulthood (Zieman, 2005, Kleigman, 2011). However, these gender-atypical young children are more likely to end up homosexual than gender typical children. Only a minority of these gender atypical children develop a transgendered identity (Dreger, 2009, Kleigman, 2011).

Transgendered The person's appearance and behavior do not conform to society's expectations for that sex. This is an umbrella term and includes transsexuals, transvestites, and intersexed.

The essence of being **transgendered** is that one's gender identity falls somewhere away from the extremes of masculine or feminine. A person may desire to dress as the other sex does, move as the "other" sex does, and be treated as though one were a member of the other sex. As a support for these individuals, The Society for the Second Self, referred to as Tri-Ess, was founded. It is a chapter-based organization with members across the United States who produces a quarterly journal filled with essays, information, and resources. The group focuses on providing support, serenity, and service (SSS) to the heterosexual cross-dresser and his/her family (Boyd, 2002).

Increasingly, college students are "coming out," so to speak, as transgendered, with campus organizations addressing LGBT issues or LGBTQIA issues. The Q sometimes stands for questioning or queer, I for intersexed, and A for ally. More openness and recognition of LGBT issues has inspired some colleges and universities to recognize gender-non conforming students by allowing transgendered students to room with their preferred gender; Going a step further, the University of Iowa has added a transgender box to the college application (Schulman, 2013).

Gender dysphoria discontent with ones biological sex or gender role

As previously discussed, the transgender group includes transsexual, those who feel their biological sex does not match who they really are as a person. Transsexuals often have **gender dysphoria** and desire sex reassignment surgery. Sex reassignment surgery, along with the array of psychiatric, hormonal, and subsequent cosmetic surgeries, represents a long and painful process. Transsexuals first must be thoroughly evaluated to ensure that gender dysphoria is the correct diagnosis. Cross-dressing is encouraged, followed by hormonal interventions to feminize male-to-female transsexuals or, conversely, masculinize female-to-male transsexuals. Changes in body hair, changes in the face, and fat deposits all move these individuals in their desired direction. These interventions are reversible if necessary and, for some, represent the extent of treatment that is both comfortable and affordable.

Surgical interventions are more complicated. The male-to-female transsexual will have the testicles and penis removed, and the skin of the penis is used to construct a vagina that can respond to sexual stimulation.

Transsexuals Members of the transgendered community who feel trapped in the body of the wrong sex and desire to have or have had a sex change

A female-to-male **transsexual** will have a complete hysterectomy and a double mastectomy and will have a penis constructed. Because the clitoris is small and behind the penis, it can be left to improve sexual response.

Transgendered communities share a variety of concerns with their gay, lesbian and bisexual peers. Issues such as coming out, violence, self-esteem, discrimination and access to health care are similar in these groups. (Maurer, 1999; Wolraich, 2007). At the same time, there are unique concerns, such as what physician to use to get comprehensive health care, perhaps hormone treatments and even sex reassignment surgery. The World Association for Transgender Health works to bring together professionals to promote health, research, education, respect, dignity and equality for transgender, transsexuals and gender variant people. This group provides a free, online data base to help patients find health care providers that promote and meet these criteria (WPATH, 2013).

Transgendered activists and those who work with transgendered clients claim that the emotional, social, and occupational stress that interferes with daily functioning is not due to the person's gender identification but is caused by society's reaction to it (Carroll, Gilroy, & Ryan, 2002; Klein, 2002; Isay, 1997). Perhaps if our society did not have such rigid expectations of how each sex must act and feel, we would have little need for the classifications we have been discussing.

The personal adjustments required of those in the LGBT are many. Some have lost friends, family, and jobs as they attempt to find personal happiness.

☙ *Emotional Wellness* ☙

The cornerstone of emotional well-being is positive sexual self-esteem. Feeling good about ourselves and accepting who we are is vital to health. What is unique about emotional health is that it derives from the other dimensions of health. Feeling good about yourself may result from others liking you, or feeling good about yourself may depend on your liking your body, or a combination of these.

All of us need to have realistic expectations about who we are. As the lyrics from "I Am Who I Am" highlight, though, "Life is not worth a damn until you can shout 'I am who I am.'" In essence, we all need to accept ourselves.

The road to positive self-acceptance is longer for some than others. If you cannot be open about who you are, secrecy and oppression take their toll. Support groups and mental health professionals trained in the area of sexuality can be extremely helpful to those who are struggling with identity issues, seeking acceptance of their orientation, and figuring out how to negotiate environments that prove to be hostile. The use of resources available in books, journals, and online can greatly add to positive sexual self esteem (Sexuality Information and Education Council of the U.S. [SIECUS], 2001).

Because our emotional health is also connected to others' behavior, we must focus attention on the need to reduce the hostility and discrimination faced by those who are perceived as "different." Improving the mental health of others and their ability to accept differences are critical factors in reducing oppression and permitting variations in lifestyle to coexist.

Personal Assessment

Messages About Gender

Our present thoughts and feelings concerning what being a man or a woman means have evolved over the years. A myriad of people and sources have contributed to our development. The purpose of this assessment is to trace the origin of many of the assumptions we all have about gender by examining the messages we received as children.

1. Describe in writing one specific message you received about expected male/female behavior during the following phases in your life that are applicable:
   a. Preschool
   b. Elementary school
   c. Junior high/middle school
   d. High school
   e. College
   f. Young adult (20s)
   g. Adulthood (30s–40s)
   h. Older adulthood

2. Describe the source of the message (parents, family, friends, and so forth) and the context (where/when it was delivered).

3. Describe the immediate impact of the message on your gender identity/role.

4. Describe the long-term impact of the message.

Thought Questions

1. How do biological identity, gender identity, and sexual orientation relate in the overall model of sexual identity?

2. How do biological and psychological factors interact to influence gender development?

3. What are some of the issues related to the process of "coming out" for lesbian, gay, and bisexual people?

4. Describe the various patterns of development and their impact on the identity of the individual.

Test Yourself!

1. Which term refers to one's psychological sense of being male or female?
   a. Gender role
   b. Sexual identity
   c. Gender identity
   d. Sexual preference

2. All but which are examples of sexual orientation?
   a. Transgendered
   b. Heterosexual
   c. Gay
   d. Lesbian

3. Which of the following body parts are considered *homologous* structures?
   a. Penis/vagina
   b. Uterus/prostate
   c. Clitoris/penis
   d. Testicles/uterus

4. Of the various aspects of sexual identity formation, which comes first?
   a. Chromosomal gender
   b. Gender role
   c. Secondary sex characteristics
   d. Sexual orientation

5. Adolescents are most likely to confront all but which aspect of sexual identity formation?
   a. Secondary sex characteristics
   b. Sexual orientation
   c. Gender role
   d. Gonadal development
6. Kinsey developed a continuum related to sexual identity that
   a. examines how adults valued their sexual behavior.
   b. categorizes how adults organized their sexual fantasies.
   c. categorizes how adults engaged in same-sex and opposite-sex behaviors.
   d. examined how adults identified themselves.
7. Before a young adult decides to "come out," it is recommended that he or she do all but which of the following?
   a. Join a college LGBT club.
   b. Be comfortable with labeling sexual orientation.
   c. Be sure there are financial and emotional supports in place.
   d. Assess the emotional climate in his or her home.
8. New research on the treatment of intersexed children recommends
   a. immediate postpartum surgery to create normal genitalia.
   b. delayed or no surgical intervention until adolescence or later.
   c. having young children switch gender roles to understand their situation.
   d. hormonal treatments to correct all imbalances.
9. Theories on the development of sexual orientation
   a. point to biological determinants as key.
   b. identify social determinants as key.
   c. identify parental dynamics as key.
   d. do not concur nor fully explain the development of orientation.
10. Body image issues for adolescents
   a. have developed primarily around weight issues.
   b. are more common among boys than girls.
   c. have been connected to a variety of unhealthy practices and interventions among teens.
   d. have little impact on emotional and social health.

Media Menu

Recommended Movies

Milk—Sean Penn won an academy award for his portrayal of Harvey Milk, a gay activist and politician. The movie does a great job of showing society's treatment of gays.

TransAmerica—Portrays a transsexual and the journey to sex reassignment surgery. It is funny and authentic.

Brokeback Mountain—A love story between gay men showing the difficulty faced by gays.

Journal article

Knight, J. L., & Giuliano, T. A. (2003, September). Blood, sweat, and jeers: The impact of the media's heterosexist portrayals on perceptions of male and female athletes. *Journal of Sport Behavior,* 26 (3), 272.

Web Resources

The World Professional Association for Transgender Health
http:/wpath.org/

The organizational goal is to promote evidence based care, education, advocacy, public policy and respect in transgender health. This group provides a free, online data base to help patients find health care providers that promote and meet these criteria.

Intersex Society of North America (ISNA)
www.isna.org

A peer support, education, and advocacy group established for intersexuals, individuals born with anatomy or physiology different from cultural ideals of male and female.

Available at this site are facts and commonly asked questions, as well as the capacity to ask your own questions as well, a library to order books on the subject of transgender, and current information on a variety of health issues.

Kinsey Institute for Research in Sex, Gender, and Reproduction
www.kinseyinstitute.org

Supports interdisciplinary research, scholarship, and study in the field of human sexuality, gender, and reproduction.

The site lists professional organizations, articles, reference resources, and a new link to Kinsey Institute Sexuality Research Information Service.

National Gay and Lesbian Task Force (NGLTF)
www.thetaskforce.org

A well-established national organization that advocates for gay and lesbian issues, along with providing information and support.

Parents, Families, and Friends of Lesbians and Gays (PFLAG)
www.pflag.org

A national, nonprofit organization supporting parents, families, and friends of lesbians and gays. The site provides resources, literature to assist in coping and to educate society to work to end discrimination and secure equal civil rights.

Renaissance Transgender Association
www.ren.org

Provides comprehensive education and support to transgendered persons and those close to them. The association offers programs and resources for cross dressers, transvestites, and transsexuals. The site offers articles from the International Congress on Sex and Gender.

National Association of Lesbian, Gay, Bisexual, and Transgender Community Centers (NALGBTCC)
www.lgbtcenters.org

Coordinates information on community centers across the United States that serve the LGBT community.

References

Bailey, J. & Benishay, D. (1993). Familial aggregation of female sexual orientation. American Journal of Psychiatry, 150, 272–277.

Bailey, J. M., & Pillard, C. (1991). A genetic study of male sexual orientation. *Archives of General Psychiatry, 48,* 1089–1096.

Bailey, J. M., Pillard, C., Neal, M. C., & Agyei, Y. (1993). Heritable factors influence sexual orientation in women. *Archives of General Psychiatry, 50,* 217–223.

Banks, A., & Gartrell, N. K. (1995). Hormones and "sexual orientation": A questionable link. *Journal of Homosexuality, 28,* 247–268.

Barlett, N. H., Vasey, P., & Bukowski, W. (2000, December). Is gender identity disorder in children a mental disorder? *Sex Roles: A Journal of Research.*

Bem, S. (1993). *The lenses of gender: Transforming the debate on sexual inequality.* New Haven, CT: Yale University Press.

Bem, S. (1995, April). *Dismantling gender polarization: Shall we turn the volume down or shall we turn the volume up?* Keynote address, 1995 Eastern Region Annual Conference, Society for the Scientific Study of Sexuality, West Atlantic City, NJ.

Bockting, W. O. (1999, October/November). From construction to context: Gender through the eyes of the transgendered. *SIECUS Report,* 28 (1), 3–7.

Boyd, R. (2002, Fall). What do you say to a college class? *The Mirror,* 27(3), 54–56.

Brody, L. (1997, Summer). Gender and emotion: Beyond stereotypes. *Journal of Social Issues,* 53 (2), 369.

Colapinto, J. (2000). *As nature made him: The boy who was raised as a girl.* New York: HarperCollins.

Coleman, E., Gooren, L., & Ross, M. (1989). Theories of gender transpositions: A critique and suggestions for further research. *Journal of Sex Research,* 26 (4), 525–538.

Diamond, M. (1982). Sexual identity, monozygotic twins reared in discordant sex roles and a BBC follow up. *Archives of Sexual Behavior,* 11 (2), 181–186.

Diamond, D., & Sigmundson, H. K. (1997, March). Sex reassignment at birth: Long-term review and clinical implications. *Archives of Pediatrics and Adolescent Medicine,* 51, 298–304.

Diamond, M., Sigmundson, H. K., & Reimer, D. (2002, November 9). *Sexual and gender identities: The significance of the John/Joan case.* Paper presented at the annual meeting of the Society for the Scientific Study of Sexuality, Montreal.

Ellis, L., & Ames, M. A. (1987). Neurohormonal function and sexual orientation: A theory of homosexuality-heterosexuality. *Psychological Bulletin,* 101, 233–258.

Ellis, L., Ames, M. A., Peckham, W., & Burke, D. (1988). Sexual orientation of human offspring may be altered by severe maternal stress during pregnancy. *Journal of Sex Research,* 25, 152–157.

Hines, M., & Collaer, M. L. (1993). Gonadal hormones and sex differences. *Annual Review of Sex Research,* 4, 1–48.

Intersex Society of North America. (2013). *Recommendations for treatment: Intersex infants and children.* San Francisco: Author.

Jenkins, W., (2010) Can anyone tell me why I'm gay? What research suggest regarding the orgins of sexual orientation. *North American Journal of Psychology,* vol. 12, No 2, 279–296.

Johnson, R., (2008). Hate crime statistics motivated by sexual orientation bias. Retrieved from http://gaylife.about.com/od/hatecrimes/a/statistics.htm

Kinsey, A., Pomeroy, W., & Martin, C. (1948). *Sexual behavior in the human female.* Philadelphia: Saunders.

Kinsey, A., Pomeroy, W., Martin, C., & Gebhard, P. (1953). *Sexual behavior in the human female.* Philadelphia: Saunders.

Klein, F. (1978). *The bisexual option.* New York: Arbor House.

Klein, F., Sepekoff, B., & Wolf, T. J. (1985). Sexual orientations: A multivariable dynamic process. In F. Klein & T. J.

Kliegman, R. (2011). Nelson Textbook of Pediatrics, 19th edition, Saunders Publishing.

Wolf (Eds.), *Bisexualities: Theory and research.* New York: Haworth.

Laumann, E., Gagnon, J., Michael, R., & Michaels, S. (1994). *The social organization of sexuality: Sexual practices in the United States.* Chicago: University of Chicago Press.

LeVay, S. (1991). A difference in hypothalamic structure between heterosexual and homosexual men. Science, 253, *Lippa, R.(2000). Gender-related traits in gay men, lesbian women, and heterosexual men and women: the virtual identity of homosexual-heterosexual diagnosticity and gender diagnosticity. Journal of Pers, 68, 899–926.* 1034–1037.

Lorde, A. (2001). Age, race, class, and sex: Women redefining difference. In P. S. Rothenberg (Ed.), *Race, class, and gender in the United States: An integrated study* (5th ed., pp. 588–594). New York: Freeman.

Marrone, N. (2001, April/May). Advice to Latino parents of GLBT children. *SIECUS Report, 29* (4).

Maurer, L. (1999, October/November). Transgressing sex and gender: Deconstruction zone ahead? *SIECUS Report, 28* (1).

Mead, M. (1935). *Sex and temperament in three primitive societies.* New York: Morrow.

Michael, R., Gagnon, J., Laumann, E., & Kolata, G. (1994). *Sex in America.* Boston: Little, Brown.

Money, J. (1999). *The lovemap guidebook: A definitive statement.* New York: Continuum.

Money, J., & Ehrhardt, A. (1972). *Man and woman, boy and girl.* Baltimore, MD: Johns Hopkins University Press.

Muehlenhard, C. (2000, May). Categories and sexuality. *Journal of Sex Research,* 37 (2), 101–107.

Pillard, R. & Weinrich, J. (1986). Evidence of familial nature of male homosexuality. *Journal of Psychiatry,* 43, 272–277.

Ryan, C., & Futterman, D. (2001, April/May). Social and developmental challenges for lesbian, gay, and bisexual youth. *SIECUS Report,* 29(4).

Sauerman, T. H. (1998). *Read this before coming out to your parents.* Philadelphia: PFLAG Philadelphia.

Savin-Williams, R. & Cohen, K. (2004). Homoerotic development during childhood and adolescence. Child and Adolescent Psychiatric Clinics of North America, 23, 529-549. Sexuality Information and Education Council of the U.S. (2001, April/May). Lesbian, gay, bisexual, and transgender sexuality and related issues: Annotated bibliography and website directory. *SIECUS Report Supplement, 29* (4).

Schulman, M., (2013) Generation LGBTQIA, New York Times.

The World Association for Transgender Health (2013). Available at: http:/wpath.org/

Vance, C. (1988). Anthropology rediscovers sexuality: A theoretical comment. *Social Science Medicine, 33* (8), 875–884 Wiederman, M. W. (2001). Orientation: What determines sexual attraction to men or women? In *Understanding sexual research* (pp. 74–81). Belmont, CA: Wadsworth/ Thomson Learning.

Woodhill, B. M., & Samuels, C. A., (2003, June). Positive and negative androgyny and their relationship with psychological health and well-being." *Sex Roles: A Journal of Research.*

Woodside, D., Blake, M., Woodside, D. B., Garfinkel, P. E., Kin, E., Goering, P., Kaplan, A. S., Goldbloom, D. S., & Kennedy, S. H. (2001, April). Comparisons of men with full or partial eating disorders, men without eating disorders, and women with eating disorders, in the community. *American Journal of Psychiatry,* 158, 570.

Wolraich, M., (2007). Developmental-Behavioral Pediatrics, 1st edition. Mosby Publisher.

Zieman, G., (2005). Gender Identity Disorder-Patient Handout [Online]. Avialable: www. Mdconsult.com.

chapter
five

Child *and* Adolescent Sexuality

Student Learning Objectives

After reading this chapter, students will be able to

- ❤ Compare and contrast a variety of theories of personality from birth through adolescence.
- ❤ Describe how the key aspects from various psychological theories impact sexual development.
- ❤ Discuss the effects of parenting practices such as bonding, toilet training, and nudity on healthy sexual development.
- ❤ Compare the biological consequences of puberty with the psychosocial aspects of adolescence.
- ❤ Describe the findings of a variety of studies concerning adolescent sexual behavior.
- ❤ Compare the adolescent sexual behavior of people in the United States with those from other cultures.
- ❤ Evaluate the positive and negative aspects of sexual activity during adolescence.

activity teaser: How do you decide what sexual behavior is right for you? Find out with the Personal Exploration Activity on page 150.

case study 5.1

Rebecca and Jake

Rebecca, 24, and Jake, 25, are white.

Rebecca and Jake became parents for the first time in their mid-20s. They both were so excited at the birth of Adam yet nervous at the same time about how to be good parents.

REBECCA: I grew up in a very puritanical household. My parents rarely touched or showed any kind of physical affection toward each other or my brother and me. I know they loved each other and us, but it just wasn't their way to express it physically, in public. Nudity also was not tolerated, and sex was never discussed. Being with Jake has taught me that the physical expression of affection and love is a natural and positive thing.

JAKE: I come from a very physical, touchy family. Our whole family loves to hug and kiss, and visitors rarely get in or out of the house without a big hug hello and good-bye. When Rebecca and I got together, differences in our attitudes about touch had to be worked out between us. I love being naked, and for me touch does not always mean "I want some sex." I felt it was really important that Rebecca commit to breastfeeding Adam . . . she knew the health benefits, but the reality of it all seemed to scare her a bit.

We often just sit and look at Adam, our precious little baby. We want him to grow up healthy and comfortable with his sexuality. We've been taking turns getting up to change and feed Adam. When it's Rebecca's turn, she gets up, goes into Adam's room, and nurses him while rocking in the chair in his room. When it's my turn, I bring Adam into our bed and then put him back in his crib after nursing. We both love the skin–skin contact we share with the baby and each other.

REBECCA: Despite how tired we both are, we know that this phase of being parents is only the beginning. There will be so many more challenges down the line. What we know for sure is that we will work together to help Adam navigate through the sexual challenges of childhood and the teen years.

Critical Thinking

Those who want to be really good at a sport or playing a musical instrument often take lessons, get coaching and read to develop and improve their skills. Why do so many people think they "just know" a skill as complex as parenting a child? What will you and your partner do to learn how to effectively parent? Are you willing to take classes together, work with your pediatrician, read books together? How do parents develop parenting strategies that bridge the gaps among how they each were raised, what they have learned to be healthy for their child, and what they are each comfortable with as parents?

As you sit here reading, you may want to ask yourself, "How did I get to be the sexual person that I am?" You look a particular way and have your own unique thoughts, feelings, attractions, and needs. Despite what is often a cultural desire to protect children from things sexual, the reality is that profound aspects of sexual development occur in childhood and adolescence. How you are as an adult stems from the varied influences and experiences you have had "growing up." And as we explore adult issues in Chapter 6, you may want to question when, if ever, development *stops*.

Psychosexual development is the process of becoming a sexual person. The term traditionally refers to the psychological aspects of sexual development. As we've mentioned throughout this text, though, to completely separate the psychological from the physical, intellectual, emotional, social, spiritual, and environmental facets of our sexuality is not possible.

Psychosexual development
The blending of sexual aspects of one's development with other psychological factors

134

Most discussions of psychosexual development present it as an outgrowth of personality, with great emphasis placed on the first years of life. Although the classic personality theorists remain important as a foundation, current theorists and critics have examined the interplay of biological, psychological, social, and cultural influences on the overall development of sexuality. In addition, debates continue as to what is truly "healthy" for children and teens.

Personality is the entire collection of one's thoughts, attitudes, values, beliefs, perceptions, and behaviors. Our personalities define how we see ourselves independently and within our environment. Personality is constantly evolving and is cumulative in nature. Your personality today is the sum total of all of the things you have experienced until this point in your life. Various theories have been proposed to explain how personality develops.

Personality The collection of values, attitudes, and behavior that make us who we are

Traditional Theories of Personality

Behaviorism: John Watson

Behaviorism, developed by John Watson (1970), proposes that personality develops as a result of responses to general and specific stimuli. Behaviorists believe that at birth we are blank slates with no predetermined attributes. Our personalities evolve as the result of myriad interactions between stimuli (people, places, events, situations, images) and the responses they evoke. Responses can be either positive or negative and vary in strength. The more powerful the response, the more likely we will either embrace (positive response) or reject (negative response) whatever stimulus prompted it.

Behaviorism A stimulus response theory of personality development grounded in the belief that human personality evolves as a result of the interaction between exposure to stimuli and the responses that this exposure evokes in the person. Watson is credited with the theory, expanded later by Skinner.

Let's use masturbation to explain how this stimulus-response model works. Imagine that when you were an infant, your mother caught you fondling yourself while lying on the rug in the living room in front of your grandmother. Your mother was upset and slapped your hand, saying, "Bad girl. Little ladies don't touch themselves down there." This negative reinforcement (slapping the hand away and saying "bad girl") in response to a stimulus (touching yourself) begins to shape how you feel toward masturbation. The specific context (in the living room, in a public setting, in front of Grandma) also contributes to shaping the behavior.

If this response is repeated over time, in similar and different contexts, it can either extinguish (get rid of) the behavior of masturbation or drive it underground and surround it with shame and guilt. The person then might practice the behavior in private and associate it with negative feelings.

Other personality theories stress developmental stages and tasks. These theories propose that personality develops in stages that build upon each other.

Humanism: Abraham Maslow

Abraham Maslow (1970) was one of the most influential humanists. The premise of **humanism** is that human beings are motivated by a desire for personal growth. Maslow believed that all humans are unique and are capable of growth and reaching their utmost potential in all facets of their lives. Humans are essentially good and are capable of making choices about the direction their lives will take. Maslow believed that all people are capable of reaching their highest potential if they progress through a series of stages

Humanism A theory of personality development proposing that human personality development is shaped by innate desire and need for maximizing personal growth

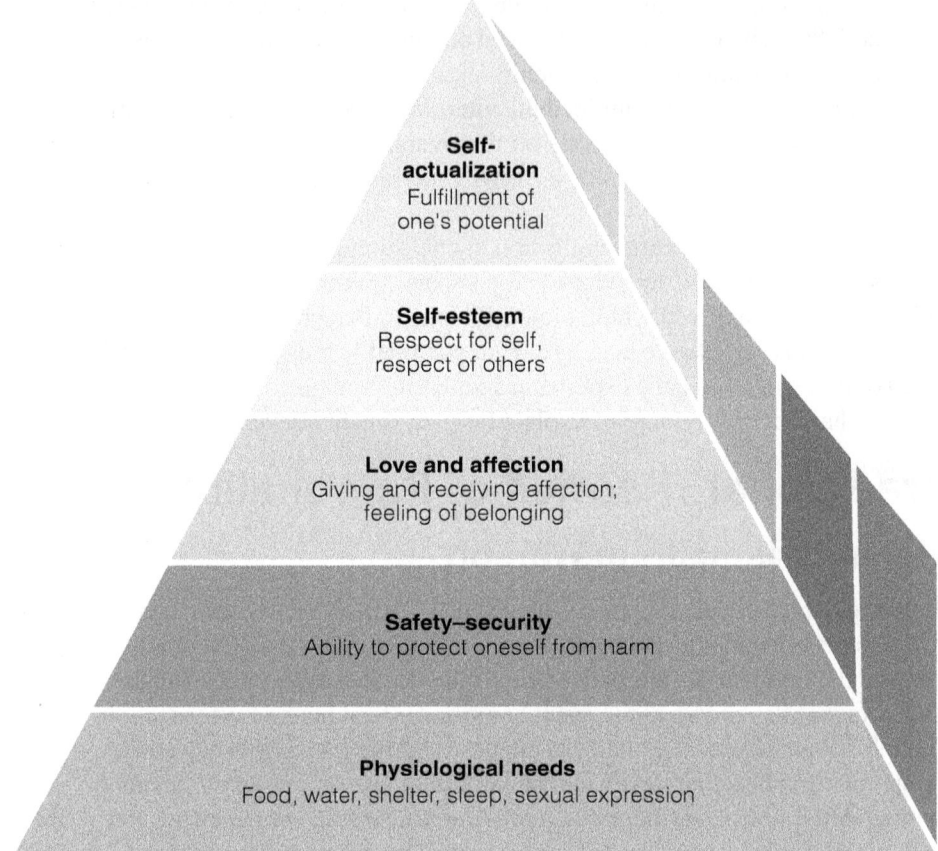

Figure 5.1 *Maslow's Hierarchy of Needs*

of development that meet various basic human needs. Figure 5.1 presents Maslow's hierarchy of needs. As you can see, they reflect the physical, social, intellectual, emotional, spiritual, and environmental domains that characterize present-day wellness theory.

Before people can develop loving, intimate relationships, they must meet their most fundamental needs for survival and safety that form the basis of the pyramid. To get to the top, one has to pass through all of the previous levels, successfully meeting the needs of each stage before proceeding to the next. The top of Maslow's pyramid, self-actualization, represents the pinnacle of human development. People reaching the top are said to be fully self-actualized.

Maslow also believed that, as we work our way up this pyramid, we often encounter "peak experiences"—moments that crystallize what it means to be fully alive, to **transcend** mere existence. He felt that these peak experiences help us feel connected to the world around us, to be one with our universe.

The following are characteristics of individuals who achieve self-actualization through transcendence:

1. Transcenders have more "peak" or creative experiences than others.
2. Transcenders are more responsive to beauty and more holistic in their perceptions of humanity and the world.

Transcend To rise above or extend beyond ordinary limits

3. Transcenders are innovators who are attracted to the unknown, embrace change, and see themselves as the instruments of their transcendence.

4. Transcenders can fuse work and play. They are less attracted by the rewards of money and more motivated by the satisfaction of being true to whom they really are and serving others.

5. Transcenders are more likely to accept others with unconditional positive regard.

Psychoanalytic Theory: Sigmund Freud

Freudian **psychoanalytic theory** purports that personality develops as a result of a struggle between conscious and unconscious forces in our lives (Hall, 1954). These forces are directed by our **ego** (the rational, thinking mind), **superego** (the conscience), and **id** (the pleasure-seeking life force). The ego is conscious and based in reality, interweaving sensory perceptions with thoughts and memories. The superego, which is partially unconscious, is judgmental; it factors in our beliefs about right and wrong.

Freud called the fuel of this life force "libidinal energy." The id does not distinguish between right and wrong, good and evil. Whatever brings pleasure is good. The superego (in concert with the ego) is supposed to keep the id in check.

Freud believed that the transference of libidinal energy has direct consequences for our psychosexual development. He outlined stages of development, each with a set of needs to be satisfied:

Oral stage. The first, or oral, stage lasts from birth to the second year of life. During the oral stage, stimulation of the mouth through sucking, biting, and swallowing is the main source of erotic satisfaction. Inadequate satisfaction during the oral stage, according to Freud, would produce an "oral personality"— someone preoccupied with mouth habits such as overeating or smoking.

Anal stage. During the second, anal phase, from ages 2 to 3, libidinal energy shifts to the anus. During this stage, the child derives pleasure from anal stimulation and being in control of defecation. This provides the child's first real opportunity to assert some independence from parental control. This stage coincides with toilet training. Freud believed it is the holding back or letting go of bowel movements (personal control) that produces physical and psychological pleasure for the child. Rushing a child through toilet training (thereby limiting the ability to derive anal pleasure) or making too big a fuss over soiling the diapers or making a mess could result in fixation at this stage. People who are fixated at this stage are either anal-expulsive (dirty, extravagant, wasteful) or anal-retentive (excessively clean, neat, cheap, and compulsive).

Phallic stage. The third phase of development is the phallic stage, between the third and fourth years. During this time, libidinal energy shifts to the genitals, and the child derives erotic pleasure through fondling and exhibitionism. Freud also believed that during this time the child develops a sexual attachment to the opposite-sex parent and becomes fearful of the parent of the same sex.

Psychoanalytic theory Also known as Freudian theory (after its founder, Sigmund Freud), describes personality development as outgrowth of interaction of id (pleasure-seeking, guilt free), superego (the conscience, influenced by society and parents), and ego (rational, analytical mind driven by logical thinking)

Ego Rational, analytical facet of human mind, according to Freudian theory

Superego The conscience, influenced by society and family, according to Freudian theory

Id Pleasure-seeking, guilt free facet of human mind, according to Freudian theory

Oedipal complex A psychoanalytical term (named after Oedipus in Shakespeare's play) that describes the internal struggle that 3- to 4-year olds face as they begin to identify more with their opposite-sex parent

Puberty Biological transition from childhood to young adulthood

Named the **Oedipal complex** (after the Greek legend in which Oedipus killed his father and married his mother), this attachment, if handled calmly and without undue concern or punishment, gradually subsides as the child moves into the next stage, latency. Psychoanalytic theorists focus on the dynamics of this phase in their attempts to explain sexual orientation.

Latency stage. Freud believed that sexuality goes into a period of latency extending from age 5 until **puberty.** At this time, the child becomes more focused on nonsexual interests such as intellectual and social issues. Modern observance of young children and preadolescents clarifies the difficulties with accepting such a concept. Sexual exploration, sex games, and, for some, mature sexual involvement makes latency an archaic idea.

Genital stage. At puberty, genital sexuality reemerges, and the adolescent becomes sexually attracted to members of the opposite sex, a prerequisite for marriage and childrearing. Freud placed marriage as the culmination of normal psychosexual development.

Freud's theory is valued more for its place in history than its current usefulness. His work brought the importance of sexuality to an understanding of personality development, yet serious questions about his methods and biases have diminished the value of his work for contemporary analysis of sexual development. From a modern perspective, Freud was sexist and heterosexist, not understanding female sexual response or the healthy development of homosexuality and bisexuality.

Eight Stages of Development: Erik Erikson

Erik Erikson (1978) constructed a model of personality development that views it as the result of a struggle between opposing forces that present themselves in a series of stages that occur throughout our lives. Figure 5.2 shows Erikson's eight stages of development. Instead of the struggle between the libidinal-driven id and the ego/superego, Erikson viewed development as a conflict between opposing psychosocial forces and qualities. According to Erikson, to continue to grow, we must resolve these crises.

Healthy personality development results from accomplishing the developmental tasks required for the stage and then moving on to the next one. In a sense, positive attributes win out over negative attributes, and the personality development moves to the next level. Inadequate task resolution results in thwarted development in that particular area. This leaves the person with a lack of certain skills and attributes that will be needed later in life.

For example, if, as an infant, one never successfully develops a sense of trust in oneself and others, the person will grow up with a stronger sense of mistrust. This stays with the person throughout life, limiting the ability to trust others, develop sustained loving relationships, and maximize the individual's potential as an adult. The inability to trust another person makes it difficult to develop intimate relationships based on faith and sharing deeply personal emotions.

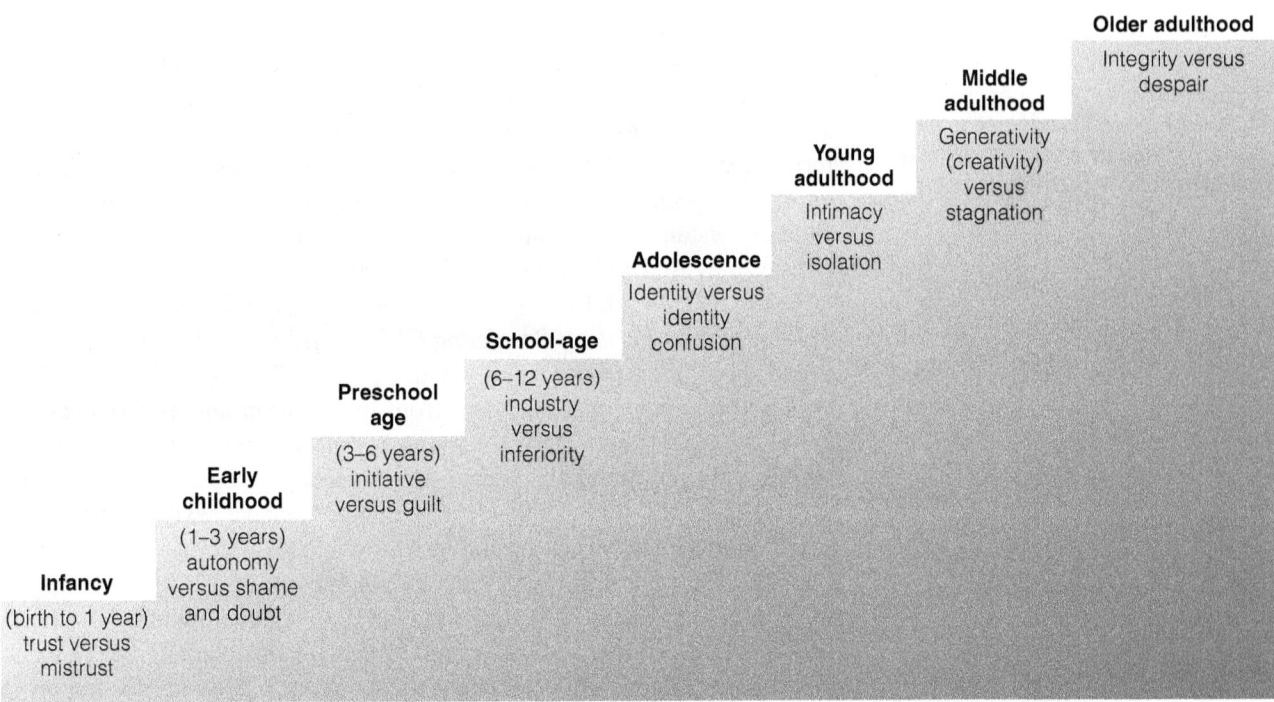

Figure 5.2 *Erikson's Developmental Stages and Conflicts*

Modern Theory

It is important to understand that certain theorists provided the basis from which contemporary work has evolved. Today, some question the very foundations of traditional personality theory. **Feminist theory,** for example, posits that personality and identity are socially constructed. What is "correct development" for boys is different from what is deemed "correct development" for girls. Judith Lorber (2001) writes, "I am arguing that bodies differ in many ways physiologically, but they are completely transformed by social practices to fit into the salient categories of a society, the most pervasive of which are 'female' and 'male' and 'women' and 'men'" (p. 48). Feminist scholars challenge the culture to reexamine the power structure, encouraging broader developmental choices for both boys and girls.

As feminism worked to increase options for girls, others brought to light the need to reexamine how boys are raised, and the limitations placed on their development as well. Michael Gurian (1996), in *The Wonder of Boys,* writes:

> *It requires pretty effective blinders these days to think as I did in the early 1980's—that boys are boys and girls are girls predominantly because of environmental forces. It is more accurate to say that much of who we are is determined by body chemicals, brain differences, hormones, and by society's efforts to honor this biology through its socializing forces. (p. 5)*

Feminist theory Theories that argue that personality and identity are socially constructed. What is "correct development" for boys is different from what is deemed "correct development" for girls.

Queer theory Theories that look to explain sexual orientation and sexual identity without relying on heterosexuality as the norm

Gurian is a firm believer that boys are hard-wired to be a particular way but can be raised to be confident, caring contributors to the culture at large.

The area of research called **Queer theory** has expanded the scholarship that examines the development of sexual orientation. In particular, those identified with this movement challenge heterosexuality as the only valid "end point" of psychosexual development. They argue for a more fluid understanding of gender and orientation, and the role that power and politics play in development (Butler, 1999).

In 2002, Judith Levine raised the ire of many with her book *Harmful to Minors: The Perils of Protecting Children from Sex.* She writes that sex is and should be a positive and wonderful part of children's lives, and that cultural attempts to protect them from information and experiences was harmful to their health and development. She was both critical of conservatives who promoted abstinence- until-marriage ideology and curricula, as well as those who were advocating comprehensive sexuality education, which in her view was doing too little, too late.

Bookstores today are filled with shelves of books on parenting. Is there one book that is the ultimate guide for the development of sexually healthy children? Our response is no. Professionals do not agree. Theorists do not agree. Even family members do not agree. However, it is important to understand that both scholarship and clinical practice have much to offer for better parenting. The American Pediatric Association and your child's pediatrician are good sources for finding valid information on parenting.

Early Development

There are some common themes related to early sexuality that influence sexual development: bonding, other expressions of physical intimacy, self-exploration and masturbation, and nudity. These critical sexual development issues surface during infancy and childhood and remain throughout life. How our caregivers initially handle these issues strongly influences the direction our development takes.

The major task of infancy, according to Erikson, is to develop a sense of trust. For trust to win out over mistrust is essential to continuing healthy psychological development in all of us.

Bonding

Bonding The close physical emotional attachment between infants and their primary caregiver(s)

One of the earliest behaviors that helps foster trust and satisfies our most primal physiological needs is bonding. **Bonding** is a process of developing a close physical and psychological relationship with one's primary caregiver. Bonding between mother and child begins almost immediately as the newborn and mother are brought together to share the first moments of life. Bonding continues as mother and child are brought together during feeding, diaper changing, and simple things such as smiling, talking to the child, and acknowledging the child when approaching him or her.

Fathers also fulfill a bonding role. They are often present at the birth of the baby and develop strong, close physical bonds with their children, sharing in their care and feeding. The increased use of the word parenting rather than mothering and fathering reflects social changes around the raising of children. Raising children as a team has advantages for both parents

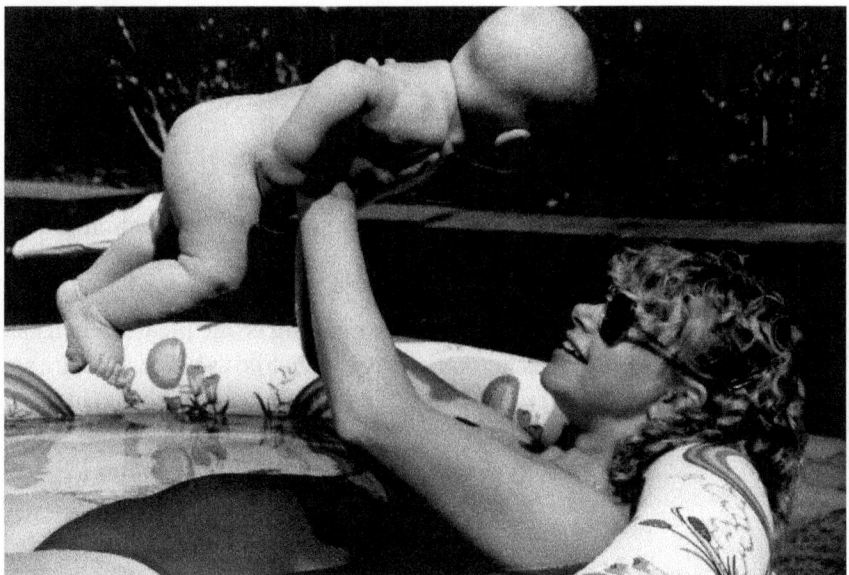

Bonding can take many forms. Here a mom plays in the pool with her child.

and their children. Parents increasingly divide child-rearing responsibilities to fit with their work schedules and time at home.

During the bonding process, infants learn to associate the mother and father with fulfilling the most basic needs for sustaining life. Trust in the world as a whole begins by trusting in mothers and fathers. Infants respond positively to touch. **Thriving**—a term pediatricians use to describe physical and psychological growth—is enhanced by touch and bonding. Failure to thrive has been noted in infants who, among other things, have been deprived of sufficient physical nurturing during infancy. As children, these infants often lack the cognitive and motor abilities of their peers.

Thriving Pattern of normal weight gain, neuromuscular development, and other developmental attributes of infants

Other Forms of Physical Intimacy

In addition to bonding as a contributor to the development of sensuality and sexuality, other forms of touch play an important part. Beyond the basic need of touch for infants to thrive, touch is related to the development of sensuality. Our entire skin surface is capable of acting as an erogenous zone. It is sensitive to touch in all of its manifestations. Babies love to be held, stroked, and rocked. Although we can't interview them, we can tell this from the cooing sounds they make, their facial expressions, and their continued responsiveness to our stroking and hugging them. Our ability or inability to respond positively to physical intimacy is believed to be rooted in the time our parents spent touching and stroking us as infants (Montague, 1986).

How we touch babies varies from generalized hugging and stroking to infant massage and baby exercise. Infant massage strokes are similar to those used with adults, but much gentler. Care must be taken to avoid sharp movements. Infants generally won't last through an entire full-body massage; they begin to wriggle and laugh. Beyond the closeness and benefits from touch that massage affords, research has identified additional health benefits that result from the effect massage has on the body. Infant massage has been found to help babies adjust their circadian rhythms and move

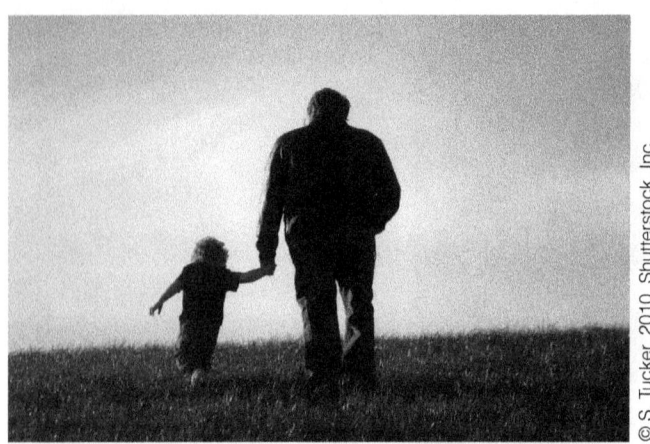

Grandparents can lavish love and attention on their grandchildren, bringing extra sources of affection.

toward better sleeping habits, as well as promote better health and development (Ferber, Laudon, Kuint, Weller, & Zisapel, 2002; Globus, 2002).

Unfortunately, many parents feel awkward or uncomfortable expressing themselves through touch and physical contact. Some of us have grown up in households where touch was withheld or minimized. Sometimes parents worry that their feelings (or their child's) are sexual, not sensual. Even though infants are capable of experiencing erotic pleasure, sensual pleasure shared with your child and sexual desire are different. Mature, parental sensual pleasure associated with hugging and stroking one's child is vastly different from sexually desiring that child. There is no intention of genital sexual contact, nor is there any desire to experience such behavior.

An aversion to touch is a learned behavior. As such, you can unlearn it and not make the same mistakes with your own children. In sharing the joys of touch with them, you can relearn the joys of physical closeness and sensuality and give them the gift of being comfortable with touch.

❧ *Spiritual and Emotional Wellness* ❧

Although we are not always cognizant of it as infants and children, we begin to develop a sense of connectedness or disconnectedness during this stage. Probably the earliest manifestation of spirituality is the bonding with primary caregivers. This is a powerful connection not only to other human beings but also to the world as a whole. Developing a sense of trust in ourselves, others, and the world as a whole begins with the skin-to-skin nurturing we receive from our parents in times of need. Parents and caregivers often describe the feeling of bonding and nurturing of an infant as one of the most profoundly spiritual feelings they have ever experienced. Many rediscover a sense of awe and faith in the power of love by connecting with and nurturing our children.

Infant and childhood emotional development forms the foundation for much of our adult emotional makeup. Basic personality constructs such as self-esteem, trust, happiness, and optimism begin to take shape during infancy and childhood. As Maslow and other developmental theorists point out, the ability to fully self-actualize as adults requires people to meet basic emotional needs early in life. It's harder to love others as adults if a person was not loved as an infant and if pieces of one's emotional development were left scattered on the floor of childhood and **adolescence. Those who were not loved as children can learn to love themselves and others, it is just more difficult.** Nurturing infants, children, and adolescents, attending to their needs, and providing a safe haven and outlet for their desires are all essential for their continuing emotional development and healthy sexuality.

Adolescence Time period representing the psychosocial transition from childhood to young adulthood

© S. Tucker, 2010. Shutterstock, Inc.

Self-Exploration and Masturbation

All infants discover the joys of genital pleasure inadvertently. They discover what it feels like to have their genitals rub against things in their immediate environment (crib, blanket, toys, diaper, clothing, their mother and father). If allowed to do so, infants between 6 and 12 months of age will touch their genitals. They will learn that they are capable of initiating the same pleasurable feelings they felt when rubbing against objects.

This behavior is not considered sexual behavior. Although it is definitely sensual and erotic, it lacks the associated sexual connotations that older children and adults have concerning genital pleasuring. These associations are learned later. This genital play should be evaluated exactly for what it is—play (Kaplan, 1974). It feels good, and children become frustrated if their hands are kept away from their genitals.

Infant self-exploration and masturbation also lay the foundation for developing a broad continuum of sexual feelings and behaviors. **Masturbation** is a normal developmental act, one of the earliest forms of sexual activity. Most children discover masturbation quite innocently as a physical, not sexual, act.

Masturbation Individual or mutual stimulation of genitalia by hand or using other objects

Boys' penile erections often occur as sexual reflexes in response to a variety of stimuli ranging from self-touching to breastfeeding. Girls experience clitoral erection and lubrication and orgasm under similar circumstances.

These earliest attempts at self-exploration teach us about our body and the potential it has for providing pleasure. Conversely, self-exploration has the potential for negatively influencing sexual development if parents overreact to their children's attempts at self-stimulation. Adults who punish children for masturbating may be denying them valuable opportunities for learning about self-pleasuring and setting the stage for negative attitudes (shame, guilt, fear) about sex. Parents who say nothing about masturbation send negative messages through their omission. Children learn that these omissions represent areas that are off-limits for discussion.

Yelling at a child, slapping his or her hand away, admonishing the child for doing something "dirty"—these adult responses to masturbation convey strong negative messages. Negatively reinforcing a behavior that is pleasurable—self-exploration —creates a confusing mixed message. If it is more related to the timing of these acts (little Billy always seems to play with his penis when Grandma is sitting next to him), gently moving the child to a crib or playpen in another room might help. When children become verbal, caregivers can acknowledge to the child that touching his/her genitals feels good but that it is a private activity and is best done is his/her room..

Self-exploration, again, is normal and healthy. It cannot be carried to excess and is self-limiting if children are left alone. Adults should view it like other forms of play. It is amusing for a while, and then the child moves on to something else. If left alone, children will not sit in their rooms all day and play with themselves. Parents who cannot accept their children's self-exploration might discuss the matter with a counselor, priest, rabbi, minister, pediatrician, or sex therapist to get help in dealing with their feelings. Exploring their sexual fears and concerns will reassure them that this self-touching behavior is healthy for their children's sexual development.

Nudity

Infants and children are nudists at heart. Most infants and young children are perfectly comfortable lying and running around the house naked. They do not associate nudity with morality. To be naked to them is simply to be without clothes. Parents and other caregivers (and, later, society at large) teach infants and children that nudity has sexual overtones.

In contrast, Scandinavian cultures have nude beaches that cater to families. Being naked with one's family is considered normal and healthy.

Unlike some other cultures that accept nudity as part of life and don't make a big deal about it one way or another, U.S. culture frowns upon most public displays of nakedness. We owe this to our Puritan heritage. When they came to America, the Puritans enacted many laws that attempted to curtail public displays of nakedness and sexual behavior. To this day, laws dating back to the early 1800s still are on the books concerning things such as proper swimming attire. The rigid views concerning sex and nudity grew out of Victorian England in the 19th century. In that formal, rigid culture, visions of naked flesh were linked to uncontrolled sexual desire and giving into the will of the devil. In an almost comical adherence to covering their exposed limbs, the Victorians went to extremes such as putting "skirts" onto the legs of pianos and chairs lest they offend and tempt their owners to engage in lewd behavior.

Given our puritanical heritage and history of opposition to nudity, most Americans, not surprisingly, feel more comfortable with their clothes on than off. This collective discomfort with nudity affects our comfort level with our own bodies and our ability to relax and be sensual and sexual with others.

Understanding nudity and how we deal with it with our infants and children has many facets. How we handle nudity plays a big part in the kind of foundation we lay for our children's psychosexual development. Bonding is enhanced by nudity. The warmth and close, physical contact that can be achieved from skin-to-skin contact is unparalleled. Even partial nudity, torso to torso, conveys a special closeness that cannot be achieved any other way. Allowing your children to be nude while establishing reasonable parameters for family nudity seems to be a prudent, middle-of-the-road approach to this issue.

Sol Gordon, renowned sexuality educator, believes that parents should take a relaxed attitude about nudity (Gordon & Gordon, 1983). Furthermore, Gordon believes that being nude with your child creates many "teachable moments"—those

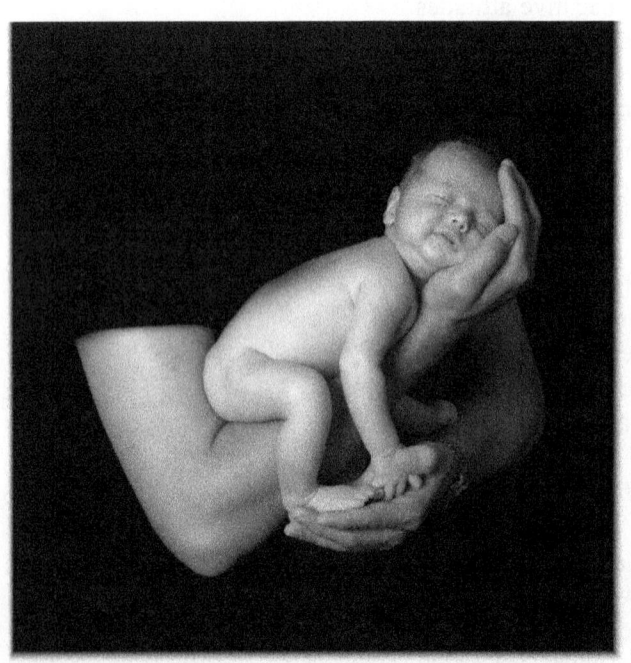

© y. van eekelen, 2010. Shutterstock, Inc.

Babies are sensual creatures. They like to be nude and feel softness and textures of things such as sheepskin throws.

case study 5.2

The Family Bath

Cara and Charles are in their early 30s; she identifies as biracial and he as African American.

Cara and Charles loved being naked and seldom wore a lot of clothes around the house when the children, Aisha and Rakeen, were little. As a couple, they had a ritual of bathing together as much as possible. Once the kids outgrew their infant tubs, each parent took turns being responsible for giving the kids a bath. Because the children were only 2 years apart, sometimes both kids were bathed together. On other occasions one parent or the other would get into the tub with the kids. Getting the whole family into the tub was just too crowded.

As a family, all four were able to enjoy being in water together when they visited the grandparents in South Carolina. Next to a small swimming pool was a tiny hot tub that fit four very comfortably. The freedom of being naked in the water, however, was replaced with the need to be in a bathing suit. Nonetheless, all four could enjoy the family time together in the water.

When Cara and Charles added a new addition to their home, they purposely spent the extra money so that a large bathtub could be installed. The ritual of bathing as a couple could now be continued without overlapping legs and arms. Even the faucet was out of the way! What was missing, however, was the family nudity. The kids, now 11 and 13, had no interest in getting in the water naked with their parents. While getting changed in front of the kids and being naked is still a pattern at home, Cara and Charles seem to be getting more unsolicited feedback about their own bodies. "Ewww . . . you have so much hair there! Am I going to get hair like that?" Or, "Mom, why do you have so many stretch marks over there? Do all moms get those?" The kids seem to have moved to greater body awareness, self-consciousness, and a general need not to see their parents naked. The family bath will have to be relegated to memory.

Critical Thinking

What are your views on family nudity? Do you think that parents and children "should" be comfortable seeing each other without clothes? Is it more appropriate to cover up at some point for healthy development?

points in time when a child's curiosity about sexuality is given a natural outlet. Children will want to know why "Mommy doesn't have a penis" or why "Daddy's penis is bigger than Junior's." These spontaneous questions provide opportunities to ask questions and explore basic sexual information and issues. In a way, it helps parents become more "askable." Capitalizing on teachable moments is a way to take advantage of children's natural curiosity and is preferable to forcing discussions about the "birds and the bees" at inopportune times. Children naturally grow out of the desire to be nude around their parents. As they move into middle childhood and pre-pubescence, they become more independent and develop a personal

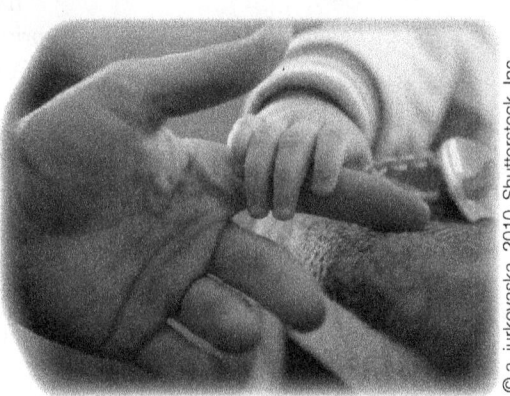

Skin-to-skin contact is something babies and adults enjoy.

© a. jurkovaska, 2010. Shutterstock, Inc.

145

healthy sex hints 5.1

Becoming an Askable Parent

Becoming an askable parent is a lifelong process. A neon sign doesn't suddenly appear during adolescence signaling approachability. Being an askable parent is a reward earned after years of sending subtle messages about the desire to listen and willingness to help. The following are guidelines on how to be an askable parent:

1. *Start early.* Body language and nonverbal behaviors concerning bonding, nudity, and toilet training send messages about approachability.
2. *Don't worry about giving too much information.* Scientific evidence doesn't indicate that too much information too soon will overstimulate children. If a child is getting too much information, he or she will simply get bored, tune you out, and change the subject.
3. *Communicate even if you're not entirely comfortable about the topic.* If you are uncomfortable with a specific sexual issue, you can still address it openly and honestly with your children. The child might respond positively to your admission that you have difficulty talking about an issue.
4. *Admit your ignorance.* You don't know it all. Even the best teachers don't know everything about their subject. If your child asks a question you can't answer, admit it and offer to look it up. Better yet, look it up together.
5. *Realize that less is better.* Concise, simple answers that address the question at hand are better than longwinded answers.
6. *Don't worry about offering information that children can't understand.* If you make a mistake by being too technical, children will extract what they need or understand, and the rest will go over their head.
7. *Don't be afraid to make mistakes.* Everyone makes honest mistakes. Handle these as you would any other mistakes: Admit you were wrong, and try to correct the mistake, if possible.
8. *Relate your values.* Children want to know how you feel about sexual matters. Take every opportunity to share relevant values with them.
9. *Have a sense of humor.* Lighten up. Sexuality education gives rise to opportunities to laugh and learn at the same time. Children feel less inhibited about an adult's talking about sexual matters if sex isn't always portrayed as a deadly serious topic. ⸾

sense of modesty. This is usually accompanied by their desire for more privacy and for other family members to be more fully clothed around the house.

Development in Early Childhood

Self-exploration continues during early childhood (ages 3 to 5) and often extends to playmates. The more mobile child now begins to interact with other children more frequently. Games such as "doctor" and "nurse" typically provide opportunities for sex play and exploration. The availability of playmates often influences the nature of play. Same-gender versus opposite-gender exploration is a function of who is available to play with rather than representing any adult sexual orientation (such as heterosexual or homosexual).

Children continue to gain freedom and begin to be exposed to a variety of people and experiences as they further explore their environment. The major task at this stage corresponds to Erikson's developmental initiative versus guilt (refer to Figure 5.2). Children's actions are more purposeful as they evaluate their own competencies and initiate behaviors consistent with these limits. Children's likes and dislikes at this stage are more firmly established, and their behavior is more purposeful. They know what they want and use their greater mobility and freedom to pursue these desires. When this pursuit puts conflicts with how significant others want them to behave, they begin to feel guilt.

Children at this level struggle with their overwhelming preoccupation with self as they are increasingly exposed to other youngsters in a variety of play and social situations. They find themselves in situations with other youngsters that force them to share, take turns, and accommodate others. This socialization is a vital and necessary developmental step that will prepare children for the kinds of social interactions necessary for their future success in school.

As we pointed out in Chapter 4, gender identity is established by age 3 so it is already strongly established by this stage. Little boys and girls know what being masculine and feminine means, and they continue to explore and refine these roles. The more freedom they are given to explore behaviors and roles, the greater opportunity they will have in moving toward a more flexible gender identity. For instance, little girls who are allowed to play with boys and engage in active, physical play and sports might find that they enjoy this type of activity. Little boys who are allowed to play house and with dolls might find this an enjoyable addition to or replacement of more traditional roughhouse activities.

Development in Childhood

Children continue to explore and mimic gender role behaviors and scripts they learn from their parents and the culture. "Playing house" is a common script for 5- to 7-year-olds. The boys play the "daddies," and the girls play the "mommies." Often these games include kissing, hugging, and cuddling. Children at this age talk about people they love and will marry someday. Children often have a "special friend" to whom they are attracted and for whom they have loving feelings. Elementary school children exchange valentines and other symbols of endearment.

Children at this age also begin to develop their own language and sense of sexual humor. Jokes about bodily functions are common. These children have a great deal of interest in sounds and smells associated with bodily functioning. Children of this age are amused by riddles and rhymes that often are crude and sexually coarse.

By 8 or 9 years of age, children begin to become more segregated in their play. Boys tend to play with other boys, and girls with their girlfriends. Although they still have the same interest in the opposite gender, the socialization process begins to segregate them more and more. Formal activities such as team sports and school-based extracurricular activities are often segregated, sometimes formally but usually informally. Little girls who might have played touch football with the guys last season may try out for cheerleading this year. Boys who played sandlot baseball with the neighborhood boys and girls may sign up for Little League, while their female counterparts sign up for softball. Leagues in some towns encourage mixed-gender participation.

healthy sex hints 5.2

Education for Children

Most parents and professional educators feel that children need to talk about sexuality issues in the home. Having the resources with which to do that in an informed way has been possible for many years. In addition, so much more is accessible over the Internet. Here is a brief list of helpful books for both parents and children.

Two by Deborah Roffman, published by Perseus Publishing:

> *Sex and Sensibility:* The Thinking Parent's Guide to Talking Sense About Sex (2001)

> *But How'd I Get in There in the First Place? Talking to Your Young Child About Sex* (2002)

One by Debra Haffner, along with her daughter Alyssa Haffner Tartaglione, published by New-market Press:

> From Diapers to Dating (2008)

One by Debra Haffner-

> Beyond the Big Talk Revised Edition: Every Parent's Guide to Raising Sexually Healthy Teens, from Middle School to College (2008)

Four by Robie Harris, published by Candlewick Press:

> *It's Perfectly Normal: Changing Bodies, Growing Up, Sex and Sexual Health* (2009)

> *It's So Amazing! A Book About Eggs, Sperm, Birth, Babies, and Families* (2004)

> *Lets Talk About Sex* (2010)

> *It's Not the Stork* (2008)

Robert Hatcher, Shannon Colestock, Erika Pluhar, and Christian Thrasher have a book designed for older adolescents and young college students:

> *Sexual Etiquette 101 and More* (Bridging the Gap Communications, 2001)

These books are honest and forthright about sexuality information. Contacting the Sexuality Information and Education Council of the U.S. (SIECUS) or Planned Parenthood Federation of America will link parents to a wide array of books and pamphlets that address how to promote sexual health. Books and pamphlets have also been developed to help families learn and talk about adoption, gay, lesbian, bisexual and transgendered youth, intersexuality, sexual assault, disability, and other related topics.

In addition to cultural influences that help shape boys and girls and influence which direction they might take regarding sports, economic and political factors play a big part. Often, funding for girls' sports and recreational activities does not equal that earmarked for boys. Consequently, girls haven't always been offered the same opportunities as boys to compete in youth sports. To attempt to rectify that, Title IX of the Civil Rights Act was passed to ensure parity in funding. The law refers to all benefits and activities available in schools. Most of the controversy regarding Title IX revolves around sports and athletic programs. Title IX has been instrumental in getting more girls and women involved in sports and athletic activities.

Development in Preadolescence

Many of the books available for children and teenagers reinforce the idea that children develop at their own pace. A new term, tweens, refers to children roughly between 10 and 12 who, although not teenagers, are confronting issues not commonly associated with young children.

Studies show that although segregation of the sexes is more pronounced during this time, feelings of desire and affection are strong. Most boys and girls of this age view relationships with other preadolescents as important and something they desire. Children in this age range are learning how to interact with members of the same and opposite sexes they find desirable. They are learning the scripts and rehearsing the behaviors necessary to make the transition from childhood to young adulthood. Adults may find some of the behavior amusing, yet the fact that we use the term social skill literally means that skill development is crucial.

Sixth-grade dances are good examples of this learning process. The room is filled with 11- and 12-year-olds who want to mix and mingle with girls and boys they are attracted to. What usually happens, though, is that boys line up along one wall and the girls the other. They horse around and act goofy but rarely cross the line and ask someone to dance. This is a transition, a rite of passage in American culture. The next year or the year after that, they will begin to cross the line and ask each other to dance. Some will even bring partners to the dance. For now, it is a stepping stone, an opportunity to try out another script. Of concern are the 6.2 % of students who engage in sexual intercourse before age 13 (CDC, 2012). Encouraging, however, is the steady decline in those having intercourse before age 13 since many believe this age group is not ready for that level of emotional and physical intimacy.

Hedgepeth and Helmich (1996), as they developed materials for sexuality educators, have noted that young adolescents between the ages of 12 and 14 are dealing with the following developmental issues:

1. They're worried about their bodies.
2. They're engaged in a search for identity, including sexual orientation identity.
3. They are very centered on the self yet influenced by peer attitudes.
4. They intellectually understand that behavior has consequences but don't necessarily think the consequences will happen to them.
5. They're fearful of asking questions of adults that may make them appear uninformed.

✌ *Intellectual Wellness* ✌

Individuals begin to learn about sexuality from the day of birth. Infants and children learn symbolically. They learn about what feels good through direct physical exploration. They learn about what is taboo by the reactions of significant others.

Children continue to grow as they become more verbal and are able to communicate by asking questions and seeking clarification. Development takes shape according to the answers received and the nonverbal messages attached to the information. If children grow up in a household where sexual questions are allowed and teachable moments are capitalized, the natural curiosity about sex is satisfied.

This learning continues through childhood and adolescence. What differs is the sheer quantity of information to which people are exposed and the sources from which it is derived. Infants and young children receive sexual information mostly from parents and other caregivers. By the time of adolescence, sexual information flows in torrents from sources ranging from parents to mass media to the Internet.

Today, more than ever before, many excellent sources of information about sexuality are available—books, recordings, educational television shows, Web sites, and more. Unfortunately, many poor sources of information and negative gender roles also bombard us daily. The ability to process all of this information and make sense of it is aided by our ever-growing intellectual development and rests on a foundation of "askable parents" and a school environment and curriculum that encourage questions and make information readily available.

Development in Adolescence

Adolescence denotes a period of years (roughly between 12 and 18). The major task associated with adolescence is to develop a self-identity (Erikson, 1978). Adolescence can be a time of great excitement and joy as individuals literally move from childhood to adulthood. During adolescence, both the body and the mind change and grow. They outgrow not only their old clothes but often their old ideas as well, and sometimes their old friends, as they struggle to come to grips with who they are and where they are going.

Experts have come to understand that the promotion of good health behaviors at this stage has a critical impact on adult lifestyles (Hatcher & Scarpa, 2002). Consequently, health programs directed at teens often focus on adolescent risk-taking behaviors with particular attention to tobacco and alcohol use, exercise and nutrition, sleep, accident reduction, and sexuality. Set up within the Centers for Disease Control (CDC), the Youth Risk Behavior Surveillance System has surveyed adolescents across the United States for the risk-taking behaviors felt to contribute to social problems, death, and disability. Its rich database has provided information from representative samples taken between 1991 and 2011 from students sampled from 50 states along with more intensive analysis of urban youth (CDC, 2012).

Puberty is the time of myriad physiological events that characterize adolescence. It is a time of profound physiological change as the body matures and becomes "reproductively ready" with fully adult genitalia, a reproductive system, and hormones coursing through the bloodstream, sending messages to the brain of arriving sexually.

Reproductive readiness Pubertal development resulting in full growth of genitalia and onset of fertility

Psychosocial readiness for sexual activity with another person takes a while to catch up to **reproductive readiness.** Adolescents become caught in a state of confusion as the body sends the mind messages about sex that the adolescent may not be ready to handle psychosocially.

Michael Carrera, a respected adolescent sexuality expert, has been working for some time to help teenagers emerge from adolescence as young adults who are strong, competent, and whole. Along with the Children's Aid Society, Carrera (2003) has developed a model for working with youth that has had demonstrable positive results on adolescent health. His program includes getting participants involved with work and money management, educational support that includes tutoring and test preparation designed to move students toward college, a family life/sex education program, involvement in the arts, and participation and development of lifetime individual sports. Simultaneously, students have access to comprehensive medical care including reproductive health care and mental health counseling. Students in his program, some 5,000 over 19 years, have shown lower pregnancy rates, delayed onset of intercourse, better sexual health behaviors, and higher graduation rates.

Today's teenagers, even those not participating in such a program, seem to be more successful at working toward healthy behaviors and healthy sexuality than those of their parents and grandparents generation. Today's teens smoke less marijuana, use fewer illegal drugs and drink less than their parent's generation. They are also much less likely to get pregnant or have sexual intercourse than their parent's generation (Parker- Pope, 2012).

❧   *Physical, Psychological, and Social Wellness*   ❧

Child and adolescent health is positively impacted by participation in exercise and organized sports. Historically, organized sports were seen as important for boys' development, yet of little interest to most girls. Title IX of the 1972 Education Amendments Act outlawed discrimination in secondary and postsecondary educational institutions receiving federal funding. Its impact on reducing gender discrimination in sports has been significant.

In 1971, 1 in 27 girls participated in high school sports compared to 1 in 2 boys. By 2001, the ratio for girls was almost the same as for boys, with 1 in 2.5 girls participating compared to the 1 in 2 ratio for boys (Lopiano, 2001). Participation in sports helps teens learn about teamwork, goal setting, and the pursuit of excellence. Physical activity can enhance self-esteem and improve body image. Research has also shown that teenage female athletes are less likely to get pregnant, delay their first sexual intercourse, and report that they had not had sexual intercourse compared to nonathletes (Lopiano, 2001).

Figure 5–3 highlights the physiological changes associated with puberty. In general, these can be grouped into changes associated with primary and secondary sex characteristics.

Primary Sex Characteristics

Primary sex characteristics are associated with the full growth and development of the sex organs. A boy's penis and testicles grow and reach full adult size by the end of puberty. The testes begin to produce sperm and androgens, and first ejaculation signals the onset of reproductive readiness.

Primary sex characteristics Growth of the sex organs

In girls, the major internal (vagina, ovaries, uterus, and fallopian tubes) and external (labia, mons, clitoris) sexual structures reach maturity. First menstruation is the sign that puberty has arrived.

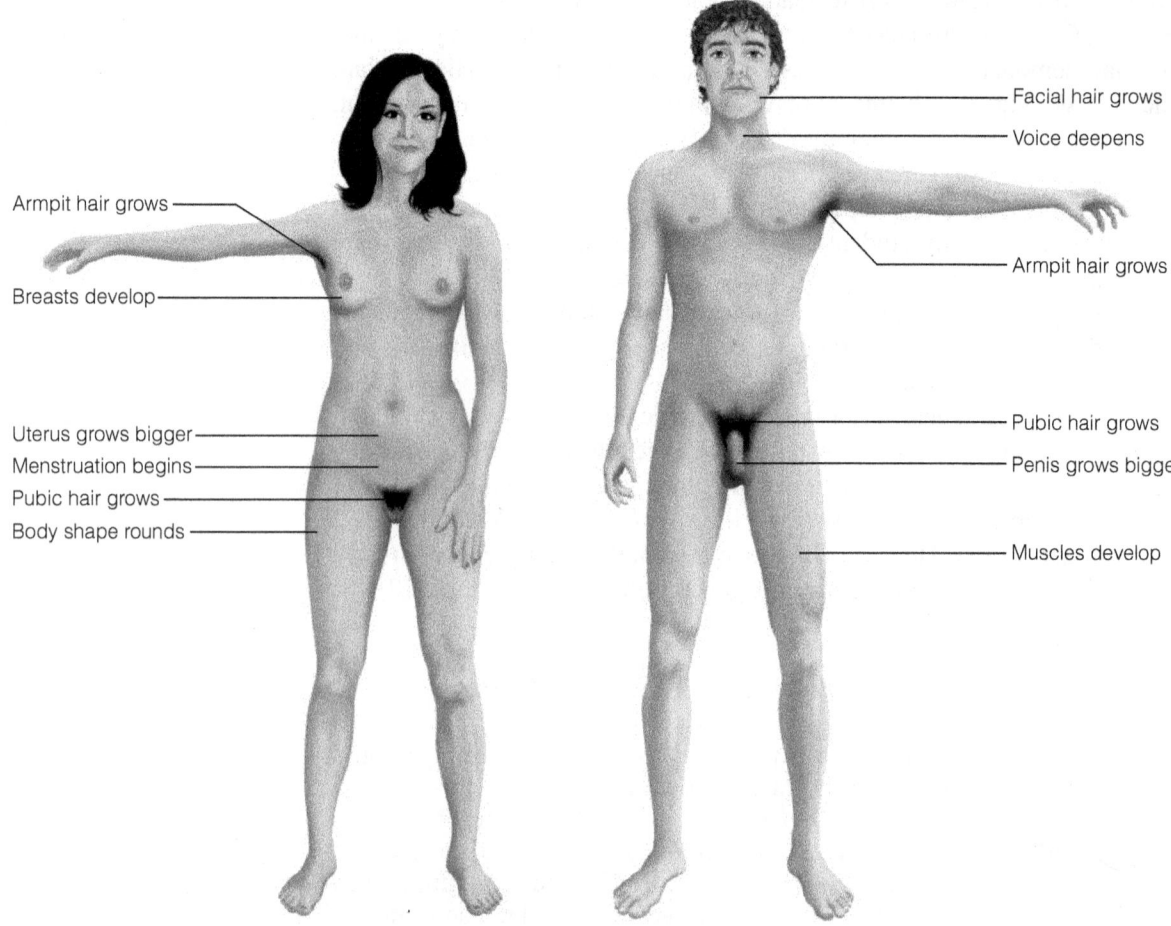

Facial hair grows

Voice deepens

Armpit hair grows

Breasts develop

Armpit hair grows

Uterus grows bigger

Menstruation begins

Pubic hair grows

Body shape rounds

Pubic hair grows

Penis grows bigger

Muscles develop

Figure 5.3 *Changes Associated with Puberty*

Secondary Sex Characteristics

**Secondary sex
characteristics** Nongenital
changes associated with puberty;
include growth of pubic, facial, and
underarm hair, breast development,
increases in height and weight

Secondary sex characteristics are nongenital changes associated with puberty. Boys and girls both experience a growth spurt and begin to attain their subsequent adult height. They both grow pubic, underarm, and body hair. Although boys characteristically grow significantly more facial hair than girls do, this generally represents a continuum with a range of possibilities for boys and girls, from relatively hairless to very hairy.

Body contours begin to develop. Girls naturally deposit more fat on their hips, thighs and breasts than boys do, but, as with facial and body hair, there is a wide continuum of growth possibilities for both boys and girls. The voice box in boys enlarges, creating a deeper, more resonating sound. The transition period involved in this change causes a squeaky quality to boys' voices.

By the end of puberty, the body has reached a stage of reproductive readiness with two major components: mature reproductive anatomy and hormonally influenced sexual desire. The sex organs are fully developed and capable of procreating as well as recreating. Not only are parts such as the penis and vagina fully mature and capable of responding to sexual desire, but ovaries and testes are also fully able to produce viable ova and sperm, respectively. This is often the time when a young girl discovers that her clitoris is capable of providing sexual pleasure.

In nature's eyes, humans are able and ready to propagate the species. Nature gives a boost in that our **gonads** (testes and ovaries), which have long been silent, now begin to produce hormones that stimulate sexual desire. **Androgens,** primarily **testosterone,** stimulate sexual receptor centers in the brain, which trigger feelings of sexual desire. All of the cold showers in the world will not quell this sexual desire because, to a certain extent, it is fueled by hormones circulating in the bloodstream.

In the physical realm, the Sexual Maturity Rating scale, sometimes referred to as the Tanner Scale (American Nurses Association, 1999), can be used to measure levels of physical maturity. The scale, as represented in Table 5.1, has five stages that allow for charting growth of pubic hair, breast development, and size and color of the penis and scrotum. Because the scale has no ages connected to it, health practitioners cannot make assumptions based on age, sex, or racial and ethnic background. Furthermore, a thorough physical exam is required which may or may not occur; some teens resist the physical inspection needed.

Adolescence has a profound impact on sexuality for the rest of our lives. Often our body image and initial impressions about our masculinity and femininity that were formed at this time color how we view ourselves for the rest of our lives. Old labels and images such as "I'm not a good dancer" or "I'm shy" or "I'm not very good-looking" influence our self-concept and can stay with us for years to come.

Gonads The primary endocrine glands in men (testes) and women (ovaries) that influence sexuality

Androgens A group of naturally occurring steroid hormones produced by both men and women

Testosterone The most notable androgen, recognized for fueling sexual desire and aggressiveness in males

Body Image Issues

Both males and females at some point during the preteen and adolescent years may become obsessed with physical appearance. So many changes are happening to the body, and comparisons to peers and "the rich and famous" can be all consuming. The media standard for female attractiveness is thin, large breasted, tall and beautiful. Males are increasingly also portrayed in an unrealistic manner as they are expected to be tall, broad shouldered, muscular and to have no body hair or odor.

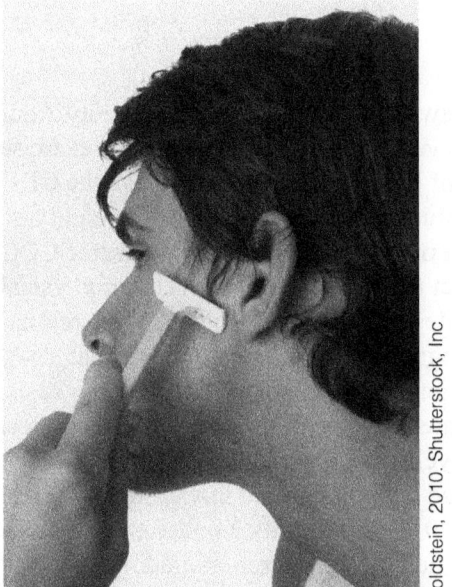

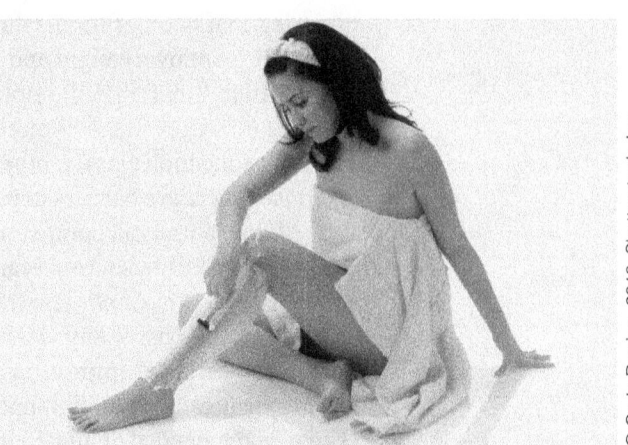

Shaving is an exciting rite of passage for teens.

Table 5.1 Sexual Maturity Rating Scale for Girls and Boys

Female		SMR	Male		
Breast	**Pubic Hair**		**Testes and Scrotum**	**Penis**	**Pubic Hair**
No development	No pubic hair	1	Testicular volume: <1.5 ml	Childlike	None
Breast bud, areola widens	Long, slightly pigmented, straight hair along labia	2	Testicular volume: 1.6–6 ml; scrotum: reddened, thinner, larger	No change	Light, downy hair laterally
Breast larger, more elevation. Extends beyond areolar parameter.	Increased in quantity, darker, more curly and coarser; present in typical female triangle	3	Testicular volume: 6–12 ml; scrotum: great enlargement	Increased length	Extended across pubis
Breast larger and more elevation. Areola and papilla form a mound projecting from the breast contour.	Hair more dense, curled, and adult in distribution but in a smaller quantity	4	Testicular volume: 12–20 ml; scrotum: further enlargement and darkening	Increased length and circumference	More abundant with curling
Breast adult appearance. Areola and breast in same plane, with papilla projecting above areola.	Abundant, adult-type pattern; hair extends to medial aspect of thigh.	5	Testicular volume: >20 ml; scrotum: adult appearance	Adult appearance	Adult quantity and distribution with hair present on inner thighs

Source: American Nurses Association (1999).

There is a major disconnect between the media's ideal and reality. Adolescents are becoming increasingly overweight, partly due to lack of exercise as well as increased consumption of high-calorie foods. In 2012 the CDC reported that 46% of high school students were trying to lose weight and that 15% were overweight and 13% obese. Not surprisingly the same CDC survey found that 50% did not meet the recommended levels for physical activity (CDC,2012). Although states mandate that students have regular physical education classes, other programs often interfere with regular, daily exercise. There are barriers to participation in organized sports such as costs, lack of transportation, competing time commitments, competitive pressures, and lack of facilities (American Psychological Association, 2002). In fact, when asked, 14% of adolescents had not participated in vigorous physical activity in the past 7 days (CDC, 2012). First Lady Michelle Obama has made a mission of improving the health of children and adolescents by promoting healthier school lunches and promoting movement and exercise. These much needed changes can go far in helping children and adolescents achieve a healthy weight and positive body image.

❧ *Fashion and Sexuality—Healthy or Unhealthy?* ❧

There are a variety of ways to change our physical appearance—some less risky than others. As a consumer, it is important to look at safety as part of our decision making. One popular option to consider is genital piercing which can occur on the head of the penis, the scrotum or the perineum for the male. Typical sites for the female are the clitoris and labia. These piercing will take 3-6 weeks to heal and make one at higher risk for transmission of an STD. If one has a piercing, a condom or dental dam should be used to protect from an STD. Additionally, there is a risk of hepatitis and HIV transmission during the piercing process(Gunter and McDowell, 2004). A seemingly harmless choice of underwear even needs careful consideration. Thong underwear act as an easy route to transport bacteria from the rectum to the vagina and bladder and thus may increase the females risk for both vaginal and bladder infections. For males, choosing to wear tight pants may even decrease his sperm count or even cause a rash (American Medical Association News, 2002). So many choices, so much to consider!

Learning to love, accept, and respect one's body is essential for becoming sexually healthy. The impacts of body image on sexual behavior and choices are numerous. Positive body image helps in expressing sexual needs and desires and facilitates sexual health. However the effects of poor body image are significant for both females and males. Females with poor body image are less likely to be assertive and ask for what they want sexually and are less likely to practice safer sex (Zamboni et al, 2006). Males with poor body image are also less likely to practice safer sex and are more likely to withdraw emotionally from their partners. However, men who are comfortable with both their bodies and women's real, not ideal, bodies have a higher level of intimacy with women and participate in more kissing, an intimate sexual activity (Schooler & Ward, 2006).

Adolescent Sexuality

" Becoming a sexually healthy adult is a key development task of adolescence…. Sexual health encompasses sexual development and reproductive health, as well as such characteristics as the ability to develop and maintain meaningful interpersonal relationships; appreciate one's own body; interact with genders in respectful and appropriate ways; and express affection, love and intimacy in ways consistent with one's own values." (Seicus, 1995, p.4). Thus begins the consensus statement of the National Commission on Adolescent Health, endorsed by well respected groups such as the American Medical Association and the American College of Obstetricians and Gynecologist. They believe adolescence is in stages, early-ages 9-13 for women, 11-15 for men; middle- ages 13-16 for girls and 14-17 for males; and late- ages 16 and older for females and 17 and older for males. During early adolescence, youth work to develop a sense of identity, connection, power and joy. If they are not supported in the development of their identity in healthy ways, sexual experimentation may be the easy way for them gain these feelings. The Commission believes that young adolescents do not have the emotional or cognitive maturity to be involved in intimate relations, especially intercourse, so parents, schools and society need to provide positive outlets. During middle adolescence, adolescents seek more independence and begin to value their peers more highly. Sexual expression and experimentation are important in their lives. In late adolescence, they begin to develop more empathetic relationships and begin to transition to adult roles. The Commission believes both families and communities have responsibility in promoting adolescent sexual health. Parents can promote sexual health in ways such as valuing their adolescents and being knowledgeable and openly discussing sexuality. The community can promote comprehensive sexuality education, community programs and accessible health care. (Siecus,1995) What the Commission advocates would bring us closer to the Dutch, German and French model where adolescents are viewed as assets, are valued and respected, and expected to act responsibly. Families in these countries have open, honest discussions with teens about sexuality and support educators and health care providers in making services available to teens. The sexual health outcomes for these teens compared to the U.S. are much more positive. The teen pregnancy rate in the U.S. is more than 5 times higher than the Netherlands and over 4 times higher than Germany. In addition, European teens are much more likely to use contraception than American teens. (Advocates for Youth, 2013). Though we in the United States have much to learn from our European counterparts, some recent trends in adolescent sexual behavior do indicate a move toward healthier behavior.

Masturbation

Conscious, erotic self-stimulation is thought to be among the most common expressions of adolescent sexual behavior, particularly for males. Kinsey and his associates discovered that the rate of masturbation was different for boys and girls (Kinsey, Pomeroy, & Martin, 1948). Among boys in that early study, the level of masturbation increased from 21 percent of 12-year-old boys to 82 percent of 15-year-old boys. Among girls, the level of masturbation increased from 12 percent of 12-year-old girls to 20 percent of 15-year-old girls. By the end of adolescence, more than 90 percent of the boys and about 35 percent of the girls had masturbated.

Compared to Kinsey's study, a 2011 study shows an increased rate of female masturbation with 58% masturbating by the end of adolescence. As in Kinsey's study, males report higher rates (74%) of masturbation than females. Masturbation is more common among 14-17 year olds than any partnered sexual behavior. There is much silence and discomfort surrounding the topic of masturbation. In 1974 when Jocelyn Elders, the Surgeon General, recommended that masturbation be included in sexual education, she was strongly criticized and eventually resigned (Robbins, Schick, Reese, Herbenick, Sanders, Dodge, & Fortenberry, 2011). This lack of openness is a lost opportunity for helping adolescents learn body awareness and healthy expression of sexual desire and experimentation. Masturbation is a way for adolescents to explore their bodies and identify what they find pleasurable. If parents encourage their children to masturbate, it may lessen the guilt they sometimes feel. As a result adolescents may be more comfortable choosing masturbation as an alternative until they are emotionally ready for sexual expression with a partner.

Sexual Intercourse

The number of teens choosing to have sexual intercourse has declined over the past 20 years. In 1991, 54% of all 9-12th grade students had experienced

personal exploration activity
What Is Right for You?

It is easy to avoid openly examining our beliefs and values concerning sexual activity. Often our sexual behavior is dictated by the moment, not by our values and rational decisions. The goal of this activity is to help you clarify the sexual behavior that is comfortable and acceptable for you, and to identify a plan for making sure you can stick to your sexual values.

Take a few minutes to really examine what you believe and respond to the following questions honestly and openly. You do not need to share this with anyone; however, you might enjoy discussing it with a close friend.

What would be some good reasons or advantages for you to choose to have premarital sex? (If you are married, substitute *extramarital* for *premarital* in each question.) *Example:* "It's fun."

What would be some good reasons or disadvantages for you to choose not to have premarital sex? *Example:* "I could get hurt."

What are some guidelines you need to follow if you choose to have premarital sex? *Example:* "Be honest with my partner about my motives for having sex."

What are some guidelines you need to follow if you choose not to have premarital sex? *Example:* "Don't drink too much."

List the reasons you might choose to have premarital sex in two columns, reasons that would make you feel guilty versus guilt-free reasons.

How can you tell when a premarital sexual relationship becomes unhealthy or harmful?

sexual intercourse and by 2011 the number had fallen to 46%. Males are no more likely to have had sex than females (Kaiser Family Foundation, 2011). The decline in sexual activity among males has been especially steep. Males are now expressing the desire to not be sexually active for the same reasons we hear expressed by females. They wait because they have not met the right person or they are in a relationship and are waiting for the right time. Contrary to popular belief, males are as emotionally invested as females in relationships (Schalet,2012). Of these sexually active teens, the majority do not have multiple partners in a given time period but instead practice serial monogamy(Kirby, 2007).

The number of teens choosing to have sexual intercourse before age 13 is 6.2%. This number is higher for males (9%) than females (3.4%) (CDC, 2012). Although the numbers are low, this is of concern since those who initiate early intercourse are not likely to be emotionally ready for that level of intimacy (Siecus, 1995). Eighty-five percent of female and 89% of males used some form of birth control the first time they had intercourse (CDC, 2011). The US has witnessed a large decline in the teen pregnancy rate, dropping from 117 pregnancies per 1000 females age 15–19 in 1990 to 39 per 1000 in 2011 (Kaiser Family Foundation, 2011). The abortion rate has also continued to decline from 24 per 1000 women ages 15–17 in 1994 to 13 per 1000 women in 2009 (Pazol, Creanga, Zane, Burley, &

Jamieson, 2012). The overall decline in teen pregnancy can likely be attributed to the decrease in sexual activity and the improved use of contraceptives. Unfortunately, accompanying these healthy behaviors comes the sobering STD estimate that 1 in 3 sexually active males and females will contract an STD by age 24. (Kirby, 2007).

First Sex Among Lesbian/Gay Youth

Sexual behavior patterns in gay and lesbian youth are more complex because of the added dimension of coming to terms with a sexual identity that is different from their heterosexual peers. Despite increased attention to gay and lesbian issues in the media, widespread acceptance still seems problematic for mainstream America. Sexual behavior seems to be the fourth step in a five-step coming-out process that involves these stages:

1. Fear and suspicion that one's sexual desires and attraction are different (although still not clearly defined)
2. Labeling of those feelings as homoerotic (sexual feelings for someone of the same sex)
3. Defining oneself as gay or lesbian
4. Having one's first gay love affair
5. Becoming involved in the gay or lesbian subculture (Herdt & Boxer, 1992; Troiden, 1988)

Having sexual feelings for someone of the same sex (homoerotic feelings) almost always precedes sexual activity by several years among gay and lesbian people. Gay and lesbian youth today recognize feelings for same-sex partners and act on them earlier than their peers of 20 years ago (Savin-Williams & Rodriguez, 1993).

Oral Sex

During the Monica Lewinsky scandal, President Bill Clinton testified before a congressional committee, "I did not have sex with that woman." He did admit, however, to having experienced oral sex. Is oral sex considered sex, is it less intimate, is it like kissing or holding hands? When asked if oral sex is real sex only 52% of men and 46% of women answered yes (Sanders & Reinsch, 1999).

The Henry J. Kaiser Family Foundation (2008), reports that over half of the males (55%) and females (54%) ages 15-19 have had oral sex with someone of the opposite sex. In 2005, the Henry J. Kaiser Family Foundation reported 21% of students age 15-17 had participated in oral sex for the purpose of avoiding intercourse with a partner.

Patterns in oral sexual behavior among adolescents have mimicked the changes of adults in the United States. In general, changes in cultural acceptance of nongenital sexual behavior have led to increasing levels of all forms of oral sex among adults (Wilson & Medora, 1999). This pattern seems similar for adolescents.

Cultural Attitudes About Adolescent Sexuality

How does U.S. society view adolescent sexuality? It seems to view adolescent sexual behavior in general, and intercourse in particular, as a "problem"

sex in society 5.1

Other Cultures, Other Ways

Over the years, researchers have studied societies that recognize and celebrate the onset of puberty in adolescent boys and girls. Ford and Beach (1951) found that more than 70 societies celebrated the onset of puberty in girls and more than 65 that in boys. In a sample of 192 societies, Schlegel and Barry (1979, 1980) found that 80 had no rites of passage, 17 had ceremonies for boys only, 39 had rites for girls only, and 46 had ceremonies for both sexes. Larger societies, with intensive agricultural and manufacturing bases, and those with more complex forms of social organizations, tended not to have initiation rites.

Of the societies celebrating puberty in girls, these celebrations usually coincide with the onset of first menses and are directly related to the sexual significance of menstruation. Schlegel and Barry found that first menses signified fertility and the tribe's continued existence.

These ceremonies often included seclusion of the young women, prohibiting any contact with men. In many instances, the ceremonies included instruction from older women in matters pertaining to sex and marriage. In some cultures, the young women were "deflowered" or subjected to piercing, tattooing, or genital adornment or mutilation. Frequently, the occasion was also marked by a feast or celebration.

Schlegel and Barry found that segregation from males at this time is usually based on avoiding contact with menstrual flow, which is feared because of its supposed ability to weaken a hunter's abilities or contaminate the tribe's meat sources.

For boys, unlike with girls' first menses, no clear demarcation indicates that puberty has begun. Generally, boys are given the rites when evidence is sufficient (usually secondary sex characteristics) that they have reached puberty. Boys' ceremonies are similar to girls' in that they usually include some form of seclusion, instruction, and ritualistic physical sacrifice (often circumcision).

The Sexual Culture of Mangaia

In the 1950s, anthropologist Donald Marshall studied the sexual attitudes and activities of the people of Mangaia, the southernmost island in the Polynesian Cook chain. There, he found, the people were exposed to sexuality from early childhood. They listened to folk stories that included detailed accounts of sex acts and sexual anatomy, and they watched sensual ritual dances.

As adolescents, males underwent *superincision,* a surgical procedure in which the tissue at the end of the penis was cut and folded back, which exposed the glans. They were taught how to stimulate a woman's genitals and breasts with the mouth, how to bring female partners to orgasm, and how to control the timing of ejaculation. Mangaian girls were taught to be responsive and to participate actively during sexual activity.

In a practice called "night-crawling," a young male would sneak into the home of a young woman with the intent to have sexual intercourse. Because most homes had a single sleeping area, this act tended to be more public than private, though the other family members feigned sleep. The parents approved of night-crawling and listened for their daughter's laughter—a sign that she was happy with her partner. The parents encouraged their children to have more than one sexual partner before marriage, to find the most sexually compatible mate.

After marriage, couples in Mangaia continued to engage in sex more often than most Western countries. The emphasis, though, shifted from the number of orgasms during a single session to a goal of copulation every night. Throughout life, the emphasis for males and females alike was on pleasing the partner (Marshall, 1971).

that will lead to negative outcomes (such as unintended pregnancy, sexually transmitted diseases including HIV, and sexual abuse, among others). Many other cultures view this matter entirely differently and celebrate this time in a young person's sexual life. Indeed, in some Pacific Island cultures, adolescent sexual behavior is encouraged, not merely tolerated. This is not to say that these cultures advocate promiscuity. Most have rules pertaining to adolescent sex.

The United States has a conservative sexual history. American culture evolved from devoutly religious, puritanical ancestors who escaped persecution for their views in Europe by coming to this country. The American patriarchal culture emphasized the family and historically has viewed sex as something that occurs within the context of a marriage, with the primary function being procreation. A strong history, institutionalized formally in law and enforced informally through cultural taboos and parenting styles, perpetuated this view. The United States is still a country where sex education is not universally taught in every school. Even when it is, it may be taught by someone who is not a trained sexuality educator and not comfortable teaching sexuality education. In some states, non procreative sexual acts, including oral sex and anal intercourse between consenting adults (whether heterosexual or homosexual), is considered sodomy and is illegal.

Besides having a moral tradition that prohibits adolescent sexual education and experimentation, U.S. culture, like that of many industrialized societies, prolongs adolescent and young adult dependency. To succeed, adolescents, in most cases, need to further their education. For most of them, this means remaining indebted to their parents and pursuing additional training and education while either living at home or remaining financially obligated to their parents. In a sense, what this does is delay the transition from childhood to adulthood, and delaying with it adult privileges such as sexual experimentation. In many other cultures, adolescents are encouraged to begin to separate from their parents earlier, and this separation is often institutionalized in a formal rite of passage.

Perhaps, a shift in American attitudes toward adolescent sexuality are long overdue. Viewing sexuality as a natural part of adolescent development is essential. Following the European model, American parents can encourage adolescents to be fully informed and to give them the rights, respect and responsibility they need and deserve. Talking openly about sexual behavior, sexual values and decisions can help guide young people in making more responsible decisions (Berne and Huberman, 1999). We can learn lessons from those teens who do choose to practice healthy behaviors. Teens who have more parental supervision, who come from two parent households and who do well in school are more likely to delay sexual intercourse until late teens or beyond (Parker-Pope, 2009).

Education and Sexual Development

Ideally, sexuality education would be infused in all parts of the developing child and adolescents life. It would begin early, with open honest discussions and questions among parents and children. The education would then continue in the pediatricians office. According to the American Academy of Pediatrics, (2001) " Children and adolescents need accurate and comprehensive education about sexuality to practice healthy sexual behaviors as adults." They believe the pediatrician has a responsibility to provide good sexuality education to his/her patients. In the churches, synagogues, mosque, and in the community, discussions on sexual values

case study 5.3

Paul and Rich: Tumultuous Adolescence

Rich and Paul, both 42, are white.

Paul and Rich met as adults and compared their experiences of going through puberty and adolescence. Even though Paul is gay and Rich is heterosexual, their adolescent years had many similarities, and both had a tremendous amount of curiosity and guilt about their sexual desires.

Rich's adolescence was a fairly typical experience for a straight, lower-middle-class young man growing up in urban America. His parents were high school graduates who worked in factories as piecework tailors. Although both were loving and attentive parents, neither was skilled at communicating openly with Rich about the issues he would face as an adolescent. Neither knew about the key developmental components of puberty and adolescence and weren't comfortable talking with Rich about these issues. Consequently, Rich's adolescence was a hit-or-miss, trial-and-error experience for which he was totally unprepared.

Rich remembers experiencing things such as wet dreams, his first "true love," masturbation, his first ejaculation, and how puzzled he was trying to figure out how male and female genitalia come together during sexual intercourse. He remembers agonizing about his first ejaculation, feeling as if perhaps he had injured himself or something had gone wrong because all of a sudden this liquid was coming out of the end of his penis. Rich had to be content with asking his friends or older brother about some of these things. Based on the responses he received, he knew that some of the answers were not the "right" ones. It took Rich several years to get over much of the guilt and shame he had about his sexual feelings and behavior during adolescence. He spent the better part of his 20s looking for the answers to unresolved questions and issues from his adolescence.

The major difference between Paul and Rich is in sexual orientation. Paul just never felt any sexual desire toward females. He played along when his friends talked about "getting laid" and carrying on with girls in general. Inside, however, Paul was troubled because he felt attracted to some of the boys in his class. In addition, Paul's church had a stated position against masturbation, which created much confusion and guilt in Paul whenever he engaged in that activity. He did not dare to discuss his sexual feelings with anyone connected with his church. Furthermore, as the only son of immigrant parents who did not discuss things of a sexual nature with him, he began to feel isolated. All through his adolescence, Paul agonized over who or what he was. He tried dating girls but found it unsatisfactory. He suspected he was gay but didn't want to admit it and believed he had no one in whom he could confide or trust while exploring this facet of himself.

Paul coped with adolescence by suppressing most of his sexual feelings. He denied that they existed and spent most of his time immersed in studying. Not until he entered college as a pre-med student did he finally give in to his urges to explore this part of himself. Later, in medical school and a steady relationship with another male student, Paul was able to work through some of the pain and confusion that had marred his adolescence.

Critical Thinking

If Rich and Paul were adolescents today, how might their stories be different?

How would comprehensive sex education have improved their lives? How could their families have made the adolescent sexual learning more positive?

sex in society 5.2

Access to the Truth

For 20 years, the Network for Family Life Education, based at the Rutgers University Center for Applied Psychology, has provided resources, advocacy, training, and technical assistance in support of age-appropriate, balanced comprehensive sexuality education in New Jersey and now nationwide. In 1994, the network asked young people if they would read a newsletter about sexuality and health written by teens, for teens. The response was an immediate and electric "Yes!" The National Teen-to-Teen Sexuality Education Program was thus established, and today it has five thriving components:

- *SEX, ETC.,* the award-winning newsletter written by teens, for teens, a free resource produced three times each year by a multiethnic board of New Jersey high school students (circulation began with 30,000 copies in 1994 and in 2003 has risen to 2.1 million copies)
- Discussion Guides designed to help adults spark lively discussions about vital health topics in each issue of *SEX, ETC.,* including a newly published teaching manual
- *The Roadmap: A Teen Guide to Changing Your School's Sex Ed,* a book to teach teens to become advocates for effective sexuality education
- Youth Media Outlets such as a monthly column on MTV.com and feature articles in *Teen People* magazine
- A Web site—www.sexetc.org—launched in 1999, that offers teens more than 300 articles written by their peers, weekly feature stories, reader polls, quizzes, opportunities to get involved, and honest and expert answers to frequently asked questions through the Ask the Experts feature. The Ask the Experts section of the Web site takes in questions from teens all over the world, and a panel of 12 experts, including health educators, physicians, social workers, psychologists, and other professionals, responds to over 350 questions a week. Each question is given a private, confidential, and individual response that is edited carefully by the experts and

returned to the teen in about 3 to 5 days. The Web site averages 350,000 teen users each month, and in 2002, it individually answered more than 18,000 teen questions.

The average age for teens writing to the site is about 15 years old, but it ranges from 13 to 21. The kinds of questions teens send to the SEX, ETC. Web site reflect their general ignorance and naiveté about most sexuality issues. The site receives a substantial percentage of questions about body image, penis size, breast size, and whether or not to shave pubic hair. In addition, the majority of questions are about what behaviors are risky for pregnancy, how to make sex more pleasurable and less painful, and how to access birth control, gynecological care, and STD testing.

The site's experts always offer honest and completely straightforward answers to all questions sent in. They also provide information about negotiating and communicating with partners, reducing risk, delaying sexual involvement, and finding alternatives to high-risk behaviors. It is clear that teens are not getting the vital health information they need at home or at school.

The popularity of Web sites that offer information about sexuality shows how greatly teens (and adults) need honest and accurate information that they can access when they need it. Many Web sites feature FAQs and Ask the Experts sections, including www.teenwire.com, www.gurl.com, and www.puberty.org. Most teens are not comfortable asking parents their most intimate questions (although the SEX, ETC. Web site encourages them to try), and most teachers in schools are ill equipped or forbidden to respond to questions about contraception, abortion, sexual response, body image, growth and puberty, safer sex, and many other topics.

Having a place where teens can find information, resources, and answers to their most pressing questions is a service that has been needed for a long time. Although the Internet can have all kinds of negative and potentially dangerous possibilities, being a source of honest, accurate information about health and sexuality is one of its best uses, especially for teens.

Source: Elizabeth Casparian, New Jersey Network for Family Life Education (2003).

and behaviors add to the sexual education of children and adolescents. In addition, sexuality education should begin early in the school career. If education is to be effective in delaying onset of intercourse it needs to be implemented by 5th grade (Frost & Forrest, 1995). However, abstinance only education has not been shown to delay onset of intercourse or increase safer sex practices (Frost and Forrest, 1995). Early comprehensive sexuality education that includes practical skills such as decision making and refusal skills should be an integral component of the early educational experience.

Fortunately, the support for sex education in the schools is at an amazingly high rate of 93% of Americans saying sex education should be taught in the schools, according to the NPR/Kaiser/KennedySchool poll (2003). The debate is really over what type of sexuality education students should receive. Fifteen percent of Americans believe in teaching abstinence only, meaning no discussion on any contraception. The majority, 46%, support abstinence plus which teaches abstinence is best but also teaches contraceptive information for those who choose not to abstain. Thirty-six percent believe abstinence is not the most important thing but that teens should be taught how to make responsible decisions. As of January, 2011, twenty states and the District of Columbia mandated sex and HIV education in the schools (Santos & Philips, 2011). This leaves far too many students without access to reliable information about sexuality provided by well trained educators.

Consequences of Teen Pregnancy and STDS

Of the unmarried adolescent females who are having intercourse, 30% will become pregnant at least once by the age of 20. The majority of these pregnancies are unplanned, with 29% of unintended pregnancies ending in abortion (Guttmacher, 2006).

The teens who maintain their pregnancies are more likely to have pregnancy related problems than women who delay childbearing until they are in their 20s. Adolescents are more likely to suffer from toxemia, hemorrhaging, and miscarriages than women who delay pregnancy. In addition, teen mothers are more likely receive poor prenatal care, have low-birthweight babies, and a higher infant mortality rate (CDC, 2000). These unmarried, teenage mothers face a harder future than their peers who delay bearing children until they are older and married. Although teen mothers are more likely to finish high school than in the past, they are less likely to go to college than their nonpregnant peers (Guttamancher, 2006). Because of the twin burdens of less education and the need for child care, these teens earn less, work in blue-collar professions and in general have a lower standard of living than their peers who delay marriage and childbirth.

These mothers are also more likely to have large families and remain single thus further increasing the likelihood that they and their children will live in poverty. The children born to these mothers are more at risk for having a less supportive and stimulating home environment and tend to have lower cognitive development. They are more likely to also experience adolescent pregnancy and the males have a higher rate of incarceration (Kirby, 2007).

The negative effects of pregnancy are not limited to the mothers but also include the fathers of these children. The pregnancy can strain the male's relationship with both the partner and his parents. Teen fathers do not go as far in school and have less income when they do work. The additional financial burden is great for the father since he is financially responsible for the child until age 18 (4 Parents.gov, 2008).

Other negative health consequences associated with adolescent sexual activity include sexually transmitted diseases. Adolescents are at greater risk than older adults for acquiring an STD due to limited access to preventive care and physiologically increased susceptibility to infection (CDC, 2003). Of those ages 15-24, twenty five percent of the population is sexually active yet they acquire nearly half of all new cases of STDs. The health costs of STD's are high- infertility, ectopic pregnancy and cancer (Kirby, 2007). The emotional cost can also be high due to the shame that is often associated with STDs. In addition to the non life threatening STD's, the CDC estimates that 61,000 young people age 13-24 are living with HIV (Kaiser Family Foundation, 2011).

Communication about Adolescent Sexuality

An open, honest and positive approach may be the best way to address adolescent sexuality. Teaching adolescents to value and respect their bodies may improve sexual decision making. If parents think their adolescent children would be better off to delay sexual intercourse or other forms of sexual activities with a partner, it is best for them to tell their children this and explain why. The healthy way to do this is to admit honestly to young people that sex is a natural, healthy but powerful force in their lives and that, as parents, you would prefer them to redirect that sexual energy from sexual intercourse into other, less risky sexual outlets, such as hugging, kissing, and masturbation. To deny the power of adolescent sexual urges or, worse, not mention it and hope the subject will never come up is unhealthy and dishonest.

Included in this open discussion should be an examination of the sexual attitudes and behaviors portrayed in the media, including film, television, music, and the internet. The media may be one of the most powerful influences on an adolescent's views of sexuality. By the time an adolescent graduates from high school, he/she will have watched more hours of television, 15,000, than hours spent in the classroom, 12,000 (Strasburger, 1993). According to a 2005 study by the Kaiser Family Foundation, the number of sexual scenes on television has nearly doubled since 1998. While the inclusion of safer sex discussions has increased since 1998 it has recently leveled off. The study found that sexual content was a part of 70% of all shows and that they average 5 sexual scenes per hour (Kaiser Family Foundation, 2005). Sexual references are common in prime time TV, music videos, and music. Educating teens to critically view the media and accept it as fantasy and entertainment is an important step in minimizing this negative influence.

Gay adolescents can face even more issues. Not only do they have to deal with the mixed messages and pressures associated with this part of their lives, but they also face a wall of silence concerning their own emerging preferences. Gay adolescents usually learn early on that discussing their attraction to same-gender partners is taboo. Few social supports and people are available to turn to for these adolescents whose school guidance counselors and other community helpers are often either misinformed about how to help these young people or homophobic and a threat to the very youth they are being paid to care for. Many school districts forbid teaching that homosexuality is an acceptable lifestyle. Local chapters of Parents and Friends of Lesbians and Gays (PFLAG) and other gay and lesbian organizations are excellent places to find help and information about resources.

Helping teens and adolescents learn to accept themselves and develop tolerance and respect for the sexuality of others remains an ongoing challenge to parents, schools and agencies working with youth.

Healthier Teens

One of the national health objectives for Healthy People 2020, a federal government plan to improve the health of Americans, is to improve the health of adolescents. The U.S. teen birthrate remains one of the highest among developed nations along with rates of STD infections. Child Trends, a nonprofit, nonpartisan research center that studies children and families, reviewed more than 150 research studies to identify the factors that contribute to improving adolescent reproductive health. Sound public policy and programming require that a holistic approach be taken, looking at the adolescent, the adolescent's family, the role of peers, the teenager's partners, the school context, and the neighborhood and community context (Manlove, Terry-Humen, Papillo, Franzetta, Williams, & Ryan, 2002). Some of the key summary findings are as follows:

1. Males are more likely than females to initiate sexual activity at an earlier age, yet for both sexes, earlier onset of puberty and an older appearance are associated with teens becoming involved in sexual activity. Adolescents who are engaged in positive activities such as sports and school and who are confident in their ability to delay activity are more likely to do so.
2. Adolescents with close family ties and good communication engage in more positive reproductive behaviors, whereas those whose mothers were teens at the time of their birth and have sexually active teen siblings are more likely to engage in risky behaviors.
3. Teens are influenced by their friends, and when their peer group engages in risky behaviors, they are more likely to do so themselves.
4. Adolescents who have experienced coercive sex and those who have much older sexual partners appear to be at greater risk for multiple partners, lack of contraception, and pregnancy.
5. There is variability in the types of sexuality programs offered in schools, with some programs associated with reduced sexual activity and increased contraceptive use and other programs associated with delayed sexual activity. It is difficult, however, to separate the school from the community context.
6. Higher rates of sexual activity, pregnancy, and birth are associated with higher rates of poverty.

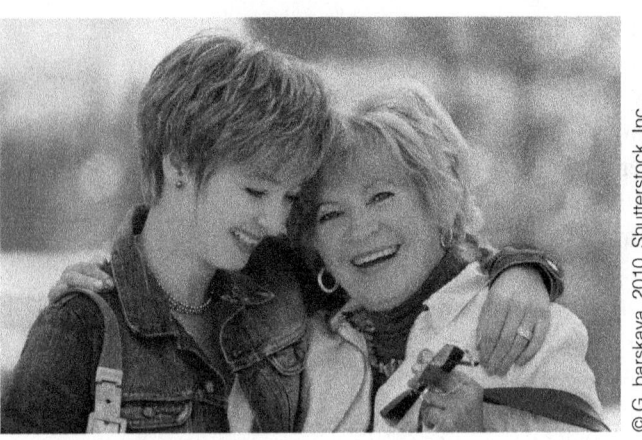

Parents can be a great source of support and information.

© G. barskaya, 2010. Shutterstock, Inc.

Overall, Manlove et al.'s (2002) analysis shows that the best programs focus on early childhood development, combine sexuality education for older children with community service activities, and send nurses to visit with teenage mothers.

Despite research findings on effective educational programs, statistical data on teen sexual activity, reports of dating violence and harassment related to sexuality, undesirable outcomes of unwanted pregnancy and infection, realities of teen parenting, and other pertinent issues, the United States has been slow in the design and implementation of comprehensive programs to meet the sexual health needs of adolescents.

Unfortunately, many pay the price for this lack of action.

Personal Assessment

Rites of Passage

U.S. culture has been criticized for lacking traditional rites of passage that help adolescents make a smoother transition from childhood to adulthood. The purpose of this assessment is to help you explore rites of passage in our culture and others by reflecting on your own experiences. This assessment will enable you to understand why adolescence is often troubling for youth in the United States.

1. Read Sex in Society 5.1, "Other Cultures, Other Ways," in this chapter.

2. Describe, in writing, your own thoughts and feelings about this reading.

3. How do you think these rites of passage would be accepted in the United States?

4. List and describe any cultural rituals that you have experienced while growing up that could be considered rites of passage, and explain how they differ from the examples in the reading.

Thought Questions

1. Describe the different psychological theories and their contributions to the understanding of healthy sexual development.

2. How do bonding, nudity, and toilet training practices affect the development of healthy sexuality?

3. What are the effects of masturbation on childhood and later adult health?

4. What are some of the key developmental issues that young adolescents confront?

5. What are the pros and cons of sexual activity during adolescence?

Test Yourself!

1. Maslow identified characteristics of those who achieve self-actualization through "transcendence." Someone who is a transcender would most likely
   a. focus on the financial rewards of work.
   b. embrace change and creativity.
   c. prefer what is familiar, tried, and true.
   d. be judgmental of others.

2. Modern personality theorists
   a. widely support the Freudian perspective that libidinal energy is the basis for sexuality.
   b. agree that biology is the primary influence on sexual development.
   c. increasingly examine social and environmental influences that help frame ideas of what is normal and expected.
   d. reject all earlier theories of development as being antiquated and irrelevant.

3. Masturbation in young children
   a. is statistically rare.
   b. should be encouraged by parents and teachers.
   c. is normal and usually self-limiting.
   d. can lead to other forms of interpersonal sexual activity.

4. A primary developmental task of adolescence is
   a. to form a sense of identity.
   b. to create close, intimate relationships with members of the opposite sex.
   c. to achieve positive self-esteem through experimentation.
   d. to separate from parents and live independently.

5. All but which of the following are considered secondary sex characteristics in males?
   a. Increased muscle development
   b. Pubic hair
   c. Facial hair
   d. Higher voice

6. The term used to describe the biological transition from childhood to adulthood is
   a. *puberty.*
   b. *transcendence.*
   c. *adolescence.*
   d. *maturation.*

7. Most research on adolescent sexual behavior has revealed
   a. little interpersonal sexual activity until the last years of high school.
   b. drastic differences in the experiences of boys and girls.
   c. increasing rates of sexual experimentation as teens age.
   d. greater experimentation among gay and lesbian students than heterosexual students.

8. Today, teens who want detailed answers to their questions about sexuality
   a. can go online to Internet sites and receive quality information.
   b. will find that the majority of school programs talk about sexuality issues in an honest, comprehensive manner.
   c. will initiate conversations with their parents
   d. complain that no resources are available to them.

9. Which statement about nudity is most accurate?
   a. All cultures react to public nudity in the same way, expecting adults to be dressed.
   b. Families are encouraged to be nude as much as possible in order to teach positive messages about the body.
   c. Young children seem to enjoy nudity and develop a sense of personal modesty as they age.
   d. Most children get upset seeing their parents naked.

10. Becoming an "askable parent" for your child's sexuality questions requires
   a. always being serious when discussing sexuality.
   b. not discussing anything that makes you uncomfortable.
   c. being careful not to make mistakes with information.
   d. letting your child know your values on a subject.

Media Menu

Film

Perceiving Gender Roles Teen, Slang for Having Sex Adolescent Body Image, Adolescent Sexual Risk Taking

Journal article

Shelby, L. (2003, February–March). Youth first: An integrated sexuality education program for pre-adolescents.

Web Resources

Here are sites where teens can write and get honest answers to their sexual health questions: www.teen-wire.com www.sexetc.org www.goaskalice.columbia.edu www.gurl.com www.puberty.org The following resources are of additional value to adolescents and adults:

Advocates for Youth

www.advocatesforyouth.org

Creates programs and promotes policies that help young people make informed and responsible decisions about their sexual and reproductive health with the purpose of preventing pregnancy and sexually transmitted diseases, including HIV. Large selection of links as well as links to minority youth sites. One section, which changes monthly, addresses contemporary issues that affect society and the way in which we live.

Coalition for Positive Sexuality

www.positive.org

A grassroots volunteer group started in 1992 to respond to the health crisis among Chicago teenagers. Teens receive information needed to make healthy decisions about sex, condom availability, and sex education. This site has FAQs with links to answers, national Web links, and information on sexuality, health issues, and birth control.

References

American Academy of Pediatrics(2001). Sexuality, Contraception and the Media, Pediatrics, 107, 191–194.

American Academy of Pediatrics(2001). Sexuality Education for Children and Adolescents, Pediatrics, 108, 498-502.

American Nurses Association. (1999). Sexual maturity rating scale [Online]. Available: www.nursingworld.org/ mods/archive/mod4/ceah2.htm.

Berne, L &Huberman, B (1999). European Approaches to Adolesecent Sexual Behavior and Responsibility. Advocates for Youth. Washington, D.C.

Billhartz, C. (2003, February 25). Teens don't realize risk of their oral sex practices. *CDC News Updates.*

Butler, J. (1999). *Gender trouble: Feminism and the subversion of identity.* New York: Routledge.

Carrera, M. (2003, October). The Children's Aid Society—Carrera Adolescent Sexuality and Pregnancy Prevention Program. Paper presented at the Network for Family Life Education's 20th Anniversary Conference, "20 Years of Great Sex(Ed): Lessons from the Past, Plans for the Future." Centers for Disease Control and Prevention. (1998, June 2). AIDS information [Online]. Available: www.cdc.gov/nchstp/hiv_aids/stats/cumulati.htm.

Centers for Disease Control and Prevention. (2012, June 6) Youth risk behavior surveillance-United States,2012.[online] Available: www.cdc.gov/Healthy Youth/yrbs/overall.htme].

Erikson, E. (1978). *Childhood and society* (2nd ed.). New York: Norton.

Elliott, V. (2002). Health risks make some fashion trends " don'ts.' American Medical News. Available: www.amednews.com.

Feijoo, A. (2001) Adolescents sexual health in Europe and the US—Why the difference?Advocates for Youth. Available : www.advocatesforyouth.com.

Ferber, S. G., Laudon, M., Kuint, J., Weller, A., & Zisapel, N. (2002, December). Massage therapy by mothers enhances the adjustment of circadian rhythms to the nocturnal period in full-term infants. *Journal of Developmental & Behavioral Pediatrics, 23*(6), 410.

Ford, C. S., & Beach, F. A. (1951). *Patterns of sexual behavior.* New York: Harper.

Forrest, J. D., & Silverman, J. (1989). What public school teachers teach about preventing pregnancy, AIDS, and sexually transmitted diseases. *Family Planning Perspectives, 21,* 65–72.

Globus, S. K. (2002, Spring). Touch me, I'm yours: The benefits of infant massage. *Special Delivery, 25*(1), 8.

Gordon, S., & Gordon, J. (1983). *Raising a child conservatively in a sexually permissive world.* New York: Simon & Schuster.

Gunter, T & Mcdowell, B. (2004). Body piercing: issues in adolescent health. Journal for Specialists in Pediatric Nursing, 9, 67-69.

Gurian, M. (1996). *The wonder of boys.* New York: Putnam.

Guttmacher Institute (2008, June) Facts on Young Men's Sexual And Reproductive Health[online] Available: www.guttmacher.org/pubs/fb/YMSRH.html

Haffner, D. (Editor) (1995). Facing Facts: Sexual Health for America's Adolescents, Sexuality Information Council of the United States.

Hall, C. S. (1954). *A primer of Freudian psychotherapy.* New York: Mentor.

Hatcher, J. L., & Scarpa, J. (2002, July). *Encouraging teens to adopt a safe, healthy lifestyle: A foundation for improving adult behaviors.* Child Trends Research Brief. Washington, DC: Child Trends.

Hedgepeth, E., & Lemich, J. (1996). *Teaching about sexuality and HIV.* New York: New York University Press.

Henry J. Kaiser Family Foundation. (2008, September). *Sexual Health of Adolescents and Young Adults in the United States* [Online]. Available: www.kff.org./womenshealth/upload/3040

Henry J. Kaiser Family Foundation (2011 January). Sexual Health of Adolescents and Young Adults in the United States. Available online: www. kff.org/womenshealth/3040.cfm

Henry J. Kaiser Family Foundation (2004). NPR/Kaiser/Kenndy School Poll-Sex education in America. Available: www.kff.org/daiserpolls/pomr012904oth.cfm

Henry J. Kaiser Family Foundation (2005, November). Number of sex scenes on TV nearly doubles since 1998. Available: www.Kff.org/entmedia/entmedai110905nr.dfm

Herdt, T. G., & Boxer, A. (1992). Introduction: Culture, history, and life course of gay men. In G. Herdt (Ed.), *Gay culture in America: Essays from the field.* Boston: Beacon.

Kaplan, H. S. (1974). *The new sex therapy.* New York: Brunner/Mazel.

Kinsey, A. C., Pomeroy, W. B., & Martin, C.E . (1948). *Sexual behavior in the human male.* Philadelphia: Saunders.

Kirby, D. (2007) Emerging Answers 2007: Research Findings on Programs to Reduce Teen Pregnancy and Sexually Transmitted Disease. Washington, D.C. National Campaign to Prevent Teen and Unplanned Pregnancy.

Laumann, E. O., Gagnon, J. H., Michael, R. T., & Michaels, S. (1994). *The social organization of sexuality: Sexual practices in the United States.* Chicago: University of Chicago Press.

Levine, J. (2002). *Harmful to minors: The perils of protecting children from Sex.* Minneapolis: University of Minnesota Press.

Lopiano, C. (2001). *Equity in women's sports: A health and fairness perspective* [Online]. Available: www.womenssportsfoundation.org.

Lorber, J. (2001). The social construction of gender. In P. S. Rothenberg (Ed.), *Race, class, gender in the United States* (pp. 47–56). New York: Freeman.

Manlove, J., Terry-Humen, E., Papillo, A., Franzetta, K., Williams, S., & Ryan, S. (2002, May). *Preventing teenage pregnancy, childbearing, and sexually transmitted diseases: What the research shows.* Child Trends Research Brief. Washington, DC: Child Trends.

Marshall, D. (1971). Sexual behavior on Mangaia. In D. Marshall & R. Suggs (Eds.), *Human sexual behavior: Variations in the ethnographic spectrum.* Englewood Cliffs, NJ: Prentice Hall.

Martinson, F. M. (1982). Against sexual retardation. *SIECUS Report,* 10(3), 3.41.

Maslow, A. (1970). *Motivation and personality* (2nd ed.). New York: Harper & Row.

McGrew, M., & Shore, W. (1991). The problem of teenage pregnancy. *Journal of Family Practice,* 31, 17–25.

Montague A. (1986). *Touching* (3rd ed.). New York: Columbia University Press.

Moran, J. (2000). *Teaching sex: The shaping of adolescents in the 20th century.* Cambridge, MA: Harvard University Press.

Newman, S., & Udry, J. (1988). Oral sex in adolescent populations. *Archives of Sexual Behavior,* 14, 41–16.

Parker-Pope, T. (2009, January 27). The Myth of Rampant Teenage Promiscuity. New York Times.

Parker-Pope, T. (2012, February 5). The Kids are more than all right. The New York Times.

Pazol, K., Creanga, A., Zane, S. Burley, K., Jamieson, D. (2012). Abortion surveillance-United States, 2009. Available :www.cdc.gov

Robbins, C. Schick, V. Reece, M. Herbenick, D. Sanders, S. Dodge, B. Fortenberry, D. (2011). Prevalence, frequency & association of masturbation with partnered sexual behaviors among U.S. adolescents. Archives of Pediatrics. Available online: http://archpedi.jamanetwork.com.exproxy.

Sanders, S. & Reinisch, J. (1999,January 20). Would you say you "had sex" if…? Journal of the American Medical Association, vol 281, no 3.

Santos, F & Phillips, A (2011, August 9). New York city will mandate sex education. The New York Times.

Savin-Williams, R., & Rodriguez, R.G. (1993). A developmental, clinical perspective on lesbian, gay male, and bisexual youth. In T. P. Gullets et al. (Eds.), *Adolescent sexuality.* Newbury Park, CA: Sage.

Schalet, A. (2012, April 6). Caring, romantic American boys. The New York Times.

Schlegel, A., & Barry, H. (1979). Adolescent initiation ceremonies: Cross-cultural codes. *Ethnology,* 18, 199–210.

Schlegel, A., & Barry, H. (1980). The evolutionary significance of adolescent initiation ceremonies. *American Ethnologist,* 7, 696–715.

Schooler, D. & Ward, M. (2006). Average Joes: Men's relationships with media, real bodies, and sexuality. Psychology of Men and Masculinity. Vol. 7, no. 1, 27-41.

Sonenstein, F. L., Pleck, J. H., & Hu, L. C. (1989). Sexual activity, condom use, and AIDS awareness among adolescent males. *Family Planning Perspectives,* 2(14), 152–158.

Strasburger, V.C. (1992) Adolescents and the media: five crucial issues. Adolescent Medicine, 4, 479-493.

The Alan Guttmacher Institute (1994) Sex and America's Teenagers, AGI, New York.

Troiden, R. (1988). *Gay and lesbian identity: A sociological analysis.* New York: General Hall.

Watson, J. *Behaviorism* (1970). New York: Norton.

Zamboni, B. Robinson, B. & Brockting, W. (2006). Body image and sexual functioning among bisexual women. Hawthorn Press.

4 Parents. Gov (2008, April). Dealing with Risky Behaviors and Other Challenges-Teen Pregnancy [online] Available:www.4parents. gov/sexrisky/teen_preg/teen_treg.html

chapter *six*

Adult Sexuality

Student Learning Objectives

After reading this chapter, students will be able to

- ♥ Describe the typical developmental tasks associated with young adulthood through older adulthood.
- ♥ Relate the findings of a variety of studies concerning the sexual behavior of college students and young adults.
- ♥ Assess a variety of living arrangements of the college years and young adulthood.
- ♥ Examine the major developmental tasks associated with adulthood.
- ♥ Assess a variety of sexual lifestyles in adulthood.
- ♥ Explain the impact of aging on sexual response and behavior.
- ♥ Describe the developmental course of long-term straight, gay, and bisexual relationships.
- ♥ Identify the major areas of discord and stress in marital and long-term intimate relationships.
- ♥ Discuss the effects of divorce and widowhood on adult sexuality.

activity teaser: What do you really need to have a successful relationship? Find out with the Personal Exploration Activity on page 196.

case study 6.1

Maria, aka Supermom

Maria, 35, identifies as white, Italian American.

Maria has been married for 15 years and has three children, ages 12, 10, and 7. Married as soon as she finished at the local community college with an associate's degree, she worked full-time for a year at an accounting office. As soon as she started having her kids, however, the idea of continuing to work and pay for day care made no financial sense. She and her husband decided she should stay home with the kids, and she could bring in some money doing child care in her home.

Once the kids were in school all day, Maria realized that she wanted to finish her own education and earn her bachelor's degree in accounting. All along she'd taken primary responsibility for the child rearing, cooking, cleaning, and chauffeuring the kids to appointments, activities, and play dates. She was an officer with the PTA, den mother for the Cub Scouts, Sunday school teacher, and all-around busy stay-at-home mom. The change of going back to school has markedly increased her stress but, in an odd way, also energized her.

Maria is finding that her relationships with her kids and husband are changing. She seems to have less time to give each the attention they want. Maria heads off for her own classes as soon as the kids are on their way. She carries a cell phone for emergencies and has been lucky that the kids have stayed well and she hasn't been beeped in the middle of her classes. Dinners aren't quite as nutritious as they had been, with more drive-through pickup meals than she'd like. She likes to get up at 5:30 A.M to enjoy the quiet of the morning before all the chaos sets in. That has been a good time for her to study while running the wash.

She and her husband find that they have to schedule "dates" now in order to be together as a couple. At the end of the week, it takes purposeful planning to keep the romance alive. It hasn't been easy, juggling the demands of motherhood, housework, and school, but everyone is adjusting. Maria feels she's making a successful passage into another phase of her life.

Critical Thinking

Can you identify some strategies Maria and her family could develop to reduce her workload and stress levels?

Intimacy A gradual process of sharing one's innermost feelings with another

The primary task we face as young adults, according to Erik Erikson (1978), is the development of **intimacy**—forming committed, intimate, loving relationships. We begin to move away from the adolescent focus on ourselves toward exploring mutually satisfying relationships. This stage emphasizes commitment, both in intimate relationships and in work.

This is an exciting time of life. We meet new friends, explore intimate, loving relationships, and test the waters for work and career possibilities. This is the first time many college students are living apart from their parents. It is a time of unparalleled freedom. Students who have mastered the developmental tasks of adolescence and childhood enter this period in their lives ready and eager to sample all that life has to offer. Maria's life, as described in Case Study 6.1, highlights the many demands of adulthood, some of which compete for time and attention.

Forming Friendships

New adult friendships form the basis of intimate relationships for many college students. Intimacy grows out of friendships as we become more trusting and comfortable with each other. In his book *Friendship,* Joel Block (1980) contends that humans are "wired" with a basic desire for contact with others. Our friendships, Block believes, are what make us whole. He says that friends enrich our existence and bond with us to form a conspiracy against the world. We like one another, understand each other, share interests, and have similar lifestyles or problems in life.

Although college literally throws people together (sharing a room or apartment, teams, class projects, and so on), what is it that draws friends together? Many friendships grow out of meeting people who share similar interests and experiences. We meet fellow students who have the same major, take the same classes, and join the same organizations. These similarities provide the initial attraction. If the attraction is strong enough, it provides the basis for spending more time together. As the friendship progresses, the friends share more time and experiences, reinforcing their commonality, deepening their bonds, and enriching their lives. Many people form their deepest friendships in college during young adulthood.

Friendship is a unique bond. Although it is fraught with entanglements that also characterize romantic relationships—competition, jealousy, and betrayal— it offers what Block calls "psychological space." Friendships are more open ended than relationships with family, mates, or lovers. Unlike these other, more intimate relationships, our friendships provide separate lives that allow time off and away from entanglements. Consequently, friends develop a greater tolerance for growth and change.

Dating and Intimate Relationships

Whereas friendships may be casual, intimacy by definition is deeply personal and trusting. Intimate relationships are characterized by sharing deep personal information. Intimacy grows out of friendship and usually is nurtured through dating.

We'll cover intimacy in detail in the chapter, "Intimate Relationships." Every society has some rituals or norms for pairing and courtship. Although the "rules" for dating and courtship vary from culture (and subculture) to culture, every society has traditions that it passes along from one generation to the next. Adults who came of age in the late 1960s and early 1970s in the United States vividly remember the differences between the rigid rules of the 1950s and the more liberated late 1960s and early 1970s. Prior to the cultural revolution of the 1960s, a young woman would not even consider asking a man out for a date. Men were expected to ask women out, pay for the evening's activities, and be responsible for picking up and dropping off their dates. Women were expected to wait for men to call them, even if a woman was interested and wanted to initiate contact. The popular media played out these and other traditional dating scenarios, and mothers and fathers passed them on to their daughters and sons. Everyone was assumed to be heterosexual, and sex was not a part of the evening's activities.

Friendships fill a special place in our lives.

© y. arcurs, 2010. Shutterstock, Inc.

The face of dating today looks dramatically different. As will be discussed in this chapter, it may be more comfortable for students to use the terms talking, *hooking up and seeing someone* rather than *date* (Crawford & Popp, 2003). Regardless of the term used, the behavior involved reflects greater role flexibility. A woman can initiate a date, pick up her date, and pay for the date. Straight, gay, and bisexual men and women have their own clubs, organizations, and dating services that make finding a partner easier and safer. In the past, bars and clubs for gay and lesbian women were disguised and subject to harassment from bullies and the police. Today they are more accepted and open, with directories available identifying various facilities, particularly in urban areas.

Although the rituals and rules of dating change over time, the purpose of dating hasn't changed much. Dating is a mechanism for developing intimate relationships. Intimate relationships, in turn, influence both sexual behavior and living patterns.

> ❧ *Emotional and Social Wellness* ❧
>
> The emotional dimension of wellness requires that we acknowledge the full range of emotions associated with our changing roles and responsibilities. Most of the major developmental tasks associated with the adult stages of our lives are part of social wellness: forming intimate relationships, committing ourselves to others and to our work, being productive—in relationships, work, and so on. Understanding our emotional responses and developing interpersonal social skills become critical as we navigate the challenges associated with adulthood.
>
> The social legacy we develop and leave behind can be one of a caring child, loving partner, and/or devoted parent. We can move through the stages of our relationships eagerly anticipating the changes and tasks that await us. We can also move through life and relationships with a self-centeredness that obscures all propensities for caring, sharing, and nurturing. Adulthood and older age may be viewed as opportunities for continued growth, reflection, and self-acceptance; for some, this stage of life may be marked by bitterness and regret. Overall health is enhanced by positive attitudes and a willingness to remain socially engaged.

College Sexual Standards

Many people equate intimacy with sexual activity and love, yet they are three separate entities. A person can be intimate and sexual with another person but not love that person. One can be in love, but with limited sexual involvement. And a person can be sexual with another but neither love nor be intimate with that person. For some the best possible combination of all three would be to be sexual with someone toward whom you feel both intimate and loving.

Research on college sexual mores has often focused on students' attitudes toward "premarital sex," defined as premarital intercourse, and "double standards" for males and females, specifically looking at how males and females engage in the same behaviors but are judged differently. Sexual

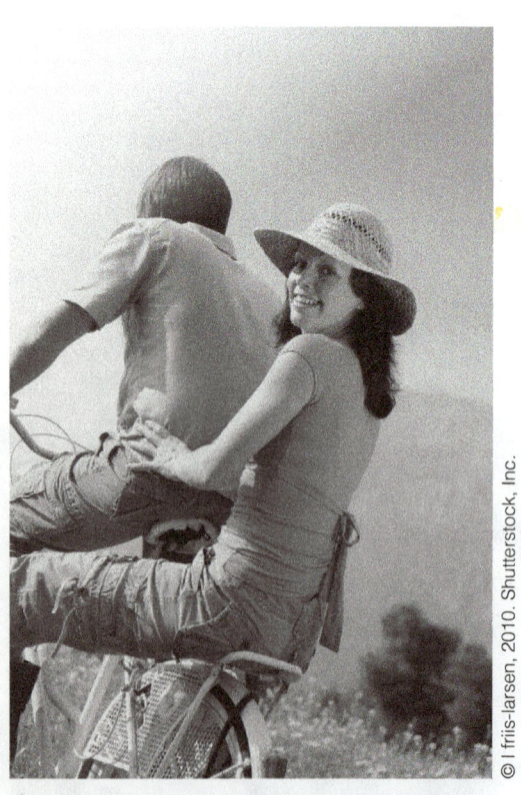

Dating provides an opportunity to get to know each other.

© l friis-larsen, 2010. Shutterstock, Inc.

standards may have been prefaced with such adjectives as *permissive* or *traditional*. The primary focus was when the behaviors took place relative to marriage or a commitment to marry.

A review of the research confirms that sexual attitudes may have become more egalitarian in recent years, yet there are still differences for males and females. Females may be judged for having had sex at an early age, having had many partners in the past, and for having sex outside a committed relationship. Males may also judge behaviors differently when seeking dating partners as opposed to long-term partners (Crawford & Popp, 2003).

Because of sampling issues, it is more difficult to assess lesbian, bisexual, and gay student mores. The process of "coming out," finding a partner, and being free to date openly is of paramount concern to the gay, lesbian, and bisexual community of students. Although working toward committed relationships may be a goal, judging behaviors as "premarital" obviously doesn't work. Like their heterosexual peers, however, gay, lesbian, and bisexual individuals may judge a potential partner's past sexual history.

All students, irrespective of sexual orientation, however, need to assess their personal levels of interest, sexual involvement, and commitment as they form pairs with others. Engaging in behavior that is consistent with one's personal values and feeling comfortable in sexual situations is essential. When our behaviors do not match our personal values, we often experience the effects of guilt. Guilt is a signal to us that we need to reevaluate our behavior and or values and make changes so that our behavior consistently reflects our values.

Hooking Up

The term **hooking up** is often used to describe a variety of sexual interactions that take place on a casual basis, often with alcohol part of the picture. Students may refer to having "hooked up" with someone over a weekend, yet the specifics of that interaction may be unclear. Two individuals may have met at a party or bar and engaged in some form of sexual behavior without the need for commitment (Lambert, Kahn, & Apple, 2003). Hooking up may be defined as "a sexual encounter between two people who may or may not know each other well, but who usually are not seriously dating" (Lambert et al., 2003, p. 129). When asked about experiences with hooking up, researchers found college students citing the occurrence of petting below the waist, oral sex, and sexual intercourse as part of the behaviors included in the definition (Paul, McManus, & Hayes, 2000). This vagueness of the term hooking up may be part of the appeal of the term. Friends can share that they did something sexual without being specific (Bogle, 2008).

In addition to the term not being specific, males and females who hook up may have differing expectations of what sexual behaviors they want to engage in. Alcohol further complicates the situation, which may lead to participation in sexual behaviors that are not desired. Students may have "bad hooking-up experiences," where the next day they regret the behavior and do not care to even talk with the sexual partner. At the most negative would be cases where the interaction involved force and qualified

Hooking up A sexual encounter between two people who may or may not know each other well and are not seriously dating

as sexual assault. One study found that college students thought their peers were more comfortable with hooking up than they themselves were. Men were more comfortable with hooking-up behaviors than women, yet men were less comfortable than women believed them to be, and women were less comfortable than men believed them to be. Overall, although it may appear that hooking up is the norm for college campuses, peer pressure and misperceptions of other's level of activity and comfort may be part of the picture (Lambert et al., 2003).

Students have also described having "friends with benefits." In those situations, a comfortable friendship exists with consensual sexual activity. There is no apparent expectation that the two will see themselves or be viewed by others as a couple.

Sexual Behavior Among College Students

Although a common perception is that hooking up is the universal behavior at colleges and universities, the data do not support this belief. A valuable source of information on sexual behavior of college students is the American College Health Association's yearly assessment of college behaviors. Data for the 2012 survey were gathered from 98,059 surveys taken at 157 colleges and universities. In 2012, almost 1 out of 3 (29%) students reported having 0 sexual contacts in the past year while almost 1 out of 2 (45%) reported only 1 contact. Less than 1 in 10 (9%) reported having 4 or more contacts. The researchers included oral sex, vaginal and anal sex as a contact. The number was similar in the 2003 American College Health Association survey when 75% of students reported having 0-1 sexual contacts during the past year. However, only 14% of students thought the typical student had only 0-1 sexual contacts in the past year (American College Health Association, 2012).

The perception that all college students have had sexual intercourse is also not accurate. Almost 1 in 3 (30%) college students report never having had vaginal sex while 1 in 2 (50%) reported having done so within the last 30 days. Similarly 27% of students have never tried oral sex while 45% have experienced oral sex within the last 30 days. The percentage of students who had never had anal sex was even higher at 76% (American College Health Association, 2012). It is common for us to believe that everyone has more sexual partner, more friends, more money and other things than we have. Examining actual data about sexual behavior of college students can help in understanding where the truth really lies.

Anal sex is included in sexual activity for some college students. In a recent study of college women, 1 in 3 (32%) of the sample had engaged in anal intercourse and almost 1 in 2 (45%) had engaged in receptive anal penetration with a sex toy or finger. Of concern is that 68% who had engaged in anal intercourse never used a condom and only 26% always used a condom. Those who engage in anal intercourse typically had their first intercourse at an early age and have a higher number of sexual partners and sexually transmitted diseases (Flannery, Ellingson, Votaw, & Schaefer, 2003). The American College of Health National College Health Assessment found that 5.0% of students report having had anal intercourse in the last month.

(American College Health Association (2012). With these numbers engaging in anal sex, promotion of safe anal sex needs to be included when discussing sexual activity. In Chapter 8, healthy sex hints 8.5 illustrates how to safely enjoy anal sex.

Living Arrangements of College Students

Living arrangements of college students vary, determined by personal finances, whether they are commuting or living on campus, whether living with a friend or romantic partner, and so forth. At some universities, the majority of undergraduates live in either dormitories or apartments. Other institutions have minimal housing for full-time students, are more accommodating to the commuting student, and have sizeable populations who attend school part time. Whereas the married undergraduate student was the exception years ago, today many students are both married and older, some with young children. Consequently, more colleges are finding the need to include day care facilities on campus. The National Coalition for Campus Childcare has surveyed campuses to determine the availability of child care for their students and employees. At the majority of institutions, students participate in the centers in a variety of ways from student teachers, paid work/study students, unpaid student observers, researchers, and other roles. As more nontraditional students are drawn to undergraduate and graduate education, the need for such facilities grows (Thomas, 2000).

Single

Many college students are single and live off-campus, either at home with their parents or in shared living environments. The current pattern where young adults remain living with parents has been tied to trends in delaying marriage, increasing percentage of never-marrieds, the poor ecomony, high cost of housing, and the need for more people to continue education.

The U.S. Bureau of the Census (2002) reports that there is a substantial increase in the proportion of "young, never-married" adults. For example, in the past three decades, the proportion of women who have never married doubled for those ages 20 to 24 and more than tripled for women ages 30 to 34 (Fields, 2001). The trend has continued with only 1 in 5 (20%) of those ages 18-29 being married. This is a major drop from 1960 when almost 2 out of 3 (59%) were married. The age of marriage has also increased with 26.5 years being the average age for women to marry and for men 28.7 (Cohen, Passel, Wang, & Livingston, 2011).

Cohabitating

Cohabitating is the most common type of relationship among women and men in their twenties and will precede more than half of all marriages (Scott, Schelar, Manlove, & Cui, 2009; Jay, 2012). The rates of cohabitation among college age people have dramatically increased in recent years. In a study by Child Trends, a nonprofit research group, 1 in 5 young adults was unmarried and living with a romantic partner (Scott et al, 2009). Of those who cohabit, half will marry within three years and if they are college

Cohabitation Living together without being married

personal exploration activity
Relationship Contract: How Much Am I Willing to Compromise?

The goal of this activity is to help you decide what you really need to have a healthy, happy, and supportive long-term relationship.

The following questions could be made into a relationship contract by which you and your future long-term partner agree to abide. Answer the questions as if you could have your ideal in the relationship. If you are in a relationship now, ask your partner to do the same and then compare your answers. This should cause a lively debate.

Freedom

Will we still maintain our outside friendships? Do we have the freedom to make new friends? Are we free to spend time with our same and opposite-sex friends without our partner? In what types of activities can we participate? Will we participate in sexual relationships outside this one?

Money

How will we make sure money is not a problem for our relationship? Will we have a budget, and, if so, what do we do if one does not follow the budget? Will we keep our own money or have a joint bank account? What will be our financial priorities?

Chores

How will we divide our responsibilities so that neither of us feels overwhelmed or taken advantage of?

Who will do the laundry, pay the bills, clean the house, take care of the yard, shop for groceries, cook, buy gifts for our families, run the errands?

Free Time

Will we spend all of our free time together? What types of activities will we do to keep the relationship from becoming boring? Will we spend most of our free time with friends, family, or alone?

Children

Will we have children? How many? What lengths are we willing to go to if one of us is infertile?

Will one of us stay home to raise the children? Will we raise them as a team?

graduates, the marriage will last at least 10 years (Roberts, 2010). Motivations for cohabitating include testing compatibility, spending more time together and sharing the financial burden. Data from one study showed very positive views toward cohabitation among those 20-24. Fifty seven percent agreed with the following statement: "It is all right for an unmarried couple to live together even if they are not interested in considering marriage" and only 25% disagreed. (Scott et al, 2009).

Married

Today, most undergraduates who plan on marriage wait until they graduate to marry. Recent data from the Child Trends study finds only 1 in 5 college age respondents were married. These low rates of marriage reflect the trend toward waiting to marry. In 1960 the median age for marriage for men was 23 and by 2006 rose to 29. A similar trend can be seen for women whose median age for marriage in 1960 was 20 compared to 27 in 2011 (Scott et al, 2009: Cohen, 2011).

Adult Sexual Behavior

We will extend the discussion of sexuality during the college and young adult years into adulthood.

The National Health and Social Life Survey (NHSLS) conducted by Laumann, Gagnon, Michael, and Michaels (1994) remains a critical source of data for understanding adult sexual behavior. Their research relied on random sampling, well constructed survey instruments, and interviews. Controversy about the "need" to study adult sexual behavior—even for its public health value—led to congressional opponents effectively stopping National Institute of Health funding for the initial survey designed in the late 1980s (Laumann & Michael, 2001). Although it would be exciting and valuable to have periodic, government-sponsored, comprehensive studies of adult sexual behavior, such efforts have not been widely funded. Therefore the data from the NHSLS study continue to provide a portrait of adult behavior.

Laumann and Youm (2001) developed a model to explain the factors that influence a person's mode of sexual expression. There are three areas where individual attributes are key. First, **individual preferences** for specific sexual activities and level of sexual interest must be considered. Great variability exists from person to person as to what they want to do and how strong their drive is to engage in a specific activity. Those preferences may be different when a college student has moved from one partner to another, changed after a negative experience, and so forth. Second, *physical health* becomes important; a person may or may not be able to participate in activities due to impaired physical and/or mental health. Depression and erectile dysfunction, for example, are two conditions that are known to interfere with sexual activity. *Social competence* as a third factor refers to the skills and resources needed to initiate and maintain social relationships. Individuals have to be able to communicate with a partner as well as be able to compete effectively for the attention of a potential partner. Social competence would seem to be a learned set of behaviors yet certainly can be influenced by how one is feeling about her- or himself at a set period of time.

Finally, the model posits that the three individual attributes jointly affect the social *opportunities* individuals confront when attempting to establish sexual relationships: who do you meet, where do you go, what are your social networks, how does geographic context affect socializing, and so on. All together, the four factors then affect what modes of sexual expression will result (Laumann & Youm, 2001).

Individual preferences Physical health status Social competence Social opportunities Sexual expression

❧ *Physical and Intellectual Wellness* ❧

As we move through adulthood, we continue to be responsible for maintaining and enhancing our physical well-being. The experiences we've had earlier on may "catch up," making physical health no longer something to be taken for granted. The choices we made, behaviors we adopted, and lifestyles we lived will either enhance or undermine our sexuality. Abusing our bodies and letting our physical well being decline will have a negative impact on our sexuality. Everything from body image to sexual response to overall energy level may decline. This will impact negatively on our social relationships with lovers, spouses, employers, and others. Better body image, sexual response, and energy level will help us meet the demands of our ever-changing sexuality. This state of wellness will not only enhance our personal functioning but also positively influence our relationships.

The ability to gather information, critically analyze it, and make good decisions is a hallmark of high-level mental functioning. Rational thinking and logical reasoning can help us understand the nature of our ever-changing sexuality as we pass through young adulthood into adulthood and older age. Having reasonable expectations about our sexuality, based on solid information, can guide us in decision making. It also can help us avoid unrealistic expectations about relationships and sexuality that are likely to lead to personal unhappiness and dissatisfaction with partners. It is important to determine the personal value of the information to which we're exposed —what relates to us, what can constructively impact our sexual health.

Masturbation in Adulthood

Laumann et al. (1994) have examined masturbation in light of its relational context. They believe that masturbation, like all forms of sexual expression, is driven by a variety of social and biological factors throughout the life cycle and can have complementary, supplementary, or independent status with reference to partnered sex. This means that masturbation can enhance partnered sexual activity. It also can be an additional source of sexual expression within the context of the relationship, and last, it can serve as a solitary source of sexual pleasure independent of partnered sex. The level of masturbation is not related to relationship status.

Rather than reinforce the stereotype that masturbation is a substitute for partnered sex, this finding shows that this isn't necessarily so. The frequency of individual masturbation is as likely to be a function of social factors and a variety of reasons as it is the availability of alternative outlets.

Sexual Intercourse Among Adults

Laumann et al. (1994) summarize the three main levels of sexual activities for adults: About 35 percent have sex with a partner two or more times per week, about 35 percent have partnered sex one to a few times per month, and the remaining 30 percent have partnered sex only a few times a year. These rates were fairly consistent across all racial, ethnic, and religious groups. About 7 to 8 percent of the respondents had partnered sex four or more times a week, and about 10 percent reported having had no sex at all during the previous year. This response, the researchers point out, paints quite a different picture of adult sexual behavior than the one portrayed in the popular media. The sexual activity of most Americans is much more modest than the frequency and expectations created by the media.

An additional finding concerning partnered sexual activity related to the number of sex partners during the past year. The number of different sex partners in the past year declines with age. In general, the largest percentage of respondents in each age cohort reported only one sex partner during the past year. Two moderating factors seem to be marital and cohabiting status. Young, single, non cohabiting men and women were much more likely than all other groups to report two or more different partners during the previous year.

Adult Relationships

One of the major developmental tasks of adulthood is the continuation and deepening of the commitment to relationships that began in young adulthood. For many Americans, this means a commitment to marriage and a family. For others, the commitment to someone else does not involve marriage but, instead, cohabitation. This is also a period frequently marked by divorce or the death of a spouse. In the remaining part of this chapter, we'll examine the changing nature of adult relationships.

Singlehood

A significant percentage of Americans are choosing to remain single for life. Reasons for remaining single include changes in sexual standards, greater financial independence for women, changing economic times, and shifting conceptions of marriage. Even being a single parent has lost much of it stigma and presently, one third of all births are to single women (Bumpass, 2004). Sometimes, postponing marriage results in an inadvertent slide into permanent singlehood (Cavanaugh, 1993). As people postpone marriage, they often realize that they can live satisfying lives being single. There is less urgency to marry, especially if they feel no desire to have children.

Regardless of the reasons, most people who chose to remain single for life reported that they were quite happy. Contrary to popular beliefs, most singles are not lonely, and they develop alternative social patterns based on friendships and non- marital love relationships. The satisfaction that singles derive from these relationships and their careers is more than adequate for their happiness (Phillis & Stein, 1983).

Cohabitation

Cohabitation in the United States has increased an amazing 1,500 percent in the last fifty years (Jay, 2012). Over half of those under age 45 have lived with someone of the opposite sex and when they marry, fifty percent of all couples have lived together. One often reads about the higher divorce rate of those who live together before marriage. Bumpass (2004) points out that during the period when cohabitation became more popular, the divorce rate remained constant. He proposes that "many of the relationships that at an earlier time would have resulted in marriage and then divorce now dissolve prior to marrying." This testing of relationships may have, in actuality, helped the divorce rate stop rising and level off (Bumpass, 2004). Others argue that cohabitating is not risk free. An important risk of cohabitating is "sliding, not deciding." Couples may go from dating and sleeping over to sleeping over more often and then to cohabitating, thus sliding into the arrangement. There is no discussion about why they want to live together and what it really means. Often the standards for a live in partner are lower than they would be for a spouse. However, after living together for some time it becomes difficult to disengage from the arrangement. Couples can spend months and years in a relationship that is unfulfilling and unhappy. To avoid this trap, couples can discuss their intentions before moving in and view living together as a step toward marriage. This change may help some couples avoid making the mistake of living with someone who does not really meet their needs. In a poll by the Pew Research Center, two thirds of Americans believed that living together is a step toward marriage. This is indeed good news since couples will be more selective in choosing the live in partner making the marriage more likely to succeed (Jay, 2012).

Unmarried adult couples who live together face similar relationship challenges of those who marry. They must learn to effectively communicate, share, compromise, argue, and make decisions about money, sex, and household labor. Parenting is also a challenge since two fifths of births to unmarried women are to those in cohabiting, two parent families (Bumpass, 2004). The reasons for adults living together but not marrying are many and varied. Generally speaking, three forms of cohabitation are casual or temporary involvement, preparation or testing for marriage, and a substitute for or alternative to marriage.

Marriage

Marriage is a life goal for the majority of those who have never been married. In fact, almost 2 in 3 (61%) of never married men and women want to get married (Cohn, 2013) However, the Pew Research Centers' analysis of the latest census data finds a record low number of adults are married, barely half. In 1960, 3 in 4 (72%) of those age 18 and older were married compared to only 1 in 2 (51 %) today. If this trend continues, in only a few years the number of married adults will be less than half. The data analysis also found a steep five percent drop in new marriages between 2009 and 2010. The poor economy may or may not be a factor in this steep decline. The same changes are also occurring worldwide in other advanced post-industrial societies. These worldwide declines continue in both good and bad economic times so are probably unrelated to the economy. Whether the young are abandoning marriage or postponing it is, as of yet, unknown. In the U.S., even the number of those never married has declined. In 1960, 85% of Americans had ever been married compared to only 72% today (Cohen, Passe, Wang, & Livingstonl, 2011).

There are so many options for living arrangements that may be more appealing than marriage to some. As we discussed earlier, more Americans are living together and also more are also living alone or living as single parents.

The expectations for marriage are much different today than for previous generations. Historically, marriages were intended to provide a stable economic unit in which to rear children. Today, people expect marriage to fulfill their social, emotional, financial, and sexual needs. When people marry, they find that many of these expectations are unrealistic and cannot be fully realized. This discovery can lead to frustration, disillusionment, separation, and divorce. They also find that marriage is hard work. Even under the best of circumstances and with a good match in a partner, successful marriage requires continual nurturing, assessment, communication, commitment, and willingness to change. Perhaps we should consider marriage as similar to driving a car. The relationship needs continual attention and small adjustments to make it healthy and strong, If neglected the small issues may become large enough to derail a good relationship just as one may drive off the road if not making small steering corrections.

The Developmental Course of Marriage

Berry and Williams (1987) propose a developmental model of marriage across adulthood. In the early, honeymoon phase, marriage is at its most intense. The two spend considerable time together, talking, sharing interests and leisure, establishing their roles within the relationship, arguing, and making up. As the honeymoon phase begins to wind down and the couple settles into a routine, the intensity of the honeymoon phase diminishes and, along with it, marital satisfaction. A big reason for this outcome is the birth of children. Children result in less time available for the mate and the relationship.

Marital happiness reaches its lowest point during the midlife phase of the relationship, which also coincides with adolescence of the couple's children. A myriad of problems—ranging from financial issues to coping with teenagers to changing roles for husband and wife—contribute to the unrest.

Happiness begins to rebound when the children leave home as adults. This frees up time and money, and the couple has rediscovered privacy to reestablish the things in their relationship that provide pleasure, as well as investigate new things together.

Marital happiness continues to rise in the later adult years and carries over into retirement. Depending on a number of factors ranging from health to retirement income, the couple continues to enjoy their freedom and in some cases relationships with their children's families and their grandchildren.

Overall, this sampling of films highlights the cultural variations around weddings. What is as important, however, is that the themes of love, family, and working through conflict are underscored. Whether the couples live "happily ever after" is a question better left to fairy tales.

Obviously, not all couples fit the Berry and Williams model. Other variables, such as physical illness, children living at home into their 30s, and loss of jobs, can strain the relationship. In some cases, children growing up and leaving the nest magnify problems in the relationship that lead to divorce. Not all relationships flourish in retirement. Sometimes work serves as a buffer between a couple and their problems.

Even with all the up and downs of marital happiness, it is well documented that married people have a significantly higher level of happiness than their single, divorced and widowed counterparts. Even throughout the lifecycle of the marriage, the happiness of the married persons remains significantly greater than their unmarried counterparts (Easterling, 2003). Economist have attempted to put a financial value on the happiness brought by different life events. They estimate that getting married brings the same amount of happiness as having an extra one hundred thousand dollars of income per year (Clark & Oswald, 2002).

Monogamy Married to only one person at a time

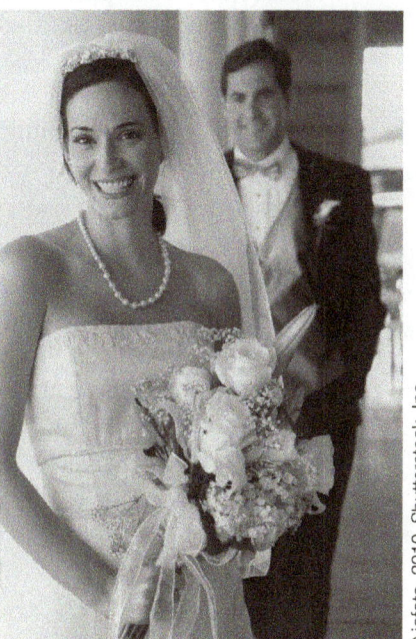

Weddings are important rituals that symbolize hope and lifelong commitment.

sex in society 6.1
Learning by Laughing at the Movies

Laughter is one human behavior that is shared by people all over the world. It represents a positive emotion, with the power to reduce stress, relieve pain, and encourage healing. Laughter stimulates the heart, alters the rhythms of breathing, and positively impacts the immune system (Hales, 2003). We can laugh at a joke. We can laugh at a situation watched on television or on the big screen. The power of creating laughter, along with making people feel good, is that wonderful lessons about life can be transmitted in a nonthreatening manner.

Many movies have been made with central themes on the institution of marriage. Some of the recent selections listed here illustrate how film can tackle various crises and sexual themes with humor, reality, and diversity.

La Cage aux Folles (1978) is a French-made film, later turned into a Broadway musical, that humorously deals with a gay couple whose son, much to their chagrin, is planning a marriage to a woman. The woman is the daughter of a conservative minister of morality for the government. Through the meeting of the parents and ensuing charades, humor is used to illustrate basic parental concern for children's happiness. Students may be more familiar with the American version of the film entitled *The Birdcage*, starring Robin Williams.

The Wedding Banquet (1997) shows the culture clash and secrecy involved when the parents of a rich Taiwanese family visit their son in New York City, not knowing he is gay and living with his partner. To help a female tenant who is an immigrant in need of a green card, a fictitious marriage is arranged. The film uses humor to address issues of love, marriage, homosexuality, and cultural traditions.

Meet the Parents (2000) focuses on the introduction of the male character to his fiancée's somewhat unwelcoming parents. The father, in particular, is very uncomfortable that his possible future son-in-law is a male nurse. The macho father views the female-identified profession negatively, not to mention the overall clumsiness of the man.

Monsoon Wedding (2001) looks at the marriage rituals among upper-middle-class Indians. Although the culture subscribes to arranged marriages, the influences of Western culture on the values of family members add to the culture clash.

Far from Heaven (2002) is not a comedy but rather an intense look at the breakup of an upper-class family as the wife learns of her husband's homosexuality. Although a "period piece," it teaches how oppressive and secretive being gay yet trying to live the heterosexual life was in the 1950s.

My Big Fat Greek Wedding (2002) depicts culture clash at its finest. A Greek American woman, hoping to break free from her overbearing family, falls in love with an upper-class non-Greek male. The differences in the families are extreme, from the Greeks being joyous and involved in every aspect of each other's lives, to the stereotypical WASP family, being overwhelmed by the outgoing, involved way of the soon-to-be in-laws.

Ingredients for a Healthy, Happy Relationship

There are many ingredients that make up a happy, long term relationship and none is more important than the choice of a partner. The romantic partner must have some of the characteristics needed to make the relationship a happy, healthy one. Once the excellent ingredients- the partner—are chosen there are some essential characteristics that help the relationship succeed. Equality between the partners will encourage them to work as a team and to treat each other with respect. Respect for one another helps couples treat each other as best friends and keeps the relationship positive. Best friends often play together, laugh and have fun, which are other key ingredients to the success of a relationship.

John and Julie Gottman have done years of research with couples and can predict with 90% accuracy which couples will have successful relationships after just three hours of listening to their interactions. They suggest seven principles to keep the relationship strong. First principle is for couples to be intimately familiar with each other's life. Each should know what their partner loves and what bothers them. Second principle is that it is essential to nurture fondness and admiration for one another. This is helpful during arguments and during the difficult times. Third, couples should turn toward one another when looking for support or humor rather than toward others. Fourth, the happiest and most stable marriages have equal sharing in power and decision making. The traditional husband role of making all the decisions may contribute to the deterioration of the relationship.

Fifth, all couples have problems that need to be solved and the Gottmans suggest good manners and the following four steps will help couples solve these issues with grace. Step one is to soften the start up- state feelings without blame. Second step is to make and accept repair attempts. This involves de-escalating the fight and expressing appreciation. Fights can bring on a flooding of emotion so step three is to take a break to sooth and distract yourself and your spouse. Finally, compromise is essential.

For the last two principles of a healthy relationship, couples need to overcome gridlock of repeated conflicts by honoring each other's dreams and goals. And finally, create customs and rituals that make you a family or a team (Gottman & Gottman, 2012).

Sexual Satisfaction and Happiness

Sexual satisfaction and happiness in marital and other partnered relationships have two dimensions: physical satisfaction and emotional happiness (Laumann et al., 1994). The relationship between the two is complex with sexual satisfaction being one of the most important components of marital happiness. (Litzinger & Gordon, 2005). Highly satisfying physical relationships usually bring with them high emotional happiness. High levels of emotional satisfaction, however, don't necessarily indicate high levels of physical satisfaction. It has been shown that when couples are good at communicating, sexual satisfaction fails to contribute significantly to marital happiness (Litzinger & Gordon, 2005). Overall, a fairly high proportion of men (47 percent) and women (41 percent) described their partnership as extremely physically pleasurable with satisfaction varying with age. Among men, the level of physical satisfaction was high to begin with and increased with age. Among women however, high levels of physical satisfaction dropped significantly after age 55. Findings are similar regarding emotional satisfaction. Laumann et al. account for this by explaining that men in their 50s and older are more likely than similar-aged women to acquire new sex partners after divorce. Equitable sharing of housework appears to improve marital happiness and the couples sex life. When husbands share housework, their wives feel more affection for them and have a higher interest in sex (Coleman, 2008).

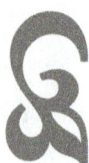

healthy sex hints 6.1

Lessons from Happy Marriages

In a happy marriage:

1. The partners find their prime source of joy in each other but maintain separate identities.
2. They are generous and giving out of love, not because they expect repayment or are keeping score.
3. The partners enjoy a healthy and vigorous sexual relationship.
4. The partners "fight" in a constructive way, airing feelings and frustrations without attacking or blaming the other.
5. The partners communicate with each other openly and honestly.
6. The partners trust each other.
7. The partners treat each other with respect.
8. Both talk about their future together. They have mutual goals.
9. The best marriages tend to be ones in which the partners are similar in these ways:
   - ethnicity
   - locality (geography; urban or rural)
   - maturity (emotional and social)
   - goals and ideals
   - intelligence levels
   - amount of education
   - economic level and financial resources
   - social strata
   - value system
   - religious beliefs

Common Marital Issues and Problems

All relationships have issues and problems that will need to be resolved to make the relationship flourish. Couples who want to resolve their problems but don't know where to start can benefit tremendously from couple's counseling. Sometimes, problems that seemed insurmountable before counseling seem workable after seeing a therapist. Early relationship counseling can help solve the problems before couples do so much damage that the relationship is impossible to repair or save. Premarital counseling can help solve issues even before the marriage begins.

The potential sources of trouble over the life span of a marriage are varied and range from loss of initial sexual passion, poor communication, to financial issues to economic instability in retirement. Some relationships are doomed from the start because they are based on an ideal that never can be fulfilled. Many expectations are unrealistic as a

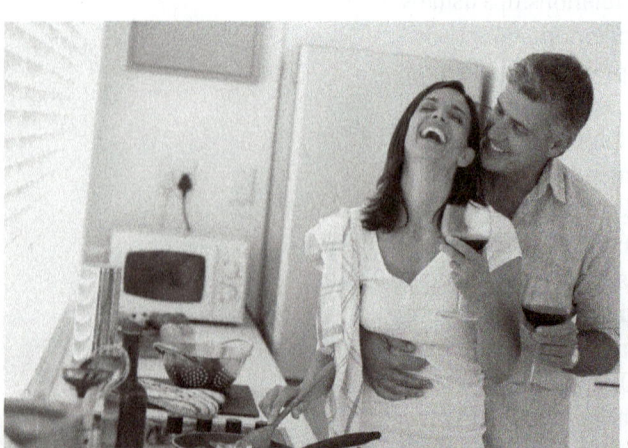

More than half of all married couples report being extremely sexually satisfied with their sexual relationship.

© y. arcurs, 2010. Shutterstock, Inc.

sex in society 6.2

Midlife Crisis or Middle-Age Myth?

You have heard the story before. A happy, successful 45-year-old businessman quits his job, leaves his wife and kids, and runs off to Tahiti with his 25-year-old personal trainer. Or, perhaps it is the 40-year-old mother of two facing the "empty nest" who jumps into her convertible BMW with her 25-year-old co-worker and heads west into the sunset in a torrid blaze of passionate sex.

These and other "midlife crises" that have been popularized by the print and film media make interesting stories and pose a romantic solution to many of the difficult issues that appear during middle age. In real life, however, relatively few people experience such catastrophic, radical changes. New information fueled by long-term research on aging is showing that middle age is the very best time of life. It is a developmental stage unlike most others, because it is not tied particularly to changes in the body, such as early childhood, adolescence, and old age. Midlife is characterized more by psychological adaptations and is reality based.

By midlife, many of the stressful questions that faced us as young adults are answered, such as, Will anyone ever love me? Will this marriage work out? Will I ever find a job? What kind of lifestyle can I afford to lead? By midlife, most people have found love. If they are married, they are more likely to stay married (the overwhelming majority of divorces occur within the first 6 to 8 years of marriage). They have settled into a job and have a pretty good idea of where they are headed (most professionals who are going to "make it" have made it by this time). They have a good sense of their earning capacity and therefore can gauge the kind of lifestyle they can expect.

Although the myth of midlife is that this period is characterized by unrest, discomfort, dissatisfaction, and upheaval, the reality is that it is a comfortable, satisfying time. It is a time to enjoy the rewards of 10 to 20 years of scuffling. It is a time to push a little easier at work, to get off a little early to watch your kid's Little League game. It is a time to focus on vacations and social gatherings, to take a class to learn how to paint or improve your backhand. It is a time to lighten up a little.

Midlife is a period of gradual adjustment, not tumultuous change. It gradually unfolds and is based on several adjustments to reality. For most people it is based in reality, not fantasy. Those most likely to experience a true crisis (about 5 percent) are people who generally have experienced similar crises in all developmental stages of their lives. Their lives are based on unrealistic (therefore unrealized) notions and expectations. One of the major criticisms of earlier studies of midlife is that they were based on small numbers of case studies of atypical populations (mostly affluent, professional, and white). In the recent cross-sectional studies of more representative samples of Americans, researchers found that the average person's midlife adjustment is based on reality. People gradually adjust their expectations to fit the reality of their lives. By the time they settle into midlife, they have learned to make the best of what they have and are not constantly longing for things that are beyond their reach.

Source: R. Blonna, *Coping with Stress in a Changing World* (3rd ed.) (Dubuque, IA: McGraw-Hill,), p. 537.

result of immature or romantic perceptions. The continuing intensity and bliss of romantic love cannot be expected to continue throughout marriage.

The early passionate, romantic love needs to evolve into mature love. Even though the early passion has cooled, mature love and long term relationships still require romance, play and adventure to flourish. Couples need to remember to treat their partner as someone who is important to them, just as they did in the early stages of the relationship. This includes playing together, having fun and laughing, and doing special things together.

As we all know, good communication is essential for a happy, healthy relationship. Communication includes not only working on issues but also sharing positive emotions with one another. Relationships can wither from a lack of expressions of recognition, caring, tenderness, and compassion. Giving positive affirmations of love and joy in the relationship helps us feel wanted and important to our partner. It is just natural to enjoy and to respond better to those we feel like us.

Communication problems can be summarized as stemming from a lack of communication skills, the lack of desire to communicate, or both. The easier problem to remedy is the skill-based one. If one or both members of the relationship do not know how to communicate clearly and effectively or don't know how to fight fairly, they can learn—assuming they have the desire. If either or both don't have the desire to work things out, no amount of skill will improve the situation.

Loss of desire to talk and work things out is a warning sign of a deteriorating relationship. Sometimes a vicious cycle begins in which a lack of skill in communicating leads to a deteriorating relationship, which feeds a loss of desire. Low levels of desire keep the cycle going by not having the interest in talking about problems in the relationship. In the last case, one or both members may want to try to communicate in general but think the problem is too difficult to talk about. Or they may want to try to communicate more effectively but lack the energy and commitment necessary to work out their problems.

Another issue, money—or, more precisely, what money means to each partner —is a major source of stress in long-term relationships. Financial counseling can be an important part of the premarital counseling and preparation for marriage. One financial firm that does premarital financial counseling has couples explore the topics of ancestry, credit, control and affluence as part of the counseling. In examining ancestry, couples look at how their parents dealt with money, how that impacts each and how that will impact the relationship. Many of our money behaviors are learned and money can become a very emotional issue. Credit history is the next order of business so credit reports are shared between the couple. Credit reports reveal past mistakes and bad habits that may need to be changed. Control of money is the third item of discussion since in a relationship money is control. The person who pays the bills has control and knows where the money is going. Who will and how will they make financial decisions is also part of the discussion. And finally affluence or how affluent do we want to be is addressed. How hard are we willing to work, how much money do we think we need to make and what are we willing to sacrifice to make this money. The answers to the affluence questions can paint a picture of what married life will be like for the couple (Lieber, 2009).

The perception of money affects everything from long-term planning to daily quality of life. It also involves the perception of gender roles as couples decide if one or both partners will work, whose job is more important, if one of them is to leave a career to take care of the children, and other issues. If one partner has a traditional gender role concerning money and the other doesn't, this could be a major source of marital discord. Couples need to discuss these issues and develop egalitarian, creative approaches to deal with their own money and the "couple's" money. Setting financial goals that both agree on, establishing a budget to lead to these goals, and sticking to the budget will help couples avoid many of the typical battles about money.

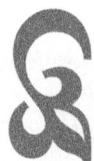

healthy sex hints 6.2

Fighting Fairly

- Use I rather than you. Instead of saying, "You're insensitive," say, "I feel hurt when you ignore me."
- Don't argue without good reason. Think before you speak.
- Don't fight in front of other people, including your children. The issue involves only the two of you.
- Don't make personal attacks—name-calling, putdowns —that you will regret later.
- Be specific. Don't generalize.
- Focus on only the issue that precipitated the argument.
- Learn to use active listening skills so your partner will know he or she is being heard.
- If you cannot agree after a "fair fight," agree to disagree or to renew the discussion later.
- Take responsibility for your own behavior. Avoid blaming.
- Obviously, do not resort to physical attacks or any form of violence.

Think of arguments as withdrawals from the bank of relationship happiness and good feelings. Make withdrawals only for those issues that really matter.

Another challenge for today's couples is finding ways to fairly share all of the responsibilities of daily living. The expectations for both males and females were clearly delineated in the traditional family. Now that both partners often work, it is essential to work toward evenly share all the chores of life whether they be parenting, cooking, or simply doing the laundry. Our society is still transitioning from the traditional style relationship to an equal relationship so the role models for making this new reality work are not always available. Therefore many couples struggle to figure out how to keep one partner from feeling "taken advantage of" and overwhelmed by what it takes to maintain daily living. On the positive side, there is some evidence that males are moving toward more shared responsibility in parenting and housework. The amount of time fathers spend caring for their children rose from 2.6 hours a week in 1965 to 6.5 hours in 2000. Mothers still spend more time than fathers but the gap has narrowed (Livingston, 2011). Males have also increased the amount of housework they do from 6 hours a week in 1976 to 13 hours a week in 2005. Women in 2005 still outpaced the men with an average of 17 hours a week. However, once these men have children, they do not look quite as progressive in their sharing of the additional responsibilities of daily living that are added with children. A mother with 3 children averages 28 hours a week on chores compared to 10 hours for the father—the same hours worked when men have no children (Mixon, 2008), Apparently the father adds no new tasks to his chore list once the children are born. It is easy to imagine the resentment these mothers must have toward a partner who is not fully sharing. Many of these mothers probably also work so the extra 28 hours adds greatly to her level of stress and fatigue. All of these are ingredients for harming the relationship and the family.

case study 6.2

Tom and Suzanne: Dealing with Finances

Tom and Suzanne, both age 30, are white.

Tom and Suzanne have an interesting way of dealing with family finances. They met at age 27 in graduate business school, where they were pursuing their MBAs. Both had lived by themselves for a few years and had several years of work experience behind them. Each had savings and checking accounts.

In discussing marriage, both were concerned about financial independence and protecting their savings, income, and spending patterns. Suzanne was a saver. She had banked well over $20,000 in savings before she met Tom, and she wanted to preserve this money. She was disciplined and always paid cash, even for her personal automobiles.

Tom was a spender. He believed in buying with credit cards, and internet shopping was a favorite pastime. Saving was something people did once they turned 50 and began to think about retirement. For as long as he could remember, he had outstanding balances on his credit accounts yet eventually would pay them off.

Being so different concerning money but so alike in a number of other ways, Tom and Suzanne decided that after they were married, they would have three separate accounts: his, hers, and ours. The "ours" account would be used for all joint bills (rent, food, joint vacations, and child rearing (if it came up). Tom had wanted other expenses covered from this account, such as car purchases and retirement savings, but Suzanne, knowing he was a spender and she'd wind up contributing more than he, did not accept this arrangement. After reviewing salaries and projected earnings, they decided that each would contribute two weeks take-home salary to the joint account, with the other two weeks kept separately. With basic expenses covered, each could then spend and/or save without guilt or explanation.

Despite some stress, things have worked out okay for Tom and Suzanne. She's still a saver and has over $20,000 in her bank account. He's still a spender and has a $15,000 car loan and credit card debts exceeding $1,000. Suzanne considered helping him out with some payments but decided against it, as she thought he might think this would be the usual. Some of their friends think they're a little eccentric and that their marriage seems more like a business than a loving partnership. In any case, for the time being it seems to work for them.

Critical Thinking

Some would argue that married couples who maintain separate checking accounts demonstrate a lack of trust in their relationships.

Others might argue that it is wise for two people with different approaches to managing money to keep some of their finances separate.

How will you approach managing money in your long term relationship or marriage?

Parenting and Relational Satisfaction

Children can be a major source of stress and change for couple's established patterns of interaction. Adding children to a marriage can be extremely pleasurable but also stressful. Unfortunately, for 40-70 percent of couples, marital happiness declines (Gottman & Notarius, 2000). As we've seen from the Berry and Williams analysis of marital happiness and adult developmental phases, satisfaction within a marriage reaches its lowest point about the time the children reach adolescence. Even though this seems to indicate that adolescents are responsible for their parents' stress, the demands of parenting pose formidable stressors at all stages of child development. However, there is some evidence that when both partners equally want to have children the relationship satisfaction does not seem to drop (Parker-Pope, 2010). This powerfully argues for couples to discuss if and when they want to have children.

Parenting requires a tremendous amount of time and effort and as a result, children decrease up to half the amount of time parents have to share activities with each other (Cavanaugh, 1993). With all the demands of parenting, remaining a "couple centered" and not "child centered" marriage is a challenge. Couples need to take time to nurture their relationship in order to maintain a healthy marriage because the marriage is the foundation of the family. If the marriage fails the family will also fail. It is essential for parents to spend time as a couple, going out alone, having date nights, talking and working on their relationship. This commitment to their marriage necessitates a balancing of all needs and time demands. Perhaps it is not as important for parents to attend all sporting and school events of every child but instead spend time improving the relationship that is the key to the family stability.

Divorce

Not all marriages progress completely through the Berry and Williams phases described earlier in the chapter. More than two fifths (43%) of all first marriages end in divorce or separation within 15 years (Peterson, 2001). Raw numbers are misleading when interpreting divorce statistics. The divorce rate, which examines numbers of divorces in relation to numbers of marriages, rose steadily for 20 years, reaching a high of 5.3 divorces per 1,000 Americans in 1981, then began declining. The divorce rate is now at its lowest level since 1970. In 2008, there were a reported 3.5 divorces for every 1,000 people, an encouraging decrease in the rate of divorce. (Cohen, 2010).

Most people marry with the hope that the relationship will last forever. Divorce, therefore, often represents a loss of this hope. This often is accompanied by the loss of economic status (particularly for low- and middle-income women), lifestyle, security, , friends, and sometimes children. The psychological effects of divorce can be compared with those of the grieving process associated with death of a loved one. First, shock sets in ("Is this really happening to me?"), followed by disorganization ("Everything feels so confused"). Volatile emotions, then guilt ("It's my fault") usually follow. Loneliness, too, often accompanies divorce. Finally, after several months to a year, these feelings are replaced by a sense of relief and acceptance. Adjusting takes time but one year after divorce both men and women are happier (Cowen, 2007).

The grieving process leads to healing, a cleansing of wounds, that allows divorced people to move on with their lives. If, after a year or so, the divorced person hasn't gotten over the divorce and begun to accept what has happened, counseling and psychotherapy may be helpful. Approximately three in four divorced persons remarry, most within 3 years after their divorce. Although most remarried people report that their second marriage is better than their first, the likelihood that this marriage also will end in divorce is greater than that among first marriages. No one knows why this is so for sure, but some of the reasons given are less willingness to stay in the second marriage when they are embittered, closer scrutiny of the second marriage, financial problems (such as alimony and child support), and the trauma of divorce being less threatening after having experienced it once.

Long-Term Gay, Lesbian, and Bisexual Relationships

Domestic partnerships
Registered relationships between gay and lesbian couples

Most research regarding relationships has related to married heterosexuals, with far less written regarding long-term gay, lesbian, and bisexual relationships. But with the many changes in same sex marriage laws there will be many more opportunities to study these long term relationships. In declaration and celebration of the relationship commitment, gay and lesbian couples are marrying or having commitment ceremonies, where vows are shared, friends and family present, and some of the rituals of marriages are repeated. In August 2002, the New York Times decided to begin publishing reports of commitment ceremonies in its Sunday Styles section. What had been the "Wedding" section became the "Weddings/ Celebrations" section, with the backgrounds of gay and lesbian couples written up in the same manner as those of heterosexual couples. The significance of that editorial decision is reflected in the fact that the New York Times has national distribution, is considered a mainstream newspaper, and is a powerful force in public opinion. On a national level, gay and lesbian activists have been working to change legislation that would enable them to marry. When Hawaii changed its laws to allow for gay and lesbian marriage, federal legislation in the form of the Defense of Marriage Act was initiated. That law passed in 1996 ensuring that if a same sex couple married in one state, their marriage did not have to be recognized in any other. It defined marriage as being between a man and a woman. According to the Human Rights Campaign (2013), the Defense of Marriage Act also denies same sex couples, regardless of their marital status, 1,100 federal rights and benefits that apply to heterosexual couples. These include filing joint taxes, taking unpaid leave to take care of a sick spouse, and receiving spousal social security benefits among many others. The Supreme Court overturned the Defense of Marriage Act in June of 2013.

The politics surrounding marriage for lesbian and gay couples relate on one level to principles of fairness, constitutional protections, and recognition of loving, committed relationships. On another level, the politics are rooted in the economic protections of legal marriage. A national campaign for "Marriage Equality" has the goal of igniting a national conversation about the power of love, fairness and equality. This media campaign includes famous actors, actresses and politicians urging the public to vote for same sex marriage in support of marriage equality. As of June, 2013, same sex marriage is legal in thirteen states; California, Connecticut, Delaware, Iowa, Maine, Maryland, Massachusetts, Minnesota, New Hampshire, New York, Vermont and Washington. It is also legal in the District of Columbia.

Gay marriage also has legal status in fourteen countries worldwide. The Netherlands in 2000 became the first nation to make same-sex marriage legal, followed by Belgium, Spain and Canada. South Africa, Norway, Sweden, Argentina, Iceland, Portugal, New Zealand, Uruguay, and France followed these early countries in legalizing same sex marriage (ProCon.org, 2013).

Support for the issue of marriage equality in the US has steadily increased in many arenas. In March of 2013, after extensive review of the scientific literature, The American Academy of Pediatrics issued a policy statement in support of same sex marriage. This esteemed organization concluded that same sex marriage is in the best interest of children since it helps guarantee rights, benefits, and long term security for children (Saint Louise, 2013).

One of the benefits of being in a same sex relationship is he absence of social norms for thus allowing the relationships to be more egalitarian as opposed to gender stereotypical. The lack of hard-and-fast gender role stereotypes forces homosexual men and women to communicate more effectively and to be more flexible and creative in meeting relationship needs. Gay men and women are more willing to communicate, experiment, and be more attentive to detail in their sexual behavior (Kurdek, 1993).

Stages in Homosexual Relationships

In one of the most extensive, long-term prospective studies of male homosexuals to date, McWhirter and Mattison (1984) followed 156 gay couples for more than 20 years. The subjects were gay couples who had been together approximately 9 years before enrolling in the study. The researchers found that gay relationships, like those of their heterosexual counterparts, went through a series of stages.

Stage 1: Blending. This stage characterizes the first year of the relationship. As with heterosexual couples, this year has the highest levels of sexual activity, strong love and passion, and a merging of personal interests.

Stage 2: Nesting. Nesting takes place during years 2 to 3, emphasizing relationship building and starting a home together. Ambivalence, problems, and doubts about the relationship are most likely to begin to surface at this stage.

Stage 3: Maintaining. The third stage is characterized by a decline in passion and frequency of sexual activity, with an emphasis on conflict resolution and reassertion of some of the individuality subverted during the initial stages of the relationship.

Stage 4: Building. The building stage occupies years 6 through 10 and is marked by increased personal productivity and independence but also enhanced collaboration and developing sense of trust and dependability between the partners.

Stage 5: Releasing. From years 11 to 20, this stage is characterized by merging of money and other assets and beginning to take each other for granted. Sexual activity drops off noticeably in this stage.

Stage 6: Renewing. The last stage extends beyond 20 years together and is marked by personal security and a restored sense of partnership based on remembering shared experiences and good times together.

Because of better planning throughout their relationship, homosexual men and women may be more prepared to deal with losses such as the death of their partner and retirement. Many homosexuals have planned for their own financial support and have consciously developed supportive social networks. They also may be better prepared to cope with hardship, having lived a life of adversity as a member of a stigmatized group. This combination of attitude, social and financial resources, and self-reliance may help gay men and women cope with the demands of aging.

Sexuality in Older Adults

In Erik Erikson's (1978) final stage, older age, our major developmental task is to maintain integrity in the face of death. This last stage begins in older adulthood with the growing awareness of the nearness of death. This is a time for facing our mortality and accepting the worth and uniqueness of our lives.

Maintaining integrity entails evaluating our lives and accomplishments. In a sense, we are verifying our existence and seeking its meaning. We do this by looking back at where we've been, what we've accomplished, whom we have touched (Erikson, 1978). This process often involves reminiscing with family, friends, and others.

Sexual Response and Aging

Sex doesn't necessarily get better or worse as we age; it just gets different. Many myths have arisen in regard to sexual response and aging. The following three are common ones that usually surface during classroom discussions in our classes:

Once you start to get older (over age 60), you lose interest in sex.

Older people aren't sexually attracted to each other.

Older people can't perform sexually or have orgasms.

Physiologically, most men and women change very little during their 30s and early 40s. The most noticeable changes in sexual response in women are associated with menopause. They begin to experience a syndrome called the **female climacteric** between 45 and 55 years of age, as a result of a drop in levels of estrogen production associated with menopause. Common symptoms are hot flashes, decreased vaginal lubrication, and declines in sexual desire. The climacteric ends with menopause, which is the cessation of ovulation and loss of fertility. About one-fourth of women experience menopause before age 45, half from 45 to 50, and the remaining fourth after the age of 50 (Kart, 1994).

The changes in sexual physiology among most men in their 40s and 50s are less noticeable. Although sperm production slows down after age 40, it continues into the 80s and 90s. Similarly, male sexual hormone levels decline gradually after age 55, and men may notice a decline in sexual desire and sexual activity as they age. These physiological changes, in men and women, which basically revolve around the sexual response slowing and the intensity of response lessening slightly, are more than offset by greater comfort about sexuality, no fear of pregnancy, familiarity with one's partner, and extending the sex act.

Female climacteric A syndrome experienced by women between about 45 and 55 years of age as a result of declining levels of estrogen production associated with menopause

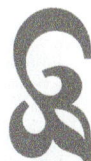

healthy sex hints 6.3

Changes in Sexual Response Associated with Aging

Women

The following changes are associated with sexual response in women who have gone through menopause:

1. The vagina is less elastic and not able to expand as much.
2. Physiological responses to sexual stimuli take more time.
3. Vaginal lubrication takes longer and may be less effective in reducing vaginal irritation.
4. The clitoris is smaller but not less responsive.
5. The intensity of orgasmic contractions diminishes slightly.
6. The ability to have multiple orgasms does not change.

Men

The following physiological changes have been observed in men older than age 55:

1. Arousal takes longer and may require manual stimulation of the penis.
2. Erections tend to be less firm.
3. Less semen is ejaculated.
4. There is less need to ejaculate to enjoy sexual activity.
5. The intensity of orgasmic contractions is slightly diminished.
6. More time is necessary to get another erection.

Changing Relationships

Older age is often affected by the changing nature of relationships and family life as the commitment to relationships that began in young adulthood continues and deepens. For some, this is a period marked by divorce or the death of a mate or lover. The case study featuring Harry illustrates that loss of a partner need not mean loss of a social and sexual life.

Although often characterized negatively as a time of loss and failed health, it also is a dynamic period in which newfound freedom, psychological and social stability, and wisdom can be a springboard to greater happiness for couples. Most older couples today have grown old together and have years of experience learning how to successfully live together. The average couple can expect at least 15 years of living together after the last child leaves. This is quite different from the turn of the century, when death affected half of all marriages before the last child left the house (Kart, 1994).

Marital Satisfaction and Aging

As married couples reach mid adulthood, happiness that was at an all-time low in their early 40s begins to rebound when the adult children leave home (Berry & Williams, 1987). The children are leaving home resulting in multiple changes for the relationship. The couple finds they have the

case study 6.3

Happy Harry

Harry, 78, is white.

Harry is living in an apartment at a newly developed senior residence. The residence is private and costs approximately $5,000 a month. Harry doesn't mind the cost because his meals are free, the staff takes care of most of his needs, and his pension, fortunately, provided nicely for his retirement. Harry's children no longer need his financial support, so he's enjoying life without worrying about taking care of anyone else.

Harry had been happily married to June, but when she passed away 5 years earlier, he decided he could no longer live in their house by himself. Little did he know how much in demand he would be once he arrived at the residence! The ratio of ladies to gentlemen is 4:1, and Harry is very popular. He knows he's not the best-looking guy, but he is agile and loves to dance, go out to movies, and generally have a good time. He's decided not to commit to any one woman, although he's had plenty of offers. At this point, being a free man with a lot of attention is just fine.

As for sex . . . well, he does have one or two special ladies with whom he spends the night. He feels a bit like a teenager again, sneaking around the residence hoping that one doesn't see him enter the room of the other.

Critical Thinking

The ratio of men to women in many adult residences is such that "partner sharing" may become necessary for heterosexual individuals.

How do you think you would react to such an arrangement? Would sharing a partner be acceptable if the alternative meant being unattached?

time, money, and privacy to reestablish the things in their relationship that provide pleasure, as well as investigate new things together. They can travel, dine in new restaurants, and learn a new hobby and other things they have been unable to fit into their lives.

Marital happiness continues to rise in the later adult years and carries over into retirement. Depending on a number of factors ranging from health to retirement income, the couple continue to enjoy their freedom and, in some cases, relationships with their children's families and grandchildren (Cavanaugh, 1993). Many who age remain healthy and active and can enjoy these retirement years enjoying the new interests and hobbies they have developed.

Along-term study of 17 happily married couples found that the most significant factor related to marital satisfaction was their ability to adapt to change and "roll with the punches" (Weishaus & Field, 1988). These couples had the ability to adapt to changing circumstances that normally might be interpreted as stressful and potentially damaging to the relationship. They might view a serious illness, for instance, as an opportunity for caring and closeness rather than anger and alienation.

Divorce in Older Couples

In many cases, marital dissatisfaction in older adulthood is not related to any age specific cause but, rather, resurfaces after years of being subordinated by issues related to child rearing. With the children grown and out of the house, old tensions and discontent surface and become a source of stress. Dependency is a key issue in the level of marital satisfaction in older couples. The extent of dependence of one mate on the other seems to be related to the strength of the relationship and its ability to last. When dependence is mutual and the level is relatively equal for both partners, relationships are strong and close. When dependence is not equal and one partner's needs are much greater than the other's, marital conflict is much more likely (Cavanaugh, 1993). When dependence is not equal or mutual, one partner may perceive normal developmental issues such as retirement and relocation as threatening, and, therefore, they become a source of resentment, discontent, and stress. Other issues that dampen marital happiness in older age include health problems, caring for sick parents and children, and financial problems.

Divorce is particularly distressing to older adults because of the long time invested in another's personal and practical life. In general, the longer the marriage, the greater is the trauma. In many cases, an elderly person's identity is closely wrapped up in being another person's husband or wife. Loss of this status often results in loss of economic status and lifestyle, friends (who often choose sides), and self-concept (Cavanaugh, 1993). Whereas younger divorced persons still have a job to report to, children to care for and interact with, and friends and family in the vicinity, elderly people often face the loss of these important connections.

Widowhood

Although a person can become widowed at any time during a marriage, it is much more likely later in life. The grieving process when someone loses a spouse can be similar to that of divorce discussed earlier. Widowhood can be stressful in a number of ways besides ending a partnership. U.S. society does not have well-defined social roles for widowed people. Therefore, they often are left alone by family and friends who don't know how to respond to them. Widowed individuals also may feel awkward as single people trying to fit into their previously coupled world.

Widowhood The period of time between loss of spouse and remarriage

❧ Spiritual Wellness ❧

Adulthood and old age are potentially a time of great spiritual awakening and renewal. For most people this is a time of developing intimate, loving relationships, making permanent (sacramental) commitments, having children, caring for sick and dying parents, and coming to terms with our own mortality. We are forced to examine these issues, all of which have a spiritual dimension. Understanding the meaning of these events, coping with them and their universality, help us develop a sense of connectedness with something other than ourselves. If we allow ourselves to look beyond the self and gain strength through connecting with others, we can enhance our spirituality, which can help us lead more satisfying and productive lives.

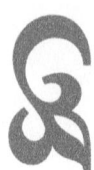

healthy sex hints 6.4

Dealing with Grief and Loss

The death of a loved one ranks at the top of life's most stressful events. The loss can impact all dimensions of our health—we may lose our appetite, feel depressed, experience a sense of emptiness in our home, not be able to concentrate, and so forth. How individuals grieve varies, with some able to cry openly while others bury themselves in tasks. Individual reactions to loss may also depend on whether a death was sudden or the culmination of a long and painful illness.

The loss of one's partner can be devastating. Individuals, who have lived decades as part of a couple, may struggle to understand how to find joy in life and live independently. Some may need to find a new partner quickly; others may feel that the lost love could never be replaced.

Grieving for a lost partner can be compounded by the relationship having been secret. It may be difficult to openly grieve and attend a funeral, for example, if your partner had never shared your existence with too many others. Long after the death of the famous aviator Charles Lindbergh, and shortly after the death of Senator Strom Thurmond, the facts of their secret "other" families came to light. Those descendents who had long been recognized as family were suddenly confronted with learning that the father they had loved had a past with which they were unfamiliar.

Whatever the circumstances, however, individuals must work through their grief. The following guidelines may prove beneficial:

- Accept your feelings, and understand that such emotions as anger, guilt, and relief are normal.
- Accept help from others, who may bring food, provide emotional comfort, and listen to you talk about your loss.
- Although grief can be private, you don't have to pretend to be strong and hold in your feelings.
- Give yourself time—grieving can be a long process.

There is no set timetable for working through grief.

There may be good days and bad days.

- Seek professional help if you remain intensely distressed for more than 6 months.

Source: Adapted from Hales (2003, p. 615).

Personal Assessment

Thought Questions

1. What are some of the major developmental tasks of college students? Compare these to the major developmental tasks associated with adolescence.
2. Compare and contrast sexual behavior during the college years with that of middle adulthood. What are the differences?
3. What is Berry and Williams's model of marital satisfaction? Identify the stages.
4. What are the similarities and differences between longterm heterosexual relationships and lesbian and gay unions of the same duration?
5. What factors contribute to satisfaction and happiness in long-term relationships?
6. What changes in sexual response are associated with aging?

Test Yourself!

1. A primary developmental task of young adults is to
   a. develop friendships with peers.
   b. form a committed, intimate relationship with a partner.
   c. learn to trust others.
   d. identify one's sexual orientation.
2. Which generalization about sexual behavior among college students is most accurate?
   a. Rates of sexual activity are similar between males and females.
   b. Fewer students participate in oral sex compared to earlier generations.
   c. There is no evidence of a double standard in values for male and female behavior.
   d. The majority of students cohabit prior to committing to marriage.
3. Couples who are happily married tend to do all but which of the following?
   a. Maintain some level of individual identity
   b. Share similar interests and values
   c. Fight effectively, laying blame where it belongs
   d. Communicate honestly
4. Berry and Williams have developed a model for the phases of adult marriage. When do couples report being the most satisfied with their marriage?
   a. At the time of the birth of their first child
   b. When their children are adolescents
   c. During the honeymoon phase, at the beginning
   d. Once children move out of the house
5. The concept of "fighting fairly" includes all but which of the following?
   a. Avoiding personal attacks
   b. Taking responsibility for your behavior
   c. Being able to discuss all the things that have been bothering you
   d. Not fighting in front of others
6. Changes in female sexual response associated with aging include
   a. loss of sex drive.
   b. less clitoral response.
   c. less vaginal lubrication.
   d. loss of orgasm.
7. Changes in male sexual response associated with aging include
   a. less firm erections.
   b. loss of sex drive.
   c. increase in semen production.
   d. loss of the ability to ejaculate.
8. Marriage is a form of relationship commitment
   a. between two consenting adults.
   b. open to gay, lesbian, and heterosexual couples.
   c. shown to endure for the majority of couples.
   d. that offers financial, personal, and health benefits.

9. Long-term gay and lesbian relationships
   a. are not possible in the oppressive culture of the United States.
   b. have been proven more stable than heterosexual relationships.
   c. go through stages similar to those in a marriage, yet with economic differences.
   d. require individuals to assume traditional roles within the relationship.

10. Which statement about widowhood among women is least accurate?
   a. Women are often better able to cope with the loss than men.
   b. Women quickly remarry after the loss of a spouse.
   c. Some women feel liberated and adopt lifestyle changes, such as traveling.
   d. Traditional widows move in with their children and become involved in raising their grandchildren.

InfoTrac Activity

Ponnuru, R. (2003, July 28). Coming out ahead: Why gay marriage is on the way. *National Review,* 55 (14).

Bradley, G. V. (2003, July 28). Stand and fight: Don't take gay marriage lying down. *National Review,* 55 (14).

Web Resources

College Sex Talk
www.collegesextalk.com

A Web site operated by Dr. Sandra Caron, certified sexuality educator and professor, where students can write in questions and receive age-appropriate responses to their concerns about sexuality.

National Institutes of Health
www.nih.gov

Typing "sexuality" into the search box will link users to numerous articles examining sexuality and health.

National Association on HIV over 50
www.hivoverfifty.org

A site devoted to older adults infected with HIV and/or those in need of information for themselves or others.

Senior Site
www.seniorsite.com

Sexual health information for older adults.

References

The American College Health Association national college health assessment (ACHA-NCHA), Spring 2012 reference group report (2012). available:www.acha-ncha.org

Bumpass, L. (2004). Social Changes and the American Family. Annals of the New York Academy of Science. 1038, 213–219.

Berry, R. E., & Williams, E. (1987). Assessing the relationship between quality of life and marital and income satisfaction: A path analytic approach. *Journal of Marriage and the Family,* 49, 107–116.

Block, B. (1980). *Friendship: How to give it, how to get it.* New York: Macmillan.

Bogle, K. (2008) Hooking Up: Sex, dating and relationships on campus. New York University Press, New York, NY.

Cavanaugh, J. C. (1993). *Adult development and aging.* Belmont, CA: Wadsworth.

Center for Disease Control and Prevention. (April, 2005). Births, marriages, divorce, and deaths: provisional data for April 2005, National Vital Statistics Report, 54(6). Available online: www. CDC. gov

Center for Disease Control and Prevention (September, 2005). Sexual behavior and selected health measures: men and women 15-44 years of age, United States, 2002. Advance Data From Vital and Health Statistics, 362. Available online: www.CDC.gov

Center for Disease Control and Prevention (2005) Faststats A-Z Divorce. Available online: www. cdc.gov/nchs/faststats/divorce.htm

Chandra, A., Martinez, G., Mosher, W., Abma, J.,& Jones, J.(2005). Fertility, family planning, and reproductive health of U.S. women: Data from the 2002 national survey of family growth. Vital Statistics, 23(25).

Clark, A.E., & Oswald, A.J. (2002). A simple statistical method for measuring how life events affect happiness. International Epidemiological Association, 31, 1139–1144.

Cohen, D'Vera (2013, February 13). Love and marriage. available:www.pewsoicaltrends. org/2013/02/13/love-and-marriage/

Cohen, D'Vera (2010, June 4). At long last divorce. Pew Research Center Publications. Available: http://pewresearch.org/pubs/1617/long-duration-marriage-end-divorce-gore

Cohen, D'Vera, Passel, J., Wang,W., & Livingston, G. (2011, December14). Barely half of U.S. adults are married-a record low. Pew Research Social & Demographic Trends. Available: www.pewspocaltrends.org/2011/12/14/barely-half- of- U-S- adults- are- married-a- record-low

Coleman, J.(2008). Parents need to get out of the house sometimes! Contemporary Families. Available: http://www.contemporary families.org

Cowen, T. (2007, April 19). Martimony has its benefits, and divorce has a lot to do with that. The New York Times.

Crawford, M., & Popp, D. (2003, February). Sexual double standards: A review and methodological critique of two decades of research. *Journal of Sex Research,* 40(1).

Easterlin, R.A. (2003). Explaining happiness. PNAS (National Academy of Sciences of the USA, 100(19), 11176–11183.

Erikson, E. (1978). *Childhood and society* (2nd ed.). New York: Norton.

Fields, J. (2001, June 29). [Report.] *U.S. Department of Commerce News.* U.S. Census Public Information Office.

Washington, DC: U.S. Government Printing Office.

Flannery, D., Ellingson, L., Votaw, K., Schaefer, E. (2003). Anal intercourse and sexual risk factors among college women, 1993-2000. American Journal of Health Behavior, 27(3), 228–234.

Gottman, J. & Gottman, J. (2013). How to keep love going strong. Available:www.gottman.com

Gottman, J. & Notarius, C.(2000) Decade Review; Observing Marital Interaction. Journal of Marriage and the Family.62. 927–947.

Hales, D. (2003). *An invitation to health* (10th ed.). Belmont, CA: Wadsworth/Thomson Learning.

Hughes, R. (2003). The demographics of divorce: United States and Missouri [Online]. Available: www.missourifamilies.org.

Jay, M. (2012, April 14). The downside of cohabiting before marriage. The New York Times.

Kurdek, L. (1993). The allocation of household labor in gay, lesbian, and heterosexual married couples. *Journal of Social Issues,* 49(3), 127–139.

Lambert, T. A., Kahn, A. S., & Apple, K. J. (2003). Pluralistic ignorance and hooking up. *Journal of Sex Research,* 40(2), 129–133.

Laumann, E., Gagnon, J. H., Michael, R. T., & Michaels, S.

(1994). *The social organization of sexuality: Sexual practices in the United States.* Chicago: University of Chicago Press.

Laumann, E. O., & Michael, R. T. (2001). *Sex, love, and health in America: Private choices and public policies.* Chicago: University of Chicago Press.

Laumann, E. O., & Youm, Y. (2001). Sexual expression in America. In E. O. Laumann & R. Michael (Eds.), *Sex, love and health in America.* Chicago: University of Chicago Press.

Lieber, R. (2009, October 24). Money talks to have before marriage. The New York Times.

Litzinger, S. & Gordon, K.C. (2005) Exploring relationships among communication, sexual satisfaction, and marital satisfaction. Journal of Sex And Marital Therapy, 31, 409–424.

Livingston, G. (2011, June 15). A tale of two fathers: more are active, but more are absent. Pew Research Center Publications. Available: http:// pewresearch.org.pubs/2026/survey-role-of -fathers-fatherhood-american-family-living.

Masters, W. H., Johnson, V. E., & Kolodny, R. C. (1992). *Human sexuality* (4th ed.). New York: HarperCollins.

McWhirter, D., & Mattison D. (1984). *The male couple.* Englewood Cliffs, NJ: Prentice Hall.

Michael, R. T., Gagnon, J. H., Laumann, E. O., & Kolata, G. (1994). *Sex in America: A definitive survey.* Boston: Little, Brown.

Mixon, B. (2008, April 28). Chore wars: Women & house work. Available: http//:www.msf.gov/discoveries/disc_summ.jsp?cnta_id=1114!

National Center for Education Statistics. (2000). *Percentage distribution of undergraduates by marital status:* 1999-2000.

Parker-Pope, T, (2010), For Better: how the surprising science of happy couples can help your marriage succeed. New York, NY: Plume,

Paul, E. L., McManus, B., & Hayes, A. (2000). Hookups: Characteristics and correlates of college students' spontaneous and anonymous sexual experiences. *Journal of Sex Research,* 37(1), 76–88.

Phillis, D. E., & Stein, P. J. (1983). Sink or swing? The lifestyles of single adults. In E. R. Allegeir & N. B. McCormick (Eds.), *Changing boundaries: Gender roles and sexual behavior.* Palo Alto, CA: Mayfield.

Reinisch, J. M. (1992). *The Kinsey Institute new report on sex.* New York: St. Martin's.

Roberts, S. (2010, March 2). Study finds cohabiting doesn't make a union last. The New York Times.

Saint-Louise, C. (2013, March 21). Pediatric group black gay marriage saying it helps children, The New York Times.

Scott, M., Schelar, E., Manlove, J., & Cui, C. (2009). Young adult attitudes about relationship and marriage: times may have changed, but expectations remain high. Child Trends Research Brief. Available: www.childtrends.org

Thomas, J. A. (2000, October 10). Childcare and laboratory schools on campus: The national picture [Online].

National Coalition for Campus Children's Centers. Available: www.campuschildren.org.

Times will begin reporting gay couples' ceremonies. (2002, August 18). *New York Times,* National Section.

Weishaus, S., & Field, D. (1988). A half century of marriage: Continuity or change? *Journal of Marriage and the Family,* 50, 763–774.

chapter

seven

Human Sexual Response

Student Learning Objectives

After reading this chapter, students will be able to

- ♥ Identify the key brain structures involved in the human sexual response.
- ♥ Describe how the nervous and endocrine systems interact during sexual response.
- ♥ Explain how psychological and physiological factors interact during sexual response.
- ♥ Describe the effects of major disabilities on sexual response.
- ♥ Compare and contrast a variety of sexual response theories.
- ♥ Diagram and describe the four phases of the Masters and Johnson sexual response cycle.
- ♥ Define **aphrodisiac** and evaluate the effects of aphrodisiacs on sexual response.
- ♥ Describe factors that enhance vasocongestion and sexual response.
- ♥ Describe a variety of theories of sexual response.

activity teaser: How do you really feel about your body? Find out in the Personal Exploration Activity on page 260.

case study 7.1

Sexual Response: John and Michelle

John and Michelle, both 23, are white.

John is working on his computer in the apartment he shares with Michelle, his steady girlfriend of 3 years. Michelle is out with friends, having agreed to give John some quiet time to work on a paper he is writing. From his desk, he can gaze out onto the street in front of his apartment. His mind is busy trying to piece together the words that ultimately will make up his paper on Shakespeare for his English literature class. His fingers move quickly over the keyboard, his eyes riveted on the screen and his attention on his work.

As he works on the computer, he senses a car pull up, its doors swing open, and someone gets out. Without taking his eyes off the screen, John senses that this might be Michelle. He looks out the window and sees Michelle. She is wearing a short, silky, summer dress that sways with her long, athletic legs. He hears her laughter as she and her friends say their good-byes as they drive off.

Michelle enters their apartment, and, although he can't see her yet, he hears the rustling of her skirt, and a trace of Michelle's perfume wafts through the door. He hears her voice call out, "John, I'm home." The sound of her voice and the smell of her perfume cause his mind to wander and his body begins to respond. He feels his penis begin to get erect. Although he tries to fight it, his mind continues to wander, drifting from his writing to his erection, to thoughts of Michelle's warm body and past lovemaking, and back to his writing again.

Realizing that he'll never finish his writing if he allows his thoughts to keep wandering like this, John focuses his attention on his paper, and his brain begins to shut down his sexual response. After about 10 minutes, Michelle enters the room and, with a sexy smile, wanders over to John's desk and interrupts his concentration.

"Interested in taking a little break?" she asks, as she takes his glasses off his nose, wraps her arms around his shoulders, and begins to nibble on his ear. He turns, gives her a kiss, and feels his body respond to her warmth and softness.

After a couple of kisses, John decides to stop trying to fight his brain's urges and allows his body to take over. He picks up Michelle, carries her over to the bed, and they proceed to make love, both deciding that Shakespeare can wait a couple of hours.

Critical Thinking

As John and Michelle have demonstrated, sexual response can often occur despite our conscious thoughts to initiate it. How does this influence our ability to control our sexual urges and behavior?

If you were to ask the average person which part of the body is the most important for controlling sexual response, the answer most likely would be "the penis" or "the vagina." Most people equate sexual response to genital functioning. In reality, sexual response begins and ends in the brain. The brain, not the genitals, is the seat of human sexual response. Human sexual response originates with the brain's perception of desire. What makes you want to respond? What allows you to become comfortable and to relax so the response will happen? In this chapter, we'll examine sexual response and try to answer these and many other questions.

> ### ❧ *Social Wellness* ❧
>
> The quality of our social relationships plays a big part in our sexual response. Being able to relax, feel secure, and trust our partner is crucial for good sex. Another key to good sex is open communication. Getting to know your partner requires time. Intimacy builds over time as a result of shared experiences and open communication about our innermost thoughts, feelings, needs, and wants. As you can see in Case Study 7.1 with John and Michelle, an intimacy, trust, and a sense of playfulness spring from this social bond between them. Their sensuality and sexuality are easy, not forced, and are a hallmark of high-level social wellness.

Physiology of Sexual Response

Sexual response is the result of a complex interaction between psychological and physiological factors originating in the brain and spreading through various body parts and systems. We'll trace the sexual response, describing the key components and mechanisms of action that control it.

The Nervous System and Sexual Response

The human nervous system is composed of two parts: the **central nervous system** and the **peripheral nervous system**. The central nervous system is made up of the brain and spinal cord. The peripheral nervous system consists of all other nerves, and connects the spinal cord to various target organs, glands, and tissue. Figure 7.1 shows the nervous system. The peripheral nervous system is made up of two divisions: the **somatic nervous system** and the **autonomic nervous system.** We'll start with a discussion of how the central nervous system works during sexual response.

The Central Nervous System (Brain and Spinal Cord)

The brain and spinal cord together comprise the central nervous system. Both the brain and the spinal cord play key roles in sexual response. Sexual arousal usually is the end result of a complex interplay among our sensations, thoughts, memories, and feelings that come together in our brains and are interpreted as being sexual. We'll begin our exploration of human sexual response with a discussion of how the brain is involved in this process.

Central nervous system Brain and spinal cord

Peripheral nervous system All other nerves connecting to spinal cord

Somatic nervous system The part of the peripheral nervous system under voluntary control

Autonomic nervous system The part of the peripheral nervous system that is automatic and involuntary

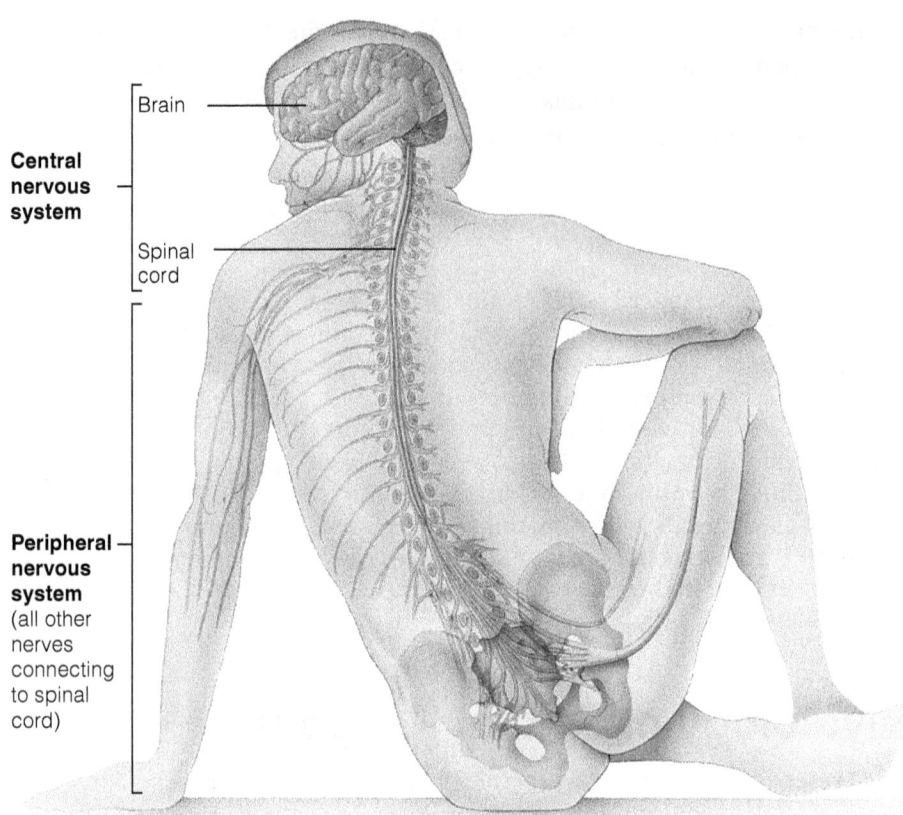

Central nervous system

Brain

Spinal cord

Peripheral nervous system (all other nerves connecting to spinal cord)

Figure 7.1 *The Nervous System* The nervous system receives and sends sexual messages electrically throughout our body.

The Brain

The brain has four major divisions (see figure 7.2):

1. Cerebrum (containing the cerebral cortex and limbic system)
2. Diencephalon (comprised of the thalamus, hypothalamus, & pineal body)
3. Brain Stem (comprised of the medulla oblongata, pons, and midbrain)
4. Cerebellum (Martini, 2005)

Cerebrum   The cerebrum is the largest and uppermost part of the brain. The cerebrum is irregularly shaped, with ridges and shallow and deep grooves, and is divided into two halves called **hemispheres.** The cerebral hemispheres form the outermost part of the brain and are divided into sections called lobes. Four of the lobes are named after the bones in the skull that they lie over. These four are; the frontal lobe, the parietal lobe, the temporal lobe, the occipital lobe. The fifth lobe, the insula, is hidden from view. The frontal, parietal, occipital, and temporal lobes of each hemisphere are responsible for controlling a variety of **motor, sensory,** and **associational** brain functions that are directly involved in sexual response. Each of the lobes controls many functions besides those related to sexual response (Martini, 2005; Fisher, 2004).

Cerebral Cortex   The surface of the cerebrum is called the Cerebral Cortex. The conscious awareness of sensations (sight, sound, smell, taste,

Hemispheres The two halves of the cerebrum, each controlling the functions of the opposite side of the body

Motor Relating to nerve impulses going out to muscles

Sensory Relating to nerve messages coming into the brain

Associational Connecting together individual sensory inputs

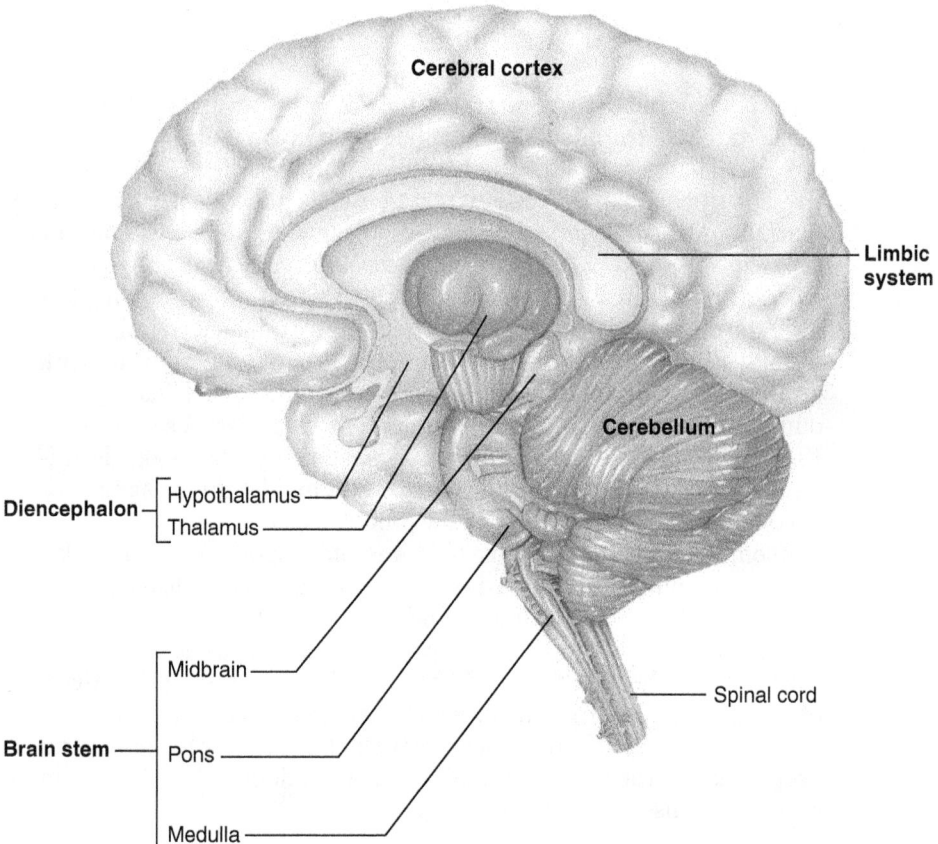

Figure 7.2 *Parts of the Brain* The brain can be divided into four main parts when studying sexuality: the cerebrum, the diencephalon, the brain stem, and the cerebellum.

and touch) is controlled by the parietal, occipital, and temporal lobes of the cerebral cortex, the thinking part of the brain. These sensations, in some combination, enter one's consciousness through the sensory areas of the cerebral cortex and are interpreted as sexual. The cortex picks up the messages, and the associational areas interpret them.

Although each sensory stimulus is entered as a distinct, separate entity, it is quickly assimilated, sorted out, deciphered, and combined with others to form a potentially "sexy" signal. This interplay relies on stored memories (whether real or imagined) of past experiences that influence one's assessment of the present incoming stimuli as sexual and one's expectations of what is to follow (Martini, 2005, Fisher, 2004).

Limbic System The limbic system is a complex arrangement of nerve tissue that links the emotional brain with the thinking, rational brain (cerebral cortex). In this way, the limbic system establishes a relationship between our thoughts and our feelings. Sometimes this relationship is clear-cut and appropriate; other times it is not. Sometimes our emotions get the best of us so we don't think clearly. We might interpret someone's verbal communication, body language, or behavior as conveying interest in having sex when they really are not. The cerebral cortex does have the ability to shut down sexual response through conscious control of behavior at any point (Fisher, 2004).

❧ *Intellectual Wellness* ❧

Knowing how our perceptions can influence our sexual response opens the door to relearning things about our sexuality that until now might have been barriers to our sexual fulfillment. If we believe in the cognitive basis of sexual response, we can unlearn negative sexual information and learn new, healthy ways of viewing ourselves and our sexuality. Knowing about the sexual response patterns in men and women and the areas that are most responsive to stimulation can make us better lovers, regardless of whether we are straight, gay, lesbian, or bisexual. Knowing our limitations and capabilities, and how to work around certain disabilities and health conditions, can help us improve our sexual response and maintain our self-respect and self-esteem. Knowing what to expect concerning sexual response can make the difference between allowing ourselves to relax and let things happen or becoming overly concerned with the process and worrying that it won't happen. Knowing that our sexual desires and responses vary from day to day will help us understand the differences, and enable us to relax and go with the changes. Understanding that our needs and responses won't always perfectly mirror our partner's can help us devise ways to work around these and other differences. Understanding the effects of drugs, fatigue, stress, and other substances on our sexual response empowers us and helps us moderate their effects. Knowledge also can prepare us for the future, by enabling us to anticipate the changes in sexual response associated with aging.

Thalamus The part of the brain that relays all inputs to the cerebral cortex

Hypothalamus The part of the brain that correlates activities between the nervous centers and the pituitary gland

Diencephalon The diencephalon forms the central core of the brain and contains the **thalamus** and **hypothalamus**. This area plays a crucial role in the continuation of sexual response that begins with the interpretation of an incoming stimulus as sexual. The thalamus, a hidden region of the brain, might best be described as the relay center for all inputs to the cerebral cortex. The hypothalamus is located directly beneath the thalamus at the end of the brain stem. Despite its small size, the hypothalamus exerts a tremendous amount of control over body functioning.

The hypothalamus works in concert with the nervous and endocrine systems to initiate sexual arousal. The hypothalamus sends both electrical

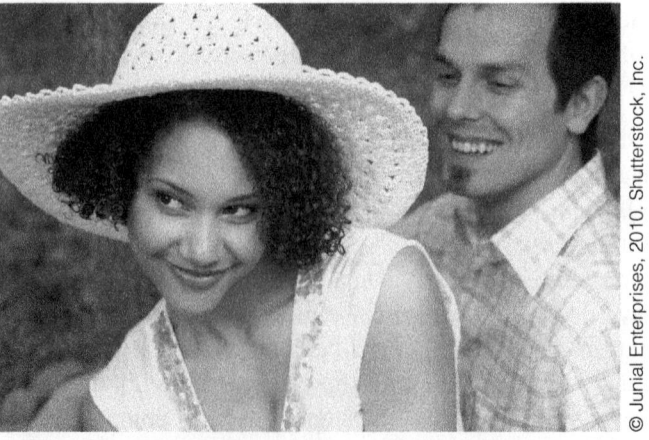

Flirting is often perceived as a sign of sexual interest.

© Junial Enterprises, 2010. Shutterstock, Inc.

case study 7.2

Jorge: Mistaken Perceptions

Jorge, 19, single, identifies as Hispanic.

Jorge is a college sophomore. He shared a story about mistaking a date's expressions of affection as an invitation to have sexual intercourse.

I'm a little embarrassed about talking about this, but I think it's exactly what we were just talking about in class. I dated a girl last semester who was really fine. I was instantly attracted to her when I saw her at the student center. I went up to her, and we hit it off, so I asked her out. We went to one of the jazz concerts on campus and hung out afterward. We walked around campus, and after a while, she kind of snuggled up against me on one of the benches by the auditorium. She smelled real good, and it felt great having my arm around her. We started to kiss and make out. Everything seemed to be going great. We were laughing and snuggling, having a great time.

It started to get late, so I suggested I walk her back to her room. Her roommates had gone home, so she invited me in, and we started making out again. I really thought she wanted to have sex. I mean, she was hot and rubbing up against me. By now I had an erection, and I started to unbutton her blouse. When I got about halfway she stopped me and said, "No." I said, "No what?" She said, "Listen, I like you a lot, but I really don't want to have sex." I must admit, I was shocked and upset. In the past I had never gotten this far without having sex.

I wasn't sure what to do. My penis was throbbing, and I really was horny. I said, "Can you take care of me?" She said "I'm really sorry. I just don't want to do this anymore. Could you please leave?" I really didn't know if she was serious or not, so I asked her, "Are you serious?" She said she was, and I got myself straightened up and left. I was surprised, but by the time I got out of her dorm and started to walk back to my place, I had lost both my erection and my desire. I found out the next week that she had just broken up with her boyfriend that day, and I guess I came along at the wrong time. I never could bring myself to call her again.

> ### Critical Thinking
>
> Has something like this ever happened to you? Have you ever either unintentionally sent sexual signals that you did not want to or misinterpreted signals sent from someone else? If given the chance, how would you handle those situations now?

(nerve impulses) and chemical (releases hormones) messages throughout the body during sexual response. These messages orchestrate a host of physiological reactions that we will describe in detail later in the chapter.

Brain Stem The structures of the brain stem produce the autonomic functions necessary for our survival, in addition to serving as the pathway for connections between the higher and lower brain functions. One of the key functions of the midbrain is the release of the **neurotransmitters serotonin** and **dopamine**, which are antidepressants that elevate mood and increase energy. These neurotransmitters, combined with the hormones epinephrine and nor-epinephrine play a major role in fueling sexual desire and arousal. We will discuss the interplay of neurotransmitters and hormones later in the

Neurotransmitters chemicals that transmit nerve impulses from one nerve to another

Serotonin a neurotransmitter that is an anti-depressant, energy and mood elevator

Dopamine a neurotransmitter that is an anti-depressant, energy and mood elevator

chapter. A key part of the brain stem, the *reticular activating system* (RAS), is a collection of neurons running through the three regions of the brain stem. It is responsible for both arousing the brain and filtering out unnecessary information. During arousal, the RAS is responsible for magnifying and increasing our awareness of specific stimuli. It allows us to hone in or focus on details of the stimulus. During sexual arousal this helps us focus our attention on important stimuli (Martini, 2005).

Cerebellum The cerebellum works with the cerebral cortex to produce skilled movement of muscles and muscle groups. It helps skeletal muscles control posture and produce smooth, coordinated, muscle movements. An example of such control would be the coordinated thrusting, grinding, and other motions associated with sexual intercourse (Martini, 2005).

The Peripheral Nervous System

During sexual response, nerve impulses travel from the hypothalamus, through the spinal cord to the peripheral nervous system, and ultimately to the specific glands, organs, and tissues involved in sexual response.

For many years it was generally assumed that sexual arousal in men and women was a simple spinal reflex located in the genital area. Figure 7.3 illustrates the simple spinal reflex arc responsible for penile erection in men. During a simple spinal reflex erection, stimulation of the penis (manual, oral, etc.) sends nerve messages along the parasympathetic nerves connecting the penis to the **erection center** in the spinal cord. The erection center sends back new nerve transmissions to the smooth muscle tissue of the arteries in the penis causing it to relax. This allows the tissue to fill with blood, causing erection. Clitoral engorgement and erection in women work similarly. When the clitoris is stimulated manually or orally, nerve transmissions travel along the **pudendal nerve** to the sacral region of the spinal cord, where it also connects to a reflex center in the spinal cord. The reflex center sends back new nerve transmissions to the smooth muscle tissue of the blood vessels in the clitoris, causing them to relax, engorge with blood, and enlarge, resulting in clitoral erection (Berman, 2000).

We now know that although initial sexual response can be the result of a simple spinal reflex, in most cases initiation or continuation of arousal involves the complex interplay between the brain and the body discussed earlier.

Erection center An area of the lowest part of the spinal cord, the sacral region, where the parasympathetic nerves of the penis connect

Pudendal nerve One of the nerves of the pudendal region of the spinal cord that encompasses the second, third, and fourth sacral regions of the spinal cord

Endocrine System

The endocrine system is responsible for the production and secretion of potent hormones that initiate and perpetuate the sexual response, in addition to a variety of other functions, ranging from the stress response to growth. The endocrine system is made up of the pituitary, thyroid, parathyroid, adrenal, pancreas, thymus, and pineal glands, as well as the ovaries and the testes.

The endocrine system works on the principle of feedback, with the hypothalamus acting as a thermostat that senses the level of a hormone circulating in the bloodstream. Just as the thermostat in your home senses the level of heat and turns on the heating or cooling system to regulate the

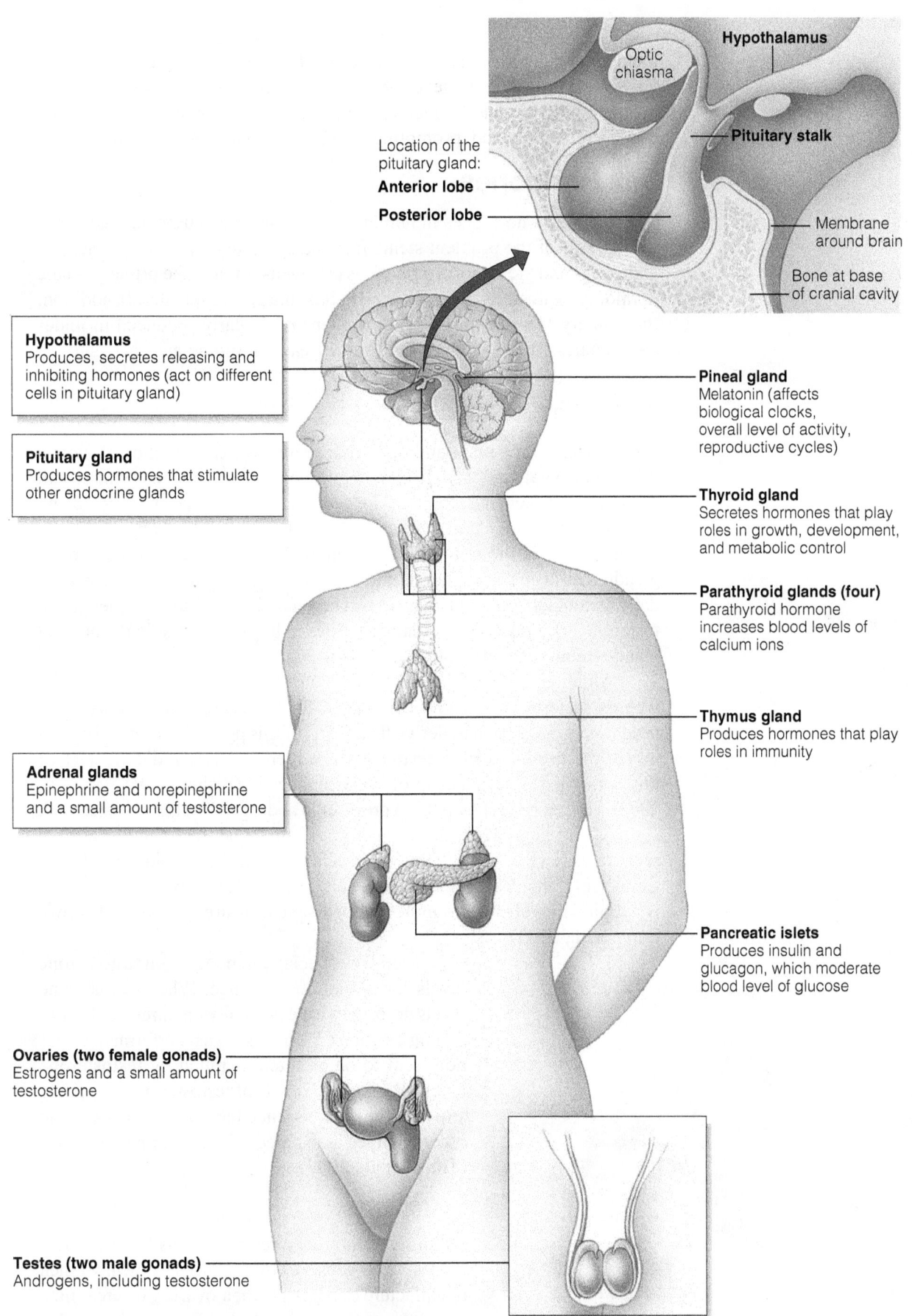

Hypothalamus
Optic chiasma

Pituitary stalk

Location of the pituitary gland:

Anterior lobe

Posterior lobe

Membrane around brain

Bone at base of cranial cavity

Hypothalamus
Produces, secretes releasing and inhibiting hormones (act on different cells in pituitary gland)

Pituitary gland
Produces hormones that stimulate other endocrine glands

Pineal gland
Melatonin (affects biological clocks, overall level of activity, reproductive cycles)

Thyroid gland
Secretes hormones that play roles in growth, development, and metabolic control

Parathyroid glands (four)
Parathyroid hormone increases blood levels of calcium ions

Thymus gland
Produces hormones that play roles in immunity

Adrenal glands
Epinephrine and norepinephrine and a small amount of testosterone

Pancreatic islets
Produces insulin and glucagon, which moderate blood level of glucose

Ovaries (two female gonads)
Estrogens and a small amount of testosterone

Testes (two male gonads)
Androgens, including testosterone

Figure 7.3 *The Endocrine System* The endocrine system sends and receives messages chemically throughout our body.

temperature, the hypothalamus senses the level of circulating hormones in your bloodstream. If the level of a hormone is too low, the hypothalamus secretes specific releasing factors that travel through the bloodstream to the target endocrine gland, prompting it to begin producing hormones.

Sex Hormones

The role of sex hormones in human sexual response is tremendously confusing. Part of the problem stems from categorizing "male hormones" as androgens and "female hormones" as estrogens. In fact, the primary "male hormone," testosterone, is produced in both males and females. In addition, the primary "female hormone," estrogen, is similarly produced in males and females. What vary are the level of each hormone and their sites of production (Lemonick, 2004; Fisher, 2004).

Androgens

Testosterone is the main androgen that seems to exert the most dramatic effect on sexual response. It is the main hormone associated with sexual desire in both men and women. The average man produces between 6 and 8 mg of testosterone daily. Most of the male testosterone (about 95%) is manufactured in the testes, and the remainder is produced in the adrenal glands. The average woman produces about 0.5 milligrams of testosterone daily, manufactured in the ovaries and adrenal glands. Prior to puberty, testosterone is produced in similar quantities in boys and girls, in the adrenal glands (Lemonick, 2004; Fisher, 2004).

Although men produce much more testosterone than women daily, women seem to have a lower threshold for testosterone sensitivity; they need less in circulation to derive the effects of this potent hormone. Regardless of the overall level of testosterone in men or women, deficiencies of this hormone result in a drop-off in sexual desire (Fisher, 2004; Bancroft, 2002). Studies have shown that a drop-off in androgen levels associated with surgery, anti-androgenic drugs, and other causes can result in diminished sexual desire (Reagan, 1999, Traish, Kim, Munarriz & Goldstein, 2002). Conversely, increasing androgen levels in men and women with diminished blood levels results in heightened sexual desire (Cama, Colleluori, Emig et al., 2003).

Men are especially dependent on testosterone levels for sexual performance. When testosterone levels drop, they have difficulty obtaining and maintaining erections. Women's sexual performance does not seem to be affected as much by testosterone levels. When their levels of testosterone drop, they still are able to experience lubrication, orgasm, and other changes associated with sexual performance (Traish et al., 2002).

Estrogens

Although commonly referred to as "female hormones," estrogens are also produced by men. Women manufacture estrogens in their ovaries, whereas men produce estrogen in their testes. Estrogen levels also

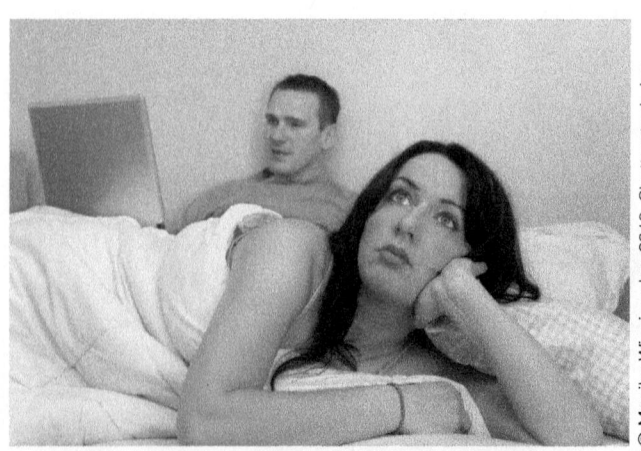
© Monika Wisniewska, 2010. Shutterstock, Inc.

Overwork can diminish one's interest in sex.

are related to sexual response. Estrogens play a role in maintaining vaginal lubrication, thus facilitating intercourse (Traish et al., 2002).

Women who have had their ovaries removed through hysterectomy and other procedures do not experience a reduction in sexual drive, although they may experience vaginal dryness and subsequent pain, which can diminish their interest and desire in sex. Women with high levels of estrogen do not experience heightened (or reduced) levels of sexual desire. Men also do not seem to be affected by too little estrogen. Excessive estrogen in men can have a "feminizing" effect that includes breast enlargement and erectile difficulties.

Progesterone

Progesterone is another major female sex hormone produced in the ovaries. It seems to play a primary role in reproduction by ensuring the viability of the endometrium. Its role in sexual desire and functioning is not understood very well. It may actually suppress the sexual interest of men and women alike (Reagan, 1999).

The Interaction Between the Nervous and Endocrine Systems

Becoming aroused may seem to be a relatively simple phenomenon, but in actuality it involves a complex interplay between the nervous and endocrine systems. The two systems work in consort with the other major systems (circulatory, respiratory, muscular, etc.) of the body to get the body ready for sexual activity. The hypothalamus sends electrical (direct nerve transmissions) and chemical (hormones) messages to switch on the body parts responsible for initiating the sexual response. The heart, responding to electrical and chemical stimulation, increases the volume of blood pumped throughout the body by raising its rate and pressure. This increased pumping of blood is necessary for supplying the extra oxygen and energy used during sexual activity. Blood vessels supplying the genitals, brain, and skeletal muscles dilate, allowing greater blood flow to the areas involved in sexual response. The lungs respond instantly by increasing the rate and depth of breathing. The airways expand, allowing maximum intake of air so its vital oxygen is mixed with the blood. The skeletal muscles began to contract and build tension (Martini, 2005, Fisher, 2004).

The Chemicals of Sex

Chemicals, neurotransmitters, and hormones interact is a variety of ways to trigger sexual arousal and keep the fires of desire ablaze. Once our brain interprets any stimuli (sensations, thoughts, feelings, etc.) as sexy, it sends nerve transmissions along our parasympathetic nervous system to the cells in our genital tissue that synthesize a complex molecule called **nitric oxide synthase (NOS).** NOS interacts with another chemical, a **nucleotide, Guanosine Triphosphate (GTP),** converting it to **Guanosine Monophosphate (GMP).** This starts a chain reaction resulting in the relaxation of smooth muscle tissue in the genitals allowing it to engorge with blood (de Tajada, 2002).

nitric oxide synthase (NOS) A complex chemical produced in genital tissue that starts a chain reaction initiating sexual arousal in men and women

Nucleotide A chemical compound that is the basic structural unit of nucleic acids (RNA, DNA etc.) that are found in all living cells

Guanosine Triphosphate (GTP) An energy-rich nucleotide necessary for protein synthesis

Guanosine Monophosphate (GMP) The converted form of GTP that is associated with the relaxation of genital smooth muscle tissue

Hormonal releasing factors
Chemicals secreted into the bloodstream by the hypothalamus. They travel through the bloodstream to specific endocrine glands and trigger them to release their hormones into circulation

In men, NOS is released in the spongy erectile tissue of the penis. In women, it occurs in the erectile tissue of the vestibular bulbs, the body and crura of the clitoris and in the tissue of the walls of the vagina. O'Connell, Sanjeevan & Hutson (2005), report that NOS causes the smooth muscle tissue of the corpora cavernosa in the penis and clitoral structures to engorge with blood, causing erection and increased sensitivity to stimulation. NOS also causes increased blood flow to the vaginal walls, resulting in lubrication.

While NOS is working its magic, the same sexual stimuli trigger the brain to release the neurotransmitters dopamine and serotonin. As we've already discussed, serotonin and dopamine are powerful antidepressants that elevate mood and increase energy. Both of these neurotransmitters have been linked to sexual arousal in men and women. When released in response to sexual stimuli, they act to increase desire and facilitate sexual arousal (Lemonick, 2004, Fisher, 2004).

While all of this is going on, a powerful hormonal response is also initiated in the brain. The hypothalamus secretes chemicals called **hormonal releasing factors** that travel through the bloodstream to the adrenal glands. These chemical messengers trigger the adrenal glands to release epinephrine and norepinephrine, powerful stimulants that speed up a host of metabolic processes including breathing, heart rate, and blood pressure just to name a few. These hormones combine with the neurotransmitters dopamine and serotonin to provide the energy that fuels sexual desire and arousal.

Circulating levels of testosterone, also play a part in sexual desire and arousal. As we mentioned previously in this chapter, testosterone is produced in the adrenal glands in women and the testes in men. New data on the effects of testosterone on vaginal and clitoral tissue shows that androgens enhance nitric oxide synthase activity (Traish et al., 2002a; Munarriz, Kim, Goldstein & Traish, 2002). While testosterone has long been recognized as the hormone of desire (Kaplan, 1974), this newer research may shed light on the specific actions of testosterone during the desire and arousal phases of sexual response.

While these findings clearly identify the chemicals of desire, the exact timing and interplay of these individual components is murky. For example, while we know that these chemicals, neurotransmitters, and hormones work together during sexual arousal we are not sure if their release must occur in a specific sequence to work properly. We also do not know if neurotransmitters can stimulate desire or if an elevated mood and more energy just set the stage for feeling sexy. Can the presence of hormones, chemicals, and neurotransmitters overcome the effects of thoughts, feelings and old memories?

As we'll see in the next section of this chapter, Models of Sexual Response, there is much controversy regarding viewing sexual desire and arousal in a purely biomedical way. While drugs like Viagra can help NOS relax genital muscle tissue and facilitate erections, many question whether this really equates to sexual desire. We'll explore this and other issues in the rest of this chapter and in Chapter 12 in the section on sexual dysfunction.

Models of Sexual Response

Four models of sexual response are discussed here. By far the best known is the one by William Masters and Virginia Johnson, pioneers in the study of sexual response.

sex in society 7.1

Participating in Sex Research

Imagine for a moment that a team of professors from your college is going to begin a study of sexual response among college students (singles and couples) at your school and on other campuses across the country. They are recruiting volunteers to participate in the study. You are curious about this and agree to be contacted by the team to see whether you meet the study's subject protocols. They give you some preliminary reading material about the study to examine before you come in for the interview.

The material explains that the team is interested in studying the sexual response of college students to see how it has changed since the days of Masters' and Johnson's research. They will be studying the sexual responses of gay and straight students under the following conditions:

> Viewing erotic films alone
> Viewing erotic films in a co-ed group

Solitary masturbation
Shared masturbation
Vaginal intercourse
Oral intercourse
Anal intercourse

The researchers explain that every attempt will be made to conduct the study under the strictest standards of confidentiality. Members of the team, however, will view sexual responses through two-way mirrors and will record the responses through various instruments including videocameras. The literature explains that this is necessary for the team to review the subjects' responses later.

Do you think you would participate in such a study? Would you participate if they paid you? How much? Do the conditions of this study create bias regarding who the subjects will be? How?

Masters and Johnson Four Phase Model

In 1966, Masters and Johnson published their ground-breaking work, *Human Sexual Response*. The book was ground-breaking for several reasons. Although previous researchers (Alfred Kinsey being the most notable) had published reports concerning self-reported sexual behavior, Masters and Johnson's was the first large-scale study of sexual response. Masters (a gynecologist) and Johnson (a psychologist) were the first researchers to study sexual response in a laboratory setting. They were the first mainstream scientists to apply the scientific rigor necessary to quantify and qualify a very private act. Their work provided a graphic depiction of the actual sexual processes in action.

Masters and Johnson invented the technology and instruments necessary for studying our most intimate body parts. They devised clear, plastic, penis-shaped cameras to photograph things such as changes in vaginal lubrication. They invented electromyographic devices to measure the most intimate of all muscular contractions, those of the penis, vagina, and anus. Many of these instruments and methods also were used to treat sexual dysfunction. The Masters and Johnson Institute in St.Louis became world-renowned for the study and treatment of sexual dysfunctions.

Besides creating the technology, they operationally defined **orgasm.** An operational definition was a prerequisite for experimental research of the phenomenon. They created a language of sexuality that included words such as *orgasm*, *vasocongestion*, *myotonia*, and others, which allowed professionals in the field to communicate with each other and disseminate their research findings.

Orgasm The stage of sexual response characterized by ejaculation in males and involuntary muscular contractions followed by relaxation in both males and females

Masters and Johnson were the first researchers to divide sexual response into phases that blend into one another as sexual response continues. They identified four phases:

1. Excitement
2. Plateau
3. Orgasm
4. Resolution

This sequence was the same regardless of the nature of sexual stimulation (masturbation, intercourse, and so forth) or sexual orientation (heterosexual, homosexual, bisexual) studied. The four stages are depicted in Figure 7.4 for women and Figure 7.5 for men.

Finally, Masters and Johnson discovered that the seat of women's sexual response is the clitoris, not the vagina. This broke new ground for understanding and conducting future research concerning women's sexual response. It opened the door for future research concerning issues such as the **G-spot,** differences in response patterns in women before and after a hysterectomy, and a host of other areas. Heterosexual and lesbian women (as well as their partners) have had the opportunity to apply Masters and Johnson's discoveries to enhance their sexual pleasure by better understanding their sexual functioning.

Excitement

During the first stage of Masters and Johnson's human sexual response—excitement—sexual arousal is initiated. Excitement can be triggered by a limitless array of cognitive and sensory stimuli ranging from viewing erotic films to listening to romantic music or getting a whiff of a familiar cologne or perfume.

The excitement stage is characterized by engorgement of erectile tissue in the genitals and a buildup of muscle tension throughout the body. The brain processes sensory and motor stimuli as being sexual in nature and passes a message to the hypothalamus, which initiates the nerve and hormonal sexual response.

Many cardiovascular changes are set into motion during excitement. The heart rate increases, and blood vessels throughout the body constrict, raising blood pressure. Blood vessels in the genitals dilate, resulting in increased blood flow to the genitalia. The increased blood flow fills up the spongy tissue that makes up this region. Blood flow into the genitals is greater than outflow. As this tissue fills with blood, it becomes engorged, enlarging in size, deepening in color, and increasing in sensitivity. Masters and Johnson called this engorgement process **vascongestion.** In men, the major changes associated with vasocongestion are erection of the penis and deepening of the color of the genitalia. In women, vasocongestion is responsible for labial swelling, deepening of the color of the vulva, vaginal lubrication, and increased size and sensitivity of the breasts.

Prior to Masters' and Johnson's research, sex researchers believed that vaginal lubrication was caused by sweat and oil glands within the vagina. Masters and Johnson discovered, and documented through special intravaginal photography, that lubrication is a by-product of vasocongestion. Vaginal mucosal tissue becomes engorged with blood and produces a clear, slippery fluid that empties from the cells directly into the vagina.

G-spot An area in the upper, rear section of the vagina named after Ernest Grafenberg, who claimed it to be an erogenous zone

Vasocongestion The movement of blood flow into the genitals resulting in a variety of responses, including erection in men and lubrication in women

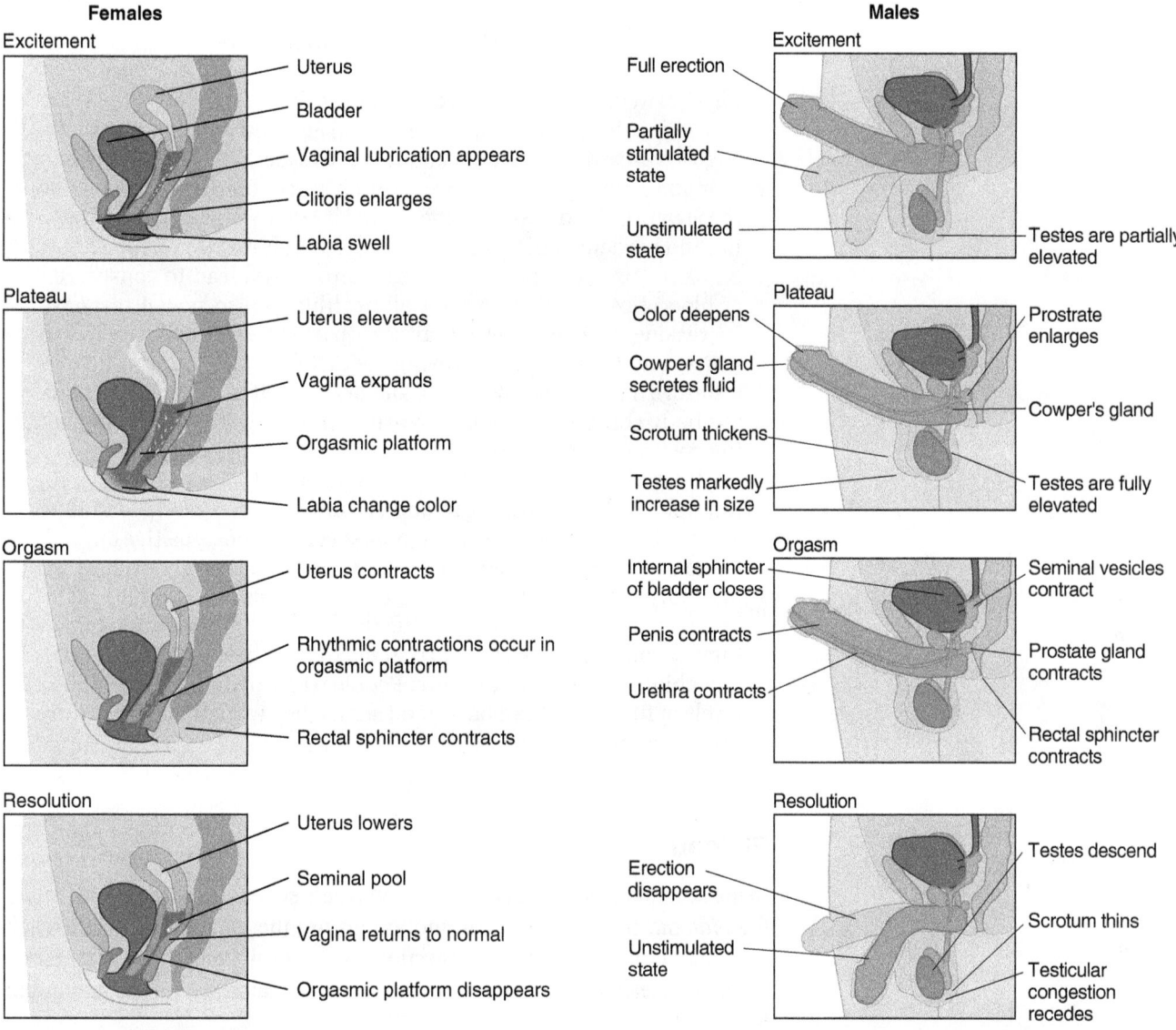

Figure 7.4 *Masters and Johnson's Sexual Response Cycle in Women* This cycle has four phases.

Figure 7.5 *Masters and Johnson's Sexual Response Cycle in Men* The cycle for men has four phases.

They called this process **transudation** and discovered that it was directly linked to the level of sexual excitement. Masters and Johnson found that insufficient lubrication is often the result of too little foreplay and low levels of excitement or high levels of anxiety.

The second characteristic associated with excitement is **myotonia,** the gradual heightened tension in the skeletal muscles throughout the body. Unlike the muscle tension associated with stress, myotonia is a gradual buildup that is progressive and pleasurable. Employing specially developed instruments and methods, Masters and Johnson were able to quantify the level of muscle tension in various parts of the body during sexual arousal. This was done by placing electrodes on strategic parts of the body to measure **electromyographic** activity during sexual arousal.

During excitement in men, the testes elevate, moving closer to the body. In women, the inner two-thirds of the vagina expand, and the uterus is pulled backward.

Transudation The production of vaginal lubrication because of sweating of vaginal tissue engorged with blood during vasocongestion

Myotonia Involuntary skeletal muscle contractions

Electromyographic Refers to measurement of muscle tension through electrical sensors at skin surface

෨ *Physical Wellness* ෨

Physical wellness contributes directly to healthy sexual response. When we are physically fit, our bodies respond and perform better sexually. High-level cardiorespiratory endurance can facilitate maximum blood flow and staying power. Vasocongestion hinges on efficient blood flow through the blood vessels to the genitals. Atherosclerosis, the narrowing and hardening of blood vessels, can inhibit maximum blood flow. Smoking also can speed up atherosclerosis and lead to constriction of blood flow. This affects overall health and also sexual response. Increasing the overall level of fitness (particularly, cardiorespiratory fitness and flexibility), improving the diet (minimizing fats and cholesterol), limiting use of alcohol and other illicit drugs, and maximizing body composition can increase overall physical well-being and improve sexual response.

Although being fit doesn't *ensure* good sex, it can enhance the physiological (body strength and endurance, increased blood flow, and the like) and psychological (higher self-esteem, positive outlook, enhanced body image) components of good sex. Conversely, having a disability or illness, or being unfit, doesn't necessarily preclude sexual satisfaction. People with disabilities and chronic illnesses that impact their sexual response can learn to maximize their sexual potentials and abilities, whatever they are. People who do not have the highest levels of fitness still can have good sex as they work their way toward becoming fit.

Plateau

In the second phase of Masters' and Johnson's sexual response cycle, called the *plateau*, processes set into motion during the excitement phase reach their maximum levels. Vasocongestion creates peak levels of engorgement, color changes, and lubrication; muscular tension also reaches its maximum level.

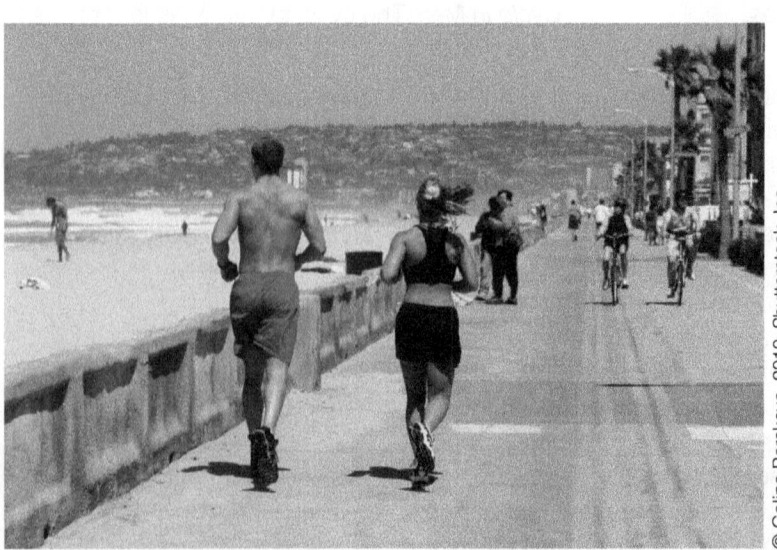

High-level cardiorespiratory fitness can enhance vasocongestion.

In men, the testes become fully elevated, and the prostate gland enlarges. The Cowper's gland releases clear, slippery, preejaculatory fluid (we will discuss the sperm-carrying capability of this fluid in Chapter 14). In women, the labia reach their maximum size, the vagina forms the "orgasmic platform," and the clitoris retracts under its protective hood. Both men and women experience a "sex flush," a rashlike reddish tinge to the skin of the chest and back associated with dilation of the blood vessels and increased blood flow in these areas.

Masters and Johnson found that the plateau was the most variable stage in terms of time. More experienced

© Galina Barskaya, 2010. Shutterstock, Inc.

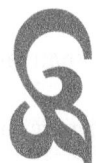

healthy sex hints 7.1

Effects of Aphrodisiacs

People are always searching for a magic potion that will enhance their sexual response and enable them to respond quicker, last longer, and become re-aroused quicker. This has enabled a multi-million-dollar aphrodisiac market to flourish. Certain foods, nutrients, and other aphrodisiacs are promoted as aids to sexual response. But do they work? The answer is yes and no.

Although no true aphrodisiac (a potion that increases desire and performance) exists, if you think it's helping, it probably is, as is the case with any placebo. Because the mind and the body work together in initiating and perpetuating sexual response, it makes sense that if a person perceives that a substance will help promote sexual response, it just might (Bergeson, 2005, Scelfo, 2002).

Physiologically, however, the effects of aphrodisiacs are mixed. In general, they can be categorized by the way they work: provide energy, increase blood flow to the genitals, decrease the sensitivity of genital tissue, and increase desire in the brain.

Various "pep pills" are promoted as increasing energy levels. These are featured in fitness and "muscle" magazines, and claim to enhance sexual desire by increasing overall energy levels. Although we believe that sexual desire is enhanced through high-level well-being, we think this should emanate from a healthy lifestyle, not a "pep pill." Other aphrodisiacs, in the form of salves and creams, claim to work by enhancing vasocongestion (firmer erections, more responsiveness)—sending more blood to the genital area. In reality, vasocongestion is a result of dilation and constriction of blood vessels and changes in blood pressure, not extra surface blood in the smaller capillaries.

Still other aphrodisiacs claim to work by decreasing sensitivity, which hypothetically allows men to "last longer." These topical creams and ointments often inflame sensitive genital tissue, creating painful irritation. Using a condom to cover the head of the penis is a better way to decrease sensitivity.

Psychoactive drugs and alcohol work by altering perception. Alcohol deadens the parts of the brain that control conscious thought. This can reduce negative thoughts and feelings that might inhibit sexual response. Other drugs, such as marijuana, heighten sensations such as touch and smell. Enhancing the ability to perceive sensations can heighten enjoyment of sexual activity and promote sexual response.

Viagra, a treatment recommended for men (and under study in women) with erectile disorders associated with impaired genital blood flow, has also been touted as an aphrodisiac. Although Viagra is very effective in enhancing blood flow in people with this problem, its utility in enhancing sexual response in men and women with adequate blood flow is questionable.

The best "aphrodisiacs," in our opinion, are summarized as the following:

> Become physically fit.
> Develop healthy eating habits.
> Reduce stress through relaxation techniques and behavior management.

couples, for instance, were able to prolong the plateau if they desired, whereas younger, less sexually experienced subjects had much shorter plateau periods.

Orgasm

The third phase of Masters and Johnson's response cycle, orgasm, is characterized by the dramatic release of tension and other physiological processes (heart rate, blood pressure, increased breathing, and so on) associated with the excitement and plateau stages. During orgasm, most of the male and female sexual structures undergo rhythmic, muscular contractions. These are responsible for the release of pent-up muscular tension in men and women, and ejaculation in men.

Masters and Johnson found that women have a one-step orgasm, whereas it is a two-step process in men. The first step in men is called **ejaculatory inevitability.** During this step, men sense the release of tension and feel the inevitability of ejaculation. During the next step, **emission** contractions of the vas deferens and other structures move sperm and other ejaculatory fluids through the vas deferens and out of the urethra. Masters and Johnson found that women did not ejaculate during orgasm.

Prior to Masters and Johnson, researchers studying sexual response used much more subjective criteria for determining whether an orgasm had or had not occurred. Masters and Johnson quantified the muscular contractions, fluid expulsions (in men only), and physiological reversals associated with the release of tension as a result of orgasm.

Resolution

The last phase of the sexual response cycle is resolution, return of the body to the unaroused state. Masters and Johnson found that after orgasm, the two key physiological processes—vasocongestion and myotonia—reverse. Orgasm triggers the brain to normalize the dilation of blood vessels, heart rate, and blood pressure, allowing blood flow to return to normal and vasocongestion to reverse. With this reversal, the erection begins to shrink, lubrication ceases, and color changes disappear. In addition, the buildup of muscular tension followed by contractions stops, and muscle tissue returns to normal.

Masters and Johnson (1966) coined the term **refractory period** to describe the time required after an orgasm before a person could enter the excitement stage again. They found tremendous variability in this time between men and women, and among individual men. They found that women did not have a refractory period. Women did not need recovery time to get excited again and reach orgasm.

Vasocongestion and lubrication could remain at optimal levels if the source and intensity of stimulation and interest in maintaining activity with the partner were to continue. The significance of this finding was that it proved that women could have multiple orgasms without a refractory period. This is both a difference between men's and women's sexual response patterns and a significant finding in terms of women's ability to extend and enjoy sexual relations if they desire.

For most women in Masters and Johnson's study, however, sexual stimulation ceased after their partner's orgasm. Often, this is because of preset agendas that couples have about trying to achieve orgasm simultaneously or a "me first, then you" pattern in achieving orgasm. In follow-up studies, Masters and Johnson (1976) found that most male partners did not realize that they could continue to stimulate their partners (if desired, through pubic contact or manual/oral stimulation), even if they were to lose their erection.

Unlike women, men need a certain amount of downtime before they can achieve another erection. The amount of time varies significantly. Among the variables related to the amount of time needed to obtain another erection, the most significant were age and time since last orgasm. In gen-

Ejaculatory inevitability The first step in male ejaculation; beginning of smooth-muscle contractions that trigger release of ejaculate

Emission The release of secretions from various organs and glands that produce male ejaculate

Refractory period The time from last orgasm to the next beginning of excitement

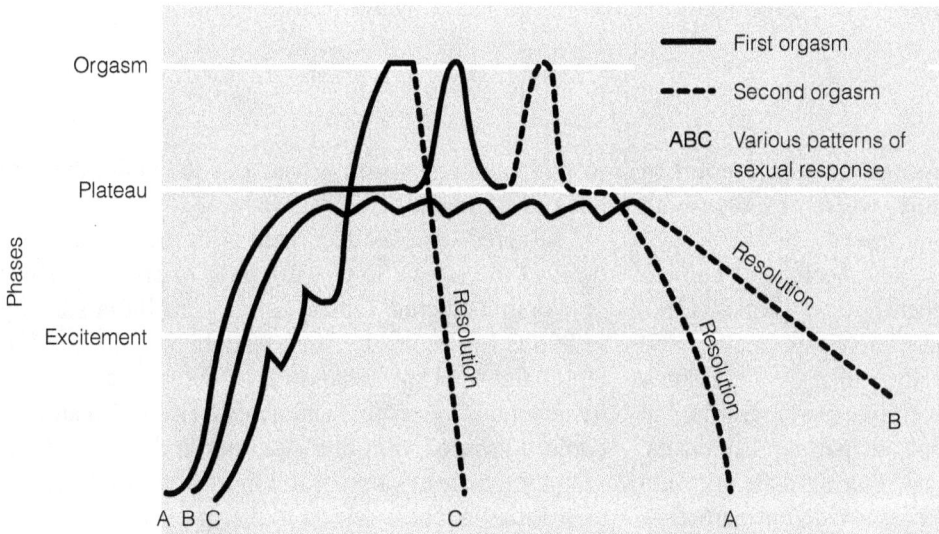

Figure 7.6 *Masters and Johnson's Sexual Response Patterns in Women* Masters and Johnson found three major sexual response patterns in women.
Source: *Human Sexual Response* by W. Masters and V. Johnson (1966).

eral, the younger the man, the shorter the refractory period. The longer the duration since the last orgasm, the shorter the refractory period. Thus, a younger man who hadn't had an orgasm in some time would become re-aroused much more quickly than an older man who recently had an orgasm. Other variables, such as overall level of health, stress, and obesity, were also found to be related to the length of refractory period.

Figures 7.6 and 7.7 show the patterns in sexual response that Masters and Johnson discovered for the men and women in their study. Figure 7.7, their classic cycle for men, shows a steady buildup in excitement followed

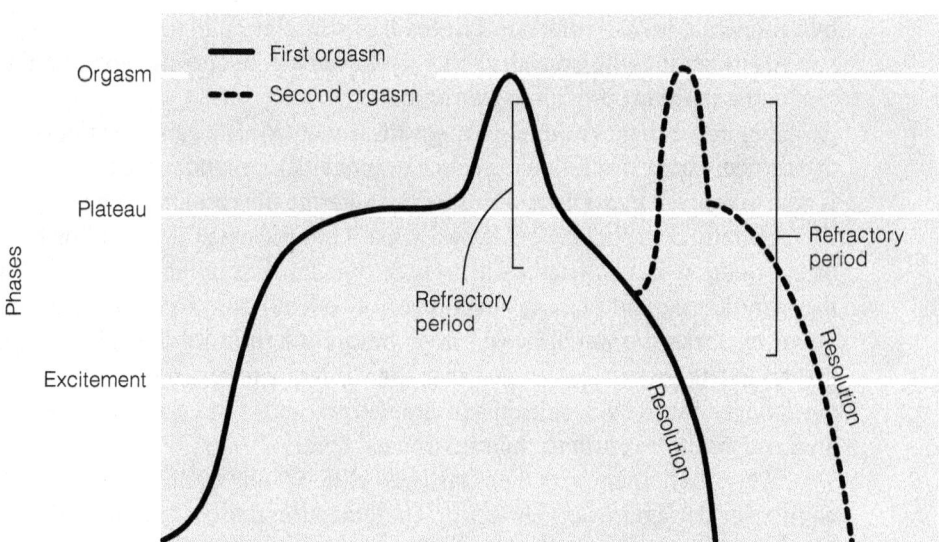

Figure 7.7 *Masters and Johnson's Sexual Response Patterns in Men*
Masters and Johnson found one primary sexual response pattern in men.
Source: *Human Sexual Response* by W. Masters and V. Johnson (1966).

sex in society 7.2
Tantric Sex

For most Americans, orgasm is the whole point of sexual activities. As a culture, we're obsessed with orgasm. We keep track of orgasms like box scores for baseball: number of at-bats (sexual encounters), number of hits (orgasms), and whether they are singles (OK), doubles (slightly better orgasms), triples (really good orgasms), and home runs (really, really, great orgasms). We are not only obsessed with our own orgasms, but we also want to know about our partner's orgasms. "Was it good for you?" we ask. Our ultimate criterion is to achieve simultaneous orgasm with our partner—the ultimate: two home runs at the same time! None of these scoring measures correlates perfectly with sexual satisfaction or healthy sexuality. Frequency, intensity, and mutuality of orgasms vary in their relationship to sexual satisfaction for people.

One can even enjoy sex without orgasm. The idea of having intercourse but intentionally not having an orgasm may seem strange, but that's exactly the point of Tantric sex: an Indian sexual/spiritual practice based on *conserving orgasm*. The origins of Tantra can be traced back over 20,000 years to markings on cave walls that resemble those still in use today in Tantric training. Tantra, originally associated with fertility worship and paganism, is based on the belief that life itself is the result of sex and love.

Sacred temples decorated with the sexual positions of the Kama Sutra were built to provide places of worship for the Tantric religion in India starting in 800 C.E.. Indian spiritual leaders taught their disciples about the spiritual power of sexual energy. They believed the energy that emanates from sexual arousal could be shared with one's partner and used to transcend the couple's sexual union to bring them closer to spiritual oneness with a higher power. Tantric sex is part of the spiritual form of yoga. The spiritual form of yoga is practiced to achieve a transcendent state of being (see www.tantric.com).

In the West, the practice of Tantra borrows liberally from Hinduism, Taoism, Buddhism, Native American spirituality, and Wiccan. Disciples view Tantric sex as a spiritual activity that unites partners in transcendence and also as a technique to enhance sexual intensity. Couples focus on sexual pleasuring, not the outcome of orgasm. This de-emphasis on orgasm allows couples to relax and enjoy the sensations without being so goal directed. Some organizations run Tantric sex training programs and retreats.

by a moderate level of plateau. The level of stimulation in the plateau stage reaches its zenith with orgasm. This is followed by the cessation of stimulation and a rapid drop-off into resolution.

Figure 7.6 diagrams multiple orgasms in women. The pattern is similar to that in men, except that following orgasm, stimulation continues and the woman is able to achieve multiple orgasms before entering the resolution phase.

Pattern B in Figure 7.6 shows what happens when the level or type of stimulation is insufficient to trigger orgasm. Excitement builds with the stimulation, and plateau is achieved. The level or type of stimulation, however, lacks the intensity (or stops before it can build to high enough levels) to trigger orgasm, which is responsible for reversing the effects of vasocongestion. This results in a protracted resolution stage until the pelvic area and genitals return to their unaroused levels.

This phenomenon in men has been called "blue balls." Although no equivalent slang term applies to women, females experience similar effects: pelvic congestion, swollen genitalia, throbbing pelvic area, and so on. Although Masters' and Johnson's findings added valuable information about the objective experience of sexual response, the analysis is physiological and is open to a more subjective interpretation.

sex in society 7.3

Rethinking the Role of the Clitoris in Sexual Arousal

Since Master's & Johnson's pioneering research on human sexual response in the 1960s the presence of penile erection and vaginal lubrication have been considered the gold standard as far as proof of sexual arousal in men and women respectively. Clitoral engorgement and erection, though noted in the literature, has not been considered to be as significant an indicator of sexual arousal in women as vaginal lubrication. Recent research findings in sexual anatomy and the physiology of sexual response are shedding new light on the nature of clitoral erection in female sexual arousal.

O'Connell et al (2005) believe that while it is appealing to use a single, simple term, the clitoris, to refer to a "cluster of erectile tissue," it can be misleading, and it de-emphasizes the complexity of female sexual response. Their research, based on autopsies of cadavers and MRI studies shows that the vascular structures of the pelvic area in women (the distal vagina, distal urethra and clitoris including the vestibular bulbs, crura, body and glans) actually form a unified cluster of structures that can be identified using MRI technology and surgical removal.

As we mentioned in Chapter 2, most of the clitoris is not visible before or during sexual arousal. The glans is exposed during sexual arousal but the underlying structures of the clitoris are not. New research suggests that these underlying structures may play a larger role in sexual arousal than previously believed. Johnson (2004) uses an iceberg analogy to explain how the glans of the clitoris is similar to the tip of an iceberg. Most of the mass of the clitoris continues under pelvic bone, turns down and surrounds the vagina from above and both sides. Starting from the exposed glans and working back are the clitoral shaft, two crura, and two vestibular bulbs. The clitoral shaft is about 2.5

centimeters long and, like the penis, contains two corpora cavernosa. The two crura (also referred to as the legs) extend back from the top, and are five to nine centimeters long, anchoring to the hip girdle. Inside of the two crura are the two vestibular bulbs.

Johnson (2004) and O'Connel et al (2005) found that the underlying structures are richly endowed with nerve endings and all, with the exception of the glans, are comprised of erectile tissue that engorge with blood during sexual arousal. Johnson (2004) and O'Connell et al (2005) have found that these underlying structures also surround the female urethra and their contractions during sexual arousal squeeze the urethra shut. Johnson (2004) believes that so-called "vaginal" or "G Spot" orgasms and female ejaculation are a byproduct of these underlying structures working in consort with the urethra and its paraurethral glands. In their findings on cadavers and on MRI analysis, O'Connell et al (2005) "did not reveal any additional structure separate from the bulbs, glans, or corpora of the clitoris, urethra and vagina that could be regarded as the G spot." Furthermore, O'Connell et al's (2005) findings clearly indicate that the erectile tissue of these interrelated vascular structures wrap around the urethra and vagina forming a midline core to the clitoris.

O'Connell et al (2005) believe that referring to this cluster of vascular structures as a unified entity with a different name would provide a new, inclusive way to describe female sexual anatomy. Such an inclusive description, O'Connell et al(2005) and Johnson (2004) believe, would end artificial discussions of female sexual response that separate clitoral from vaginal orgasms and highlight individual areas within this region such as the "G Spot" that are actually interrelated.

For instance, even though an orgasm, according to Masters' and Johnson, is characterized by a certain number of muscular contractions at a certain intensity and other physiological parameters, a person could have an enjoyable sexual experience without having an official Masters and Johnson orgasm.

What operationalizing a concept such as orgasm does is to allow us to study it more rigorously. For instance, if researchers want to study the effects of alcohol on orgasm, their research will be easier and more accurate if they are able to operationally define orgasm. The same kind of rigor need not enter into our human relations.

Kaplan's Triphasic Model of Sexual Response

Helen Singer Kaplan (1974) disagreed with Masters' and Johnson's four-phase sexual response cycle. She argued that the model neglects the importance of sexual desire in human sexual response. Furthermore, she agreed with others in the field who claimed that the plateau stage is really indistinguishable from excitement and that the two stages would more appropriately be merged together.

Kaplan's original model had two stages: excitement and orgasm. She modified it, however, after her work with dysfunctional individuals and couples revealed that many of them had problems with low levels of interest in sex. She then proposed a triphasic model of sexual response that included the phases of desire, excitement, and orgasm (Kaplan, 1985). She placed most of the emphasis on desire and the role of the brain in initiating sexual response.

Desire

During the desire phase, some activating thought, emotion, fantasy, or sensation arises in the cortex or limbic system and triggers the activation of neural and hormonal sexual stimulation. The emphasis here is on the key role the cerebral cortex plays in initiating sexual response, and the subjective, emotional nature of arousal. As we mentioned at the beginning of this chapter, the brain is the sexiest organ in the body and plays the key role in determining whether the sexual response continues.

Excitement

Kaplan accepted Masters' and Johnson's findings concerning the physiology of sexual arousal. She agreed that vasocongestion is the key physiological process involved in excitement. She disagreed, however, with the idea of separating the plateau from excitement. She argued that the plateau is really nothing more than end-stage excitement or culmination of the excitement phase. When excitement peaks, the person reaches the plateau, or level of maximum arousal. As such, however, to clinically distinguish plateau from excitement is next to impossible, and, therefore, the two phases should be merged.

Orgasm

Once again, Kaplan accepted Masters' and Johnson's findings concerning the physiology of orgasm. She also described orgasm as the one phase that is clearly distinguishable for most people. Unlike the transition from desire to excitement, which is hard to pinpoint, the onset of orgasm is an event most people readily identify.

Criticisms of Kaplan's and Masters' and Johnson's Models

Although Kaplan's model of sexual response is important because it expands Masters' and Johnson's conceptualization by adding the dimension of desire to the cycle, it still left gaps in fully understanding the nature of sexual response in men and women.

Lieblum (2000), a renowned sex therapist and educator, notes how Kaplan's model doesn't always match up to women's experiences of sexual response. Lieblum describes how many women do not have spontaneous feelings of sexual desire, and for those who do, it doesn't always lead to arousal. She found that most women rely on their male partners to initiate sexual activity, and they may or may not participate, depending on a host of sexual and nonsexual factors, such as intimacy.

Lieblum adds that for many women *and* men, arousal comes *before* desire. A man's morning erection may trigger feelings of desire and interest in initiating intercourse with a partner. The feeling of pleasurable genital sensations or touch may ignite feelings of desire in women. In other words, the order of the response is reversed from what Kaplan found.

Lastly, Lieblum (2000) found that Kaplan's and Masters' and Johnson's models do not take subjective feelings of sexual satisfaction into account. A purely physiological explanation of sexual response is inadequate, according to Lieblum, because it doesn't attend to the subjective feelings of satisfaction or dissatisfaction, which contribute greatly to future desire and arousal. For many women, satisfaction with sexual activity with their partner did not necessarily revolve around whether or not they had an orgasm (as it usually does with men).

❧ *Emotional Wellness* ❧

Good sexual response hinges on our emotional well-being. As Lieblum, Basson, and the other sexual response theorists in this chapter point out, our sexual response involves both physiological and psychological variables. We have to be in the right frame of mind for vasocongestion to happen. When we are nervous, angry, sad, worried, or in a number of other negative emotional states, we have trouble relaxing enough to allow our brain to trigger efficient vasocongestion. Even if we allow ourselves to become sexually excited, we may not be able to have an orgasm. The best sex is usually when we are able to let down our guard, free our mind, and relax. High-level emotional wellness allows us to do this. We are in control of our emotions; they don't control us. We feel good about ourselves and about our partners, and we trust ourselves and our partners enough to relax and let the sexual responses happen.

Expanding Your Perception of Lovemaking and Orgasm

Sex is a goal-oriented activity for many people. It seems they view sex as a race, with both partners competing to see who crosses first with an orgasm. Even better, both partners cross at the same time and have the ultimate prize—mutual orgasms. The prize is the perfect orgasm, achieved together. The ultimate victory is the quest for perfect sex. Is this really the best sex? Is sex best viewed as a competition, a race? We like to think of sex as more of a multicourse gourmet meal. With each course the couple anticipates something special, a unique taste delight.

A before-dinner aperitif sets the mood for the evening and whets the appetite for the next course, appetizers. Appetizers delight the palate. They come in an infinite variety, each with its own special ability to please.

Next comes a soup, followed by a special salad. Each tickles the taste buds and is savored for its uniqueness. Between these courses we pause and have a refreshing sorbet to cleanse the palate. We stop and sit back, savoring the exquisite gastronomical delights we've already sampled, and we eagerly anticipate the rest of the meal to follow. We enjoy good conversation and admiring looks.

The entree comes next—not too much food, just enough to satisfy our cravings and delight our palate.

We pause again to savor our meal before dessert is served. Dessert provides just a taste of sweetness to round off our meal.

Finally, we sit back, sipping our after-dinner brandy. This brings our meal to a close.

When we eat a meal such as this, who can argue that the entree is the only or most important part of the meal? Sometimes the entree isn't as special as the other parts of the meal, and we only sample it. We can view lovemaking as a feast, a multicourse meal that first involves the buildup of desire through kissing, hugging, massage, and noncoital foreplay.

The lovemaking continues with a variety of techniques including oral sex, vaginal intercourse, and so on, extending the plateau as long as we desire. We pause frequently to talk, laugh, touch, have a drink, and the like. We continue into and through orgasm, and we finish by staying coupled and basking in each other's pleasure until we go limp.

If we envision sex as a feast for the senses rather than as a race, perhaps we will enjoy our orgasms more when they occur, and not feel as though we've missed something if we don't have them once in a while.

Stayton's Spiritual/Theological Model

William Stayton (2002), a Baptist minister, has an interesting spiritual/theological perspective on sexual response and pleasure. In 1965, in his early years as a minister, Stayton was asked by his church's youth group to develop an education program on sexuality. He admits to have been both excited and scared by the prospect. He was excited because he felt such information was needed and who better than the church to provide it to the congregation. He was afraid, however, because sex was very controversial, and he was not sure how his congregation would view his program.

❧ *Spiritual Wellness* ❧

By definition, spirituality revolves around transcending ourselves and connecting with something greater than ourselves. Whether we believe our spirituality connects us with God, some higher power, or all other living things, transcendence of the self is the key to spirituality. We've often heard people describe orgasm in terms of feeling "uplifted," "out of this world," or "at one with the universe." We believe the transcendence that orgasm offers is inherent in our sexual response and not totally reliant on our emotional connections to another. We also believe, however, that sex and orgasm with someone we love and are committed to gives a heightened level of spirituality. Sharing an intense orgasm with another person can, at times, make you feel instantly at one with the universe. If one positive human experience is capable of linking all of us together, it just might be orgasm. Humans and other animals seem to share the ability to respond sexually to one another. Sexual activity with a partner, by its nature, connects us to someone else in a unique way. A high level of spiritual wellness can help us form sexual relationships based on caring and mutual respect, instead of exploitation and disrespect.

His fears were assuaged when 60 young people, parental permission slips in hand, showed up for his first session. His program was such a success that the local school district asked him to develop a curriculum for the Glouchester, Massachusetts, Board of Education.

Stayton's basic premise is that it is not by coincidence that sexual response is undeniably pleasurable. The theological significance of sexual pleasure and response is that God created humans in such a way to respond to sexual pleasure. He cites Masters' and Johnson's discovery of the clitoris as the center of sexual response in women as evidence that God intended humans to be sexual creatures and enjoy this blessing. Why else would he make such an organ that has no other function except to provide sexual pleasure?

Stayton uses sexual research about sexual response as proof that God created humans with the ability to derive extreme pleasure from loving each other. In fact, Jesus' core teachings were about love. Stayton explains that Jesus, God's son, never, even in his teachings of self-denial, condemns sexual pleasure. Jesus' primary teachings revolved around love, not condemnation of pleasure. Stayton's "theology of sexual pleasure" is that love, spirituality, and sexuality are inextricably bound together and that God created people who are sexual in the fullest sense of the word. To be fully sexual in God's world is to be both physical and spiritual.

Love, Stayton believes, has both sexual and spiritual dimensions. Why would God create in us the ability to feel such intense sexual pleasure if it were not his intention to connect it to the pursuit of love? Doesn't "making love" have a strong spiritual component that transcends the act of sexual intercourse with the loved one? Aren't we truly at one with the universe when making love to another person?

Stayton believes that God intended sex researchers to continue his mission by guiding them to understand more about this gift he bestowed

case study 7.3

Steve and Tracy: What Good Sex Means to Us

Steve, 26, identifies as African American; Tracey, 23, is white.

Steve is a senior majoring in small business administration. He took some time off after high school and worked in construction before starting college. Tracy is an education major and a fifth-year senior, having worked her way full-time through college.

STEVE: Good sex to me is being able to relax with my partner. With Tracy, I don't have to worry about anything. I trust her.

TRACY: Yeah, that's it—trust. Before I met Steve, I went through a lot of one-night stands or real short relationships where I think the guys just wanted to get laid. I never felt I could trust any of them.

PROFESSOR: What do you mean by "trust them"?

TRACY: I guess I mean trust them about *anything*. Would they respect me and my wishes? Would they have my interests at heart or just their own? I also was worried about pregnancy and disease. Could I trust them to be disease-free, wear a condom, those sort of things? Oh, yeah, I also wanted to be able to trust that they'd respect my privacy. I didn't want them to go bragging to their friends about me or tell other people the most intimate aspects of my sex life.

STEVE: I feel the same way. I like to be able to let down my guard in order to enjoy sex. I guess you could say that, for me, it's sexy to be vulnerable with a woman. With Tracy, I can tell her about my desires, concerns, and fears, and trust her to act in my best interests. I remember telling one woman I had sex with that I liked it when she played with my anus during sex but that I always worried that this might mean I was gay. I later found out she had told this to a sorority sister, and before long everyone in the house knew, as well as some members of the fraternity they were little sisters to.

PROFESSOR: How does trust affect your sexual response?

TRACY: For me, it allows me to let down my guard and relax. I trust Steve completely, and that allows my mind and body to relax. I've never been as responsive with anyone else as I am with Steve. I can get sexually aroused and have an orgasm with very little effort.

STEVE: I feel the same way. With Tracy, I feel so relaxed that things just naturally happen. I remember with other women worrying that I might not perform up to their standards, and that made it real difficult to get excited and erect. I know I can please Tracy, and even if I have an off-night, she'll understand and not use it against me.

TRACY: I hope I don't make it seem that because I'm so relaxed, there's no spark or sexual tension between Steve and me. Nothing can be farther from the truth. Even though I'm completely relaxed in bed with him, I can get aroused just thinking about sex with him. I hope this never changes.

Critical Thinking

How has trust, or lack of trust, in a sexual partner influenced your enjoyment of sex with that person? What role would trust play in your future sexual relationships?

on us. Like theologians who interpret God's word through studying the Bible, sex researchers interpret God's gift of sexual pleasure by studying sexual response.

Lastly, Stayton believes that when people combine love, sex, and spirituality, God's intentions are born anew in the world. Sexual pleasure is not a hindrance to God's mission; it is part of it. He cites "creation" as something God did for humans but also as something God intended to create us to be able to derive sexual pleasure through our love for each other and to create new life.

Basson's Model

The newest sexual response model was developed by Rosemary Basson, a sex therapist, in 1999. Basson's (2000) model is both similar to and different from those that preceded it, and grew out of her work as a sex therapist. As we will see in Chapter 12, traditional diagnostic criteria for sexual dysfunction are based on the widely accepted sexual response phases of Masters and Johnson (arousal, and orgasm) and Kaplan's (desire) models. Basson does not believe that these models hold the key to treating women with sexual dysfunction. A new model of sexual response in women was needed, one that would serve as the basis for treating women's sexual dysfunction.

Basson does not take issue with the physiology of sexual response. She doesn't dispute the physiological processes involved in arousal, orgasm, and resolution. Her dispute is with the interplay of psychosocial and physiological factors during sexual arousal, and the lumping of men's and women's sexual response patterns together.

Basson also believes, like Walen and Roth (1987), that cognitive factors continually mediate the physiology of sexual response. Positive thoughts and feelings (trust, caring, happiness) about one's partner are necessary for intimacy to exist and for sexual response to occur. Negative thoughts and feelings (anger, fear, unhappiness) can sabotage intimacy and make desire and arousal difficult, if not impossible.

Basson's model also revolves around the premise of gender-based differences in sexual response between men and women. Basson believes that emotional factors and intimacy issues are central to understanding sexual response in women. She feels that female sexual response doesn't begin with desire or arousal as it does in men; it begins with intimacy. Basson believes that for many women, the starting point for the sexual response cycle is not the desire for sex (physical sexual release) but the desire for intimacy (being close emotionally and physically with one's partner).

The desire to initiate intimate contact could occur either for positive reasons or to avoid negative consequences. For instance, a woman could initiate an intimacy because she wants to hug and talk, to get close to her partner (positive reason). She might also initiate intimacy because she feels she has neglected her husband (or vice versa), and she doesn't want this to create any anger, resentment, or displeasure in her relationship with him. In either case, the primary motivation isn't a feeling of sexual tension and the desire for sexual release. It was a desire for intimacy.

The woman herself may have no conscious feeling of need of sexual release (desire) to initiate an intimate connection with her partner. Once the intimate connection is made, however, classic stimuli (internal and external) for sexual arousal are introduced.

case study 7.4

Alyssa: A Case of Fear and Mistrust

Alyssa, 20, white, identifies as lesbian.

Alyssa is a college junior. She recently broke up with Carla, her girlfriend of 2 years. She and Carla had been having sex for about 1.5 years. Alyssa has had little sexual desire and some problems having an orgasm ever since she broke up with Carla about 3 months ago.

COUNSELOR: Tell me about what's been troubling you.

ALYSSA: I've been having a hard time having an orgasm lately when I have sex. I seem to be able to get excited, but something seems to keep me from being able to come.

COUNSELOR: Have you ever had this kind of problem before?

ALYSSA: No, I never had problems coming when I was going out with Carla.

COUNSELOR: When did you break up with Carla?

ALYSSA: About 3 months ago.

COUNSELOR: How many times have you had sex since then?

ALYSSA: I still masturbate about twice a week, but I've had sex only four or five times—once with a woman I met at a party and the other times with a gal from one of my classes. In each case, I didn't have sex on the first date, only after we went out a couple of times.

COUNSELOR: Do you achieve orgasm when you masturbate?

ALYSSA: Yes. Always.

COUNSELOR: Tell me about your feelings toward these two women.

ALYSSA: The first woman, Jill, is fun to be around. She's a real party gal, likes to dance, go to karaoke bars. . . . We have a good time together, but I worry about her past. I try to talk to her about her past sex life, but she kind of blows it off. It's hard to talk about this stuff. One of my girlfriends told me that she heard that Jill was bisexual and has had a lot of different sexual partners in her life. This worries me. I don't want to get AIDS.

COUNSELOR: What are you doing about this?

ALYSSA: I insisted that we practice safe sex until we got to know each other better. It basically worked. We didn't go down on each other and got off other ways, but I got the sense that she really wasn't into it. She's never said as much, but I could pick it up from her attitude. It didn't make for great sex. I kind of anticipated that it was going to be a problem, so it put a damper on things for me. I never really relaxed. I didn't come.

COUNSELOR: Tell me about the other woman.

(continued)

Critical Thinking

How is the issue of trust in lesbian and gay relationships similar to and different from that in heterosexual relationships? What special trust issues might gay and lesbian people face that heterosexuals don't?

Case Study 7.4—Continued

ALYSSA: The other woman, Luz, is very nice. I know her from class last year, and she's in my psychology class this semester. She asked me out when she found out I broke up with Carla. She was very tender and understanding. She encouraged me to talk about Carla and get a lot of things out. We've had sex a few times, but I still haven't been able to come.

Luz has a real temper. I've seen her almost lose it a couple of times over silly things like getting cut off by another driver on the highway. She seems to respect me, but I worry about her going ballistic on me if I ever get on her bad side. I can't fully relax around her when we're in bed. I've heard of date rape, and I'm afraid if I ever refuse her because I'm not in the mood for sex, she might force me. Not a real good way to start a relationship, huh?

The woman's partner may tell her he finds her attractive, desirable, and the like (internal stimuli). They may hug, listen to music, or share a bath (external stimuli). Desire and arousal emerge from these elements of intimacy between them. In many cases, the woman makes a conscious decision to become aroused.

Basson (2004) points out a problem with using the same models and evidence of sexual arousal in men and women. Studies in men traditionally have pointed to erection and other physiological changes as evidence of sexual arousal and desire. While this is adequate in most cases for studying men because most men equate physical arousal with desire, it may not be suitable for use as the model and evidence for studying sexual response in all women. Basson (2004) feels that while women might show *evidence* of sexual arousal (vaginal lubrication and clitoral engorgement) this may not be an accurate indicator of their true arousal. Using the latest magnetic resonance imaging (MRI) technology, Basson (2004) found that women's *subjective* experience and description of arousal does not always correlate with her *objective* physiological (vaginal lubrication, clitoral structures engorged with blood, etc.) *evidence* of arousal. What this research suggests is that even though women show genital physiological evidence of sexual arousal, this doesn't always correlate with their thinking about and feeling desire and arousal in their brain.

Another difference in Basson's theory is her belief that desire *follows* arousal and results in greater levels of arousal. Because the two are so closely related, it is often difficult to distinguish when one starts and the other ends. Basson believes that sexual response in this sense is more circular than linear. A woman doesn't move from intimacy to arousal and then to desire, and then to orgasm, and so forth. Intimacy leads to arousal, which sparks desire, which leads to greater feelings of intimacy, which leads to higher levels of arousal and therefore more desire. The cycle could end in orgasm, but it doesn't have to in order for the woman to feel satisfied and desire more intimacy. At every point in the cycle, cognitive factors (positive or negative) affect what is going on. Levels of desire, arousal, and satisfaction are always mediated by the subjective perception of cognitive factors such as trust, mistrust, fear, anger, and so on (Basson, 2002).

Another key difference is the reference to an end point of sexual response other than orgasm or resolution. Basson believes that a subjective end point relating to satisfaction is critical to understanding women's sexual response. Many women, she found, report enjoying a sexual encounter, even if it didn't end in orgasm. Men typically equate satisfaction with orgasm, but Basson found that for many women, that wasn't the case. Rather than equate "good" sexual response with achieving orgasm, Basson feels that sexual response should be evaluated on whether the person enjoyed the experience. In fact, attaining orgasm may not always be related to an enjoyable sexual encounter. Lieblum (2000) found that men and women can go through an entire sexual response cycle (including orgasm) while reporting that the encounter wasn't enjoyable. Consequently, Basson feels there should be some end point such as feelings of satisfaction, disappointment, frustration, and so on, that characterizes the cycle rather than just the presence of orgasm.

Disability and Sexual Response

Perhaps the most misunderstood aspect of persons with disabilities is their sexual response. People with disabilities are often viewed by the nondisabled as either asexual or lacking in the ability to respond sexually and in the capacity for normal and satisfying relationships (Chance, 2002).

In fact, most people with disabilities are not asexual. They have both the desire and the ability to respond sexually, seek outlets for their desire, and seek to establish satisfying sexual relationships with others. As we have learned, there are a variety of ways to define sexual response. We will examine a few different types of disabilities to illustrate how the sexual response manifests itself for persons with these conditions.

Spinal Cord Injuries

The effects of spinal cord injury on sexual response are directly related to where the injury is located. In a spinal cord injury, neural functions above the lesion tend to remain intact. Functions dictated by areas below the injury change and often cease. The lower the injury, the greater the chance the person will be able to experience some type of sexual stimulation and response.

Another variable related to how a spinal cord injury manifests itself in sexual response is *when* the injury occurred in the person's sexual life cycle. The older a person is when the injury occurs, the more they can draw on past sexual memories, associations, and behaviors. Being born with a spinal cord injury, having one occur during childhood, or becoming disabled in the prime of one's sexually active period all manifest themselves differently in the individual's sexual response.

Desire

As we previously mentioned, there is no physical relationship between spinal cord injury and sexual desire. Alexander, Sipski, and Findley (1993) found that most men with spinal cord injuries return to sexual activities within 12 months of their injury. Although most of the subjects reported lowered sexual satisfaction postinjury, their level of sexual desire did not change significantly. A key factor influencing the subjects' sexual desire was the level of desire of their partners. The highest levels of sexual desire were correlated with high levels of partner sexual desire.

personal exploration activity

How Do You See Yourself?

How we feel about our bodies can either enhance or inhibit sexual response and pleasure. Our society places an incredible emphasis on looks, thus often leading us to have very unrealistic expectations about how we should look. The goal of this activity is to encourage you to take a realistic look at your body and accept who you are.

Take a full sheet of paper, and cover the entire page with a drawing of your body. You do not need to be an artist, but be as realistic as possible. Make your drawing a nude one of yourself. Once you have drawn your body, put an X over the parts of your body that you think need work and a star over the parts of your body that you like or that inspire pride. Once you have finished, your entire body should be clothed in X's or stars. Take a minute and write a short analysis of what has influenced your view of your body and how this view affects the way you respond in a romantic relationship, both physically and psychologically. Conclude by making a contract with yourself to work on the parts that you are really willing to change, or accept yourself as you are and like who you are. Lack of body acceptance has a very negative impact on our sexuality, so eliminate this by loving and accepting who you are.

Arousal

Spinal cord injury usually results in the inability of men to achieve erection through thoughts and emotions alone. "Reflex" erections occur in over 90 percent of men with spinal cord injury. These erections can be brought on through nonsexual functions such as catheter changes and having a full bladder, or through direct stroking of the penis, particularly the glans and frenulum (Geiger, 1981). Although the erection is present, the man usually cannot feel it because of the absence of sensation below the spinal injury. Reflex erections are typically more difficult to maintain than tradition erections, although penetration and intercourse can be achieved with the help of special rings and other devices that trap blood flow (Chance, 2002).

Sensations above the injury usually remain undisturbed. During arousal, sexual thoughts and feelings can initiate sexual excitement above the injury that manifests itself in all of the classic indicators: increased heart rate, respiration, blood pressure, and so forth. Women with spinal cord injuries lose the ability to produce vaginal lubrication due to the lack of vasocongestion. This problem can be alleviated through the use of water-soluble vaginal lubricants.

As with men, sensations above the injury usually remain undisturbed among women with spinal cord injuries. In addition to increased heart rate, respiration, and blood pressure, women experience breast engorgement and nipple erection.

Sex flush occurs, and pleasure is derived, through sensations associated with stimulation of erogenous zones about the injury. Many report an intensification of pleasure associated with kissing, breast and nipple stimulation, and stimulation of the spine in the area of the injury (Chance, 2002).

sex in society 7.5
Redefining Orgasm

Researchers are always trying to "operationalize" the variables they study so they can minimize bias in their research. Because of this, terms such as *orgasm* have been qualified and quantified to such a degree as to include such components as the frequency and intensity of contractions of the anal sphincter muscles. This is of crucial importance when studying orgasm in the laboratory. It would be almost impossible to study the effects of an independent variable (such as alcohol use, sleep deprivation, hormone levels, and so forth) on orgasm without first operationalizing the term.

In the real world, however, such precision doesn't exist and may not be necessary. Most people don't necessarily know or care about the frequency and duration of anal sphincter muscle contractions when experiencing what they would characterize as "orgasms." This point is especially true in understanding sexual pleasure and the release of sexual tension in people with disabilities.

Many disabled persons who are unable to have genitally based orgasm can experience a sense of building excitement and climax through (a) the stimulation of nongenital body parts, (b) the integration of these sensations with fantasy and memories of preinjury experiences, and (c) a sense of connection and excitement with their partners (Chance, 2002; Tepper 2001). Rather than exclude people with disabilities from the joy of sex and orgasm because they don't "measure up" to a nondisabled conceptualization of this experience, we need to embrace the diversity and richness of their experiences. By including disabled persons and inviting them to share their experiences and perceptions of sexual response and orgasm, nondisabled persons can get a better understanding of "human" sexual response.

Orgasm

The greatest variability in sexual response among those with spinal cord injuries is associated with orgasm. As we've discussed, orgasm traditionally is associated with ejaculation in men and a series of muscular contractions, changes in heart rate, respiration, and blood pressure in men and women. Ejaculation is a relatively rare occurrence in men with spinal cord injuries, as is contraction of the various muscles of the pelvic area.

As we've noted time and time again in this chapter, orgasm involves much more than genital contractions and the expulsion of body fluids. Orgasm is a very subjective experience involving the whole body and mind, as well as one's relationship with one's partner. Many people with spinal cord injuries report a buildup of excitement and release of tension through climax despite not experiencing ejaculation or vaginal contractions.

Cerebral Palsy

Cerebral palsy is a motor function disorder caused by a permanent, nonprogressive brain defect present at birth or shortly thereafter. It manifests itself in a range of motor functions, including (a) seizures; (b) stiff, awkward movements; (c) spasmodic movements of facial muscles, hands, arms, and fingers; (d) abnormal breathing, sucking, and swallowing patterns; (e) slurred speech; and (f) hearing difficulties—to name a few of the major abnormalities (Anderson, 1994).

Although the effects of cerebral palsy present many challenges, the disorder has few direct effects on sexual response. Cerebral palsy has no direct physical effect on sexual desire in either men or women. Desire disorders associated with cerebral palsy usually originate in psychosocial issues involving the person with the disorder and his/her partner(s). Living with a person who has cerebral palsy can be a daunting challenge and place incredible nonsexual demands on partners.

Additionally, engaging in sexual activity with a partner who has cerebral palsy requires special accommodations not normally present with partners who do not have the condition. These can place a strain on the relationship, and can tax communication skills to the limit. If these issues are not resolved, they can diminish the desire for sex in the person with cerebral palsy as well as the partner.

Sexual arousal and excitement are also not directly affected by cerebral palsy. Vasocongestion can occur, resulting in erection and vaginal lubrication. Behaviors associated with arousal ranging from holding hands, fondling, kissing, and talking are affected to some degree. Sexual behaviors can also be affected because some positions and activities may be difficult or impossible to consummate.

The ability to experience orgasm is generally not affected by cerebral palsy. The key mediating aspect regarding "traditional" genital orgasms is whether the person or his or her partner can sustain sufficient (duration and intensity) clitoral and penile stimulation to trigger orgasm. Once again, expanding the conceptualization of orgasm can help alleviate this issue. Persons with cerebral palsy and/or their partners might also find that mechanical devices such as vibrators and dildos can help moderate the duration and frequency of genital stimulation necessary to trigger orgasm (Sexual Health.com, 2003).

✎ *Environmental/Occupational Wellness* ✎

Feeling secure and being safe are essential to healthy sexuality. Our sexual response depends on a safe and comfortable environment. If we can't relax and feel safe and secure, we won't be able to relax enough to let the sexual response flow.

Have you ever been in a strange house as a guest and felt uncomfortable having sex? Think about being in a strange environment (your boyfriend's/girlfriend's fraternity/sorority house, a tent in a campground, a bed and breakfast with thin walls, your partner's parent's house) and how it feels to try to relax fully and let your sexual response flow. Even meeting potential sex partners requires a safe environment.

Think about going out to a bar, club, or other public place and feeling that people there don't like you or want you around, or having to suppress your natural urges to hold hands, dance, or make out. This is what many gay and lesbian people face every day in trying to meet potential friends and lovers. This environment may also include the work site.

Personal Assessment

Things That Turn Me On

People become aroused in a variety of ways. Each of us has our own unique sights and sounds that get us in the mood. The purpose of this assessment is to help you take a personal inventory of your personal turn-ons and give you the opportunity to share them anonymously with your classmates.

Describe in detail the things that turn you on in the following categories: Sights (visual images that are arousing to you): Sounds (types of music, words, conversation that you find stimulating): Tastes (food, drink, body fluids, or other tastes that are arousing): Smells (perfume, cologne, body smells, other odors you find stimulating): Touches (types, body parts, motions you find stimulating):

Thought Questions

1. How do the various regions of the brain process potentially arousing sexual stimuli and initiate sexual response?

2. How do the nervous system and the endocrine system work during sexual response?

3. What are some of the things that made Masters and Johnson pioneers in the field of sexual response?

4. What are *vasocongestion* and *myotonia*?

5. Compare and contrast the physiological changes in men and women during Masters' and Johnson's sexual response cycle.

6. Compare Masters' and Johnson's model of sexual response to the other models presented in this chapter.

7. Describe Basson's major criticisms of traditional theories of sexual response.

8. Evaluate the effectiveness of common "aphrodisiacs" on sexual response.

Test Yourself

1. Sexual response begins and ends
   a. in the genitalia.
   b. in the brain.
   c. in the rectum.
   d. in the vasocongestive tissues.
2. Which best describes the role of the brain in controlling sexual response?
   a. It is central in triggering its onset but has little influence after that.
   b. It can shut down sexual response at any time.
   c. It cannot shut down sexual response without orgasm.
   d. It plays a limited role in sexual response.
3. Which statement best characterizes male and female sex hormones?
   a. They have completely opposite effects.
   b. They complement each other.
   c. Men and women produce some of the same hormones.
   d. They act as antigens in the wrong body.

4. Testosterone is primarily associated with ____ in men and women.
   a. acne
   b. antisocial behavior
   c. sexual desire
   d. fertility
5. The role of estrogens in sexual response is mostly related to
   a. vaginal lubrication.
   b. rectal lubrication.
   c. vaginal vasocongestion.
   d. clitoral vasocongestion.
6. Which of the following is *not* a phase of the Masters and Johnson sexual response cycle?
   a. arousal
   b. plateau
   c. resolution
   d. erection

7. *Sex flush* refers to
   a. embarrassment felt over sexual desire.
   b. blood flow to the genitals during arousal.
   c. blood flow to the skin's surface during plateau.
   d. the feeling of swelling in the genitalia following arousal.
8. One of Basson's major criticisms of Masters' and Johnson's sexual response cycle is
   a. men and women respond differently to sexual stimuli.
   b. men and women respond the same to sexual stimuli.
   c. most women don't respond to the same stimuli as men.
   d. most men don't respond to the same stimuli as women.
9. The main goal of Tantric sex is
   a. to meditate on orgasm.
   b. to speed up and intensify sexual response.
   c. to achieve simultaneous multiple orgasms.
   d. to deemphasize orgasm and focus on the union with your partner.
10. Walen and Roth's and Basson's models of sexual response add a cognitive component that relates to
   a. multiple orgasms.
   b. the resolution phase.
   c. arousal and sexual satisfaction.
   d. sexual abuse.

Web Resources

Sinclair Intimacy Institute
www.bettersex.com/t-bsu-university.aspx

A database for information concerning sexual response and other areas of sexuality, written by the Sinclair Intimacy Institute staff. Provides answers to frequently asked questions through an up-to-date sexuality database with access to additional online resources.

The Church of Tantra
www.tantra.org

The home page for the Church of Tantra. It has, as its base, the belief that sexuality is a spiritual force and a pathway to direct spiritual experience. Sexuality "is the vehicle, not the destination."

The Sexual Health Network
www.sexualhealth.com

The Sexual Health Network is dedicated to providing easy access to sexuality information, education, mutual support, counseling, therapy, health care, products and other resources for people with disabilities, illness, or natural changes throughout the life cycle and those who love them or care for them.

Sex Smart Films
www.sexsmartfilms.com

This online archive features sexuality videos from the last 60 years.

References

Alexander, C. J., Sipski, M. L., & Findley, T. W. (1993). Sexual activities, desire, and satisfaction in males pre– and post–spinal cord injuries. *Archives of Sexual Behavior, 22*(3), 217–219.

Anderson, K. N. (1994). *Mosby's medical, nursing, and allied health dictionary* (4th ed.). St. Louis: Mosby.

Bancroft, J. (2002, February). Biological factors in human sexuality. *Journal of Sex Research, 39*(1), 15–21.

Basson, R. (2000). The female sexual response: A different model. *Journal of Marital Therapy, 26,* 51–65.

Basson, R. (2002). Are our definitions of women's desire, arousal and sexual pain disorders too broad and our definition of orgasmic disorder too narrow? J Sex Marital Ther. 2002 Jul–Sep;28(4):289–300.

Basson, R. (2004). Recent advances in women's sexual function and dysfunction. *Menopause.* 2004 Nov–Dec;11(6 Pt 2):714–25.

Bergeson, L. (2005). The Big Organic O. Utne Reader no. 129 (May/June 2005) p. 20–1.

Cama, E., Colleluori, D. M., Emig, F. A., Shin, H, Kim, S. W., Kim, N. N., Traish, A. M., Ash, D. E., Christianson DW. (2003). Human arginase II: crystal structure and physiological role in male and female sexual arousal. *Biochemistry*. 2003 Jul 22;42(28):8445–51.

Chance, R. S. (2002). To love and be loved: Sexuality and people with physical disabilities. *Journal of Psychology and Theology, 30*(3), 195–209.

deTejada, I. S. (2002). Molecular mechanisms for the regulation of penile smooth muscle contractility. *International Journal of Impotence Research* 2002 (14) Supplement 1, pp 6–10.

Fisher, H. (2004). Why we love; the nature and chemistry of romantic love. New York: Henry Holt and Company.

Geiger, R. C. (1981). Neurophysiology of sexual response in spinal cord injury. In D. G. Bullard & S. F. Knight (Eds.), *Sexuality and physical disability.* St. Louis: Mosby.

Johnson, J. (2004). Exposed at last; the truth about your clitoris. pp 387–389. In Worcester N., Whatley, M. H. (2004). *Women's Health: readings on Social, Economic, and Political Issues.* Dubuque IA: Kendall/Hunt Publishing.

Kaplan, H. S. (1974). *The new sex therapy.* New York: Times Books.

Kaplan, H. S. (1985). *Comprehensive evaluation of disorders of sexual desire.* Washington, DC: American Psychiatric Press.

Ladas, A., Whipple, R., & Perry, T. (1982). *The G-spot.* New York: Holt, Rinehart, & Winston.

Lemonick, M. (2004). The Chemistry of Desire. Time, Jan 19th, 2004, pp 62–68.

Lieblum, S. R. (2000, November). Redefining female sexual response. *Contemporary Obstetrics and Gynecology, 45*(11), 120–131.

Martini, F. (2005). *Fundamentals of Anatomy and Physiology*, 5th Edition. San Francisco: Benjamin Cummings Publishing.

Masters, W., & Johnson, V. (1966). *Human sexual response.* Boston: Little, Brown.

Masters, W., & Johnson, V. (1976). *The pleasure bond.* New York: Bantam.

Munarriz, R., Kim N. N., Goldstein, I., Traish, A. M. (2002). Biology of female sexual function. *Urol Clin North Am.* 2002 Aug 29(3):685–93.

O'Connell, H. E., Sanjeevan, K. V., Hutson J. M. (2005). Anatomy of the clitoris. *J Urol.* 2005 Oct;174 (4 Pt 1):1189–95.

Reagan, P. C. (1999, Spring). Hormonal correlates and causes of sexual desire: A review. *Canadian Journal of Human Sexuality, 8* (1), 1–29.

Scelfo, J. (2002). Bored with sleeping? Sleep and Sex. Newsweek v. 140 no. 3 (July 15 2002) p. 45

Sexual Health.com. (2003). Possible effects of cerebral palsy or CP on a person's sexuality [Online]. Available: www.sexualhealth.com/content/read.cfm?ID_6&theTopic_Disabilitypercent20orpercent20Illne. . . .

Stayton, W. R. (2002, April–May). A theology of sexual pleasure. *SIECUS Report, 30*(4), 27–30.

Tepper, M. (2001). Sexual healing with a disability [Online]. Available: http://www.sexualhealth.com/content/read.cfm?ID_90&theTopic_Disability percent20or percent20Ill. . . .

Traish, A. M., Kim, N. N., Munarriz, R., & Goldstein, I. (2002, October). Biochemical and physiological mechanisms of female genital sexual arousal. *Archives of Sexual Behavior, 31*(5), 393–400.

Traish, A. M., Kim, N., Min, K., Munarriz, R., Goldstein, I.(2002a) Role of androgens in female genital sexual arousal: receptor expression, structure, and function. Fertil Steril. 2002 Apr;77 Suppl 4:S11–8.

chapter
eight

Sensuality and Sexual Behavior

Student Learning Objectives

After reading this chapter, students will be able to

- Compare and contrast sensuality and sexuality.
- Compare and contrast celibacy and abstinence.
- Describe a variety of non-penetrative sexual behaviors.
- Know how to give a sensual massage.
- Evaluate the myths associated with masturbation.
- Compare and contrast a variety of positions for vaginal intercourse.
- Identify the factors associated with healthy anal sexual behavior.
- Describe a variety of oral sex behaviors.
- Explain the effects of spinal cord injury on sexual behavior.

activity teaser: Is your arousal boost an arousal block to your partner? Find the answer in the Personal Exploration Activity on page 278.

case study 8.1

Delores: Sex in Pregnancy

Delores, 26, identifies as African American.

Delores is a 26-year-old nontraditional sophomore. She is married and the mother of a 6-month-old son, Greg. Delores describes her sexual experiences during her pregnancy.

Before I got pregnant, I was very concerned about the effects it would have on my sex life with my husband, Joe. We were married for 3 years and had a very satisfying sex life. I was worried about that changing. I've always liked sex, and I've kept in shape through running and lifting weights. I was concerned about gaining weight and my body changing shape. But I decided that I wouldn't limit my weight gain and make the baby suffer.

During the first trimester, my sex drive dropped a lot. I wasn't as horny as I normally was, and I had terrible morning sickness. Actually, I had morning, afternoon, and evening sickness and could hardly keep any food down. Other than that, though, nothing much changed. The frequency of sex dropped in half, but the kinds of things we did—positions—didn't change.

During the second trimester, my morning sickness disappeared, and I felt much better. I had put on some weight, but it really didn't affect our intercourse. I was concerned about bouncing around too much and things like rolling off the bed, but for the most part we didn't change our behaviors. The good news was that my sex drive returned to normal.

During the third trimester, things changed again. I had put on over 20 pounds and had a big belly. I was really concerned about deep penetration. I worried that it might hurt the baby, but my doctor reassured me that everything would be OK. I didn't have much energy, so we made love less often. We couldn't use any man- or woman-on-top positions. I've always liked the woman-on-top position with me sitting on my husband's lap, and I had to give that up, too.

I found that the only position we could use was the spoon [side-by-side] position. That allowed us to have full-body contact without putting pressure on my belly. It also allowed my husband to massage my breasts and belly. I had no desire for him to perform oral sex on me, but sometimes I liked to satisfy him that way, particularly on those days when I didn't have much energy. Overall, I think our sex life survived my pregnancy very well.

Critical Thinking

Pregnancy is a time of physical, emotional, social, and other changes. Pregnant women and their partners react to these changes in a myriad of ways in regards to sexual response and desire. If you have never been pregnant, how do you think being pregnant will influence your sexual desire and response? If you have been pregnant before, how did it influence your sexual response and desire? How can pregnant women and their partners maintain or enhance their sexual desire and response during this period?

As Delores has shown us, one's sensuality and sexual behavior manifest themselves in many ways. In this chapter, we'll start by examining sensuality and how it is related to sexual behavior. Then we'll consider the full range of sexual behaviors, starting with celibacy.

Sensuality

As we discussed in Chapter 7, sexual response originates in our brain and senses. But what *is* sensuality? What makes a person sensual? Is it the richness and texture of her features (thick, long hair; distinct, angular nose; high cheekbones; long, exotic nails; tantalizing perfume/cologne; self-assured body language)? Is it his attitude (a deep thinker, caring/loving personality, down-to-earth simplicity)? Could it be her appreciation of life (enjoys great food, appreciates music, likes nature, enjoys physical activities)? We will answer these questions and provide hints on how to enhance and develop one's sensuality since it is the basis for all sexual response and behavior.

Although they are intimately related, sexuality and sensuality are different. **Sensuality** is the quality of being sensual, of experiencing life fully through all of the senses. **Sexuality,** you will remember, is a broad term that refers to all aspects of being sexual, encompassing a variety of biological, psychological, and cultural variables.

Sensuality is a part of our sexuality. People who are very sensual have a heightened awareness of sight, sound, taste, touch, and smell. They use this increased awareness to experience life through all of these senses whenever possible. They approach each experience, every day, through this context or frame of reference. A walk in the woods or down a bustling city street is a symphony of sounds, colors, scents, tastes, and textures (Spayde, 2001).

This increased sensitivity to and appreciation of all sensory stimuli carries over into their sexuality and lovemaking. The heightened awareness of all the senses enhances lovemaking. Sensual lovers delight in all aspects of their partners and their surroundings, making sex a feast for the senses. Sex isn't just a genital-driven quest for orgasm. It is a five-course gourmet meal that may include climax as the entree.

Sensuality Experiencing things through all five senses

Sexuality Broad term that refers to all aspects of being sexual

Developing Sensuality

William Burnham, a pioneering educational psychologist, believed that all humans are born as sensual creatures (Burnham, 1932). As newborns, we experience life through all of our senses. Burnham referred to this as being "fully integrated." Little separates our intellect and our senses. A good example of this integration is how children play in the grass.

Think about how toddlers play in the grass. They roll around in it, close their eyes, lie back in it, and listen to the sounds the wind makes as it blows through the high blades. They pull out handfuls of grass, throw them up in the air, and watch the blades fall to earth. They take a blade of grass and examine it carefully, rolling it around in their fingers, maybe even against their cheeks with their eyes closed. As they squeeze the grass between their fingers, they notice that oils are secreted. They smell this oil and taste it. Satiated with the grass, they move on to the next activity.

How many of us as adults take the time to get into the "grassiness" of life anymore? Have we lost our ability to revel in the "grassiness," or do we still have it but don't utilize it? We authors believe that we still have the ability to be fully integrated with the Here and Now of our lives but do not take advantage of it as often as we could. Along the course of our lives, most of us, for many reasons, stop experiencing life with all of our senses. We pay less and less attention to anything other than sight and sound (the primary senses we need to get through our work day). Of course we still occasionally remark about "how good something tastes" or how "nice something smells," but these observations are more often than not isolated and not part of our overall orientation to life.

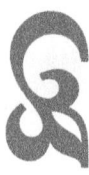

healthy sex hints 8.1

Becoming a More Sensuous Person

Becoming more sensual starts with acknowledging the need to and giving yourself permission to *indulge* your senses. For some people this will involve unlearning some of the prohibitions and inhibitions you were raised with (Spayde, 2001). It's OK to pamper yourself.

Sight: Enhance Visual Sensations

Most of us take our sight for granted and don't look at visual detail as something we can develop and expand. If something beautiful passes through our lives, we acknowledge it and move on. Try the following tips to develop and enhance the sights in your life.

1. Discover *flowers;* keep flowers on your desk, in your kitchen, and elsewhere in your home.
2. Immerse yourself in art (pictures, posters, photographs, drawings).
   - Paint/shoot/draw them yourself, buy art books, or cut works of art out of Magazines.
   - Visit art galleries, museums, and online art sites (such as www.art.com).
   - Don't worry about what you don't know about art; focus on *what you like* and *surround yourself* with it (Marrone, 2002).
3. Take a good look at nature (sunsets, sunrises, natural beauty).
   - Star gaze.
   - Watch the sun rise and set.
   - Become an ardent cloud watcher.
   - Watch the waves crash, the tides move in and out, a local brook/stream tumble over rocks and cascade over cliffs (Eiseman, 1999).
4. Explore minienvironments.
   - Scoop a handful of sand where the water meets the shore, and spend 30 minutes examining it.
   - Take a close look at snowflakes, icicles, and frost on leaves.
   - Spend a half an hour exploring a tide pool (Eiseman, 1999).
5. Add color to your life.
   - Open your shades and let the sun shine in.
   - Drape colorful sun shades over your windows—pale orange will help trigger an endorphin release (Eiseman, 1999).

Touch: Enhance Tactile Stimulation

1. Try massage.
   - Take turns giving and receiving foot and hand massages.
   - Your feet contain over 7,000 nerve endings. Stimulating them sends pleasurable electrical impulses coursing throughout your body (Bender, 1999).
   - There are over 40,000 nerve endings in the palms waiting to be rubbed, scratched, and tickled (Kemp, 2000).
2. Knead dough.
   - Try making bread by hand, and/or throwing pottery. Nothing beats these two nonsexual activities for developing an appreciation of touch.
   - Kneading dough or clay is one of life's most enjoyable tactile delights. It slows you down, stimulates the more than 40,000 nerve endings of the palms and hands, and is great practice for massage.

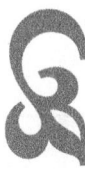

3. Give/receive shampoos.
   - There is nothing quite like having someone else wash your hair slowly and lovingly with warm water and lots of shampoo.
   - Practice on your pet. He or she will love you for it, and you will derive tactile joy from doing it.
   - Combine a long, gentle shampoo with a sensual bubble bath or shower. Take time to wash your partner with lots of soap, bubbles, and shampoo. Use a wash towel or sponge to add different textures to the experience.
4. Pet your pet.
   - Snuggling into the furry comfort of your pet's luxurious fur/hair is a sensual pleasure you both will enjoy.
   - Try to brush/comb your pet's coat at least once a week. It will slow you down and help you learn to relax and appreciate the luster of beautiful fur/hair.
5. Indulge yourself with different fabrics to wear.
   - Treat yourself to something that feels good: silk underwear; satin sheets; fleece scarves and mittens; a cashmere or angora sweater; a flannel nightshirt; leather pants, vest, or blazer. Soft, supple leather has always had a sexual appeal, as does soft, well-worn denim.
6. Be naked more.
   - Sleep naked, swim naked, run outside in the rain naked, sunbathe naked (of course, do this in places where you won't get arrested for indecency).
   - Start slowly. Sleep naked beneath clean satin, flannel, or Egyptian cotton sheets. Feel the sensations on your flesh.

Smell: Enhance Olfactory Delights

1. Use perfumes, colognes, soaps, and other scents.
   - Scientists have finally found the existence of pheromones in humans.
   - Perfumes, soaps, and other products that contain human pheromones switch on parts of the brain (hypothalamus) and increase feelings of well-being and self-confidence (Kraus, 2000; Brand, 2001).
   - Scents range from very light to heavy and from musky to fruity, to floral.
   - Goins (2001) suggests rubbing your partner's favorite scents on parts of your clothing, like your shirt collar, so he or she can smell it as you give him or her a good-bye/hello hug and kiss.
2. Light candles.
   - Use candles to set the mood (candles combine scents with color to heighten both visual and olfactory sensations).
   - Use candles in the bathroom when you take a bath.
   - Use them at night to serve as sensual night lights while you watch TV.
   - Use candles to add to the joys of a special meal.
   - Use seasonal candles to add the scents of the season to your day. For instance, pine candles have always been associated with the winter holidays (Bender, 1999).
3. Try sachet bags.
   - Use sachet bags of your favorite scent to liven your room, closet, office, or car.
   - Make your own sachet bags by using leftover pieces of cloth, cuttings from your favorite plants, pine needles, or flower petals.

(continued)

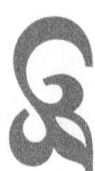

healthy sex hints 8.1 *(continued)*

4. Buy or pick flowers.
   - Flowers help develop and maintain your olfactory senses.
   - Flowers such as lilac can provide a gentle scent, while others, such as honeysuckle, can sometimes be too overpowering. Your local florist can help you identify flowers that meet your sensual demands.
5. Experience nature.
   - Walk or bicycle more. You'll be amazed at the different smells that surround you if you get out of that protective cocoon (your car).

Sound: Listen to the Environment

1. Make music a part of your day.
   - Music can relax you, help you forget your problems, reduce stress, recharge your batteries, and even turn you on.
   - Certain rhythms and beats mimic your body's natural tempo during sex.
   - Matching music (such as Caribbean or Latin) to the movements of your lovemaking can enhance the response (Goins, 2001).
2. Listen to nature.
   - Listen to the wind blow through the trees, the waves crash on the shore, the stream trickle through the rocks.
   - Walk in the woods; listen to the birds.
3. Become comfortable with silence.
   - Build "quiet time" into each day.
   - Allow your mind to unclutter by shutting out auditory stimuli for 20 minutes each day.
   - Listen to your partner's breathing (holding your partner or being united in intercourse and listening to his or her breathing can be both a sensual delight and a sexual turn-on).

In general, try to *slow down* and *pay attention* to the interplay of your five senses in whatever you are doing whenever you can. This will increase your awareness of how the senses work together and will reinforce the importance of becoming more sensual.

Taste: Sample Your World

1. Taste your partner.
   - Experience your partner with your mouth.
   - Experience all parts of his or her body.
   - Take a shower together and drink the water from his or her flesh. Lick the beaded water off your partner's nipples and body.
   - Experiment with oral sex.
   - Play with sensual eating.
   - Put together a sensual snack feast of fresh fruits, cheeses, and a bottle of wine.
   - Put it on a big platter with some crackers, and spend an hour eating it slowly in bed while you feed each other and toast your good fortune.
   - Some people like to play with things such as whipped cream or chocolate syrup in bed and lick these delights off each other (the authors have found this to create a sticky mess that can often put a damper on rather than heighten the sensual experience).
   - Try mixing tastes when you can. Moving from a tart to sweet or mild to potent taste sensation can awaken your taste buds.
   - Slow down and take smaller bites. Savor rather than devour your food, and enjoy the process of eating as well as the outcome.

What transforms the sensual child into a constrained adult? Why does this happen? Are we afraid of what others would think if they were to see us rolling in the grass at age 18 or 28 or 48 years? Or have we "been there, done that?" Are we too jaded to enjoy the simple, free, sensual delights that surround us? We've asked our students these questions, and the results are very interesting. Often, students will just stare at us like we are crazy and then say, "Yeah, right, I can just see myself rolling around the grass like a baby, pulling up handfuls of grass." When pressed about what they would feel, they admit that such behavior would make them "feel weird" or "self-conscious." Many said, "What would other people think?" Many fear that such behavior could get them labeled by other people as "crazy" or at the very least "strange." Some even worry that a neighbor might think they are on drugs and call the police.

We asked them to think of other, less conspicuous scenarios such as sitting on the beach and playing with a handfull of sand (chosen because of the diversity of the size, colors, and textures of things found within it), watching a sunset, making bread from scratch, giving someone a shampoo, and listening to the wind blow through the trees on a brisk autumn day. In most cases the opposition to these activities was the same, but two other major issues were time and familiarity. "Who has the time?" and "Been there, done that" were often their refrains.

Often, it's not until we make the connection between their sensuality and their sexual pleasure that they begin to take the topic seriously. Losing the ability to be sensual can greatly affect our ability to experience sexual pleasure and experience eroticism through all of the senses. In many cases it can lead to dysfunction (in Chapter 12 we describe "sensate focus," a technique used by sex therapists to help dysfunctional people relearn how to be sensual). Our advice is to *make the time* now to enhance your sexuality and prevent dysfunction. By slowing down and integrating all of your senses into your daily experiences, you are setting the stage for doing the same thing in the boudoir.

Types of Sexual Behavior

One way to present the many forms of sexual behavior is to place them on a continuum from celibacy to oral/anal sex. This presentation is useful in understanding safer sex options, as well as choices in fertility control.

Celibacy and Abstinence

Celibacy is defined as abstaining from sexual intercourse. Although the formal definition of celibacy refers specifically to abstaining from sexual intercourse and never marrying, many people assume that celibacy and abstinence mean total avoidance of all forms of sexual release and the absence of sexual desire. Celibacy may or may not include masturbation and fantasy as forms of sexual release.

Celibacy Abstaining from sexual intercourse

Celibate people also have varying degrees of sexual desire. Not all celibate people lack sexual interest and desire; they merely choose to channel that energy and desire into different avenues of expression.

Celibacy is usually associated with a spiritual or religious sacrifice and is considered to be a lifelong commitment. Priests and nuns, for instance, declare a vow of celibacy so they may devote themselves fully to serving

God and never marry. It is a conscious, willful diversion of sexual energy into nonsexual activity. Kathleen Norris (1996) uses the phrase "celibate passion" to describe how celibate monks are able to transform sexual energy into a sense of deep caring and love that she found to be unique among celibate people.

Not all people who choose celibacy, however, do so as part of a religious commitment. Actually, all of us choose to wait before we engage in intercourse. Many people choose celibacy because they are not ready to begin having intercourse, and they satisfy their sexual needs through other behaviors. We all develop at our own pace, and some of us are simply not ready as soon as others are.

We sometimes choose celibacy because we need time to recover or grieve from relationships that have ended. We need time to heal emotionally and are not interested in forming sexual relationships at the time. Others choose celibacy because they do not have the time or energy to sustain a commitment (sexual or otherwise) with another person. They think they need all of their energy for school or work, especially if they are beginning a new career or starting school. They don't want to divert time and energy from these areas. Some students find being celibate helps them focus more attention on their schoolwork and improve their academic performance (Rajen, 2004). Netting & Burnett (2004) found that about 30 percent of the students they studied in a 30-year prospective study in British Columbia, Canada were celibate.

Abstinence Self-restraint or self-denial, as in not engaging in sexual activity

The generic definition of **abstinence** is self-restraint or self-denial. Sexual abstinence, therefore, refers to self-restraint or self-denial of sexual activities (Foston, 2004). Many people assume that abstinence means denial of all forms of sexual behavior. Actually, one can choose to abstain from unprotected intercourse but not other forms of sexual behavior. Abstinence usually is not discussed as a lifelong spiritual or religious commitment. It is more situational; a person can abstain for a day, a week, a month, a semester, and so on. It doesn't have to be an all-or-nothing proposition. Most of us have voluntarily chosen to abstain from sexual intercourse at various times during our lives. Once abstinence is viewed as a situational choice and not a lifetime commitment, it becomes easier to accept and understand as a viable sexual option. We also believe that although abstinence is a valid option for people, it is not the only option.

Non-Penetrative Sexual Activity

Non-penetrative sexual activities offer a wide variety of pleasurable behaviors that can be carried out to the point of orgasm and involve little risk of pregnancy or disease. This activity has been called "outercourse" and includes options ranging from kissing and hugging to using sex toys. To us, non-penetrative sexual activity includes any sexual behaviors that do not involve genital-to-genital, mouth-to-genital, or insertive anal sexual contact.

Kissing

Kissing can provide intense sensual and sexual delight. The sucking, licking, rubbing, and tongue probing associated with kissing is pleasurable and carries no risk for pregnancy. Volumes have been written about kissing.

case study 8.2

Susan: Choosing to Be Celibate

Susan, 31, divorced, identifies as bisexual.

I've been celibate for the past year and a half. I'm 31 years old, have a 5-year-old daughter, work full-time, and go to school full-time. Things just never worked out with my daughter's father, and ever since I've been back to school, I haven't had the energy to even think about sex. My schedule is crazy, and I don't have much free time. When I have time off, I prefer to spend it with my daughter.

I don't have the time to spend on cultivating a relationship. I really want to finish school and get good enough grades to get into graduate school someday. I don't miss intercourse. It's not that I don't like sex. Before I got married, I used to really get off on sex with both men and women. My sex life with my daughter's father was really great, and eventually I stopped having sex with anyone else but him and got pregnant. Things between us were never the same after that, and since we split up, I've just been burned out on the idea of starting a new relationship. I masturbate a couple of times a week and prefer to deal with my sexual needs that way. I can see this changing someday and hope to meet a woman who can love and satisfy me and love my daughter. For now, though, I'm not looking for a relationship.

Critical Thinking

Think about your own life and periods where you have chosen voluntary celibacy. What were the circumstances surrounding your choice? Did you view this as situational abstinence or long-term celibacy? Was it the right decision for you? If you have never chosen celibacy, describe a future situation where this strategy might work for you.

As we age, we seem to become more genitally focused and lose some of our interest in kissing. Kissing becomes an ancillary activity associated with the real objective—orgasm—rather than a satisfying activity in and of itself (Gulledge, Stahmann, Wilson, 2004: Gulledge, Gulledge, Stahtmann, 2003).

Hugging/Rubbing

Kissing is usually associated with hugging and rubbing. These activities, once commonly called *petting,* can take on new meaning if we can visualize them as viable forms of sexual expression. Hugging and rubbing, even with one's clothes on, can be intensely pleasurable and can be carried to the point of orgasm with no risk of pregnancy or disease. These activities also can serve as a prelude to other non-insertive forms of sexual activity such as masturbation and use of sex toys.

A delightful way to use rubbing as a safe sexual release is to rub against your partner to the point of orgasm. Typically this is done with both partners fully clothed. You rub your penis or vulva against your partner's groin, leg, arm (or another convenient body part) to the point of orgasm.

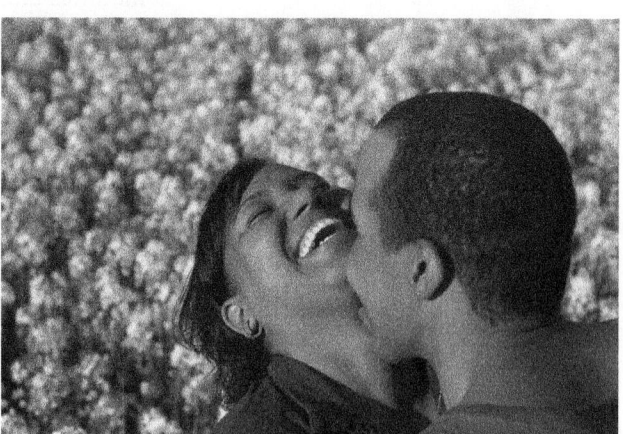

Kissing is an almost universal form of sexual expression.

© Htuller, 2010. Shutterstock, Inc.

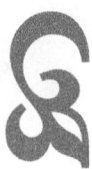

healthy sex hints 8.2

10 Good Reasons for Choosing Abstinence

Abstinence has gotten a bad rap over the years. It's almost politically incorrect to talk about abstaining from sexual intercourse (and penetrative sex, if you're gay or a lesbian). Here are 10 good reasons to choose abstinence:

1. To retain your virginity for someone special
2. To get to know your partner better (you want to become more comfortable with your partner and come to trust him or her)
3. To ascertain your partner's STD/HIV status (you'd rather wait to have intercourse but might consider safer-sex options)
4. To wait to be in the mood (you'd rather be doing something else)
5. If you're heterosexual, to avoid pregnancy if neither of you has contraception (you might consider a low-risk sexual outlet other than intercourse)
6. To find a suitable partner (sure, you've had offers, but no one turns you on)
7. To recuperate from an illness or surgery (you're not feeling very sexy or are feeling downright lousy)
8. To get a medical opinion on unusual genital symptoms (these might represent an STD)
9. To get some sleep (you're tired and need sleep, not sex)
10. To adhere to your personal moral code (regarding premarital, extramarital, and other sexual taboos that make up your personal code of ethics)

What other good reasons for abstaining from intercourse can you come up with?

You control the pressure, rhythm, and intensity. Although students sometimes call this "dry humping," it doesn't have to be either. You can enhance your enjoyment by doing it with your clothes off and adding oil or lotion to the equation. Try spreading lotion on your partner's breasts or chest. Take your clothes off, lie on your back, and let your partner rub your penis or vulva back and forth and up and down between her breasts or his chest until you come. Try spreading some lotion or oil on your partner's buttocks and the small of his or her back. Straddle the backside and ride back and forth to the point of orgasm. If this seems too messy, try rubbing your penis or vulva through your partner's hair and against his or her head and neck. You can use hugging and rubbing in many ways to enjoy a highly erotic sexual episode without fear of disease or pregnancy.

Massage

Non-genital massage is one of the greatest sensual delights you can share with your partner. Massage can be a stand-alone sensual activity or can be part of activities culminating with orgasm. Sex therapists often prescribe non-genital massage for clients as a way to help them reestablish touching each other's bodies again. Massage allows us to explore every nook and cranny of our partner's bodies in a relaxed, sensual way.

Separating our sensuality from our sexuality is sometimes difficult when it comes to massage. The only time many of us touch others in such an intimate way is when we are being sexual. Massage is not an inherently sexual activity. It *is* sensual, though. Kneading, stroking, and manipulat-

sex in society 8.1

Variations on Kissing

We asked our students to talk about kissing—their likes, dislikes, the role it plays in their relationships. Here's what they had to say:

Marcia 19, single, freshman, identifies as Latina.

I love kissing. I especially like long, deep, French kissing with my boyfriend. I really enjoy deep tongue thrusting—you know, like when he tries to run his tongue all the way down my throat. What a turn-on.

Mary 18, single, freshman, identifies as Italian American.

I like gentle kissing. I like lighter pressure—soft pecks, nuzzles, gentle tongue probing. I hate it when a guy tries to ram his tongue down my throat. It's disgusting. Oh, and I hate hickeys. Why do some guys feel compelled to leave their mark on my neck? I never go out with a guy again if he tries to lay a hickey on me. How gross.

John, 20, single, junior, identifies as Asian American.

I like kissing. It's kind of like a game, tongues darting back and forth, in and out. There's almost a rhythm or method to kissing. I like to work my tongue around my girlfriend's whole mouth.

Sonja, 20, single, junior, identifies as African American.

I personally think French kissing is overrated. I prefer lip action. I like to nip and suck, just using my lips. I like it when my boyfriend nibbles on my lips and when we just use the tips of our tongues around our lips and the outer parts of our mouths. I find this kind of darting tongue action preferable to all of that deep tongue thrusting. That makes me gag.

Glen, 41, married, nontraditional senior, identifies as African American.

At this point in my life, I find that my wife and I are more gentle in our kissing. We still get into all the deep French kissing every once in a while, but most of our kissing is more affectionate than passionate. Don't get me wrong—our sex is great, and intercourse is usually pretty passionate. We just seem to kiss more as an expression of love and affection. Kissing during sex is less frequent than when we were in our 20s.

ing another person's flesh require us to be in tune with the sensation of touch. We must be acutely aware of pressure and motion when we give a massage. Also, many of the massage oils available are scented and bring into play our sense of smell. Visually, the sight of exposed flesh has the potential for arousal.

The ability to enjoy giving and getting a massage and viewing these as sensual delights that don't have to lead to sexual activity may take time. Of course, giving a massage with the intent to arouse your partner sexually is a natural way to initiate erotic activities if that is the intention. Being able to give and receive sensual pleasure without sexual release is excellent training in becoming a compassionate lover.

Giving a massage is a natural behavior. Instinctively, we believe that if it feels good to us, it will feel good to the person we are massaging. Usually, giving a massage is easier if you use some form of lubricating oil. Some people prefer powder to reduce friction, and they like the sensation of powder. Most people, however, prefer oil. Oil should be warm or at room

personal exploration activity

Boosts and Blocks to Arousal

There are so many differences in what each person finds sexually arousing and what blocks each person's arousal. Too often we don't even recognize what are our own boosts or turn-ons and our blocks or turn-offs to being aroused. Remember that arousal does not just happen as a prelude to sexual intercourse. Arousal can happen while we are walking across campus and notice a great body. The goal of this activity is to help you recognize what is sexually significant and important to you.

To identify your own personal boost and blocks to sexual arousal, keep a diary for 1 week where you list all the little things that sexually arouse you. Include not just physical but social and psychological factors that arouse you. (You can keep this in code if you don't want anyone to know what you are doing.) Notice all the little contributors such as reading an erotic passage in a novel, having someone you find attractive brush your hand, how you respond when you are being kissed, and so forth. When the week is finished, examine your list and star the ones that are the most effective in arousing you. These are the things you want to enhance in your sensual activities to increase your arousal. Next put an X by those that most effectively block your arousal, and try to eliminate these factors when possible. If you have a partner, you may want to share what you discovered about yourself and suggest he or she keep a diary for a week. Your partner can then share the findings with you. The two of you can use your list to enhance what is really important to both of you in your sensual life together.

temperature. Cold oil on the skin can get the massage off to a bad start. The oil should sit at room temperature or be warmed in the container under hot water in the sink before starting. The oil should be poured into the hands and rubbed onto the body rather than squirted directly onto the person's skin (Good Arts, 2003).

Massage should be done with sufficient room to get completely around the person without having to lean on or jump over him or her. When straddling a person, you should not sit directly on him or her. You should be able to position yourself over the person so you can apply firm pressure during some strokes. A massage table or high bed is ideal because it allows you to stand while giving a massage. You also could kneel next to the person receiving the massage. It allows the person to lie comfortably with the face down, facilitating easy access to the neck, shoulders, and head. A professional table isn't necessary. You could place a pillow under the person's head for support and have him or her rest the head gently to the side.

Most important in giving a massage is to take your time. The other person will sense if you feel obligated to do this and are rushing through it. Giving a massage is an act of kindness and must be done slowly, lovingly, with no expectations for getting anything in return.

Several types of strokes can be used in giving a massage. All of them require maintaining contact with the partner as much as possible while moving from one body part and stroke to the next. The strokes should merge to form a sense of continuous motion with the muscles. A visual image of the muscular system may help (see Figure 8.1). The strokes should be rhythmic and symmetrical, and will get better with practice. The whole hand should be used to master all of the strokes effectively. The fingers,

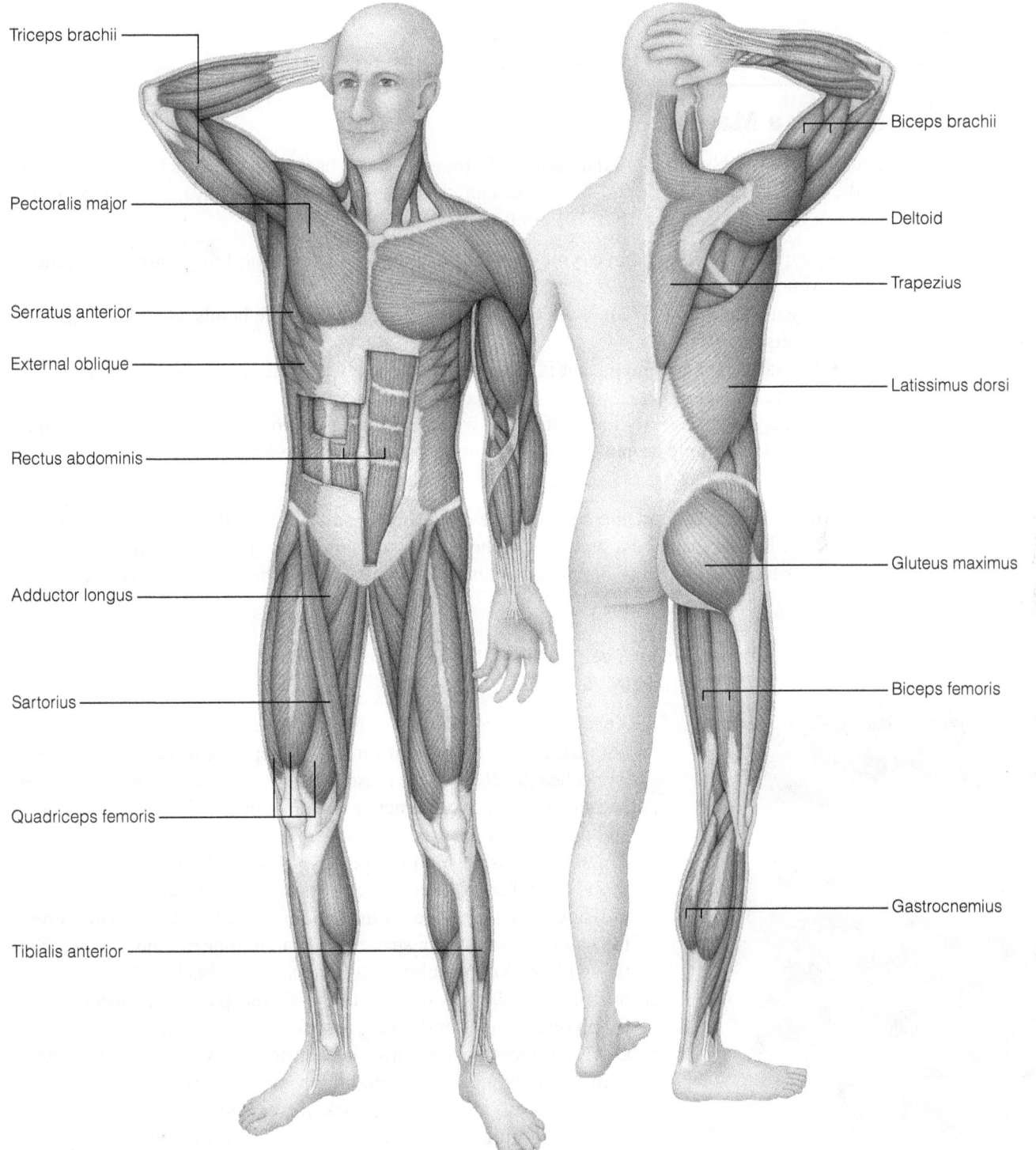

Triceps brachii

Pectoralis major

Serratus anterior

External oblique

Rectus abdominis

Adductor longus

Sartorius

Quadriceps femoris

Tibialis anterior

Biceps brachii

Deltoid

Trapezius

Latissimus dorsi

Gluteus maximus

Biceps femoris

Gastrocnemius

Figure 8.1 *Muscular System* Knowledge of the muscular system can help you when giving a massage.

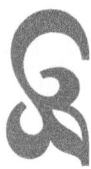

healthy sex hints 8.3

Giving a Massage

You can give full-body or partial massages. Sometimes just a back massage or a foot massage will do the trick. At other times, a full-body massage, complete with scented candles, is preferred. When giving a full body massage, try these pointers:

- Start anywhere. Wherever you start, move in the direction toward the heart to facilitate venous blood flow.
- If you start with the feet, work up to the head, and finish at the hands. Or work in the reverse order.
- Or start at the abdomen, as it is the center of the body and, when stressed, is the place where blood pools.
- Cover the entire body in a systematic way. Finish a part thoroughly, then move on to the next. Don't jump around from feet to head to toes. Massage both hands/arms or feet/legs before moving to the next body part.

After a massage, allow the person some quiet time to savor the results—and maybe even to reciprocate. Massage can be a prelude to other forms of sexual activity. In sensual massage, the focus shifts to providing more direct contact with the genitals and other erogenous zones.

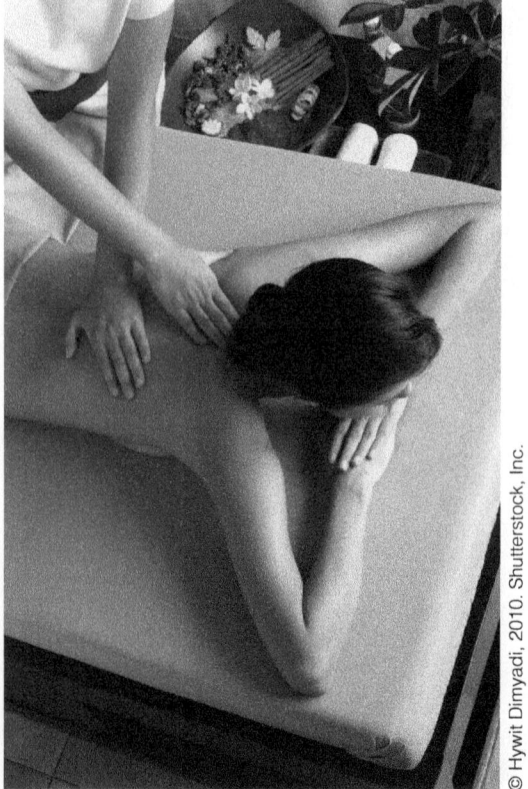

Kneading the back is a classic massage technique.

© Hywit Dimyadi, 2010. Shutterstock, Inc.

palm, heel, and fist all come into play. The types of strokes are as follows (Inkeles & Austin, 1992):

1. *Kneading.* In kneading, you grasp the flesh with all four fingers of both hands and rotate your thumbs in opposite directions. Kneading works beautifully with the muscles of the arms, legs, hands, feet, back, and shoulders. You can practice kneading by making homemade bread and working on the dough.

2. *Pressing.* Pressing involves pushing against the body with the heel of the hand. For extra pressure, you can use your other hand to apply pressure against the heel of the hand involved in the pressing. Pressing can be used in long strokes or in a circular motion, and is effective with thicker muscles such as those in the back.

3. *Stroking.* Stroking is done with the fingertips, either pushing away from you in circles or drawing toward you. Stroking also can employ all five fingers gently drawing flesh toward you. Stroking is good with the scalp, neck, and inner thighs and also works well as a long continuous motion along the back, torso, arms, and legs.

4. *Pulling.* Pulling is similar to stroking toward you except that it involves more pressure. Whereas stroking movements glide over the skin, pulling involves grabbing hold and gently tugging. You can pull with just your fingers, an entire hand, or both hands. Pulling is well suited for the head, hands, fingers, toes, feet, arms, and legs.

5. *Lifting.* In some cases, actually lifting a part of the body, such as the head, torso, or leg, and supporting it in your hands is relaxing. When lifting, the hands are cupped to cradle the part being elevated.

6. *Pounding.* Making a fist and gently pounding a body part can release accumulated tension. Pounding isn't for everyone or every body part. It is most effective on the back.

case study 8.3

Chrissy and Ken: Sensual Massage

Ken, 23, is white; Chrissy, 22, is white.

Chrissy and Ken are single and in their senior year of college. They have been dating and having sex for 2 years and are planning to get engaged sometime before graduation in June. They have worked massage into their sexual lifestyle.

KEN: We got into massage as a way to relax and enjoy the sensual part of it. I didn't want Chrissy to think the only time she'd get a massage was when I wanted to have sex.

CHRISSY: We talk about what our needs are. If we want just a massage, we know this going into it, and that's what we do. If we're feeling sexy, we sometimes use massage to feel more sensual and get excited. We spend a lot of time massaging each other's erogenous zones.

KEN: I really get excited when Chrissy uses oil to massage my toes. I also love it when she uses long, slow strokes up my inner thighs and gently kneads the skin there.

Chrissy: I really go wild when Ken uses small, circular strokes around my temples or kneads the base of my skull. I start to get wet when he spends a few minutes doing that.

Critical Thinking

How does your own background and upbringing affect your ability to give and receive sensual massages with your partner? How does this influence your use of professional massage services? Does the gender of the massage therapist matter when seeking professional massage services?

Masturbation

One of the first activities linking our sensuality to sexual behavior is **masturbation.** Masturbation usually evolves out of sensual exploration of our own body. We notice that it feels good when we unintentionally or intentionally rub (or rub up against) our genitals. In her book *Liberating Masturbation*, feminist writer, artist, and sex educator Betty Dodson (1996, p. 11) describes masturbation as "our primary sex life, our sexual base." According to Dodson, all other forms of sexual expression are a result of socialization. The expression of healthy sexual relationships between individuals begins with self-exploration of sensual and sexual pleasure from the time of birth.

As described in Chapter 5, most of us learn the joy and security of cuddling, hugging, and warm, caring touch early in our lives, from contact with our parents and other caregivers. Although our earliest bonding experiences with our mother and father are not sexual in nature, they provide a sensual connection that leads to healthy sexuality.

Besides laying the foundation for developing trust and self-esteem, physical bonding with, and nurturing by, parents sets the stage for recognition and acceptance of our own body as a potential source of pleasure. Solitary sexual behavior, or masturbation, provides our first, and usually lifelong, source of sexual pleasure. Too many of us, however, associate masturbation with sinful, inappropriate behavior.

Masturbation Individual or mutual stimulation of genitalia by hand or using other objects

Masturbation can be a solitary sexual behavior or can be enjoyed with a partner. As a solitary behavior, masturbation may or may not be accompanied by sexual fantasy and other autoerotic activity. Many people combine masturbation with viewing erotic material or engaging in simulated sexual activities with someone online (Daneback, Cooper, Mansson, 2005). Couples can masturbate each other simultaneously, take turns pleasing each other, or masturbate themselves simultaneously.

Female Techniques

Masters and Johnson noted that women exhibit much greater variation in masturbatory behavior. Even when women had a similar style of stimulation, the tempo, timing, and approach to masturbation varied. The most common form of female masturbation is to stimulate the clitoris, labia, and mons by hand through stroking, pulling, or rubbing (Hite, 1976).

Most women prefer to masturbate while lying on the back. A smaller percentage chooses to sit or stand while stimulating the genitalia. Between 5 and 10 percent of women prefer to masturbate while lying on their stomach, either placing a hand between their legs to stimulate the clitoris or rubbing the vulva against a pillow or some other object (Hite, 1976). Figure 8.2 illustrates female masturbation.

Masters and Johnson reported the following patterns of masturbatory behavior in order of preference: (1) manually stimulating the vulva, (2) using a vibrator to stimulate the clitoris/vulva, (3) inserting something into the vagina, (4) rubbing up against an object, (5) pressing the thighs together, (6) using water massage, and (7) all other methods. About half of the younger women reported using sex toys (vibrators, dildos, or other devices) to masturbate, choosing either to insert these or to use them to apply external vibration. A smaller percentage of women report using these devices in a similar fashion to stimulate the anus during masturbation. The variety and complexity have increased markedly as more women (and their partners) express interest in these products.

Male Techniques

In her study of male sexuality, Shere Hite (1981) reports the following male masturbatory techniques in order of preference: (1) stimulating the penis by hand, (2) lying down on the stomach rubbing against a bed, and (3) with water in the shower.

Few men choose to masturbate using sex toys such as vibrators, dildos, plastic sleeves,

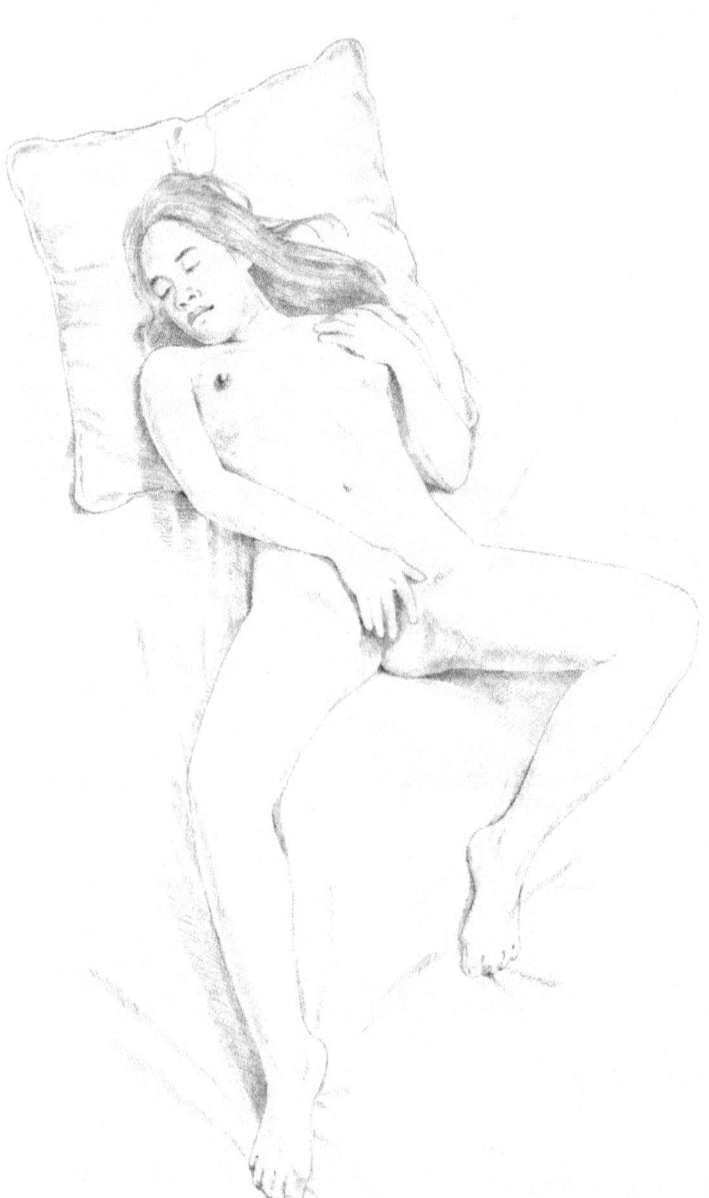

Figure 8.2 *Female Masturbation* Lying on the back and massaging the genitals with one hand is a common position for masturbation.

penile pumps, and inflatable dolls, although these devices are readily available. Though still relatively uncommon, proponents of these sex toys claim that they can enhance sexual pleasure, provide a change of pace from routine masturbatory practices, and add variety to safe-sex options.

Masters and Johnson found that many men masturbate by rubbing, stroking, or pumping the shaft of the penis with one hand (Masters, Johnson, & Kolodny, 1996). The tempo of movement usually builds gradually in response to the increase in arousal. Slow, deliberate touch gradually gives way to more forceful, rapid movements, often accompanied by increases in pressure and tension. A small percentage of men studied spend time stimulating the frenulum on the underside of the glans of the penis. Uncircumcised men seem to spend more time stimulating the glans and frenulum through pulling the foreskin back and forth. Ejaculation varies more, some men preferring to slow down and relax their grip and others desiring to increase pressure, squeezing out the last drops of semen. Figure 8.3 illustrates male masturbation.

Because the male penis is not lubricated, and masturbation usually involves a buildup of heat and friction, most men use some form of lubrication while masturbating. Body lotion and baby oil are two commonly used lubricants.

Health Aspects of Masturbation

Early critics of masturbation posed pseudoscientific charges that masturbation was neither "healthy" nor "normal." There is no evidence to support the claim that masturbation has adverse health consequences. In fact, recent studies indicate just the opposite. Several recent studies have shown that masturbating on a regular basis may decrease one's risk for prostate cancer. It does not cause any physical problems. It carries no risk for any physical or psychological illness. Most safe sex educators encourage their students to masturbate to relieve sexual tension or to enjoy an orgasm whenever they want one. It is also an excellent way to learn what feels good and how their bodies respond.

From a physiological perspective, a person cannot masturbate to excess. It is a self-limiting behavior; we ultimately lose our interest in it. As long as people follow basic hygienic precautions (clean hands, toys, and so on) and have adequate lubrication, they can masturbate as often as they want to. Rather than being a source of problems, masturbation is a healthy outlet for sexual desire, can reduce risk for sexually transmitted diseases in people who don't have safe sexual partners, and is an alternative to having sex with prostitutes or anonymous partners.

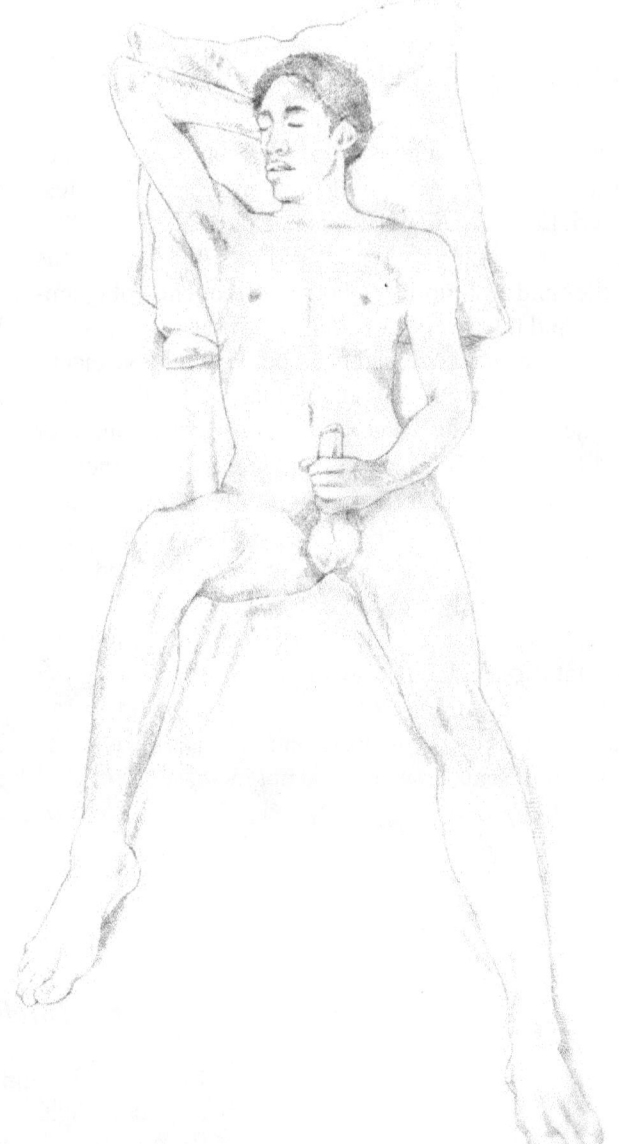

Figure 8.3 *Male masturbation*

sex in society 8.2

An Orgasm a Day Keeps the Cancer Away

Recent research suggests that frequent orgasms can reduce risk of developing prostate cancer (Giles, Severi, English, Credie, Borland, Boyle, Hopper, 2003; Leitzman, Platz, Stamfer, 2004; Fox, 2003). Previous studies and assumptions about the frequency of ejaculation and the risk of developing prostate cancer were based on the use of sexual intercourse to achieve ejaculation. These studies assumed that as the frequency of ejaculation increased so did the subject's number of different sexual partners. Increased frequency of ejaculations through intercourse with multiple sexual partners actually increased the risk of prostate cancer. The increased risk was believed to be associated with increased sexually transmitted disease risk. Studies that correlated the number of ejaculations with the number and status of sexual partners found that increasing the number of ejaculations per/week was not related to increased risk for prostate cancer as long as the number of different sexual partners did not increase (Leitzman et al., 2004).

Giles et al (2003) studied the prostate cancer risk associated with ejaculations from all sources, not just those associated with sexual intercourse. In their study of over 2000 men Giles et al (2003) found that for men between the ages of 20-50 the *more often* they ejaculated, the *less likely* they were to develop prostate cancer. The prostate glad produces fluid that contributes to the make-up of semen. Giles et al (2003) propose that ejaculation cleanses the prostate and prevents carcinogens from building up. Men who masturbate to ejaculation had a lower incidence of prostate cancer than men who climaxed through partnered activity. Giles et al (2003) report that men who had high-frequency ejaculations through sexual intercourse with multiple partners or a single partner had a 40 percent increased risk of prostate cancer compared to the men who masturbated.

Perhaps, rather than viewing masturbation as childish behavior and something to be avoided, it will promote the idea that masturbation can be perceived as an adult, prostate cancer risk-reducing behavior (Fox, 2003; Bean, 2004).

❧ Intellectual and Emotional Wellness ❧

Intellectual wellness provides the objective basis for understanding sexual behavior. It allows you to separate fact from fiction, truth from myth, science from theology. It empowers you to gain access to information and make informed choices that are free from dogma and outside pressures. Emotional wellness allows you to understand your emotions about the information without being overwhelmed by them. Perhaps nothing illustrates this interplay more than the topic of masturbation.

Centuries upon centuries of misinformation based on religious dogma, pseudoscience, and Puritanism have clouded the truth about masturbation and shrouded the topic in a veil of shame, guilt, and punishment. While the scientific "truth" about the behavior (it is a harmless outlet for sexual tension and a viable sexual behavior in itself) is well documented, the emotions it arouses often makes it difficult for people to deal with masturbation honestly and openly. People with high-level intellectual and emotional well-being about masturbation realize that it is a normal, healthy sexual behavior, and they try to work with their emotions regarding it rather than to suppress them or feel worse because of them. They talk about these issues with their partner(s) and seek help if they need it.

Patterns of Masturbatory Behavior

Masturbation is a form of autoerotic behavior. **Autoeroticism** is the dimension of the sex life defined by sexual desire or gratification, or both, experienced by a person without the direct participation of another (Laumann, Gagnon, Michael, & Michaels, 1994). Even though autoerotic activities lack a sex partner, sexual fantasies always include the imaginary presence of another person. In addition, autoerotic activity follows a specific social script appropriate to the individual, even if he or she never wishes to act out the fantasy.

Autoerotic activities differ from partnered activities because they do not require coordination with another person, can avoid many of the reality-based features of sex with a partner, and are limited only by the person's imagination. A surprising finding of Laumann et al was the lack of imagination and repetitiveness of pornographic and fantasy themes. Table 8.1 describes women's top 10 favorite fantasy themes. These common themes permeate various autoerotic media (adult books and magazines, films, CD-ROMs, videos, telephone and computer sex) and behaviors (use of sex toys, vibrators, dildos). Table 8.2 illustrates the use of autoerotic materials by gender.

Even though the content of sex fantasies is similar for men and women, the most important finding in this area by Laumann et al is the great disparity in levels of autoerotic activity between men and women. Men are much more likely to engage in autoerotic activities and to associate masturbation with these activities. They attribute this to the continuing social context of masturbation among men. Masturbation is a socially acceptable concept among adolescent males and almost completely absent in the social context of adolescent females.

Autoeroticism The dimension of the sex life defined by sexual desire and/or gratification experienced by a person without the direct participation of another

Table 8.1 Women's Top 10 Fantasies Gender

1. Sex with current partner
2. Sex with another man
3. Sex with another woman
4. Sex in embarrassing places/situations
5. Receiving oral sex
6. Romantic sexual scenarios
7. Forced sex
8. Being found irresistible by a man
9. Working as a prostitute
10. Sex with a stranger

Source: Tracey Cox, *Hot Sex*. New York: Bantam, 1998. (Cox is a former associate editor with *Cosmopolitan* and a freelance writer.)

A final finding of Laumann et al concerning autoerotic activity is the lack of association between autoerotic behavior and not having a primary sex partner. In fact, higher levels of autoerotic activity were associated with higher levels of partnered sexual activity. Rather than being a way to compensate for the lack of a sex partner, autoerotic activity seems to be a source of additional sexual pleasure.

Laumann et al found that individuals with higher levels of autoerotic activity were more likely than those with lower levels to engage in a broader range of sexual activities. In a sense, they have a much more elaborate set of sexual scripts. The development of sexual scripts or scenarios is influenced by a variety of sources of information, including autoerotic activities.

Autoeroticism is highly correlated with an increased incidence of techniques such as fellatio, cunnilingus, and anal intercourse (Lauman et al., 1994). Men and women who reported the highest levels of autoerotic behavior were more likely to engage in these behaviors than their peers who had lower levels of autoerotic activity.

> ❧ *Social Wellness* ❧
>
> The quality of social relationships plays a big part in sexual behavior. The foundation of social well-being is a solid relationship with your sex partner. This relationship is built on caring, trust, mutual respect, equality, and openness. Within this type of relationship, sexual communication and experimentation will flourish. It allows you and your partner to explore and understand your sexuality in a safe, caring, disease-free way.

Sexual Intercourse

Many people think that being a good lover means being particularly adept at sexual intercourse. Actually, being a good lover means having certain skills (knowing how to arouse your partner, using various sexual behaviors, and so on), as well as having good psychosocial skills (knowing how to communicate, when to initiate, and the like). In this section, we will focus on a variety of intercourse positions.

Vaginal Intercourse

Coitus Vaginal intercourse

Vaginal intercourse, also known as **coitus,** is one of the most common forms of heterosexual sexual activity, although sexual paraphernalia (strap-on or hand-held dildos and the like) allow lesbian women to penetrate their partner's vaginas if they desire. The three starting points for vaginal intercourse are face-to-face, side-by-side, and rear entry. We call these starting points rather than positions because each starting point offers a limitless array of positions, depending on how you place the rest of your body (arms, legs, torso, and so on).

sex in society 8.3

Masturbation—Student Reports

Although masturbation is a generally accepted form of sexual expression for our students, their feelings about it vary considerably. Some are completely accepting and open about their masturbatory behavior. Others still feel guilty masturbating and hide their behavior from their partners and friends. Here are a few reports from our students concerning masturbation:

Susan, 21, senior, is white and identifies as lesbian.

I masturbate a couple of times a month, usually when I'm stressed out. I used to feel a little guilty about it, but I've found I can deal with things a lot better if I can get rid of my tension. Usually my lover and I make love when we see each other on the weekend, but sometimes she's away on business and we miss a week. I'll usually go home and take a nice bath, relax, and make myself come. My parents were very strict when I was growing up, and masturbation was a definite no. I don't think they could imagine that I do it, and I guess that's why I still feel guilty about it.

Tom, 18, freshman, single, identifies as African American.

I would say I masturbate once or twice a week. I'm a little nervous masturbating in my room because I can't really relax, having a roommate. I'm never sure when he's going to walk in. When I go home on weekends, I enjoy it more because I can lock my door, look at my magazines, and "get off" in private. My parents have never said anything, but I think they know I do it.

Edwardo, 25, senior, engaged, identifies as Hispanic.

I masturbate about two times a week. Sometimes my fiancée and I will watch X-rated films and then masturbate each other. She'll do me, and then I do her. Other times, if either one of us isn't horny, we'll masturbate the other to orgasm. Sometimes we won't even have intercourse. We masturbate each other and finish off with oral sex. I never have had any inhibitions about masturbation. My parents always told me it was normal and OK as long as I keep it private. I don't view it as second best to intercourse, just different.

❧ *Spiritual Wellness* ❧

A key component of spirituality is the sense of being connected with something beyond the self. In one sense, a person can't become more "interconnected" with another human being than through sexual intercourse. When our sexual relationships are based on respect, mutuality, and caring, our union with another person creates something that we cannot experience as individuals. In contrast, when our sexual relationships are based on exploitation, power, mistrust, fear, or other destructive intentions, we become disconnected from others, mere sexual mercenaries, out for ourselves only. Regardless of whether we are religious, we each have a moral code, a sense of right and wrong that can enhance our connectedness to others or destroy it. Those with high-level spirituality view their sexual relations with others with integrity and morality.

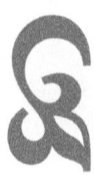

healthy sex hints 8.4

Safe Fantasy

Sexual fantasy serves several important functions. Fantasies help us expand our sexual scripts. They help us explore and expand our sexual repertoire. Sexual fantasies are a healthy sexual outlet. Coupled with masturbation, they provide a safe, exciting release of sexual tension. Sexual fantasy provides a "practice arena" to work through sexual scripts and encounters that we eventually may want to enact in real life. This safe practice carries none of the interpersonal or health risks of an actual encounter. Fantasies allow us to experience activities that turn us on but are not things we want to experience in real life. Fantasies do not necessarily represent what we really want in reality.

Sometimes, however, the lure of living out our sexual fantasies is strong. When is turning a fantasy into a reality a good idea? The following criteria may help you determine when you may appropriately cross that line:

1. The nature of the fantasy
2. The strength of the turn-on
3. The social context of the fantasy
4. The nature of your partner(s)
5. Your level of control over the specific situation
6. Whether the person is willing to lose the fantasy (sometimes living out a fantasy makes it lose its fantasy appeal)

The nature of the fantasy refers to how unusual, bizarre, or dangerous the fantasy is. The more bizarre or dangerous the fantasy, the more cautious you should be about wanting to turn it into a reality. If you can control for some of the other variables (items 3, 4, and 5) and safety, you might want to act it out. If you can't control these variables, you're probably better off leaving it as a fantasy.

The strength of the arousal exerts a powerful influence on whether to act out the fantasy. If a strong desire isn't there, you may not want to turn it into reality at this time.

The social context of the fantasy refers to the setting in which the fantasy plays out. For example, many people are turned on by the fantasy of having sex in a public place. Public places range from semi-deserted beaches (where the likelihood of discovery is minimal) to the elevator at your favorite hotel (where the chance of discovery is high). Combining the risk of exposure with the consequences of being discovered (being arrested, losing your job or public stature, and the like) will help you evaluate the social context of acting out the fantasy.

The nature of your partner(s) will help you evaluate the safety and confidentiality of acting out your fantasy. Asking your wife to tie you to the bedpost and then acting out a dominatrix scenario in the safety of your own bedroom is vastly different from going downtown to Mistress Helga's illegal place and allowing her to put manacles on you. Fantasies acted out with a well-known partner whom you can trust are much safer than those with strangers and prostitutes.

Some fantasies are based on giving up control. The turn-on with dominance and submission lies in being vulnerable and letting someone have control over you. Other fantasies are more amenable to control. The greater the control, the safer is the fantasy. In general, the less control you have in the situation, the greater is your need to act out the fantasy with a trusting partner in a familiar, safe environment.

The last warning concerns losing the turn-on after you act it out. Some sexual experiences are better left as fantasies and not acted out. These fantasies provide a strong turn-on that is satisfying. When you turn this into reality, however, you run the risk that the reality won't be as exciting as the fantasy. When this happens, the fantasy often loses its appeal and its ability to turn you on.

Face-to-Face

Face-to-face positions have two variations: man on top and woman on top.

Woman on Top. The woman-on-top position, shown in Figures 8.4 (heterosexual couple) and 8.5 (lesbian couple), allows women greater control in the depth, pace, and motion of her partner's thrusting. It allows the woman on the top the greatest control in clitoral stimulation and is the easiest intercourse position for manual clitoral stimulation. Orgasm rates for heterosexual women are better for this position than any other. This position is also good for helping heterosexual male partners control premature ejaculation. The woman can get to this position in two ways: She can start with her partner on top and roll over into this position or start with her partner on his or her back and move on top. In the latter case, the partners must have enough room on the bed so they won't find themselves rolling off the bed and onto the floor.

When starting with the man on his back, the woman kneels over him with one knee on either side of his legs. Either partner can part the vaginal lips as the woman lowers herself onto the erect penis, guiding it in with a free hand.

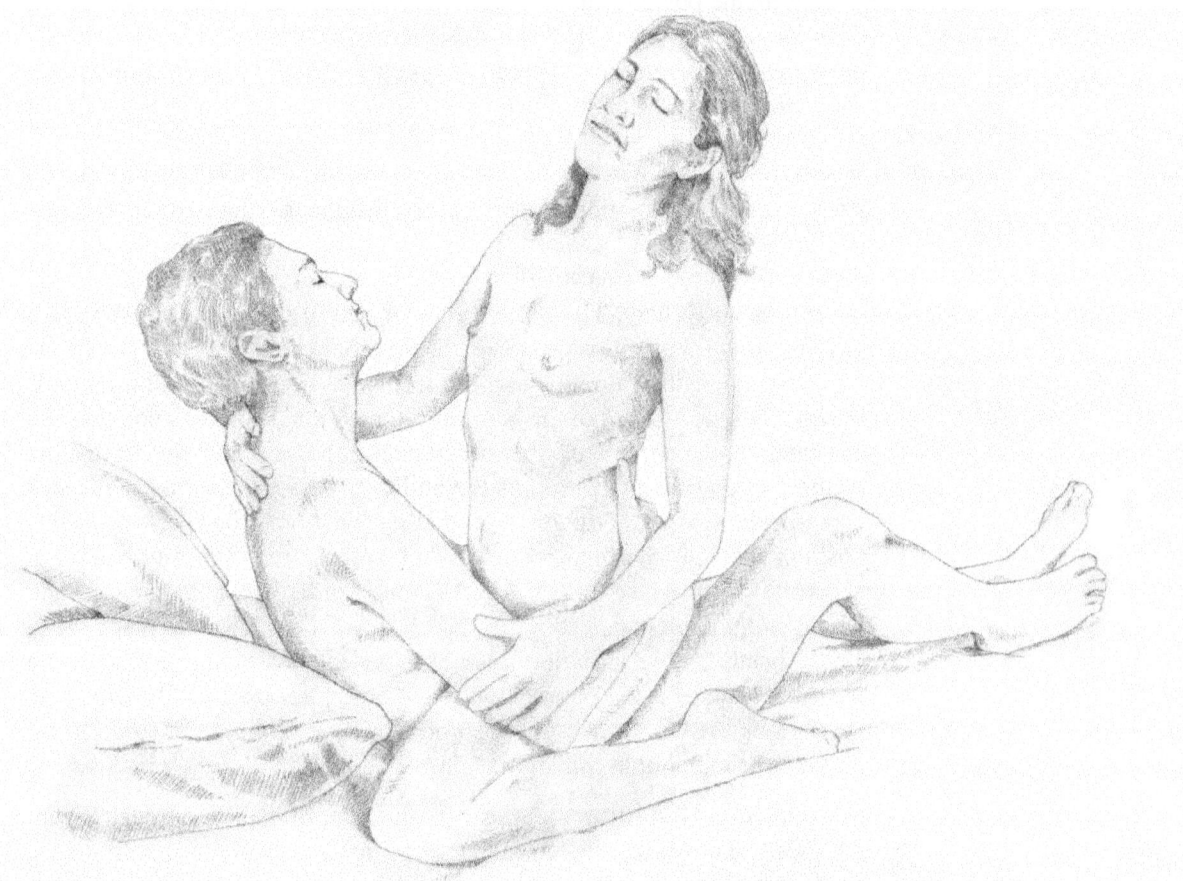

Figure 8.4 *Woman on Top Sitting: Heterosexual Couple* This position allows for the partner on the bottom to use his hands to massage his partner's breasts and upper body.

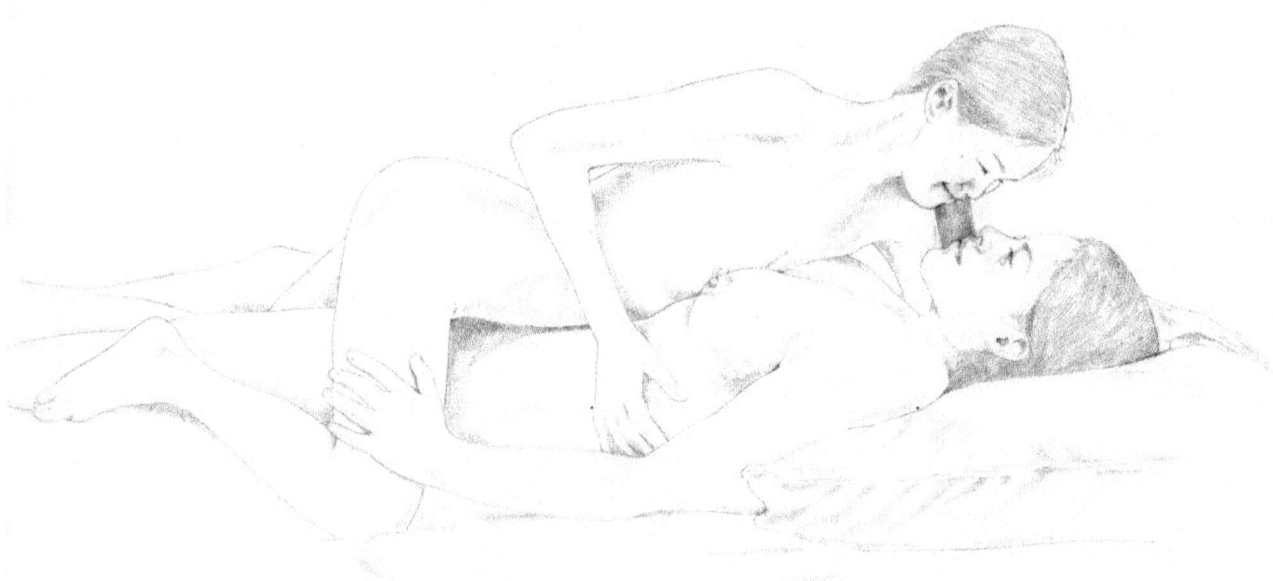

Figure 8. *Woman on Top Lying; Lesbian Couple* Lying on top of one's partner while facing her allows both partners to kiss as they make love.

With the penis inside, the woman can rock or thrust her hips or move them in a circular fashion. The rocking and thrusting motions allow maximum penile penetration, whereas the circular grinding motion stimulates the clitoris more directly. Each of these three creates entirely different sensations.

Lesbians can use this position in a similar fashion with the aid of a strap-on dildo. The motions, activities, and benefits are the same as those for heterosexual couples. The partner on the bottom can be passive and allow the woman on top to control all movements or move with her, synchronizing motion with hers. The bottom partner can also initiate thrusting and grinding if the woman on top becomes tired or desires it.

In this position the woman also has more freedom to use her hands in ways similar to those of the man-on-top position. From this position she can caress and manipulate either her partner or herself. One option that the woman-on-top position offers is the ability to rotate her torso, while still being penetrated by her partner, so that her back is to her partner. In this position she can lean forward or sit back and achieve different depths of penetration and sensations. Her partner can fondle her buttocks and back while maintaining penetration.

An interesting variation of the woman-on-top position is to move from kneeling or lying on to actually sitting on her partner. By sitting on her partner, the woman-on-top position affords maximum penetration and intimacy as the couple can embrace, kiss, and talk.

Man on Top (Missionary). The man-on-top position, illustrated in Figure 8.6, is also known as the "missionary position." It is the most commonly used intercourse position in the United States. In this position, the partners stimulate each other until they are sufficiently aroused. The man then moves on top of the woman. Either partner spreads the female's vaginal

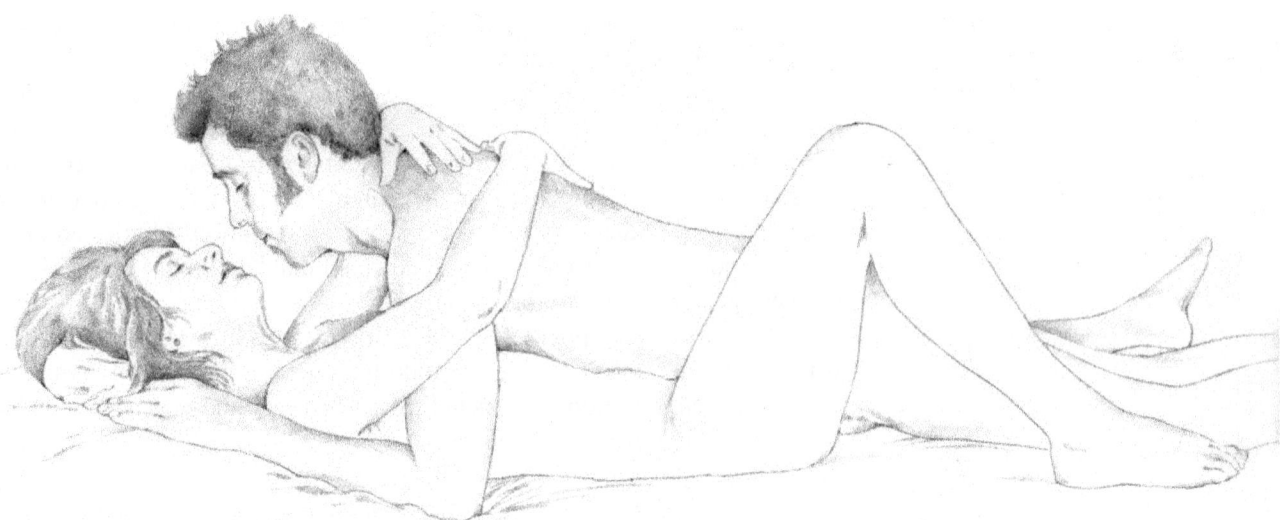

Figure 8.6 *Man on Top, Heterosexual Couple* The man-on-top position is commonly referred to as the "missionary position" and is the most common heterosexual intercourse behavior.

lips and inserts the penis into the vagina. The man supports his weight on his elbows, hands, knees, or across his partner's entire body as his penis moves in the vagina.

The most typical penile movements involve thrusting in and out as the female either remains still or moves her hips in concert with her partner's thrusting. These motions provide direct sexual stimulation of the male's penile nerve endings (on the shaft, glans, and corona). The woman's clitoris usually is stimulated as the clitoral hood (top of the labia minora) pulls back and forth over it or the man's pubic area rubs against it. The vagina is stimulated as the penis slides in and out. The deeper recesses of the vagina (cervical area) may or may not be stimulated depending on the depth of the strokes and the positions. An option to thrusting in and out is a circular motion, known as *grinding,* which involves more pubis-to-pubis contact and stimulates the female's clitoris differently. This provides more direct and intense stimulation of the clitoris and the base of the man's penis and can be done even if the man has ejaculated. If he hasn't withdrawn the penis before it has become limp, he can continue stimulating his partner with the circular motion. Sometimes this can go on through his refractory period, and he can achieve another erection without removing his penis. This allows his partner to be stimulated and have additional orgasms even though he has climaxed. Many men find this type of stimulation enjoyable even though they have a limp penis and already have had an orgasm.

Variations of this starting point involve changing the position of the legs and arms. The woman on the bottom can experience a variety of different sensations and depths of penetration by wrapping her legs around the partner's ankles, legs, or waist. Or she can throw her legs over her partner's shoulders as he thrusts in and out, which affords the deepest penetration.

One of the advantages of this position is that it allows the partners to look into each other's eyes and communicate. It also allows the partners to rub and caress each other's chest and shoulders. Furthermore, it allows use of the hands to enhance stimulation by touching or rubbing the partner's genitals during intercourse.

The woman may enjoy stretching her arms over her head, arching her back. This allows her partner better access to caress the breasts and nipples. She may enjoy having the partner pin her arms back over her head. This mild form of domination/submission allows her to "lose control" in a safe way. Individuals should participate in domination/submission only with someone they trust and must understand that "no means no" if either partner wants the activity to stop.

The missionary position can also be used by lesbian women if the partner on top is using a strap-on dildo to penetrate her partner's vagina. The positioning, motions, and benefits are similar to those experienced by heterosexual couples.

Rear Entry

The rear entry starting point (Figure 8.7) is also known as "doggie style" because it is the way in which dogs and most other animals have intercourse. In rear entry positions, the partner enters the woman's vagina from behind. This usually is accomplished with the woman kneeling on her hands and knees and the man kneeling behind her, either between or straddling her legs. Either partner parts the vaginal lips and guides the penis in. This position creates deep vaginal penetration but little direct clitoral stimulation. For this reason, either the man or the woman stimulates the clitoris manually.

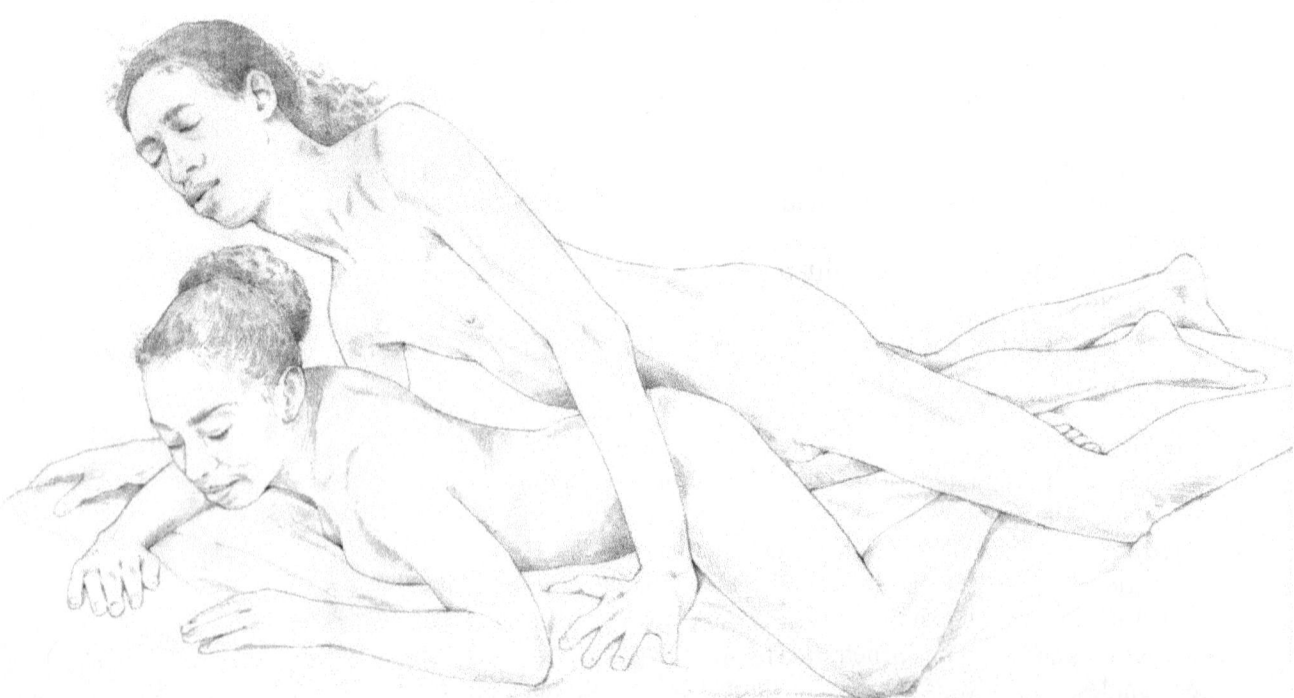

Figure 8.7 *Rear Entry, Heterosexual Couple* The rear-entry intercourse position is commonly referred to as "doggie style."

This position also offers stimulation of the anus and perineum through pressure and friction from the man's pubis rubbing or grinding against it. Once engaged, the woman can lower her head and raise her hips higher to achieve maximum penetration. The rear-entry position can also be used by lesbian women with the aid of a strap-on dildo for vaginal penetration. The positioning, motions, and benefits are similar.

Two other rear-entry position variations are (1) the couple can lie down with the man on top of the woman, or (2) they can lie on their sides. The latter is commonly known as the "spoon" position. One disadvantage of this position is that the partners do not face each other, which makes communication and kissing more difficult.

Side-to-Side

The side-to-side vaginal intercourse can involve face-to-face positioning (Figures 8.8 and 8.9) or rear-entry positioning. Because neither partner is bearing the full weight of the other, the side-to-side position is ideal for leisurely lovemaking or the rest period between more vigorous sessions. The easiest way to get into the side-to-side position is by rolling into it from the man-on-top or woman-on-top or the rear-entry position.

Besides being a comfortable position for leisurely lovemaking, the side-to-side variation has many advantages. It also is good for obese people, as it minimizes weight-bearing. The rear-entry variation (Figure 8.9) is good for pregnant women whose developing fetus and protruding abdomen make the man-on-top position impossible. The side-to-side position also facilitates

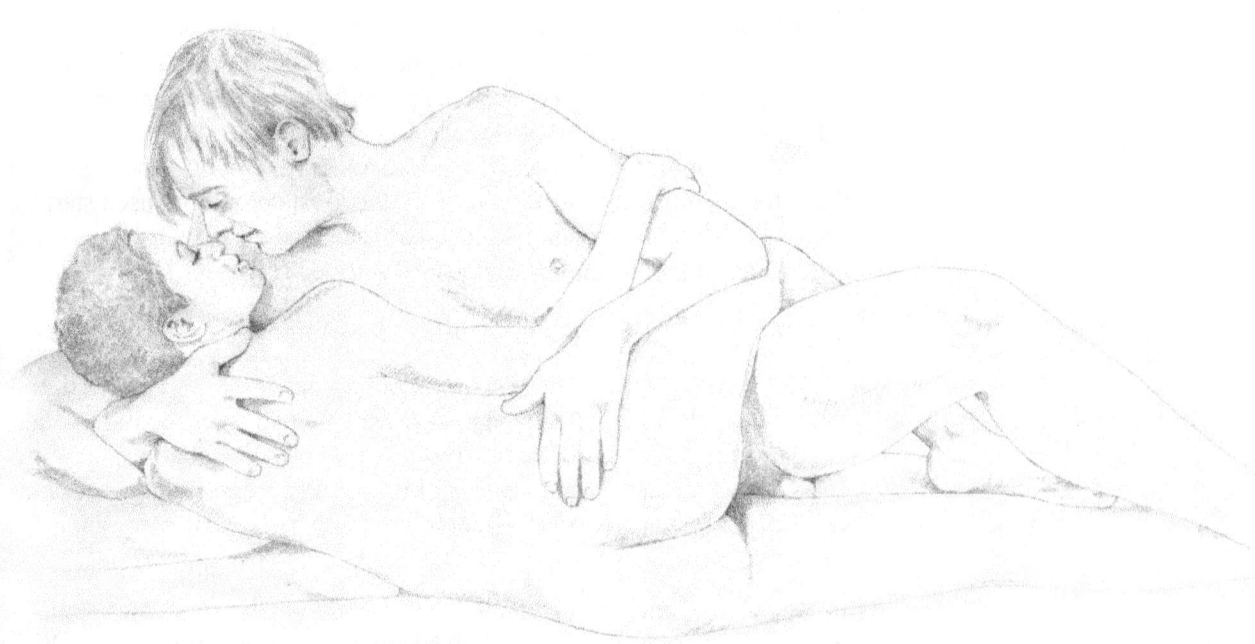

Figure 8.8 *Side-by-Side, Heterosexual Couple* The side-by-side facing and rear-entry intercourse positions are very comfortable and are often used to relieve pressure on the partner.

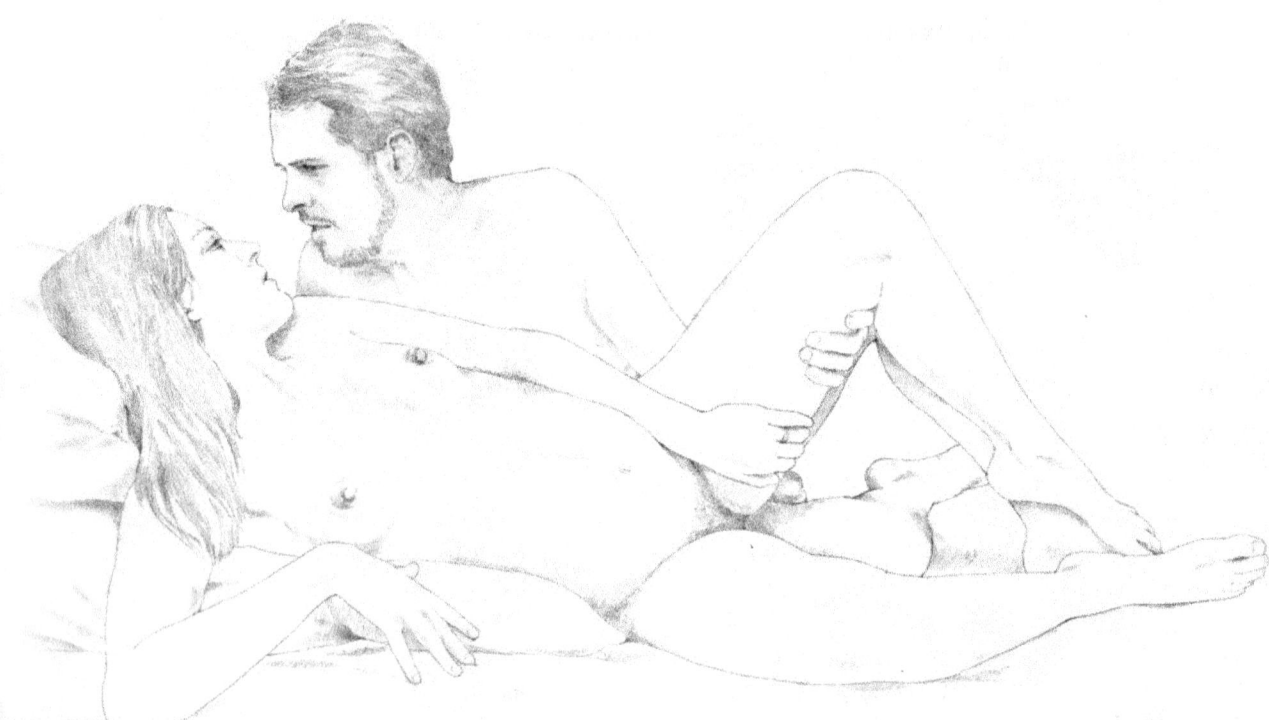

Figure 8.9 *Side-by-Side, Pregnant Heterosexual Couple*

good communication and kissing while leaving the hands free for hugging and forms of manual stimulation.

Anal Intercourse

In anal intercourse, a man inserts his penis into his partner's rectum. Heterosexual and homosexual couples both practice anal intercourse. Like vaginal intercourse, anal intercourse can take place from the three starting points: side-to-side, rear-entry, or face-to-face. The advantages and disadvantages associated with these starting points for vaginal intercourse are similar to those for anal intercourse. Rear-entry is the most commonly used starting point for anal intercourse, although anal penetration can be accomplished through all of the positions previously described (Figure 8.10).

Oral Sex

Oral sex, also known as oral-genital sex, mouth-genital sex, giving head, and going down, is the stimulation of the partner's genitals with the lips, mouth, tongue, and face. The three main types of oral sex are fellatio (mouth-to-penis contact), cunnilingus (mouth-to-vulva contact), and anilingus (mouth-to-anus contact). All three are common forms of sexual expression for straight, gay, lesbian, and bisexual people.

Fellatio Oral stimulation of the penis

Fellatio Also known as a "blow job," **fellatio** involves licking and sucking a man's penis. The term is derived from the Latin word *fellare,* which means "to suck." During fellatio, the partner begins by licking and sucking the flaccid penis while holding it. As the penis begins to grow, a man usually enjoys having his penis move in and out of his partner's mouth. The

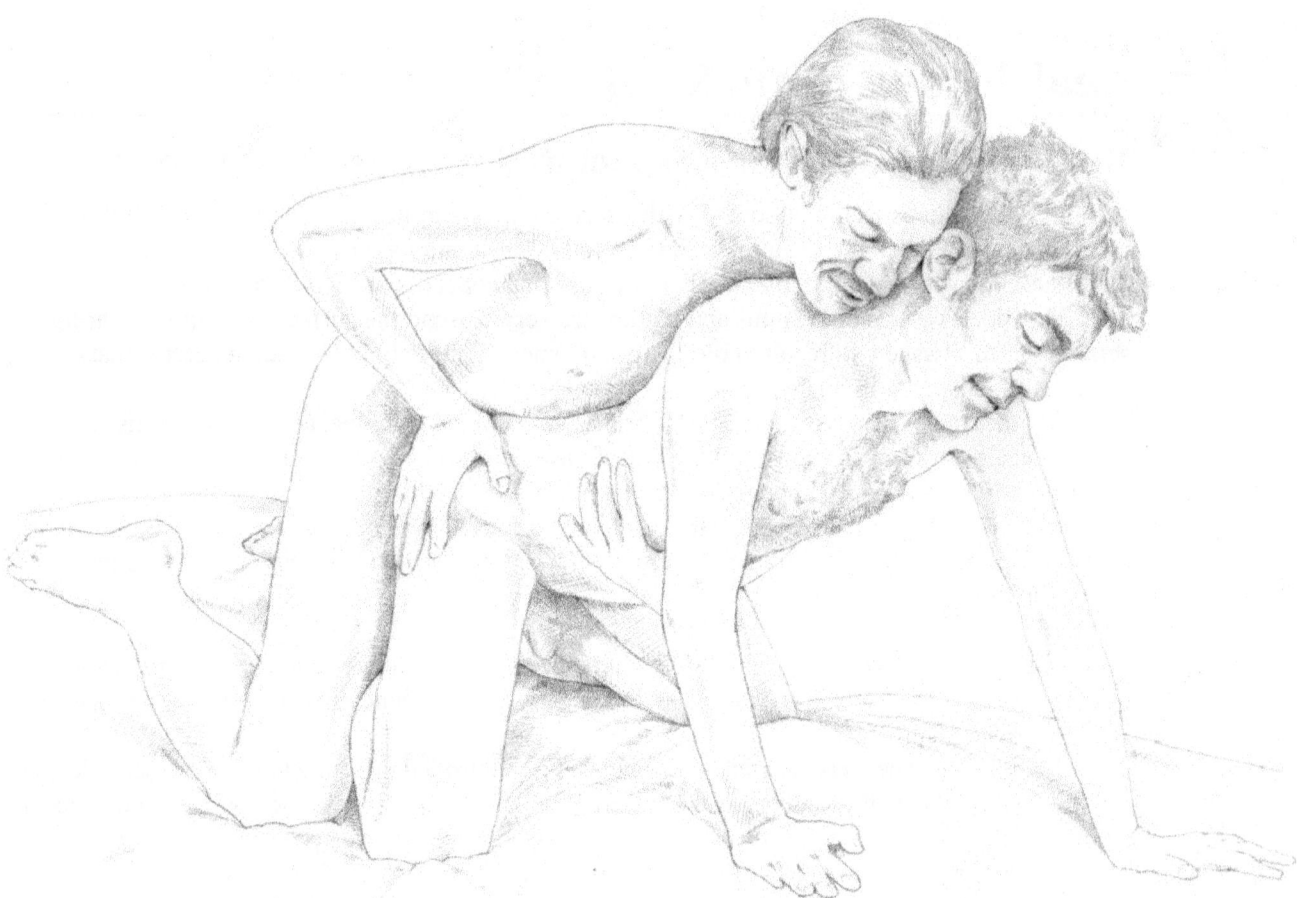

Figure 8.10 *Rear Entry Anal Intercourse, Gay Couple* The rear entry position is commonly used by gay couples.

man can accomplish this by gently thrusting his hips, driving the penis in and out of his partner's mouth. The partner can do this by moving his or her head up and down, moving the penis deeper into the mouth and then letting it slide back again.

The sliding motion is accompanied by sucking, which can vary in intensity depending on the man's preference. The tongue is used to lick, flick, or swirl around the penis as it moves in the mouth. Using these tongue motions to stimulate the glans and the coronal ridge (particularly the underside where the shaft meets the glans) provides maximum stimulation for the man.

These movements, if continued, usually provide enough stimulation to trigger orgasm. Many men find that a combination of oral and manual stimulation is necessary to provide enough stimulation for orgasm. The partner can grasp the penis at its base or along the shaft and pump it while simultaneously stimulating it with the mouth and tongue. Grasping the penis in one hand while licking and sucking it can also give the partner a sense of control over the depth and intensity of the man's thrusting.

When the penis is thrust into the throat, it typically initiates a gag reflex, which can be minimized by using your hand to control the depth of the partner's thrusting. To minimize this, the partner can relax the throat muscles and control the depth of thrusting by holding the penis.

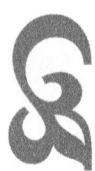

healthy sex hints 8.5

Reducing Health Risks Associated with Anal Intercourse

Although the anus is richly endowed with nerve endings and has erogenous potential, it differs from other body parts and requires a few special considerations. One major difference between the tissue of the anus and rectum and that of the vagina concerns the blood vessels that supply the area. The blood vessels of the anus and rectum are very close to the surface. Any minor tearing or scraping of this tissue will result in bleeding and exposing these blood vessels to germs that could enter the bloodstream in this way.

Another major difference involves lubrication. Unlike the vagina, anal and rectal tissue does not produce natural lubrication as a product of vasocongestion. Therefore, care must be taken to adequately lubricate the anal opening and rectum with some other product. Saliva or a commercial water-based sterile lubricant is advisable. Saliva is not as slippery as most commercial products, such as K-Y Jelly, but it is free and can be used at any time. Because petroleum-based products can erode the latex in condoms, these products, such as Vaseline, should not be used in conjunction with a condom.

Lubricants should be spread liberally on the penis and the anus. Gently inserting a lubricated finger into the rectum will lubricate this area and relax the sphincter that keep the anus closed. (Make sure your fingernails are trimmed!)

The lubricated penis is inserted gently and begins controlled thrusting to work the penis deeper into the rectum. Once the penis is inserted comfortably into the rectum, the couple can decide on the nature and intensity of pelvic thrusting. From this rear-entry starting point, couples can try most of the positions described in the section on vaginal intercourse.

Sex involving the anus and rectum also carries an increased risk for transmitting a range of infections ranging from hepatitis B to HIV. Organisms that are transmitted through contact with fecal matter or blood are easily transmitted through insertive or receptive anal intercourse or anilingus.

To reduce the likelihood of disease transmission and increase sexual response associated with anal stimulation:

1. Do not engage in anilingus or anal intercourse with an anonymous (don't know at all) or a casual (don't know that well) partner.
2. Before engaging in anal activities, be sure your sex partner is HIV-negative and free of other STDs. This means getting to know your potential partner better and, sometimes, being tested.
3. With disease-free partners, shower normally with soap and water before having sex to provide adequate hygiene.
4. Always use a water-based lubricant when anal penetration is involved.
5. Do not insert foreign objects (other than specially designed dildos, vibrators, and the like) into the rectum. Be careful not to let things you insert slip past the anal sphincter muscle. The object can get "lost" in the rectum and may require surgical removal.
6. If your partner's STD/HIV status is unknown, use a condom for anal intercourse.

Couples need to discuss their feelings about ejaculation. As discussed in Chapter 3, the male ejaculate is typically about 1 teaspoon of fluid when he comes. The ejaculate is milky-white in color, has a slippery texture resembling egg whites, and leaves a salty aftertaste. Most men enjoy the sensation of ejaculating into the partner's mouth. This also can be enjoyable to the partner. If the partner finds swallowing ejaculate distasteful, an

> ❧ *Environmental Wellness* ❧
>
> In this chapter, we openly discuss sexual behaviors from a scientific/ health perspective. We discuss the pros and cons of such things as oral and anal intercourse, heterosexual, homosexual, and bisexual variations on these behaviors, and how to engage in them with minimal health risks. We realize, however, that people don't engage in these behaviors in a vacuum. There are still places in the United States where century-old statutes regarding *sodomy* (a term that can be broadly interpreted to include such things as oral sex between consenting marital partners) laws are still enforced. You need to know what laws are still on the books regarding sexual behavior in your city, town, county, and state. This is vital information that can help you make informed choices about your sexual behavior and lifestyle.

alternative is fellatio to the point of orgasm, then to withdraw the penis and ejaculate outside the partner's mouth, or to switch to some other form of sexual behavior prior to the point of orgasm.

Cunnilingus

The oral stimulation of a woman's vulva through licking, sucking, and nibbling or rubbing with the face is called **cunnilingus**. It is a common sexual practice of straight, lesbian, and bisexual men and women. Although cunnilingus (from the Latin words *cunnus* [vulva] and *lingere* [to lick]) by definition refers to oral stimulation of the vulva, often the perineum and outer parts of the vagina are also stimulated during this act.

Cunnilingus Oral stimulation of the vulva

Cunnilingus typically begins as the partner kisses and licks the partner's inner thighs, abdomen, and mons area. The partner then gently parts the labia majora and uses the tongue to lick, flick, or swirl around the vaginal lips, clitoris, and introitus.

Pressure can be applied by pressing the tongue against the vulva with greater force. Circular motions are often used to stimulate the vulva in a somewhat different fashion. Care must be taken not to apply too much pressure directly to the clitoris, as it is the part of the female sexual anatomy that is most richly endowed with nerve endings.

The mouth can be used to gently suck on the vaginal lips and clitoris. Gently sucking one or more lips into one's mouth can provide intense pleasure. The clitoris also can be sucked on gently. Some women find it arousing to have their partner gently nibble the vaginal lips and clitoris. The tongue also can be used to penetrate the vagina with thrusting motions.

The face (chin, cheeks, and forehead) can become involved in cunnilingus while the mouth and lips are busy providing stimulation. A partner can intentionally use the face to provide additional stimulation through direct pressure or circular motion. For instance, the bridge of the nose can provide clitoral stimulation while licking or sucking on the labia.

As with fellatio, cunnilingus can be performed with or without manual stimulation. Many women derive pleasure from having their partner insert a well lubricated finger into their vagina or anus while performing cunnilingus. Saliva or vaginal lubrication can be used to make the fingers slippery. The partner also can stimulate the woman's clitoris with manual stimulation while licking or sucking on another part of the vulva.

Anilingus

Anilingus Oral stimulation of the anus

Although it isn't as common as fellatio or cunnilingus, **anilingus,** also known as *rimming,* is another form of oral sex practiced by people of all forms of sexual orientation. During anilingus, a person kisses, licks, or sucks the partner's anus. The motions and activities of anilingus are similar to both cunnilingus and fellatio.

Performing anilingus affords a good opportunity to stimulate the perineum, an area richly endowed with nerve endings. Some men and women enjoy having their partners insert their tongues into their anus during anilingus. Others prefer that their partner insert a well-lubricated finger into the rectum. When performing anilingus on a woman, care must be taken to avoid spreading *Escherichia coli* bacteria into the vagina. The tongue or fingers never should be inserted directly from the anus to the vagina without first being washed.

Another concern is the spread of hepatitis and other STD organisms through anilingus. We do not recommend performing anilingus with a casual sex partner or someone whose STD status is unknown, as this could result in ingesting disease-causing organisms. (This topic is discussed in greater detail in Chapter 15.)

Mutual Oral Sex

Mutual Oral Sex The term used to describe simultaneous cunnilingus and fellatio is sixty-nine.

Heterosexual **Mutual oral sex** is often referred to as *sixty-nine* because of the shape couples form when engaged in it. This usually is accomplished in the side-to-side starting point, with each partner's head at the other's genitals (see Figures 8.11 and 8.12). From this position, both partners have easy

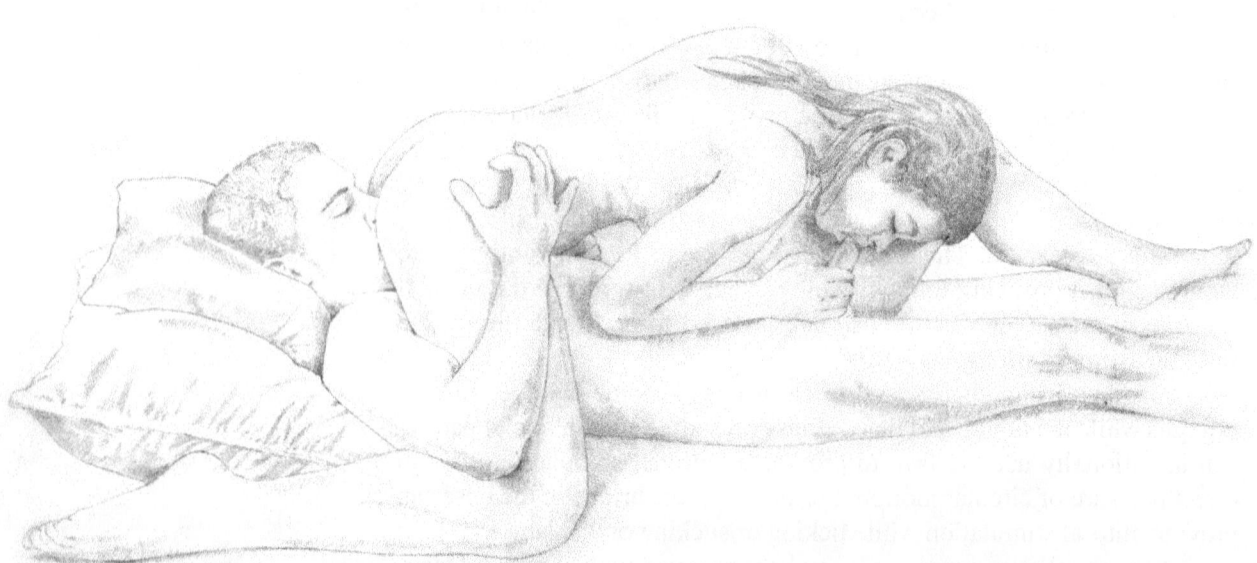

Figure 8.11 *Mutual Oral Sex Heterosexual Couple* Mutual oral sex is often referred to as sixty-nine because of the shape couples form when engaged in it.

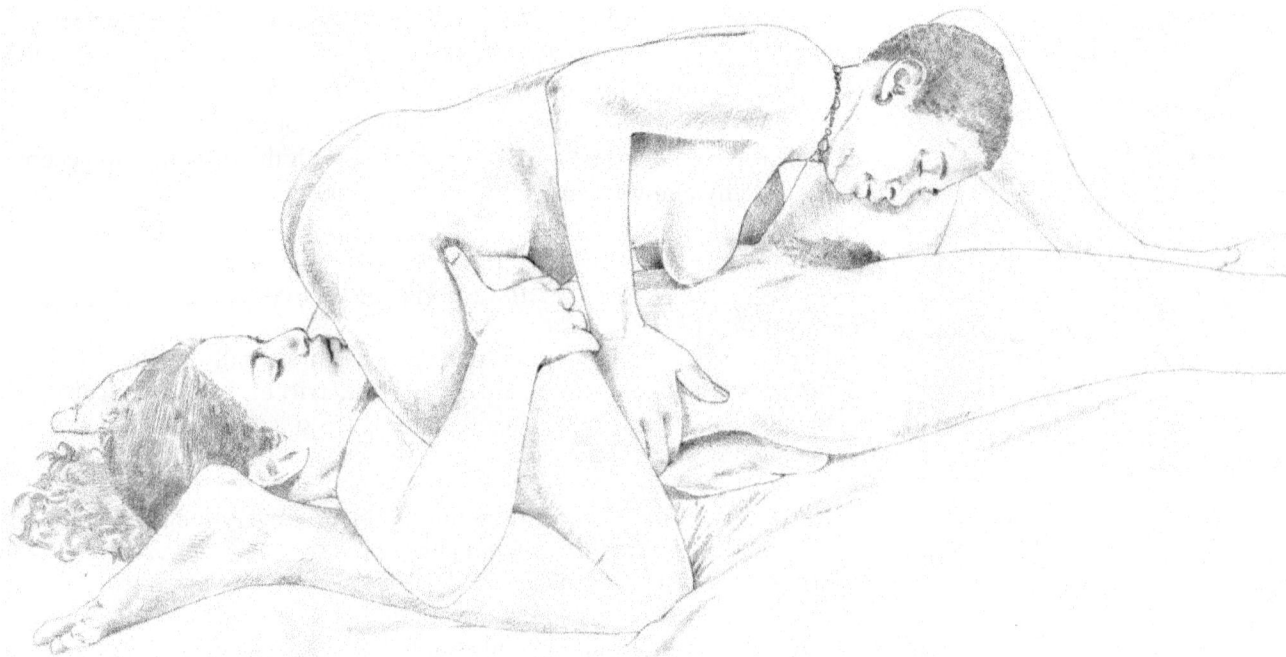

Figure 8.12 *Mutual Oral Sex, Lesbian Couple*

access to their partner's genitals. From the side-to-side starting point, it is easy to roll into the man or woman on either the top or bottom positions. By being on the top or the bottom, a person can control for deeper penetration of the tongue when performing cunnilingus, or the penis during fellatio. Mutual oral sex is enjoyed by heterosexual, gay, and lesbian couples.

Sexuality and Disability

Physical disabilities can manifest themselves across a broad spectrum of afflictions. People who are physically or developmentally challenged can maximize their sexual potential by being creative despite their limitations. They experience sensual and sexual pleasures the same way people without disabilities do. Although they may have some restrictions concerning what they can and cannot do, they still can enjoy robust sexual activity and satisfying relationships.

Disabilities, Body Image, and Self-Esteem

For some people with physical disabilities, the main obstacles to sexual activity are social—finding and attracting partners and overcoming self-imposed or societal attitudinal barriers to sex. For these people, sexual behavior is affected very little by the actual physical disability. Their disability affects their body image and their perception of themselves as desirable. Their disability doesn't create a physical barrier to engaging in specific sexual acts or behaviors. Rather, it is their perception of the disability that creates the barrier (McCabe, Taleporos, Dip, 2003; Hingsburger & Tough, 2002).

Ostomy is the perfect example of this and will be covered in greater detail in Chapter 11. A *colostomy* can be described as a resectioning of the colon to a stoma that empties the contents of the colon into a bag attached to the abdominal wall.

This procedure does not normally affect sexual response, and it doesn't impede engaging in a variety of sexual behaviors ranging from oral sex to different forms of intercourse. However, learning to manage these and other sexual activities while wearing a colostomy bag (or temporarily removing it) depends on the willingness of the person with the disability to accept the colostomy and work around it (Chance, 2002).

❦ *Physical Wellness* ❦

Physical well-being implies the absence of sexually transmitted diseases, which can severely curtail sexual activity and pleasure. It also includes daily hygiene and health behaviors, both of which play a role in enjoying sexual behavior. High-level physical fitness can enhance sexuality, and nowhere is this more evident than in relation to sexual behavior. High-level physical wellness enhances everything related to sexual behavior. It influences our ability to perform sexually. Although the goal is not to become a sexual acrobat, a high level of fitness will increase our strength, flexibility, and endurance—all elements that can enhance sexual ability and creativity.

People with physical disabilities or illnesses may not be able to achieve the same levels of fitness as those who are not disabled or ill. However, they can strive to get the most out of their abilities and maximize their individual fitness level to achieve their sexual potential despite their limitations.

Disabilities and Physical Barriers

For others, the disability directly affects sexual behavior. Arthritis and low-back injury/ pain can be used to illustrate this. A woman with arthritis in her hands, for instance, might find masturbation difficult and have to adjust, perhaps enlisting the aid of a vibrator, dildo, or the willing help of a partner. The pain in her hands and fingers, her limited range of motion, lack of strength, and physical deformity (depending on the severity of her arthritis and her ability to control it with a therapeutic regimen) all affect her ability to stimulate herself sufficiently through masturbation.

A man with a lower-back disc-related injury can experience chronic pain, which makes certain sexual behaviors impossible. For example, positions that require him to support his partner's weight (partner-on-top vaginal intercourse, partner sitting on top while seated on a chair, and so forth) would be difficult, if not impossible, to accomplish. He might have to substitute side-by-side, rear-entry vaginal intercourse, or mutual oral sex, behaviors that don't require him to support the full weight of his partner.

Neurological Disabilities

Some disabilities such as spinal cord injuries (covered in detail in Chapter 7) and Parkinson's disease will actually affect the transmission of nerve messages that trigger sexual response. Men with spinal cord injuries or Parkinson's disease rarely achieve erections except through reflexive

case study 8.4

Charlotte: Spinal Cord Injury

Charlotte, 30, single, identifies as African American.

As a young woman, Charlotte was a promising athlete. She was a multifaceted track star who at 20, while on spring break, got into a serious automobile accident that put her into a coma for 4 days and left her paralyzed from the waist down.

I was very bitter for several months following the accident. I didn't want to talk to anyone and was angry all of the time. I broke off my engagement and retreated into a world of antidepressant drugs and disability checks. I hated rehabilitation and didn't work hard at all. I couldn't accept myself without my legs. They had been the source of my greatest accomplishments, and my best feature.

After about 6 months, we had a guest lecturer at the rehabilitation center. A social worker spoke to us about redefining our selves, including our sexual selves. I hadn't even begun to think about redefining myself let alone redefining my sexuality. She made me realize how much I missed my partner and the intimacy and sex we had. I really used to love oral sex (giving and receiving) and how my partner kissed and caressed my breasts when we made love. I really began to wonder whether I could really recapture that again with another man.

I slowly came around and began to take my rehabilitation seriously. I also started paying attention to myself as a whole person, capable of satisfying myself and someday my partner. I started taking night classes again and eventually went back to college full-time where I met my present husband. He was a graduate student in the counseling department, and it took me a long time to believe that he really loved me and wasn't just looking to "help" some poor cripple out.

I'm glad I gave him a chance because he is the best thing that ever happened to me. He helped me rediscover the intimacy, passion, and sex in my life. Sure, there are things I can't do sexually any more, and I can't have vaginal orgasms like I used to, but that is becoming less and less important in my life.

We've adopted a little girl, and I am thoroughly enjoying motherhood and hoping I can still teach her a thing or two about running high hurdles.

neural activity, and they lose their ability to ejaculate. This makes vaginal intercourse difficult, if not impossible, for them. However, these men might find that although they can no longer get erections, they can still enjoy cunnilingus and other forms of nonpenetrative sexual pleasuring (Yang, 2000; Alexander, Sipski, & Findley, 1993). Chance (2002) reports that some men with spinal cord injuries pride themselves in their abilities to satisfy their partners orally.

Chronic Lifestyle Diseases

Chronic illnesses such as cardiovascular disease, obesity, and diabetes can affect sexual behavior. These and other chronic diseases, besides influencing body image and sexual desire, impact strength, endurance, and coordination. People with these conditions can find themselves unable to sustain sexual activity for a sufficient duration to achieve orgasm. They might also find certain sexual positions unattainable because of excess body weight.

Redefining Sex

The major challenge for people with disabilities is redefining sexual activity and the goal of sexual behavior. Most people in American culture define sexual activity as genital intercourse and orgasm as the goal of sexual behavior. For certain people with physical disabilities, however, that activity and goal are unattainable (Chance, 2002). It is essential, then, that people with physical disabilities set their own activities and goals for sex and not evaluate their happiness in terms of societal expectations.

We have seen that activities such as massage, masturbation, and oral sex, with or without orgasm, can be as satisfying as penile-vaginal intercourse. In some cases, people with physical disabilities develop new levels of sensitivity and sensuality. Research has shown that people with spinal-cord injury can develop new erogenous zones and are more than able to become aroused when stimulated (Chance, 2002).

Persons with developmental disabilities usually do not face the same limitations as those with physical disabilities. Rather, their greatest challenge is protecting themselves from unintended pregnancy, disease, and abuse. Care must be taken not to lump all developmentally disabled people together, because their abilities vary across a broad spectrum. Many are able to make informed decisions about their sexuality and risk reduction.

In this book, we cannot describe all of the potential variations in lovemaking associated with a full range of physical disabilities. We suggest that people with disabilities use the information in this chapter as a starting point to experiment with different forms of sexual behavior. They may find that accessories such as chairs or stools can be helpful when trying various positions. Communication with the partner is of primary importance, to ensure that the erotic and safety needs of both are being met.

Personal Assessment

Online Sensuality Test

Take an online sensuality assessment developed by Discoveryhealth.com. The test is one of many contained on its Web site (see Web Resources). Go to http://discoveryhealth.queendom.com/sensuality_abridged_access.html.

Favorite Sexual Behaviors

People satisfy their sexual needs in a variety of ways. We each engage in unique activities and behaviors to satisfy our sexual desire. The purpose of this activity is to illustrate how different positions satisfy different sexual needs. This will enable you to take a personal inventory of your personal turn-ons and have the opportunity to exchange them anonymously with your classmates.

1. Which autoerotic sexual activity do you find most enjoyable, and why? (If you do not engage in autoerotic activity, simply state this.)

2. Which partnered sexual activity do you find most satisfying? Why? (You could also include masturbation in this category.)

3. Describe your favorite sexual position within this category (for instance, if you enjoy vaginal intercourse most, which starting point and position do you find most enjoyable?).

4. Describe your favorite sexual fantasy. (If you do not fantasize, simply state this.)

Thought Questions

1. What is sensuality? What does "sensual lover" mean?

2. What is Burnham's concept of integration? What contributes to adults losing this capacity?

3. What are some guidelines for giving a massage?

4. What is the difference between celibacy and abstinence? When are each appropriate?

5. What are five non-penetrative forms of sexual activity?

6. What are the pros and cons of the man-on-top and woman-on-top intercourse positions?

7. What are the advantages of the side-by-side and rear-entry intercourse positions?

8. Describe how a person with disabilities might "redefine" sexual behavior and the goal of sexual activity.

Test Yourself

1. Burnham's concept of "integration" refers to
   a. interracial sex.
   b. a merging of the senses and the intellect.
   c. acting childlike in response to sexual stimuli.
   d. integrating childish things into sensuality.

2. Which of the following best characterizes the relationship between sensuality and sexuality?
   a. They are the same.
   b. Sexuality is an important part of sensuality.
   c. They are completely different.
   d. Sensuality is an important part of sexuality.

3. The major distinction between abstinence and celibacy is
   a. celibacy is something that only involves the clergy.
   b. celibacy is very rare while abstinence is much more common.
   c. abstinence is usually viewed as a situational choice, not a lifetime commitment.
   d. abstinence makes the heart grow fonder.

4. Which of the following is generally *not* considered outercourse?
   a. mutual masturbation
   b. sensual massage
   c. coitus
   d. use of sex toys
5. Most health experts would agree that masturbation
   a. is an acceptable sexual outlet for children and teens only.
   b. can be carried out to excess and needs to be controlled.
   c. is not acceptable adult sexual activity.
   d. is an acceptable sexual outlet for people of any age.
6. Laumann et al found that adults who masturbated on a regular basis
   a. had higher levels of sex with their partners.
   b. had lower levels of sex with their partners.
   c. did not have steady partners.
   d. preferred solitary sex to partnered sex.
7. Which of the following statements best characterizes how sexual health experts perceive anal sexual intercourse?
   a. It is a source of STDs and should be avoided.
   b. It can be a pleasurable sexual activity if care and extra lubrication are used.
   c. It is similar to vaginal intercourse because of the naturally occurring lubrication.
   d. It is a homosexual activity.

8. Which response best characterizes sexual intercourse during pregnancy?
   a. Should be avoided.
   b. Should be avoided after the first trimester.
   c. Can be facilitated through side-by-side or rear-entry intercourse positions.
   d. Is best accomplished using the man-on-top position.
9. Which answer best describes people with physical disabilities such as multiple sclerosis and Parkinson's disease?
   a. Are almost always unable to engage in sexual intercourse.
   b. Are uninterested in sexual intercourse.
   c. Can't make the necessary adjustments to enjoy sexual intercourse.
   d. Can enjoy sexual intercourse if they are able to make the necessary adjustments.
10. Which answer best describes people with developmental disabilities such as Down's syndrome?
   a. Are too immature to have sexual intercourse.
   b. Do not respond sexually the way "normal" people do.
   c. Have the same desires as people without such disabilities.
   d. Can't be trusted to have sex and not get pregnant.

Web Resources

My Pleasure
http://www.mypleasure.com/education/index.asp

This is a comprehensive site for all of your sexual pleasuring needs. It contains excellent articles on a myriad of topics related to sexual pleasure. There are links to a full line of sexual products and services.

Good Vibrations
www.goodvibes.com

This is the definitive site for all of your sexual aids. The site offers an online catalog for sexual toys, book, films, and related materials and information from the sensual to the erotic.

Discovery Health
http://health.discovery.com/tools/assessments.html

This is the Discovery Channel's health Web site. It contains a variety of assessments related to health.

Intimacy Institute Sexuality
http://www.bettersex.com/?searchengine=1&cm_mmc=VSM-_-NA-_-Google-_-%5Bsinclair%20intimacy%20institute%5D&sc=7PG&ad=1591354189

This is the home page of the Sinclair Intimacy Institute. It provides products and information on sexual response and a host of other topics.

National Abstinence Clearinghouse (NAC)
www.abstinence.net

An alliance of nationally known educators formed to promote the practice of abstinence. The NAC provides a resource center and training for educators and parents. Many links are provided for related topics in the area of abstinence.

The Kama Sutra
http://www.bibliomania.com/2/1/frameset.html

The Kama Sutra, by Vatsyayana (1883), online and translated by Sir Richard Burton. The timeless Indian sex manual that merges yoga, spirituality, and sex.

Tracey Cox.com
www.traceycox.com

This is the home page for Tracey Cox, writer of *Hot Sex* and other self-help sex books.

References

Alexander, C. J., Sipski, M. L., & Findley, T. W. (1993). Sexual activities, desire, and satisfaction in males pre- and post spinal cord injury. Archives of Sexual Behavior, *22*(3), 217–229.

Bean, M. (2004) Cancer-Proof Your Prostate. Men's Health, 19 (2) pp. 100–101.

Bender, M. (1999). The secret to living a sensuous life. Cosmopolitan, 227, 236–242.

Brand, H. (2001). Sexual chemistry (the use of pheromones) Soap, Perfumery & Cosmetics, *74*(9), 19.

Burnham, W. H. (1932). *The wholesome personality.* New York: Appleton Century.

Chance, R. S. (2002). To love and to be loved: Sexuality and people with disabilities. Journal of Psychology and Theology, *30*(3), 195–209.

Cox, T. (1998). *Hot Sex.* New York: Bantam

Daneback, K., Cooper, A. L., Mansson, S. A. (2005). An Internet Study of Cybersex Participants. Archives of Sexual Behavior v. 34 no. 3 (June 2005) p. 321–8.

Dodson, B. (1996). *Sex for one: The joy of selfloving.* New York: Crown.

Eiseman, L. (1999). *Colors for your every mood.* New York: Capitol.

Foston, N. A. (2004). Is Celibacy The New Virginity? Living The Single Life Without Sex. Ebony v. 59 no. 3 (January 2004) p. 118, 120, 122.

Fox, D. (2003). Can masturbating each day keep the doctor away? New Scientist v. 179 (July 19, 2003) p. 15.

Giles, G. G., Severi, D. R., English, M. C., Credie, M. R., Borland, R., Boyle, P., Hopper, J. L. (2003). Sexual Factors and Prostate Cancer. BJU International 92, pp 211–216).

Goins, L. (2001). 5 secrets for making sex supersensual. Cosmopolitan, *230*(4), 156–160.

Good Arts. (2003). *Sensual massage* [Online]. Available: www.goodarts.com.

Gulledge, A. K., Gulledge, M. H., Stahmann, R. F. (2003). Romantic Physical Affection Types and Relationship Satisfaction. The American Journal of Family Therapy v. 31 no. 4 (July/September 2003) p. 233–42.

Gulledge, A. K., Stahmann, R. F., Wilson, C. M. (2004). Seven Types of Nonsexual Romantic Physical Affection among Brigham Young University Students. Psychological Reports v. 95 no. 2 (October 2004) p. 609–14.

Hingsburger, D., Tough, S. (2002). Healthy sexuality; attitudes, systems, and policies. Research & Practice for Persons With Severe Disabilities 27 (1) Spring 2002, pp 8–17.

Hite, S. (1976). *The Hite report: A nationwide study of female sexuality.* New York: Dell.

Hite, S. (1981). *The Hite report on male sexuality.* New York: Knopf.

Inkeles, G., & Austin, K. K. (1992). *The new sensual massage.* Bayside, CA: Arcata Arts.

Kemp, K. (2000). How to touch a naked man. Cosmopolitan, 228 (4), 194–206.

Kraus, D. K. (2000, October 27). Realm of the senses. San Francisco Business Times, pp. 29–33.

Laumann, E. O., Gagnon, J. H., Michael, R. T., & Michaels, S.(1994). *The social organization of human sexuality: Sexual practices in the United States.* Chicago: University of Chicago Press.

Leitzman, M. F., Platz, E. A., Stampfer, M. J. (2004). Ejaculation Frequency and Subsequent risk of Prostate Cancer. JAMA 291 (13) April 7, 2004, pp. 1578–1586.

Marrone, S. (2002). Indulge your sensual side: Eat a mango, sniff some cinnamon, and other fun, fast ideas for putting more pleasure into your life. Redbook, *198*(5), 84–86.

Masters, W. H., Johnson, V., & Kolodny, R. (1996). *Human sexuality.* New York: HarperCollins.

McCabe, M., Taleporos, G., Dip, G. (2003). Sexual self esteem, sexual satisfaction, and sexual behavior among people with physical disability. Archives of Sexual Behavior, 32 (4) August, 2003, pp. 359–369.

Netting, N. S., Burnett, M. L. (2004). Twenty Years of Student Sexual Behavior: Subcultural Adaptations to a Changing Health Environment. Adolescence v. 39 (Spring 2004) p. 19–38

Norris, K. (1996, September–October). Celibate passion. *Utne Reader,* 51–53.

Rajen. P. (2004). T*he Times Educational Supplement* (October 29 2004 Friday supp) p. 20

Spayde, J. (2001). Hear sensuality, think sex? Utne *Reader* no. 108 (November/December 2001) p. 57–58

Yang, C. C. (2000). Female sexual function in neurologic disease. Journal of Sex Research, *37*(3), 205–208.

chapter
nine

Sexual Variations

Student Learning Objectives

After reading this chapter, students will be able to

- Distinguish between the following sexual variations; normative sexual behavior, atypical sexual behavior, and paraphiliac sexual behavior.
- Describe the four typical measures used to assess normalcy.
- Assess their own attitudes, values, and beliefs about what is normal.
- Describe the key characteristics of a variety of paraphilias.
- Evaluate the paraphiliac risks associated with the Internet.
- Evaluate the health risks associated with body piercing.
- Differentiate transvestic fetishism and transsexualism (gender dysphoria).
- Describe the origins of atypical sexual behavior and paraphilias.
- Evaluate various ways of treating atypical sexual behaviors and paraphilias.

activity teaser: Discover your true feeling about different sexual behaviors in the Personal Exploration Activity on page 322.

case study 9.1

Greg: Exhibitionism or Mooning?

Greg, 20, single, is white.

Greg was the first client assigned to Dr. Blonna during the supervised clinical training component of the master's degree in counseling. Greg was on probation as a first-time sex offender convicted of exhibitionism. As a condition of parole, Greg had to seek counseling for a prescribed period of time. In Dr. Blonna's words:

I'll never forget Greg. I was a 25-year-old man, not too much older than Greg. I was still working through issues related to my own sexuality and found Greg quite a challenge. He was referred to counseling because he had been arrested for exposing himself to a young woman.

It was hard for me to understand the significance of exhibitionism. I had been raised as a typical man of the 1950s and 1960s and viewed exhibitionism with amusement more than a clinician's understanding of it as a paraphilia. Indeed, I was only a few years removed from engaging in mooning and streaking as fraternity pranks. In time, my work with Greg crystallized the significance of his behavior and the furtive nature of exhibitionism.

Greg was a reluctant client at first. He did not want to be in counseling, and the first couple of sessions were almost totally devoid of any conversation. Gradually we began to establish a relationship, and Greg started to talk about his exhibitionism. It became quite evident after that point that Greg's behavior was vastly different from mooning and other juvenile sexual behavior that, although offensive, has an entirely different motivation. Mooning, streaking, and other prank public displays of nudity are not intended to serve as sexual come-ons. Greg's behavior had an entirely different purpose.

Greg was immature—both socially and sexually retarded. He was painfully shy, could not communicate with women effectively, and had limited dating experience. His sexual experience was limited to autoerotic activities and a handful of sexual liaisons with prostitutes. He lacked self-esteem and self-confidence, and had a hard time maintaining eye contact. He also admitted, while in counseling, that he was a voyeur and had masturbated several times while watching a few women in his neighborhood get undressed. He had a couple of peeping vantage points that allowed him to peer into the windows of apartment buildings in his neighborhood.

After seeing Greg for several sessions, it was obvious that exposing himself was his way of coming on to women sexually. He really believed that women, upon seeing his nakedness (and throbbing erection) would literally throw themselves at his feet and perform oral sex on him or ask him back to their place to have intercourse. He believed that his "manhood" would speak for itself and make traditional forms of establishing a sexual relationship unnecessary. In reality, Greg lacked the conversational and other social skills necessary to meet women and establish a sexual relationship.

Critical Thinking

Many people experiment with a host of sexual behaviors and participate in sexual pranks such as "mooning." When you read Greg's case study, however, it becomes obvious how Greg's behavior varies from these more typical sexual activities. What makes Greg's behavior exhibitionistic instead of a prank? How does Greg's exhibitionism impact the rest of his life?

As we can see with the illustration of Greg, sometimes there is a fine line between what is considered "normal" sexual behavior and what isn't. Normative behavior can be classified as sociological, biological, psychological, and statistical. Sexual behavior that is *sociologically* normal falls within the laws, mores, and customs of a society. Most of this behavior is culturally defined and passed from one generation to the next as a result of socialization. *Biologically* normal behavior is characterized as healthy and natural, and helps perpetuate the species in positive ways. *Psychologically* normal sexual behavior is sexual activity that does not result in emotional distress or in neurotic or psychotic functioning. Finally, behavior that is considered normal *statistically* is sexual behavior in which the majority of people engage.

Given these four categories of "normality," defining abnormal sexual behavior might seem easy. Anything falling outside the parameters established by these four categories would be considered "abnormal." The words *normal* and *abnormal* are commonly used labels because they characterize sexual behavior in easy-to-understand, stereotypical patterns. Furthermore, dichotomizing normal and abnormal makes it easier to stigmatize and discriminate against people who are not in the norm. A more commonly accepted term to describe behaviors that the majority of the population does not practice is atypical sexual behavior. Atypical sexual behavior is described as behavior that is not statistically typical. It could also be referred to as a sexual variation. The terms atypical sexual behavior or sexual variations do not carry the same pejorative tone as abnormal (Levinson, 2003).

Paraphilias

Paraphilias are atypical or unusual sexual behaviors that become the focal point for an obsessive preoccupation or need. The paraphilia is almost always the central focus of the person's sexual repertoire, and arousal and orgasm are difficult, if not impossible, in the absence of the paraphilia.

Paraphilia An unusual or atypical sexual behavior that becomes the focal point for an obsessive preoccupation or need

Paraphilias generally revolve around three common themes: (a) nonhuman objects, (b) suffering or humiliation involving oneself or one's own partner, and (c) children or other nonconsenting persons. In addition, to qualify as a paraphilia, a behavior has to occur over a period of at least 6 months and cause clinically significant distress or impairment in social, occupational, or other important areas of functioning [American Psychiatric Association (APA, 2013)].

The fourth edition, text revision, of the *Diagnostic and Statistical Manual of Mental Disorders* lists eight categories of paraphilias and one catchall category. The eight officially recognized categories are: exhibitionism, voyeurism, fetishism, frotteurism, pedophilia, sexual masochism, sexual sadism, and transvestic fetishism (APA, 2013). The catchall category "not otherwise specified" includes the following paraphilias, which are less common and don't meet the criteria to be included in any of the other eight categories: telephone scatologia (obscene phone calls), necrophilia (sex with a corpse), partialism (focus on certain parts of the body), zoophilia (sex with animals), coprophilia (contact with feces), klismaphilia (enemas), urophilia (undue attention to urine) (APA, 2013).

A person often exhibits more than one paraphiliac behavior (APA, 2013). Also, someone who exhibits true paraphiliac behavior and someone who casually experiments with atypical behavior are different. True paraphilia creates almost obsessive recurring, intense sexually arousing fantasies, urges, and behavior, and it is the main focal point for sexual arousal.

In addition, the person recognizes that the paraphilia causes significant enough emotional, social, occupational, or other distress to interfere with daily functioning. Someone who casually experiments with episodic paraphiliac behavior (such as occasionally liking his lover to tie him to the bedpost) and does not suffer negative emotional or other consequences is considered a person who simply enjoys occasional atypical sexual behavior.

Exhibitionism

Exhibitionism deriving sexual arousal by exposing one's genitals to unsuspecting strangers

The paraphiliac focus of **exhibitionism** involves deriving sexual arousal by exposing one's genitals to unsuspecting strangers. The overwhelming majority of people with this paraphilia are men between 18 and 40 years of age. Sometimes the person masturbates while exposing himself or fantasizing exposing himself (APA, 2013). Often the sexual gratification is derived from the sheer shock value of the act and the reaction from the victim. The greater the reaction, the more the person has proven his masculinity.

Men who reveal exhibitionism tend to be shy, passive, and sexually inhibited. Exhibitionism is generally perceived to be unrelated to rape or sexual assault. In some instances, the man with this paraphilia believes that his victim will be sexually aroused by his nakedness and that it will provoke a sexual encounter with her.

Exhibitionism is often confused with "mooning" (baring one's buttocks to unsuspecting passersby). Generally, those who moon do not derive sexual gratification from the act, and it usually is a prank typically associated with adolescents.

In a sense, exhibitionism is culturally disparate. Male and female exotic dancers get paid to expose themselves. Nude or partially nude dancing and other forms of exotic entertaining are designed to be sexually arousing and are legal, yet streaking, which is not sexual, is illegal.

Voyeurism

Voyeurism Deriving sexual pleasure from observing unsuspecting individuals undressing or engaging in sexual activities

The paraphiliac focus of **voyeurism** is exactly the opposite of exhibitionism. The voyeur derives sexual excitement and pleasure from observing unsuspecting people (usually strangers) who are naked, disrobing, getting dressed, or in the act of having sex. The pleasure is derived from the act of "peeping" and is not intended to lead to an encounter with the unsuspecting stranger. Sexual release usually occurs through masturbation either while peeping or later with the voyeuristic memory of the encounter. The person may fantasize having sex with the stranger (APA, 2013).

Voyeuristic behavior can be depicted along a continuum. At the extreme is the person who can achieve sexual release only by observing others having sex. At the other end of the continuum is the person who watches others to augment sexual pleasure with a partner. This person might get turned on by watching exotic entertainers to fuel a sexual episode with a partner.

Fetishism

Fetishism Deriving sexual pleasure from inanimate objects

The paraphiliac focus of **fetishism** is deriving sexual arousal and gratification from nonliving objects. The overwhelming majority of people with fetishes consists of men who derive sexual pleasure from items of women's clothing such as underwear, bras, stockings, shoes, and boots. Typically, the man with paraphiliac fetishism masturbates while holding, stroking, smelling, or licking the object. To a lesser extent, the person may ask his partner (or pay a prostitute) to wear the item of clothing while they engage in sex or while he masturbates (APA, 2013).

A person with a true paraphiliac fetish usually strongly prefers and needs the object to experience sexual desire. Often, a person with a fetish is unable to obtain or sustain an erection without the object being present. Fetishes often are linked to significant childhood experiences and are in place by adolescence (APA, 2013).

Frotteurism

The paraphiliac focus of **frotteurism** is deriving sexual arousal and pleasure from rubbing one's genitals against an unsuspecting, non-consenting person. The male rubs his genitals against his victim's buttocks and thighs while simultaneously fondling her breasts or genitalia, or both. This typically occurs in crowded public places such as busy sidewalks, subways, buses, and other public places where the perpetrator can make a quick escape and avoid arrest (APA, 2013).

Frotteurism Deriving sexual pleasure from rubbing up against unsuspecting and unwilling victims

❧ *Environmental/Occupational Wellness* ❧

The overwhelming majority of paraphiliacs are harmless, and as long as their behavior is private and with consenting adults, it does not represent a threat to society. In other instances it does. Legislation was passed in New Jersey and a host of other states to protect children from sex offenders in their communities. The New Jersey legislation, "Megan's Law," was enacted in response to the brutal murder of a young girl, Megan Kanka, by a neighbor who was a known sex offender. Essentially, the new law requires that neighbors be notified that a convicted sex offender has moved into their neighborhood. The hope is that such notification will enable parents and other neighbors to protect their children by keeping them away from the sex offender. In 1994, 12 new laws were enacted in California specifically targeting sex offenders. Provisions of these laws include, among others, a state-maintained toll-free phone number that alerts people to registered sex offenders living in their area, stiffer penalties for first-time offenders convicted of child molestation or rape, and the barring of unsupervised visits of sex offenders to their children.

The workplace can present many challenges to persons with atypical behavior. Transsexuals, and those with certain paraphilias such as fetishism, face daily stress (and often outright discrimination) as they struggle to earn a living and cultivate a career while living with atypical sexual desires and behavior.

Pedophilia

The legal aspects of **pedophilia** are discussed in detail in Chapter 16. The paraphiliac focus of pedophilia is fantasizing about engaging in sexual activity with a prepubescent child. Those sexually attracted to girls, in general, prefer 8- to 10-year-olds. Those attracted to boys favor slightly older

Pedophilia Engaging in sexual activity with or fantasizing about prepubescent children

sex in society 9.1

The Internet and Pedophilia

The Internet and the World Wide Web have become a major source of concern for law enforcement officials around the world trying to stem the tide of child pornography and pedophilia-related abductions and murders that originated in chat and other services available on the Web. The cases of Marc Dutrox of Belgium and Ronald Riva of California are just two of many that have brought attention to the problem of pedophilia and its many manifestations on the Internet.

Dutrox was convicted of kidnapping and murdering young girls in Belgium. The suspected head of a Europe-wide pedophile sex ring, Dutrox used the Internet to meet and lure his victims.

Riva, an unemployed truck driver, former prison officer, and father of four, was discovered when the mother of one of his victims (a 10-year-old girl) pressed charges of child abuse against him. The girl claimed that Riva had abused her when she stayed overnight at a slumber party for one of his daughters.

The case broke wide open when detectives discovered that Riva's house contained equipment (similar to that used in videoconferencing) that was set up to broadcast live "photo shoots" on the Internet. Police also discovered computer files containing child pornography and links to another man, Melton Lee Myers, who had similar equipment.

The investigation ultimately linked the two to a worldwide pedophile ring with members based in the United States, Finland, Australia, and Canada. The group was abusing children as young as 5 years old and broadcasting pictures and live child-sex shows on the Internet (Cusack, 1996).

The Web and Internet have made it almost impossible to control kiddie porn, and the number of federal "cybercops" (federal agents who scour the Internet for such material) has increased from a handful to more than 100 operating in the United States alone (Kaplan, 1997). Besides having a voracious appetite for pornography, which has contributed literally tens of thousands of child sex visual images to the Internet, pedophiles and child molesters have taken advantage of sophisticated broadcasting techniques to stay ahead of the law. Child pornographers often "morph" the head of one child onto the body of another, making identification of the child and proof of sexual abuse almost impossible. The naked images of adults in child pornography are limited almost exclusively to shots from the torso down.

Additional obstacles to tracking pedophiles, child molesters, and child pornographers include the sheer volume and worldwide scope of their activities. Keeping abreast of new sites, linking perpetrators, and identifying victims are indeed difficult. Often, just as investigators are making progress, a site closes down and relocates with a new Web address or country of origin.

One potential inroad being explored is forcing service providers to sever relationships with sites that have been known to contain child porn. A key component of the Communications Decency Act, which the U.S. Supreme Court struck down as unconstitutional in 1997, was the provision to hold providers (such as America Online) liable if their customers could gain access to obscene and indecent material. At present, a global effort is under way to come up with a way to control access of child pornography via the Internet.

children. The two subtypes of pedophilia are (a) exclusive (individuals who are sexually attracted to children only) and (b) nonexclusive (individuals who are sexually attracted to both adults and children) (APA, 2013). A pedophilia arousal pattern refers to the act of fantasizing about and becoming aroused by thoughts of sexual contact with children. A pedophilia behavior pattern refers to acting on the arousal (Oliver, 2005).

Individuals with pedophilia show a wide range of sexual activity with their victims. Not all pedophiles are child molesters. According to the law, a pedophile is an individual who fantasizes about sexual contact with children, whereas a child molester actually commits that act in some form (Davis, McShane, & Williams, 1995).

Most pedophiles masturbate while watching their victims undress, fondle themselves, or engage in sexual activities with another child or an adult. These activities can be live (paying children to perform in person or observing live sex shows broadcast over the Internet) or available through print (magazines, newspapers, and the like) and other electronic media (including movies, videotapes, and CD-ROMs).

Child molesters engage in a variety of sexual activities with their victims. This may consist of rubbing or fondling the child. Other child molesters penetrate the child's mouth, vagina, or rectum with their fingers, penis, or a foreign object. Some people with pedophilia obtain these sexual favors by gaining their victims' trust, affection, or loyalty. Others use physical force and psychological pressure and terror to obtain sex and control their victims.

Numerous state and federal laws have made the possession of any sexual image of kids under age 18 illegal. Nonetheless, the underground market for all forms of child pornography and prostitution is thriving (Kaplan, 1997). Pedophiles have victimized their own children, stepchildren, foster children, or relatives' children. Less often victims are children adopted through foreign services, bought through underground slave trade, or exchanged with other pedophiles.

People with pedophilia have been known to use extraordinary means to obtain child pornography or actual live victims. In recent years, several pedophiles have made headlines by arranging encounters with children while posing as adolescents in Internet chat rooms.

Pedophilia usually is chronic and is more difficult to treat than other paraphilias. The recidivism rate for men attracted to boys is more than twice that of men attracted to girls (Davis et al., 1995). Public outrage and increased law enforcement efforts directed toward child sex offenders has resulted in a wealth of information regarding the association of pedophilia to sexual offenses against children. Despite advances in this type of knowledge, much remains to be learned about pedophilia, including its prevalence in the general population, cross-cultural manifestations, and etiology (Seto, 2004).

Sexual Masochism

The paraphiliac focus of **sexual masochism** is deriving arousal and pleasure through being beaten, bound, humiliated (physically or mentally), or made to suffer in some other fashion (APA, 2013). Although fantasizing about being the victim of masochistic acts is common, true paraphilia involves engaging in the behaviors.

Sexual masochism Deriving sexual pleasure from being humiliated or forced to suffer pain

Many different masochistic acts typically are sought with a partner. These include being bound (physical restraint involving being tied, strapped, taped, chained, or handcuffed), spanked, bitten, paddled, whipped, beaten, shocked with an electrical current, cut, or pierced/pinned (infibulation). Another common masochistic desire is to be humiliated by being urinated or defecated on, to be forced to crawl and bark like a dog, and to be verbally abused. **Infantilism** involves being treated like an infant and forced to wear a diaper.

Infantilism Deriving sexual pleasure from being treated like an infant

The last category of masochistic paraphilia involves **hypoxyphilia** (also known as *autoerotic asphyxia*), or oxygen deprivation, by noose or wire (ligature), chest compression, plastic bag, mask, or chemical (such

Hypoxyphilia Deriving sexual pleasure from activities that involve oxygen deprivation

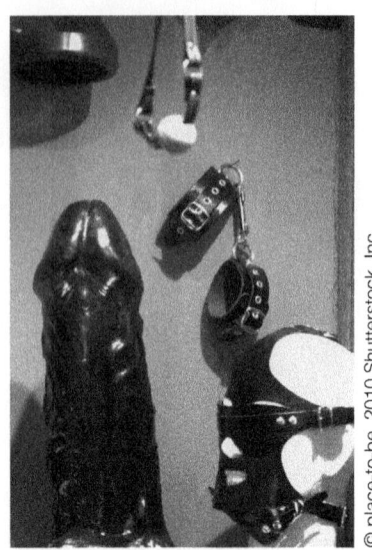

Many sex shops cater to sexual paraphernalia associated with sadism and masochism.

© place-to-be, 2010.Shutterstock, Inc.

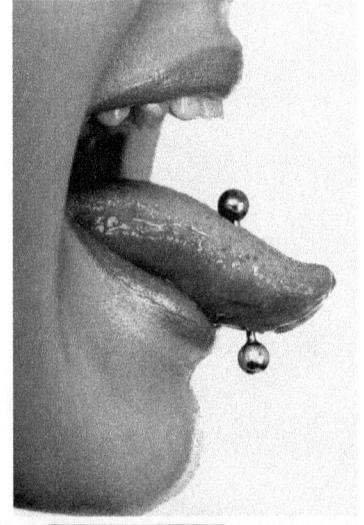

© Shalimov Sergii, 2010. Shutterstock, Inc.

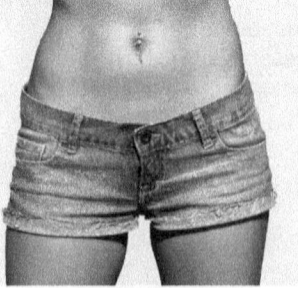

Piercing has become so popular that many states have adopted guidelines for ensuring the health and safety of the practice.

© Jose AS Reyes, 2010. Shutterstock, Inc.

Sexual sadism Deriving sexual pleasure from inflicting pain or humiliation

as amyl nitrate, a powerful vasodilator that reduces the flow of oxygen to the brain). This behavior is particularly dangerous because mishaps in applying these procedures for sexual arousal could result in death. Little is known about this behavior, since information about individual cases is usually derived from postmortem physical and psychological evaluations of the victim. Investigation is made even more difficult by the victim's family attempting to cover up the sexual nature of the death (Downing & Nobs, 2004).

It does not seem that hypoxyphilia is attempted suicide (Hickman, 2002). Rather, in most cases it is accidental, a result of ritualized auto-eroticism where oxygen deprivation is part of the sexual attraction and risk-taking. Most people who engage in autoerotic asphyxia are males with a history of sexual abuse, physical abuse, choking behavior (sometimes associated with asthma), exposure to traumatic family experiences, and other risk-taking (Downing & Nobs, 2004).

Sometimes, individuals with sexual masochism engage in masochistic acts by themselves. They self-inflict pain and humiliation through pinning, binding, shocking, or engaging in hypoxyphilia. Men with sexual masochism often concurrently have fetishism, transvestic fetishism, or sexual masochism (APA, 2013).

The practice of body-piercing has an interesting historical association with sexual masochism. Body-piercing gained prominence during the 1970's as it became increasingly popular among the punk, gay, and sadomasochist subcultures in the United States and England. Fashion designers incorporated piercing with punk and sadomasochistic clothing and personal adornment styles, and the three merged to create a trademark look among music and film stars (Stirn, 2003). Over the years this look mainstreamed into popular American culture. Most body-piercers, however, have the procedures done for personal adornment, a reflection of style [Association of Professional Piercers (APP), 2002].

❧   *Physical Wellness*   ❧

The continuum of atypical sexual behavior, as we've discussed, ranges from the relatively benign (occasional use of a fetish object) to the very dangerous (sadomasochistic beatings and torture). As we've mentioned throughout this text, healthy sexuality promotes physical well-being and behaviors that enhance health. Engaging in many of the atypical sexual behaviors can put your physical health in jeopardy. It is crucial to follow all of the warnings associated with these behaviors. There are ways to reduce the physical health risks associated with atypical sexual behavior.

Sexual Sadism

The paraphiliac focus of **sexual sadism** involves deriving sexual arousal and pleasure by inflicting physical or psychological pain and suffering on another person. The person may engage in sadistic activities with either a willing victim (usually someone with sexual masochism) or a nonconsenting victim (APA, 2013). Sexual sadism incorporates a range of acts, including

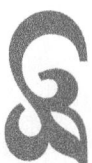 healthy sex hints 9.1

Reducing the Health Risks Associated with Body-Piercing

Body-piercing, like other forms of adornment such as tattooing, branding, and ear-piercing, carries some risk. The risks vary and are related to the body part being pierced, the piercing equipment, sterilization procedures used (or lack thereof), and the skill of the provider. The following hints can help reduce the risks associated with body-piercing:

1. Think long and hard about your motivation for getting your body pierced. Make sure you understand the risks associated with the procedure.
2. Talk with people who have had piercing done. Ask what kind of experiences they had.
3. Before getting pierced, ask your physician about vaccination for hepatitis B, a blood-borne infection passed through contaminated needles.
4. Do not pierce yourself or let an inexperienced person (such as your best friend, who pierced her own ears) pierce you.
5. Go to a reputable piercing parlor that has been in business for some time. Ask for references from former customers.
6. Make sure the piercing parlor you choose uses an autoclave (a tabletop sterilizing device that uses heat and pressure to kill germs) to sterilize equipment. Ask to see the certificate verifying that the autoclave has been recently inspected. If only boiling water is used to clean equipment, head for the door.
7. If a tattoo artist uses individually sealed, sterile needles, ask him or her to open these in front of you. Request the same for the containers of ink being used for your tattoo.
8. Talk to your physician to learn about special considerations concerning the body part being pierced. Particularly risky parts (because of increased likelihood of infection or permanent damage) are the eyelids, the tongue, the nipples, the clitoris, and the frenulum of the penis.
9. Don't have piercing done if you are pregnant or nursing.
10. Follow after-care instructions to the letter. If you suspect infection, consult a doctor immediately.
11. Wear only jewelry that is 14K gold, niobium, or surgical-grade stainless steel. These contain fewer alloys and are less likely to cause allergic reactions.

Source: Association of Professional Piercers (2002), *Procedure manual* (Chamblee, GA: Author).

all of those discussed previously under the topic of sexual masochism. In extreme cases, people with sexual sadism seek sexual arousal through extreme brutality, torture, mutilation, and murder.

Typically, they engage in such behavior with nonconsenting victims and have had the condition for several years. The fantasies of sexual sadism usually are present in childhood, and the behavior begins in early adulthood and becomes chronic.

Transvestic Fetishism

Transvestic fetishism differs from other forms of fetishism in that the fetishist derives sexual arousal by cross-dressing (dressing up as a female or wearing an article of female clothing). The transvestic fetishist typically masturbates to orgasm while dressed in that clothing.

Transvestic fetishism Deriving sexual pleasure from wearing women's clothing

> ❧   *Emotional Wellness*   ❧
>
> The difference between someone who engages in atypical sexual behavior and the true paraphiliac is in the emotional distress and social dysfunction the latter experiences. An individual or couple can engage in almost all of the atypical behaviors of paraphiliacs without this representing a paraphiliac sexual condition. A person can be emotionally healthy and still enjoy an occasional walk on the wild side. Actually, some people engage in atypical sexual activities to add a spark to their sex lives. When the behavior becomes an obsession, however, and carries with it emotional distress and social dysfunction, it becomes a paraphiliac sexual disorder.

The disorder is known only in males. It runs the full spectrum of behavior from routinely wearing a single item of female clothing (such as silk panties) under the male clothing, to spending thousands of dollars on customized gowns and makeup and participating in the transvestic subculture (APA, 2013).

Men with transvestic fetishism do not have gender dysphoria (think they are really females), and most are heterosexual in sexual orientation. When not cross-dressed, men with transvestic fetishism look like the average man. Men who do not have transvestic fetishism but occasionally like to put on articles of female clothing often do so with the willing participation of their female partners.

Gender Dysphoria

Up until the release of the fifth edition of the DSM , the term "gender identity disorder" has been used to diagnose people who are transgender. In the DSM V (APA, 2013), people whose gender at birth is contrary to the one they identify with will be diagnosed with "gender dysphoria." The new diagnosis aims to avoid stigma and ensure clinical care for individuals who see and feel themselves to be a different gender than their assigned gender. It is important to note that gender nonconformity is not in itself a mental disorder.

In addition to viewing oneself as having a different gender than their assigned one people diagnosed with the new condition must also demonstrate:

- persistent discomfort with his or her sex or a sense of inappropriateness in the gender role of that sex;

and

- the behavior has to occur over a period of at least 6 months and cause clinically significant distress or impairment in social, occupational, or other important areas of functioning (APA, 2013).

case study 9.2

From James to Jenny

Jenny, 46, is white.

James Finney Boylan was living an idyllic life. He was a successful novelist and a professor of creative writing at Colby College in Maine. He was a loving husband with two sons. There was just one thing wrong. Since childhood, James felt he was living the wrong life. James had a secret: He was a woman trapped in a man's body.

In her book, *She's Not There: A Life in Two Genders,* Jennifer Finney Boylan chronicles her journey to womanhood. In 1998, James accepted the reality of his situation and began the process of transition, including psychotherapy, hormone treatments, electrolysis, and voice coaching. She underwent gender reassignment surgery in 2002.

Boylan began his transformation by telling his wife "Grace" about the psychological torment he was enduring because of his gender identity issues. In one particularly poignant moment, Boylan apologizes to his wife for all that she is enduring as they are watching the first *Lord of the Rings* movie: In the words of Bilbo, "I am sorry. Sorry you have come in for this burden, sorry about everything." Boylan's children seem to take the metamorphosis in stride, even inventing a name to call her that makes sense: "Maddy," a combination of *Mommy* and *Daddy*.

Boylan takes a leave of absence from his duties at Colby, announcing to his colleagues via a letter that when he returns he will be Jennifer Finney Boylan. Boylan's close friend and colleague at Colby, Pulitzer Prize–winning novelist Richard Russo, initially cannot accept his friend's decision and evokes him to "be a man." Eventually, however, Russo comes to support his friend's decision and even accompanies Boylan and Grace to Wisconsin for the surgery.

Now Boylan notices that as a female her moods are more wide-ranging; she often feels more vulnerable, and cries easily. She also deals with body image issues, being more conscientious about ordering a salad rather than the slab of ribs James would have requested. She also says that she is now attracted to men.

Today Jenny and Grace are in a new kind of relationship. Not husband and wife, or lesbian partners, but something different. They are still legally married and are committed to being partners in parenting. They are not currently seeking relationships with other people. At the end of this particular personal journey, Jenny Boylan is finally enjoying the life that she always felt was meant to be.

Critical Thinking

Think about you life so far. Imagine that you have felt you have been living a lie and are actually someone of the opposite gender and decide to go through with sexual reassignment. How would your life change in positive and negative ways? How do you think your family and friends would react to the "new" you?

sex in society 9.2

The Underground World

In the 1970s Lou Reed, an avant garde artist and the lead singer for the Velvet Underground, sang about taking a walk on the wild side. The wild side in this case was the underground world of transsexuals—a world replete with its own bars, clubs, magazines, and clothing outlets.

Today you still can experience this underground world on certain streets in every major city in the United States, from New Orleans to New York City to San Francisco, and find a world filled with all of the transpeople—transsexuals, transvestites, and the transgendered. You'll find boutiques catering to transsexuals that carry everything in "women's" clothing from panties to feather boas in sizes designed to fit the average truck driver. You'll also find shoe stores that cater to spiked heels in sizes 10, 11, and 12 in every

width. At night these districts come alive as clubgoers of all sexual persuasions flock to see their favorite female impersonators, although some of the actors and actresses already have gone through sex reassignment surgery and can hardly be called impersonators.

The World Wide Web has opened the globe to the transcommunity. You now can view entire catalogs of merchandise on your computer and shop from the privacy of your own home. There are social organizations, self-help groups, political action committees, legal aid societies, chat rooms, list serves, travel clubs (they find the best places for transpeople to vacation), auto clubs, discount purchasing cooperatives—and the list goes on and on. The amazing thing is that most of these people, places, and services operate outside the realization of mainstream society.

The Origin and Treatment of Atypical Sexual Behavior

There are many different theories regarding the causes and treatment of atypical sexual behavior and paraphilias. Implied in "atypical" is the need to fix something that is wrong. Therefore, we reemphasize the difference among individuals who occasionally engage in behaviors that are atypical and cause no harm to another person and individuals who have paraphilias that cause themselves and others pain and suffering. The difference lies in the psychological distress and impairment in social, occupational, and other functioning between the two types of behavior.

Ethical Considerations

Society has an ethical and moral obligation to protect paraphiliacs and their victims from harm, even if they do not realize they are at risk. A sexual masochist, for instance, should be protected from the violence and suffering that may coexist with that paraphilia.

The need for treatment is less clear with problems such as Gender Identity Disorder. Is this really a psychological disorder? Is the condition really a problem that requires treatment, or should their desire to be the other sex be respected?

Many question the essential duality of maleness and femaleness. As mentioned in Chapter 4, gender is best viewed as a continuum rather than an absolute value (100% male versus 100% female).

The ethics of sexual reassignment surgery (surgically removing the genitals and reconstructing the genitalia of the desired, opposite sex) has

sex in society 9.3

Jan Morris: A Conundrum

Jan Morris started out in life as John Morris, later to be knighted and become Sir John Morris. John Morris—man, husband, father, athlete, soldier, explorer, writer, world traveler, climber of Mount Everest—was the epitome of every man's fantasy. He had power, prestige, wealth, and fame. Beautiful women wanted to be around him. He held the world in his hands.

John Morris had everything he wanted, except for one thing: he really wanted to be a woman. He'd gladly have given it all up (and did) to become the woman he always wanted to be. In the book *Conundrum,* one of the first of its genre, Jan Morris explains the crux of what being a transsexual means—feeling as though nature made a mistake. Morris recalls early recollections of feeling literally trapped within the wrong body. Her whole life, up to the point of having sex-reassignment surgery, consisted of trying to do things to convince herself that maybe she actually did belong in that body. Ultimately she realized that she didn't, and she had the surgery necessary to become a female.

been the subject of much debate. Should people who have GID be allowed to have sex reassignment surgery? Would it make more sense to try to help these people learn to accept both the fact that they have the genitalia of one gender and the identity of another? Why do we have to fit them into only one neat niche? These and other questions related to the diagnosis and treatment of atypical and paraphiliac sexual behavior are still being debated and may never be fully resolved.

> ## ৯ *Spiritual Wellness* ৯
>
> When discussing spiritual wellness, we must take care to separate people who engage in occasional atypical sexual behavior from paraphiliacs. Spirituality, as we've mentioned throughout the book, emphasizes the interconnectedness of people and treating all people with respect and dignity. Paraphilias such as sadism, masochism, and pedophilia are based on seeking gratification by inflicting pain, humiliation, or dominance over another. Hurting others represents an absence of spirituality.

Etiology

Many explanations have been set forth for the causes of atypical sexual behavior and paraphilias. Three of the more commonly accepted views revolve around (1) a psychoanalytic appraisal, (2) a behaviorist explanation, and (3) an eclectic etiology.

Psychoanalytic Appraisal

A classic psychoanalytic explanation for atypical or paraphiliac sexual behavior is the fixation of libidinal energy at a specific point in development. An individual becomes "stuck" and, with advancing age, constantly regresses to that point in psychosexual development. The immature level of sexual development is a result of not having been allowed the full expression and passage of libidinal energy at the age-appropriate stage.

Sexual masochists' need to be humiliated by having their partner urinate or defecate on them, for instance, is attributed to unresolved issues at the anal stage of development. Perhaps this person was rushed through toilet training or belittled for soiling his underpants. Whatever the specific issue, the unresolved transition through this period results in the fixation of sexuality at this stage of development.

Behaviorism

The behaviorist focuses on some facet of learning, and argues that atypical sexual behavior and paraphilia stem from some associative learning experience. Perhaps it was extremely harsh parental punishment for some minor sexual act such as observing Mom in the shower or being caught masturbating. Or it may be pairing an act (observing a woman undressing, for instance) with a pleasurable sexual experience (such as masturbation) that is positively reinforcing. This type of behavior is likely to be repeated.

Eclectic Perspective

John Money (Money & Lamacz, 1989) offers an eclectic explanation to atypical sexual behavior and paraphilia. He has developed a biosocial theory of sexual and gender development (see Chapter 4) based on what he called "lovemaps" ("templates" in the brain for patterns of eroticism and love). These templates, according to Money, are developed between 5 and 8 years of age as a result of biological and psychosocial forces.

During this period of development, Money believes children begin to link sex, love, and lust. The child usually develops a normal, healthy connection between romantic love and lust (sexual desire). Each of us has a unique lovemap based on a combination of biology (genetic inheritance, gonadal and hormonal influences) and psychosocial learning (parental and other models of love and affection). Healthy lovemaps are imprinted in our brain and create our idealized lover, love affair, and erotic imagery.

Atypical sexual behavior and paraphilia, according to Money, are a result of a distorted or "vandalized" lovemap that does not make a healthy connection between romantic love and lust. Love and lust are imprinted as disparate entities.

Because the two are not linked, sexual desire (lust) is not attached to normal romantic involvements but, rather, becomes attached to the inanimate objects, humiliating behavior, and the like, that evolve into paraphilias. Sexual desire is something apart from intimacy and affection. Lovemaps can become distorted for a variety of reasons including incest, physical abuse, extremely harsh parental punishments for normal sexual activity in childhood, repressive parental attitudes, and lack of displays of affection between parents.

Treatment

Most paraphiliacs enter treatment as a result of being arrested for their behavior. They do not seek treatment on their own or enter willingly. Paraphilias are extremely difficult to treat, and "cure rates" are low. Regardless of which view one holds regarding the etiology of paraphilias, most experts agree that atypical and paraphiliac behavior originates early in life, manifests itself in fantasy and desire, and evolves into full-blown behavior and lifestyle by young adulthood. As such, the person has a long history of behavior that has been reinforced over time through pleasure (masturbation or other sources of orgasm). The prognosis for eliminating such behavior is not good. In a study of 435 juvenile sex offenders, Zolondek and colleagues (2001) found that 10 percent to 30 percent were involved in exhibitionism, fetishism, frottage, voyeurism, obscene phone calls, and phone sex.

Biomedical and Surgical Treatment

One way to treat people with paraphilia is to attempt to lower their level of sexual desire through chemical (drugs) and surgical (castration) procedures. Drug therapy consists of administering drugs that either inhibit the production of testosterone or block its effects on the brain. As we discussed in Chapters 2 and 3, testosterone is the main androgen linked to sexual desire in men and women. Drugs such as cyproterone acetate (CPA) and medrohxyprogesterone (MPA-Depo-Provera) interfere with the effects of progesterone. They have been shown to have limited effectiveness in treating pedophiles, rapists, and other male sex offenders (Wincze, Bansal, & Malamud, 1986; Cooper, 1986). Until the 1980s, castration was used to reduce the sexual desire of sex offenders. The surgical removal of the testicles eliminates the production of most testosterone but does not prevent sexual excitement and erection (Nobre, Wiegel, Bach et al., 2004).

Although decreasing testosterone levels lowers sexual desire, it does not eliminate desire entirely. Also, no evidence is available to show that reducing testosterone levels, and thus sexual desire, has any permanent effect on the focus of sexual behavior. Testosterone is linked with sexual desire, not sexual orientation or the focus of sexual activity. Drug therapy seems to work by lessening the compulsion to engage in paraphiliac behavior (Walen & Roth, 1987). It doesn't eliminate the desire but, in conjunction with other approaches invoking the patient's support system, helps control the desire enough to allow intervention.

Treatment for transsexualism (gender identity disorder) often involves surgically reconstructing the patient's genitalia. The overwhelming majority of transsexual surgical reassignments involve male-to-female transitions. In male-to-female transsexual-reassignment surgery, a new clitoris, vulva, and vagina are constructed from penile and scrotal tissue. Internal structures remain the same.

In female-to-male surgery, a penis and scrotum are constructed from vulval and vaginal tissue. In this case, artificial testes (with implants) are constructed, and removable penile implant rods can be inserted into the structure to achieve an erection.

Transsexual-reassignment surgery is part of a four-part treatment process that also involves psychotherapy, hormone therapy, and living as the other gender. The goal of psychotherapy is to help the client readjust in his/her new role. The client begins taking hormones of the new gender to either "feminize" (in male-to-female reassignment) or "masculinize" (in female-to-male reassignment) the client's body. Lastly, before surgery is performed, clients must live as the new gender (complete with cross-dressing) for a year to learn what it is like to function as a member of society in one's new gender (Meyerowitz, 2002; Money & Wiedcking, 1980).

Behavior Modification

Behavior modification is used to desensitize paraphiliacs to their paraphilias and sensitize them to new, aversive stimuli. **Aversion therapy** is a behavior modification technique that pairs an aversive stimulus (such as electric shock) with the behavior that is targeted for change (Hermans, Dirikx, and Vansteenwegenin, 2005). Covert sensitization is a type of aversion therapy sometimes used with paraphiliacs. In **covert sensitization,** an aversive fantasy (not behavior) is paired with the paraphiliac fantasy in an attempt to extinguish it. For example, a voyeur is asked to visualize a past fantasy that accompanied one of the voyeuristic episodes. As the person visualizes the pleasing fantasy (say, peeping on an unsuspecting woman), the therapist introduces an aversive fantasy image (such as vomiting uncontrollably). By pairing the new aversive image (the vomiting) with the previously arousing image (peeping at the victim), the therapist links the negative image to the paraphilia.

Aversion therapy A behavior modification technique that pairs an aversive stimulus with the behavior targeted for change

Covert sensitization A type of behavior modification in which an aversive fantasy is paired with the paraphiliac fantasy in an attempt to extinguish it

❧ *Intellectual Wellness* ❧

High-level intellectual functioning can help a person know when an atypical behavior pattern represents a true paraphilia. Knowledge can help people understand that they have a problem and how to seek help in dealing with it. Paraphilias, however, tend to have such a strong hold over people that knowledge alone usually isn't enough to motivate them to seek help. Even so, knowledge can play a part in helping them learn how to live with their obsession and channel it into more acceptable forms of expression.

Skills Training

The focus of skills training is to enhance interpersonal skills. Paraphiliacs often rely on the paraphilia because of their inability to engage in satisfying interpersonal sexual relationships. Often they lack the self-esteem, confidence, and behavioral skills to meet potential sex partners and cultivate sexually satisfying relationships.

In skills training, they learn a variety of behaviors ranging from communicating (how to initiate conversations, meet new people, and the like) to coping with stress. As individuals become more proficient with these skills, they can learn to rely less and less on their paraphilia for sexual arousal (Zilbergeld, 1992).

✎ *Social Wellness* ✎

People who engage in atypical sexual activity (particularly partnered activities) can be socially healthy. They may engage in atypical activities to add spice to their sex lives. Most people with full-blown paraphilias, however, are not doing well socially. Their paraphilia often originated from disordered social functioning and learning. The paraphilia takes the place of functional adult social and sexual relationships. Many paraphiliacs experience sexual release through solitary masturbation in the presence of their paraphiliac object of desire.

Personal Assessment

Values Continuum

Instructions: For each of the 15 sexual behaviors listed here, mark the appropriate spot on the continuum indicating your level of approval/disapproval.

1. Consensual sexual behavior other than vaginal intercourse

   1   2   3   4   5
   strongly disapprove   neutral   strongly approve

2. Being tied to a bed, chair, or other structure during sex

   1   2   3   4   5
   strongly disapprove   neutral   strongly approve

3. Being spanked or paddled during sex

   1   2   3   4   5
   strongly disapprove   neutral   strongly approve

4. Being pinched or bitten during sex

   1   2   3   4   5
   strongly disapprove   neutral   strongly approve

5. Masturbating or having sex with the aid of a special object (a shoe, for example)

   1   2   3   4   5
   strongly disapprove   neutral   strongly approve

6. Being totally submissive during sex (must follow your partner's instructions or be punished)

   1   2   3   4   5
   strongly disapprove   neutral   strongly approve

7. Being totally dominating during sex (your partner must follow your instructions or be punished)

   1   2   3   4   5
   strongly disapprove   neutral   strongly approve

8. Being humiliated during sex (your partner does something humiliating such as urinating on you).

   1   2   3   4   5
   strongly disapprove   neutral   strongly approve

9. Humiliating someone else during sex (you do something humiliating to your partner such as urinating on him/her)

   1   2   3   4   5
   strongly disapprove   neutral   strongly approve

10. Secretly watching someone else (or a couple) get undressed or have sex

    1   2   3   4   5
    strongly disapprove   neutral   strongly approve

11. Openly watching someone else (or a couple) get undressed or have sex while you masturbate.

1	2	3	4	5
strongly disapprove		neutral		strongly approve

12. Intentionally getting undressed in public view (with shades open, etc.)

1	2	3	4	5
strongly disapprove		neutral		strongly approve

13. Intentionally having sex in public view (with shades open, in a public place etc.)

1	2	3	4	5
strongly disapprove		neutral		strongly approve

14. Masturbating while looking at pictures of children or young teenagers

1	2	3	4	5
strongly disapprove		neutral		strongly approve

15. Masturbating while looking at pictures of people engaged in paraphilias (S & M, acts, etc.)

1	2	3	4	5
strongly disapprove		neutral		strongly approve

There are no absolute right or wrong answers to these questions from a *sexual health perspective*. However, from a *legal perspective*, in cities and towns across America, engaging in some of these behaviors is against the law.

Remember, for any of these (or other) sexual behaviors to qualify as a paraphilia, it has to occur over a period of at least 6 months and cause clinically significant distress or impairment in social, occupational, or other important areas of functioning [American Psychiatric Association (APA), 2000].

By examining your position on the 15 different continua, you will know where your values lie regarding sexual variations. The important point is understanding your values and sharing them with your sex partner. You may wish to have your partner take this assessment and discuss your results with each other.

Thought Questions

1. What are some of the many facets of "normal" sexual behavior?

2. What does "atypical" sexual behavior mean?

3. Compare and contrast the sexual behavior that is abnormal, atypical or a variation.

4. When do atypical sexual behaviors and sexual variations become paraphilias?

5. How do a person's morality and ethics influence their participation in sexual variations?

6. How have the media treated some of the more common paraphilias such as voyeurism and exhibitionism?

7. What is the difference between a true transsexual and someone with transvestic fetishism?

8. What are the origins of paraphilias?

9. What are three treatment approaches for paraphilias?

10. Describe the controversy associated with sexual reassignment surgery.

Test Yourself

1. Which of the following is *not* considered a category of normative sexual behavior discussed in this chapter?
   a. Biological norm
   b. Anthropological norm
   c. Statistical norm
   d. Sociological norm

2. *Abnormal behavior* is generally considered
   a. an outdated term, replaced by *atypical behavior.*
   b. an outdated term, replaced by *nonnormative behavior.*
   c. an acceptable term synonymous with *atypical behavior.*
   d. an acceptable term still widely used by most experts in the field of human sexuality.

3. Atypical sexual behaviors and sexual variations becomes paraphilias when
   a. they are the major recurring theme in the person's sexual fantasies.
   b. they are obsessive and interfere with a normal sex life.
   c. they become repetitive and obsessive.
   d. they cause obsessive preoccupation or need, and interfere with daily functioning.

4. Occasionally tying your lover to the bedpost to simulate loss of control during sex is an example of
   a. a fetish related to rope.
   b. a sexual variation or atypical behavior.
   c. a paraphilia.
   d. an abnormal sexual behavior.

5. Which behavior is often mistaken for mooning or other forms of consensual public sexual activity with a partner?
   a. voyeurism
   b. frottage
   c. urophilia
   d. exhibitionism

6. A sexual sadist is someone who derives sexual arousal and pleasure from
   a. inflicting pain and/or humiliation on sexual partners.
   b. experiencing pain and/or humiliation at the hands of sexual partners.
   c. "snuffing" a partner with no direct sexual involvement.
   d. torturing a partner with no direct sexual involvement.

7. A sexual masochist is someone who derives sexual arousal and pleasure from
   a. inflicting pain and/or humiliation on sexual partners.
   b. experiencing pain and/or humiliation at the hands of sexual partners.
   c. "snuffing" a partner with no direct sexual involvement.
   d. torturing a partner with no direct sexual involvement.

8. The best answer to describe the major differences between transsexuals and transvestites is
   a. transsexuals derive sexual arousal and pleasure from cross-dressing.
   b. transvestites derive no sexual arousal and pleasure from cross-dressing.
   c. transvestites feel they are members of the opposite gender and are "trapped" in the wrong body.
   d. transsexuals feel they are members of the opposite gender and are "trapped" in the wrong body.

9. John Money's "lovemaps" theory of atypical sexual behavior and paraphilia says that paraphilias develop as a result of
   a. neurolinguistic programming that distorts lovemaps.
   b. unhealthy lovemaps that link love and lust.
   c. unhealthy lovemaps that imprint love and lust as distinct entities.
   d. people who vandalize other people's lovemaps.

10. The prognosis for treatment of people with paraphilias is
    a. excellent over time using conventional behavioral modification.
    b. fair using short-term aversion therapies such as electric shock.
    c. not good regardless of the treatment modality.
    d. pretty good if the patient is highly motivated.

Web Resources

The American Psychiatric Association (APA)
www.psych.org/index.cfm

American specialty society recognized worldwide. Its 37,000 U.S. and international member physicians work together to ensure humane care and effective treatment for all persons with mental disorder, including mental retardation and substance-related disorders. The APA is the voice and conscience of modern psychiatry and envisions a society that has available, accessible quality psychiatric diagnosis and treatment.

Above & Beyond
www.abgender.com

This site is a smorgasbord of resources (everything from shopping to emotional support) devoted to the transgender community.

Transgendered Suite
www.tgni.net

A major site for transgender information, support, and services. It provides everything from general information to a transgender dating service.

The Association of Professional Piercers (APP)
www.safepiercing.org

An international nonprofit association dedicated to the dissemination of vital health and safety information related to body-piercing to piercers, health care providers, and the general public. The group believes that it is the obligation of all professionals in the field to assume responsibility for their continued education. The organization dedicates itself to enabling this responsibility to be met.

References

American Psychiatric Association (APA). (2013). *The diagnostic and statistical manual of mental disorders* (5th ed.) Washington, DC: Author.

Association of Professional Piercers. (2002). *Procedure manual.*Chamblee, GA: Author.

Cooper, A. J. (1986). Progesterone in the treatment of male sex offenders: A review. *Canadian Journal of Psychiatry, 31,* 73–79.

Cusack, J. (1996). The murky world of Internet porn: The "Orchid Club" shakes up the law. *World Press Review, 43*(11), 8–10.

Davis, L., McShane, M. D., & Williams, F. P. (1995). Controlling computer access to pornography: Special conditions for sex offenders. *Federal Probation, 59*(2), 43–48.

Downing, L., Nobus, D. (2004). The Iconography of Asphyxiophilia: From Fantasmatic Fetish to Forensic Fact. *Paragraph*, Oct 2004, Vol. 15 Issue 3, pages 265–280

Friedman, R. C. (1998, January 19). Gender identity. *Psychiatric News: Viewpoints* [Online]. Available: www.payxh.org/pnews/98-01019/gender.html.

Hickman, W. (2002, August 8). A real swinger—Part IV (autoerotic asphyxiation cases). *Mondau Business Briefings.*

Hermans, D., Dirikx, T., Vansteenwegenin, D. (2005). Reinstatement of fear responses in human aversive conditioning. *Behaviour Research and Therapy* v. 43 no. 4 (April 2005) p. 533–51

Kaplan, D. E. (1997). New cybercop tricks to fight child porn: Police struggle against an online onslaught. *U S.News & World Report, 122*(20), 29.

Levinson, J. (2003). Sexual Perversity. *The Monist* 86 no1 30–54 Ja 2003

Meyerowitz, J. (2002). *How sex changed: A history of transsexuality in the United States.* Boston: Harvard University Press.

Money, J., & Lamacz, M. (1989). *Vandalized lovemaps.* New York: Prometheus.

Money, J., & Wiedcking, C. (1980). Gender identity/role: Normal differentiation and its transpositions. In Nobre, P. J., Wiegel, M., Bach, M., Weisberg, R. B., Brown, T. A., Wincze, J. P., Barlow, D. H. (2004). Determinants of sexual arousal and accuracy of its self-estimation in sexually functional males. *J Sex Res.* Nov 2004:41(4):363–71.

Oliver, B. E. (2005). Thoughts on Combating Pedophilia in Non-Offending Adolescents. *Archives of Sexual Behavior* v. 34 no. 1 (February 2005) p. 3–5.

Seto, M. C. (2004) Sexual Offenses Against Children. A*nnual Review of Sex Research* v. 15 (2004) p. 321–61

Stirn, A. (2003). Body piercing: medical consequences and psychological motivations. *Lancet,* 0099-5355, April 5, 2003, Vol. 361, Issue 9364.

Wolman & J. Money (Eds.), (1998). *Handbook of human sexuality.*Englewood Cliffs, NJ: Prentice Hall.

Walen, S., & Roth, D. (1987). A cognitive approach. In J. H. Geer & W. T. O'Donohue (Eds.), *Theories of human sexuality.* New York: Plenum.

Wincze, J., Bansal, S., & Malamud, M. (1986). Effects of medroxprogesterone acetate on subjective arousal, arousal to erotic stimulation, and nocturnal penile tumescence in male sex offenders. *Archives of Sexual Behavior, 15,* 293–306.

Zilbergeld, B. (1992). *Male sexuality: A guide to sexual fulfillment.*Boston: Little, Brown.

Zolondek, S. C., Abel, G. G., Northey, W. F. (2001). *Journal of Interpersonal Violence* v. 16 no. 1 (January 2001) p. 73–85.

chapter

ten

Intimate Relationships

Student Learning Objectives

After reading this chapter, students will be able to

- Describe the key elements of healthy relationships.
- Identify issues related to meeting potential partners.
- Describe ways to meet partners safely online.
- Define intimacy and trace its development in relationships.
- Define love and describe how it develops in relationships.
- Compare a variety of theories regarding love.
- Evaluate a variety of barriers to intimacy.
- Describe various techniques used to overcome barriers to intimacy.
- Identify characteristics of unhealthy relationships.
- Become aware of markers for abusive relationships.
- Examine a variety of ways to end unhappy relationships.

activity teaser: The couple that laughs together, stays together. See the Personal Exploration Activity on page 307.

case study 10.1

"Fitting In and Finding My Niche"

Lily, 20, identifies as biracial.

For some reason, the questions about "What are you?" at times are more frequent here at college than they were in high school. I notice people looking at my eyes, more than my skin tone, and wondering. My dad is white; my mom is Thai. So, am I "Asian American"? "Thai American"?

When I got here, there were two clubs for Asian students; one was Chinese American, and that didn't fit. The other was Asian American, yet at the meetings most of the students were of Indian descent. I didn't really feel like I fit there, either.

I find myself hanging with the African American students most. White students see me as different, and while my black friends know my background, they don't seem to care. I have a black boyfriend right now, and his friends accept me. My parents don't know about him, though. I don't think they'd approve. Funny . . . they're a mixed-race couple, yet some groups are more comfortable for them than others.

I've joined a sorority and have friends there. My boyfriend and I are in a good place, so I'm just taking one day at time. He hasn't tried Thai food with me yet, but I'm working on it!

Critical Thinking

Do you think there are many students on your campus who choose not the cross the racial line when socializing? How important are issues of race for you when choosing friends? Romantic partners?

Intimacy Connectedness to another person characterized by respect, equality, mutual caring, openness, self-disclosure, honesty, attentiveness, sharing, commitment, trust, empathy, and tenderness

Intimacy can be a confusing concept with many uncertainties as the following questions outline. What is intimacy and how do we know when we have achieved intimacy in our relationships? Is intimacy a part of friendships and family relationships or only possible in romantic relationships? How important is intimacy to our lives? Our quality of life depends to a large extent on the types of relationships we develop. Relationships define our connectedness to others and provide opportunities for **intimacy.** Intimate relationships are characterized by respect, equality, identity, honesty, caring, sharing, trust, commitment, empathy, and tenderness. Intimacy requires us to self disclose and be vulnerable and open in order to have this richer level of affection. (Lewis, 2010) This can be somewhat scary since we must trust the other person enough allow ourselves to be vulnerable.

Intimacy is often linked with being sexual with another but in reality there others forms of intimacy. Cognitive intimacy happens when we exchange opinions and ideas freely. Experiential intimacy is the sharing of activities. Having a variety of these activities is essential for preventing boredom in relationship thus blocking intimacy. Excitement in a relationship promotes closeness (University of Michigan, 2009). In emotional intimacy we try to

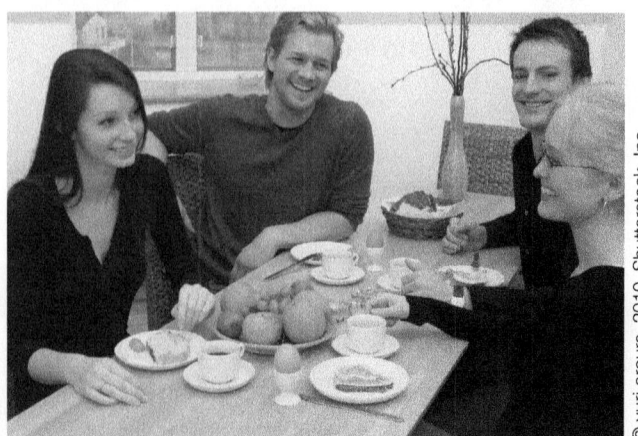

College provides opportunities to meet a wide variety of people.

© yuri arcurs, 2010. Shutterstock, Inc.

understand how the other feels. And finally is sexual intimacy which is the physical part of intimacy. This physical form of affection includes not only intercourse but activities such as hugging and holding hands. (University of Florida, 2013).

Forming healthy relationships with others is a skill a person develops and practices. For relationships to be intimate, we have to be ourselves and let others be who they are. Good relationships derive from good role models and require giving thought to the outcome of our actions. As Lily explained in the case study, her social comfort was connected to her race to some degree. For others, connections may be stronger along gender lines or sexual orientation.

As we age, we form social relationships with others on many levels including family, friends, working colleagues, neighbors, and partners. Although this chapter focuses primarily on partner relationships, we have to realize that becoming sexually intimate with someone does not necessarily mean that we automatically have an emotionally intimate relationship.

We learn patterns of relating to others from our families, friends, and past experiences. Some people are extroverted and outgoing, and they enjoy having many different types of relationships. Developing relationships is easy for them. Other people are introverted and enjoy doing many things alone. They develop fewer relationships in their lives and may have difficulty forming new relationships. Regardless, human contact is essential for health and wellness.

❧   *Intellectual and Social Wellness*   ❧

College affords many opportunities to meet and learn from different types of people. Many of us grow up in communities where those around us are of similar race, religion, and social class. Institutions of higher learning commit themselves to meeting the needs of diverse students and enabling the exchange of a variety of perspectives. Challenging opinions, listening to the views of others, and learning about difference all contribute to greater intellectual well-being.

Dating and being in relationships provide opportunities to broaden one's social network, to meet new people and make new connections. Being with others and forming intimate relationships is critical to social well-being. We all need people we can count on, who are our friends, and who see us through the good times and bad. Sharing activities with others is part of social health. Lifelong friendships may develop in college, and for some college also becomes the source for one's lifelong romantic partner as well.

Establishing Relationships

The dynamics of forming close, intimate relationships with friends are different from the dynamics of developing intimate relationships with sexual partners. A look at the shelves of a bookstore quickly reveals rows of books offering advice on how to find a partner, keep a partner, satisfy a partner, and be satisfied with a partner. But you won't find rows and rows of books on how to make and keep friends. The same holds true for music. The lyrics of country, rock, and blues passionately describe the ups and downs of emotions related to love relationships. The intensity of feelings related to platonic friendships just doesn't compare.

Friends share activities, thoughts, and feelings. They help each other out. When a life experience tests a friendship, we often hear the comment "That really let me know who my true friends are!" A healthy romantic relationship, one that is founded on intimacy, requires the same expectations as a friendship, yet we may find ourselves not being authentic with our thoughts and feelings, second-guessing the other person, and sometimes tolerating behaviors we would never accept from our friends. The erotic piece of the puzzle is what changes the interaction. We often become self-conscious in ways we hadn't anticipated, and we might lose our identity in pursuit of the relationship. Healthy relationships are based on being able to clearly identify who we are, what we want, how we want to be treated, how we want to live, and recognizing that we deserve to have a relationship that meets our needs.

Meeting People

The first step toward developing an intimate relationship is connecting with a potential partner. People can meet in many ways, not all equally comfortable or familiar. College is sometimes viewed as an ideal place to meet someone and form an intimate relationship, yet some students graduate without experiencing a serious dating relationship. Unlike years past, students today are likely to feel less pressure to be married upon graduation. Even when students do not have marriage as a goal, they may have the desire to form intimate relationships.

Much of the research that examines partner and mate selection has been conducted on samples of college students using laboratory experiments and questionnaires; such research has limitations and may not explain how the population at large develops couple relationships (Wiederman, 2001). For example, young adults who don't go to college may choose partners in different ways and from different social situations than those who attend college. Important partner characteristics and strategies for meeting people may change as one ages. A typical, college student may have important criteria that do not match those who are divorced, have children, and may be in their 30s or 40s. Furthermore, the process of attraction and partner selection often includes socializing with someone on multiple occasions and evaluating how that "chosen person" reacts to expressed interest. Being part of a college community may afford opportunities to see a partner regularly, yet exposure to and participation in the types of situations that test relationships over time may be limited. Overall, it is important to distinguish between what may be reported as a "preference" for a partner and what goes on in actual social experiences.

Before looking at issues of where and how to meet a prospective partner, people have to be ready for a relationship. Are they open to a relationship? Are they comfortable with themselves? If they were hurt in a previous relationship, they may not have let go of the pain and hurt. Too often people approach a new relationship with defensiveness, negative past associations that become expectations with a new partner, and patterns of relating that prevent new relationships from developing. A healthier response is to look at past relationships as a learning experience. We are better able to decide what we need and what is important to us in a partner and a relationship when we experience ones that are not ideal for us.

Meeting people and forming relationships are social skills and are behaviors that are modeled, taught, and practiced. People have to feel comfortable enough with themselves to believe they are worth getting to know, a fundamental aspect of self-esteem. People who consider themselves "shy" may find social settings very intimidating. They may not be able to identify the behaviors and words needed to make social contact with others.

Shyness

Zimbardo's (1977) classic work on shyness provides a framework for understanding what is a nearly universal experience of being shy at some point in one's life. More than 80 percent reported feeling shy at some time, 25 percent described themselves as chronically shy, and 4 percent described themselves as being shy all the time, in all situations, with virtually all people. Since that classic work, the percentage of people who describe themselves as chronically shy has risen to 48% (Marano, 2005). Some believe the changes in our society such as the focus on electronic communication, telecommuting, the internet, e-mail, cell phones, and the fast pace of life, have all contributed to this increase (Carducci, 2000). The ability to overcome shyness is essential to forming relationships.

Shyness is revealed in a number of ways. People who are shy may experience or demonstrate one or more of the following characteristics:

Overly concerned with themselves: how they look, how others perceive them

Speaking softly

Not making eye contact

Being reticent/reluctant to relate to others

Blushing

Experiencing "butterflies" in the stomach

Feeling embarrassed

Feeling self-conscious

Although everyone has those experiences and feelings at times, shyness becomes a problem when the level and frequency of those experiences impede the development of relationships. Shy individuals may see themselves as unacceptable and unworthy, and they typically lack the social skills of knowing how to initiate conversation and make connections. Zimbardo found that overcoming shyness is possible if individuals are willing to work on making changes in the way they think about themselves and others and in how they behave.

Shyness can become painful enough that professional intervention may be warranted. Individuals may choose to avoid social situations, cancel out at the last minute, avoid pleasurable activities, and/or choose to spend the majority of time at the computer rather than in face-to-face interactions. Additionally, chronic low moods, use of alcohol and drugs to manage social situations, or excessive time spent on academic work and professional activity to the exclusion of socializing can be symptoms of painful shyness (Henderson, Zimbardo, & Rodino, 2001).

Approximately 12% of those who are shy use alcohol to help themselves feel comfortable in social situations. Since drinking interferes with cognitive functioning, they are less likely to improve their social skills through good practice. In addition, they are likely to over consume alcohol, making it not a surprise that a significant number of problem drinkers are shy (Carducci, 2000).

Another impediment to forming intimate relationships is the fear of being rejected. Some people enter social situations with an expectation that they will be rejected. They become anxious about being rejected, expect to be rejected, and overreact to what may be ambiguous behavior in others (Downey & Feldman, 1996). Again, having a frame of mind that allows one to approach others in a positive way, without worrying about rejection, is more likely to lead to better interactions and a possible friendship or relationship.

Where and How to Meet People

As our lifestyles become busier, "meeting that special someone" can become a project in and of itself. Individuals may purposely go to a social event in the hopes of finding a prospective partner. Friends may purposely invite a range of people to a party—some single, some coupled—hoping that additional pairing occurs. Although it may not be productive to set purposeful goals to meet someone, and it can be frustrating when a social event doesn't introduce a new potential partner, individuals have to put themselves in social situations where potential opportunities exist. An essential strategy for meeting people involves widening the scope of one's activities.

College offers a comfortable social environment in which to form relationships. Academic classes, coed sports, clubs, exercise classes, parties, religious organizations, sorority and fraternity functions, rallies, student newspapers, student government and the like, involve students in activities while simultaneously providing environments to meet others with similar interests.

If similarities in race, culture, or religion are important, campus organizations whose members align themselves with the relevant similarities may be places to meet. Because of issues of "coming out" and the added burden of attempting to determine someone's sexual orientation, lesbian, gay, and bisexual students may want to meet through organizations in which sexual orientation is the foundation for the group.

Our culture has started to redefine and pay attention to settings where developing romantic attachments is deemed inappropriate and adds unhealthy complications. For example, although dating someone in your class can become awkward if the relationship doesn't work out, dating someone with whom you work can be more complicated, as work situations often involve competition and power. Sexual harassment laws and policies usually define the prohibitions associated with work-based relationships, with policies against romantic and sexual involvement most directed at power imbalances. Specifically, prohibitions and sanctions focus on relationships that could develop with a professor or supervisor; such individuals have the

sex in society 10.1

Finding That Special Someone on the Internet

The strategies available for meeting a potential partner have become more complicated than in decades past. Although college still provides a very social environment, the expectations of the "real" world after graduation may increasingly lead to organized searches for a partner through dating services and the Internet. Some people are in search of a long-term partner, while others focus on finding partners for sexual behavior without commitment. Parties, personal introductions, bars, and other venues may still lead to romance, yet for the very busy, the Internet may become a tool for organizing one's own social life. With work expectations, commutation, and other demands on one's time, the possibilities afforded by a system that is available 24 hours a day, every day, become very attractive.

There are many possible sites such as Chemistry.com, Match.com, eHarmony.com, and Zoosk.com, Individuals can create personal profiles, rewrite them over time, read and reread profiles of potential partners, take personal assessments that identify interests and better matches. Some sites require a membership fee; others are free. Approximately twenty-two million Americans subscribe to online dating sites yielding substantial industry revenues. In 2010, Match.com and Chemistry.com alone generated $343 million (Boostin, 2010).

While the increased availability of personals in newspapers and magazines provides one mechanism for meeting, the Internet increases the amount of information that can be transmitted. Many sites allow members to place their photographs online. Readers can react to a photograph and decide whether someone seems attractive. Pictures can be deceptive, however, and real face-to-face meetings potentially disappointing. Someone could easily be older, heavier, or shorter than what was conveyed in a photograph; even if those qualities are of minimal importance, there is still the issue of sexual chemistry and whether a potential romantic relationship will develop. On the positive side, by the time a couple decides to meet for the first time, they may have already established good lines of communication and a friendship.

Overall, healthy relationships form with people, not computers. The technology may change some of the dynamics of meeting and communicating, but in the long run being with someone who is right for you is the goal.

power of determining grades, promotions, graduate school recommendations, hiring, transfers, salaries, or firings.

Outside the school environment, you may find that dating becomes more of a project than you had anticipated. Work hours, busy schedules, and a desire to avoid looking for a partner in bars have led to technological interventions for dating. Personal advertisements, which used to be a feature in select newspapers and magazines, now have worked their way into mainstream newspapers (see Figure 10.1), cable television, and the Internet. Sophisticated video dating services, in which registered members can review tapes of people they might want to meet, have flourished in some areas. Hefty membership fees and promises made by some dating services, however, have sometimes resulted in dissatisfied consumers suing for fraud.

Finding a partner via the Internet allows people of all backgrounds to do some initial screening from the privacy of their own homes. Since there has been no friend or family member who introduced this new person and who knows who they really are, caution is advised when meeting someone

Females Seeking Males	Casual Only
Call 1-000-000-0000 **$2.39 per minute** You must be 18 years of age or older to use this service.	SWM 34, 5'11", lives in XXXX County, seeks a well-built, clean-shaven, SM, 21–45, who likes to have fun, for discreet relationship. Ad #0000
Prince Charming Educated professional SWM 40, 6', 180 lbs. Likes movies & nature. Seeking SWF, 20–40. Ad #000	**Hardworking** Personable, humorous SWM, 37, 5'11", self-employed, seeks sensitive slender SWF, under 32, to share a serious, loving relationship with. Ad #XXXX
Try Bi Disease-free W couple, 30, seeks bi-GWM, 30+. Ad #XXX	

Figure 10.1 *A Sample of Personal Ads Personal ads usually are coded for age, race, and sex of the desired partner.*

for the first time. Healthy Sex Hints 10.1 outlines guidelines for safe online relationships.

Choosing a Partner

What is it that attracts us to someone? Some generalizations have been formed based on the research on partner choice and attraction. Most people are drawn to partners from similar backgrounds and form relationships with people who are close in age, race, ethnicity, and social status. The National Health and Social Life Survey (NHSLS) conducted by the National Opinion Research Center (NORC), found that race, education, age, and religious background were similar in a significant number of couples (Michael, Gagnon, Laumann, & Kolata, 1994).

The authors reported that about 90 percent of couples were of the same race. Having similar educational backgrounds was also the predominant pattern as individuals chose sexual partners. Men who had less than a high school education seldom had a partner who had gone to college, and men with a college degree almost never reported having sex with women who had much less or much more education than they did (Michael et al., 1994). Religion and age comparisons also yielded choices based on similarity. The authors of the NHSLS study concluded that couples with more marked differences in background tend to be the exception rather than the rule. Most people choose partners and marry someone who is the same race, same educational background, same religion, and within 5 years of their age. Our society tends to be structured in segregated ways. Consequently, where you live, work, and with whom you socialize have an influence on your choice of partner (Michael, et al., 1994).

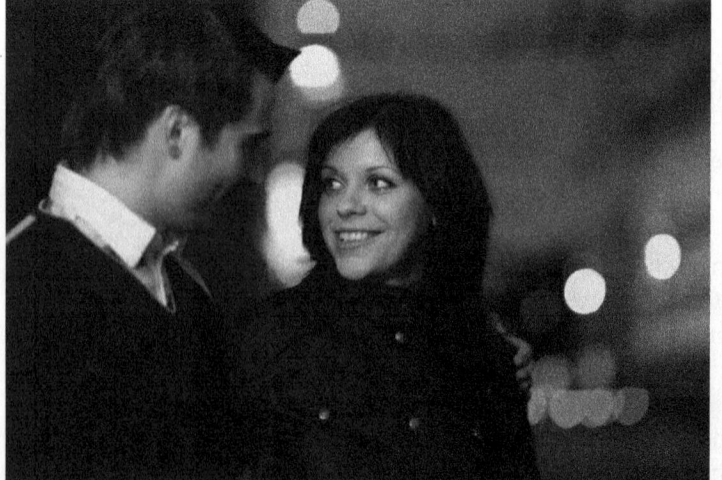

Figure 10.2 *Attraction is based on a variety of physical and personality attributes.*

© k, stutyagin, 2010. Shutterstock, Inc.

Attraction

Researchers have long concluded that people prefer romantic partners who are physically attractive and that there is some cultural consistency in what is deemed attractive (Berscheid & Walster, 1974; Dion & Dion, 1987; Hatfield & Sprecher, 1986). An image of the ideal female and male physique emerges from the media and advertising, and though it may be hard to attain in reality, the standard is set in many people's minds. How we each think we measure up to cultural ideals also may influence our sexual self-esteem. Are we acceptable? Are we attractive? We have found in our classes that just as students can identify what they find attractive

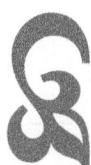

healthy sex hints 10.1

Guidelines for Safer Online Relationships

Meeting people online can be fun and exciting. Unfortunately, it can also be very dangerous, as evidenced by news reports of predators and children. Recommendations for teens may differ from those for college students and older adults, yet some basic guidelines prevail:

Do not use your real name in your e-mail address or disclose it, or disclose your address or telephone number to someone you have only met online.

Do not give details about yourself, such as the state in which you live or other information that would make it easy for someone to find you.

If after chatting with someone you decide to meet them in person, here are additional guidelines to follow:

Ask the person to give you information that will help you determine whether he or she is "for real," such as any employers, name of his or her school, or other references.

Ask the person to send a picture so that you will recognize him or her. Remember, too, that any information provided can be easily faked.

Meet in a public place like a mall or restaurant.

Bring a cell phone with you so that you can call for help if needed.

Consider taking a friend with you when you meet, and have the friend stay throughout the entire first meeting. It would also be a good idea to have a friend call you on the cell phone during the meeting to make sure that everything is OK. Be sure your friends know where you are so that they can send help if you need it.

Never go to this person's car or anywhere else alone and out of view of others.

Tell a friend or other trusted adult where you are going and who you are meeting. Tell that person you will call when you get home. (Have that friend be prepared to call your parents and the police if you do not call by the specified time.)

If you plan to meet a second time, introduce the person to family and friends.

Any person who cares about you and is interested in a real relationship with you will be more than willing to make you feel safe and secure about the relationship, and they will not mind the precautions that you are suggesting.

Anyone who refuses to meet in public, or who refuses to meet your parents or friends, is not someone you can trust, no matter how wonderful they might seem.

Source: Prepared by E. Casparian, New Jersey Network for Family Life Education, New Brunswick, NJ, 2003.

in others, they can identify aspects of themselves they deem attractive, as well as characteristics they do not like. Individuals will become sexually healthier when they can accept themselves or make constructive changes that allow them to interact in a healthier way. It is helpful to assess what you like about your body and what you think needs work. Following this

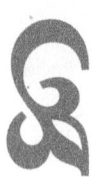

healthy sex hints 10.2

Tips for Assessing the Health of a Relationship

- Are you comfortable with yourself—know who you are, what you want, what you believe in? This is a critical first step toward being able to relate to others.
- Are you able to communicate freely and openly without being criticized for your thoughts and feelings ?
- When you're with this person, do you feel good about yourself? Do you feel appreciated and important? Do you feel you receive a lot of support?
- Are you treated as an equal? Do you respect and show respect for one another ?
- Is your relationship based on shared interests? Are your personal values close enough in perspective to allow for becoming close?
- Can you tolerate differences? If you two are different, are those differences critical? For example, can your relationship surpass differences in age, race, philosophy about money, and political outlook?
- Can you maintain a sense of individuality within the relationship?
- Do you laugh and have fun when you are together ?

assessment, make a decision about what you are willing to do to improve your body and do the work needed to improve. If you find that you are really not willing to make changes, then accept and love your body just the way it is. It is essential to stop being critical if you are not willing to work to improve your body. It is also important to accept the body of your partner and celebrate and enjoy each as they are.

Research on attraction has indicated different values between the sexes. Males place more emphasis on physical attributes than females do. Females value interpersonal warmth, personality, and earning potential over appearance (Bailey, Gaulin, Agyei, & Gladue, 1994; Nevid, 1984; Sprecher, Sullivan, & Hatfield, 1994; Wiederman & Allgeier, 1992). Regardless, looks alone do not define attractiveness, nor can looks sustain a relationship. Most of us have admired someone for their looks only to discover that this person had a personality that detracted from their appearance and values that we found objectionable, making that person unappealing after all. Over time, looks diminish in importance, as we develop loving feelings toward our partners and fully accept them for who they are.

Social psychologist Donn Byrne (1971) developed a theory of attraction focusing on rewards and punishments. He postulated that we tend to like people who reward us by making us feel good about ourselves and tend to dislike people who punish us and are nasty. Researchers have also documented that people tend to be attracted to those who share similar attitudes on issues (Smith, Becker, Byrne, & Przybyla, 1993). Relationships can develop and function well when we get along with our partners. Although this point sounds like common sense, too many people invest time and energy in relationships that are not working, with people who do not treat them well, and where they do not feel good about themselves.

> ❧ *Environmental/Occupational Wellness* ❧
>
> People today seem to spend more and more hours at work. Many students juggle classes and jobs. Consequently, the people one meets and spends a lot of time with can be classmates, coworkers, teachers, and employers. What continues to be a thorny question is whether people should become romantically involved with those at work. Prohibitions about workers becoming involved romantically may be included in sexual harassment policies. Colleges and universities also have such policies, dictating the acceptable parameters of romantic relationships. At work, romantic involvements may be permitted as long as the two involved are not in the same division or unit. At the university level, professors are not to get involved with those they grade and mentor. In reality, the prohibitions do not always prevail.
>
> For LGBT (lesbian, gay, bisexual, transgendered) individuals, romantic relationships become more complicated. If one is "out" at work and school, secrecy and fear of reprisals can be minimal. Job discrimination based on gender and sexuality is outlawed in many states, yet harassment still occurs both overtly and subtly.
>
> Our overall health is enhanced when we can share and be open about the positive love relationships we have.

Sexual Chemistry

Many times friends and family offer to "fix up" a person with someone they're "sure you'll like." A man may be told, "She's attractive, very nice, interested in a lot of different things." Or a woman may be told, "I have just the man for you! He's smart, handsome, talented, and has a great sense of humor." So, with such glowing testaments, they agree to a blind date. They go out. They have an OK time but can't see anything romantic developing. They don't disagree about their date's attributes; he or she is objectively attractive, has a nice personality, and so on, but just doesn't excite the other person. The explanation to the matchmaker is "Well, there was just no chemistry—no spark." Despite a host of attractive traits, chemistry may be lacking.

People respond to the smell of others, and bad breath may turn us off. Certain colognes, perfumes, and aftershaves are designed to turn us on. On an unconscious level, we may be responding to **pheromones,** which are sex-attractant chemicals, more familiar in lower animal forms. For example, a female dog "in heat" puts out an odor that male dogs can pick up from some distance. Even though human attraction is not grounded so heavily in reproductive issues, odors may have a larger role than we recognize (Kohl & Francouer, 1995).

Studies have begun to look at the impact of chemicals in male sweat and female vaginal secretions, examining their role in increasing attraction between a male and a female; their role in same-sex couples has yet to be assessed. The intense feelings associated with the early phases of a relationship, when we feel excited and caught up with the newness of the relationship, may have a chemical connection to higher levels of phenylethylamine (PEA) and possibly dopamine and norepinephrine, stimulants the

Pheromones Body chemicals that attract potential sexual partners

body produces. As a consequence, we literally can be on a "romantic high" that can be explained through chemistry (Botting & Botting, 1996).

An online matchmaking service has taken a new, creative approach to finding the right chemistry between two people. Chemistry.com uses neuroscience to find just the right person for each subscriber. Subscribers answer a lengthy questionnaire to uncover their individual brain's "love map." This profile is then run through a computer algorithm to find the ideal match for each person (Arnst, 2005).

Compatibility

In the long run, what makes a relationship work is how compatible the two individuals are. A healthy relationship allows two people to be who they truly are, with no attempt to change their partners. The values and lifestyles of the two, therefore, must mesh closely.

Popular books abound, offering advice on finding the right partner and making the relationship work. Although the advice is plentiful, those providing it may base their guidance not on solid information but rather on their own perspectives. Clinical psychologists, for example, may develop advice after working with a variety of clients on their problems. Likewise, identifying patterns of behavior drawn by surveying college students has limitations.

Nonetheless, some of the "popular" authors can provide helpful, down-to earth, practical advice. One author whose approach works well from a wellness model is Barbara DeAngelis (1992), author of Are You the One for Me? Knowing Who's Right and Avoiding Who's Wrong. DeAngelis advises her readers to develop a compatibility checklist along 10 dimensions, identifying qualities that are important to them in each category. When two people are in an actual relationship, assessing compatibility takes time, as some things are learned early in a relationship and others over a period of months, if not longer.

Maintaining Healthy Relationships

In plain language, a healthy relationship is one that is good for you. Finding a compatible partner is part of the process, yet the number of relationships that break up and marriages that end in divorce indicate that initial assessments can change or be wrong in the first place. It is essential to identify fully the characteristics we need in a partner and our relationship and then choose our potential partner very carefully.

Relationships that are good for you make you happy most of the time. They are fun, serve as sources of strength and support, and provide connections that improve the quality of your life. You can be who you are and be appreciated for your uniqueness. If you are unhappy, depressed, sad, and feeling that you are hiding your true self, those feelings should serve as a barometer to the health of the relationship. As with Jessica, in Case Study 10.2, it is not easy to recognize what is really going on between two people. Putting your needs and self aside to "keep a relationship going" is not good, as it fosters imbalance of power and interest in the relationship. Other people often can identify relationships as unhealthy when those in the relationship cannot.

sex in society 10.2

Compatibility List

According to author Barbara DeAngelis (1992), "Your Compatibility List can help you understand what is and what isn't working between you and your mate, and make it easier to decide whether it's time to separate. If you're looking for a new relationship, your Compatibility List acts like a shopping list, directing you toward partners who are right for you and helping you avoid partners you don't need and who will be a waste of time." Here is her list:

Directions: Use the following 10 categories to identify qualities you possess and those you want in a partner. Being as specific as possible will make the list more useful. When comparing results, you need to keep in mind how flexible you can be, how frequently you need traits to be exhibited, and which aspects of a relationship may work even if you two don't match.

1. *Physical style:* appearance, eating habits, personal fitness habits, personal hygiene
   Example: I exercise regularly. I would want a partner who likes to work out and exercise.
2. *Emotional style:* attitudes toward romance and affection, expression of emotions, approach to relationships
   Example: I'm very affectionate and need a lot of support. I would want a partner who would be affectionate and care about my interests.
3. *Social style:* personality traits, ways of interacting with others
   Example: I'm very outgoing and love to have family and friends around. I would not want a partner who only wanted to be with me and stay at home.
4. *Intellectual style:* educational background, attitude toward learning, world affairs
   Example: I'm a college graduate and read the newspaper daily. I also love books, both fiction and nonfiction. I would want a partner who is aware of what is going on in the world and also loves to read. My partner would have to at least have an associate's degree, although I would prefer someone who has finished a 4-year college program.
5. Sexual style: attitudes, skill, ability to enjoy sex
   Example: I love to try new things and be adventurous. I would want a partner who enjoys sex and is creative.
6. Communication style: patterns of communication, attitude toward talking, other forms of expression

Example: I know that I tend to scream when I'm angry.
7. My family is a bunch of screamers. While I may need to work on that behavior, I'd need someone who would understand that the screaming is more style than substance and wouldn't let the volume get to him [her].
8. Professional/financial style: relationship with money, attitudes toward success, work, and organizational habits
   Example: I work hard and budget my money carefully, never owing more than a couple hundred dollars on a credit card. I couldn't be with someone who gambles and is always in debt. Personal growth style: attitudes toward self-improvement, ability to be introspective and change, willingness to work on a relationship
   Example: I tend to think a lot about what I value and how I came to be who I am. If a relationship is important to me, I would do anything—even seek professional help if necessary—to make it work. I wouldn't want a partner who couldn't look at how we were getting along and work on the relationship.
9. Spiritual style: attitudes toward a higher power, spiritual practices, philosophy of life, moral views
   Example: I'm very involved with my church, working with youth groups and helping at local shelters. My partner wouldn't have to be exactly the same faith but would have to respect my beliefs and have a sense of his or her own.
10. Interests and hobbies
    Example: I love to travel, and I do my best to take at least one exciting vacation to some place new each year. I would want a partner who also likes to travel, or at least would be willing to travel.

After reviewing your list, think about how open you are to changing any of your answers. If you are without a partner, thinking about your interests becomes valuable in assessing how well you two match. As you get to know someone, finding dissimilar answers and styles in too many areas highlights a lack of compatibility. Most important, not all areas are equally important.

Source: From Are You the One for Me? by Barbara DeAngelis Ph.D. Used by permission of Dell Publishing, a division of Random House, Inc.

Relationships enhance physical and emotional wellness in a variety of ways. Being in love energizes a person and may actually boost the immune system. Because the partners want to please each other, they may take better care of themselves. Emotional health is aided by involvement with others. As young children, most of us learn to trust and form loving relationships. As we get older, we have the opportunity to develop our own partner relationships. Having someone with whom to share thoughts and feelings, who will love us for who we are, who can give constructive feedback and support—all contribute to emotional well-being.

Having intimate relationships usually means that someone is physically there for us, sharing daily experiences and also caring for us. Traditional marriage vows speak to "in sickness and in health"; couples in commitment ceremonies also vow to be there for each other in the good times and bad. A partner can help the other be healthier as well as manage challenges that come along.

Plenty of evidence also indicates that unhealthy relationships can have a negative impact on physical and emotional well-being. Being stressed about a relationship, depressed about a partner, being the recipient of anger, and so forth, affect not only mood but our physical bodies as well. Individuals may find that they have difficulty eating, sleeping, and concentrating, and in order to find solutions to relationship problems, they need to seek out professional help, in the form of both counseling and medication.

Jealousy

Healthy relationships are based on trust and respect. Unfortunately, many believe the destructive myth that jealousy shows how much someone loves the other person. Jealousy is neither a sign of love nor a healthy way of showing love but instead results from a number of factors: low self-esteem, fear of loss, bruised pride, insecurity, and, in some cases, a sense of "lost property" (Hatfield & Rapson, 1996). Individuals may react with feelings of jealousy in response to behaviors they find threatening. For example, a woman may get upset at seeing her boyfriend be kissed by a female friend. Another woman may not care about gestures of affection but not be able to handle a current boyfriend even having a cup of coffee with a woman he used to date. Jealousy, particularly if allowed to become out of control and increasingly intense, can spell the end of a relationship.

Men and women have been found to respond to feelings of jealousy in different ways. Jealous women are more likely to focus on the emotional involvement of their partner with another person, whereas men may focus on the sexual activity of their partner with another person. Researchers continue to find gender differences in how distressing infidelity becomes to the relationship, with women identifying emotional infidelity as the most distressing and men choosing sexual infidelity (Cann, Mangum, & Wells, 2001; Buss, Larse, Westen, & Semmelroth, 1992). Men are more likely to respond with rage and violence, and women are more likely to blame themselves and display more possessive behavior (Hatfield & Rapson, 1996).

316

personal exploration activity
Let's Have Some Fun Together

An important element of a healthy relationship is laughing and having playful, fun times together. Some experts believe that when a couple stops laughing together, this signals trouble in the relationship. Doing new and unusual things together activates the brain's reward system flooding it with the same chemicals released in early love (Parker-Pope, 2010). Laughing and playing together helps couples strengthen their bond. It takes creativity and work to make sure you do interesting activities that strengthen a relationship. The purpose of this activity is to develop a creative list of interesting things to do with a date or your partner so you can keep the joy and excitement in your relationship.

Your goal is to make a list of 30 activities that you would enjoy doing with a date or partner. They should not be expensive and should be easily accessible—you should not have to travel great distances to do these. First, list as many as you can think of that you would enjoy. Once you have exhausted your own ideas, start interviewing your friends and acquaintances to see what they can add to your list. Only add those that you would really like to do. When you have interviewed as many people as possible, share your list with your partner and put a check by those activities your partner would also enjoy doing. Decide which ones you want to do first and try to add one new activity each week. If you are not in a relationship at the present time, try these with your dates or with your friends. You should experience more laughter and enjoyment in your times together.

When asked in a classroom setting, college students have voiced the opinion that some amount of jealousy is good for a relationship and shows love for the partner. In actuality, the foundation for jealous feelings is not based on love, and these feelings are not healthy for a relationship. Couples can learn healthy ways of dealing with jealousy to strengthen their relationship. Some communicate openly about the triggers for jealous feelings and together develop a strategy to minimize the triggers. For example, if Trent feels jealous when Sara talks to an old boyfriend at parties, she could start including him in the conversations. Each partner can also decrease jealous feelings by working to improve his/her confidence and self esteem. Honest, open communication and working on strategies to decrease jealousy will turn the destructive force of jealousy into a way to strengthen the relationship.

Love

Love is tied closely to our expectations for a relationship and has long been a topic for songwriters and researchers. Studies on love have attempted to classify, develop theory, examine love styles, make cross-cultural comparisons, and recognize the complexity of love. The need to love a partner is important for individuals, regardless of sexual orientation.

Finding a comfortable definition of love is not easy. Some advise of the need to differentiate "love" and "lust." Others talk about being able to tell the difference between "love" and "infatuation." Hatfield and Rapson

Passionate love Feelings characterized by intense longing for another, infatuation, ecstasy when reciprocated, and emptiness when not shared by the other

Companionate love Feelings that include deep attachment, commitment, and intimacy

(1996) distinguish between **passionate love** and companionate love. Passionate love has an intense quality, in which the individual can feel lovesick, head-over-heels in love, and totally infatuated. There is an obsessive focus, intense longing, and, if reciprocated, a sense of fulfillment and ecstasy. When the lust or passion dies, as it always does, some assume they have fallen out of love. Actually, they are now able to move to the next stage which is developing a mature love, companionate love.

Companionate love is what we ideally experience as relationships endure. It is characterized by feelings of deep attachment, commitment, and intimacy. Companionate love encompasses feelings of affection and tenderness we feel for those with whom our lives are deeply connected.

Theories of Love

In his classic book, The Art of Loving, Eric Fromm (1956) asserts that before we can love another, we must learn to love ourselves. It is important not to confuse self love with conceit, which is actually a result of a lack of self love. A person who does not love him or herself spends much time trying to convince him or herself and others how amazing he or she is. When we truly learn to love and accept ourselves, we have no need to convince other of our "greatness" and are capable of fully giving to another. Loving someone who has no self love is similar to having a relationship with a vacuum. This person will take all they can from you (vacuum you) in an attempt to fill him or herself with love and will give you little or nothing in return. Fromm also believes love is a decision, not a feeling or emotion. We decide who and when we will love. Since love is a decision, we will not just fall out of love with someone but will decide to continue loving or to stop loving someone. There are many reasons we choose to stop loving someone including betrayal, loss of trust, lack of intimacy, and not having our needs met. It is very reassuring to know that love will not just disappear suddenly.

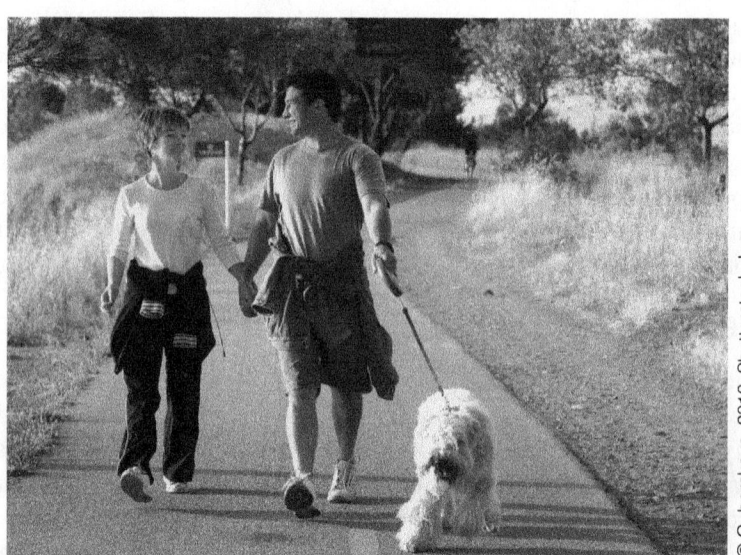

Shared interests are important to a relationship.

case study 10.2

Jessica: "Finding My True Love"

Jessica, 31, is white.

Jessica, now engaged to be married, shares the journey of finding the right partner:

I used to be a real romantic. There was one true love "out there somewhere" for me. I am much more grounded in the realities of relationships today than I used to be, but there is still nothing to match those intense feelings of love for someone.

My first true love was Tim. We met at a party senior year of high school and dated each other exclusively from that moment on, spending Christmas with each other's families, going out alone or with friends every weekend, and sharing a very romantic senior prom. Graduation was both joyous and sad, as we had to face the prospect of separation, with each of us going away to different colleges.

We talked about our feelings for each other and decided we wouldn't date anybody else at our respective schools. We called frequently, saw each other on vacations, and spent the summer together. I still get knots in my stomach thinking about the summer after junior year. One week Tim said he loved me. The next he wasn't sure. We would fight. I would cry. He would apologize.

We'd be fine for a while, and then the cycle would start up again. My parents tried not to interfere, but they could see how miserable I was. At the end of August, we decided to break up and date other people.

Tim and I became one of those on-again/off-again couples. I always loved him and hoped we'd get married. He was never sure. After college he accepted a job in California and asked me to live with him. I followed him west, attended graduate school, and was sure that our being together would solidify the relationship. We had our ups and downs, but I kept thinking that things would work out. He was transferred to Chicago, and after I graduated, I followed him there. We lived together for a year, and then Tim broke off the relationship. I had really been miserable with him for a long time, taking a lot of emotional abuse and neglect. I had few friends, low self-esteem, and most of the affection I received was from our dog.

That was a few years ago. The memories are very strong, yet finally the anger has subsided. I was angry at Tim. And angry with myself. As the saying goes, I "couldn't see the forest for the trees." I invested a lot of time with one person and lost myself too much in the process.

I am now with Mark. We, too, have had our ups and downs, a temporary hiatus from being a couple, but now we're engaged. I am honest about my feelings, I am independent yet want to be part of a couple, we each have our own and shared group of friends, and we truly want the same lifestyle.

Am I still a romantic? In some ways, yes. But I've also learned that good relationships don't "just happen." Both people work at it.

Critical Thinking

When couples get into a cycle of an on-again/off-again relationship, what can help them figure out whether to stay together? What criteria can one use to decide if the relationship is really what one needs and wants it to be?

Robert Sternberg (1986) has developed a theoretical model for examining love. Shown in Figure 10.3, love is conceptualized as a triangle with three faces: passion, intimacy, and commitment. Each person within a love relationship brings his or her triangle to that relationship, albeit with varying dimensions. When two people are well matched, they tend to find satisfaction within their relationship.

Sternberg identifies six different kinds of love that evolve in response to the varying dimensions:

Liking—Intimacy only, such as may be found between friends

Infatuation—Passion only, with high physical and emotional attraction

Romantic love—A combination of intimacy and passion, similar to liking with the addition of physical attraction

Companionate love—A combination of intimacy and commitment; may have had romantic components, but the key element is the emotional bond between the two people.

Fatuous love—A combination of passion and commitment, which may lead to two people quickly living together but over time realizing that they lack a deep, emotional intimacy

Consummate love—Ideal love, combining passion, intimacy, and commitment.

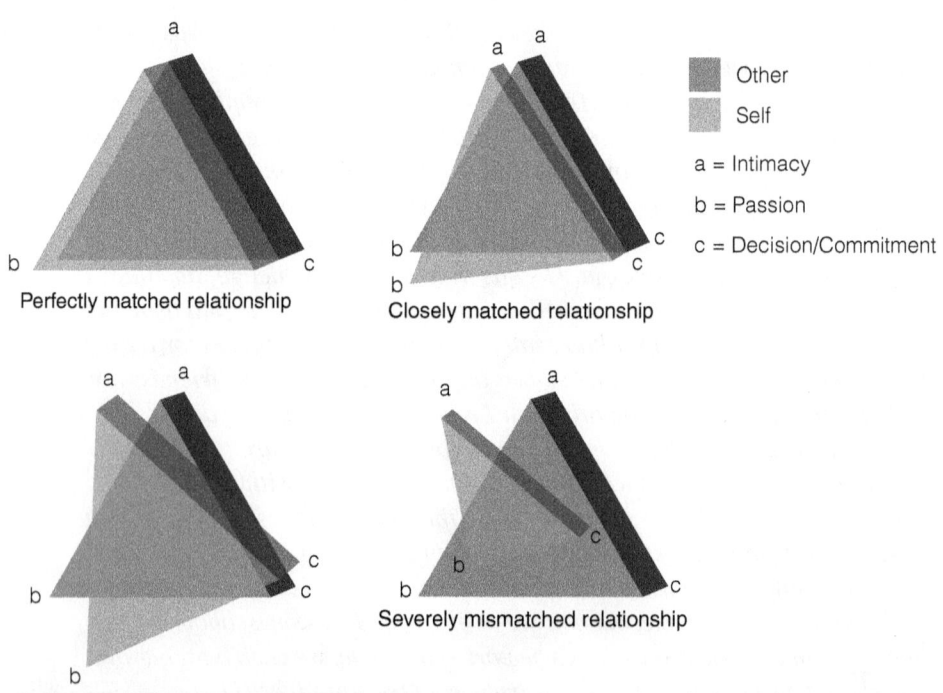

Figure 10.3 *Sternberg's Triangular Theory of Love*

Source: Sternberg, R. (1986) A triangular theory of love. Psychological Review, 93, 119–35. Sternberg R. (1988) Triangular love. In R. Sternberg and M. Barnes (eds.) The Psychology of Love. New Haven, CT: Yale Univ. Press.

Though we may strive to achieve this, it is hard to sustain over time and takes much nurturing of the relationship. However, with work long term relationships can maintain the intensity, interest and sexuality that characterize early relationships. The passion and excitement does not necessarily die as the relationship matures (Acevedo &Aron, 2009).

Another typology for examining styles of love is credited to John Lee (Lee, 1974). Recognizing that some styles can be combined, Lee describes six styles of love:

Eros—Focuses on physical beauty and has a strong sensual component

Mania—Characterized by a lot of roller-coaster emotions, with anxiety and ecstasy at the extremes

Ludus—Love for fun and play—nothing too serious

Storge—Marked by much affection, gradually deepening into love

Agape—Type of love that is undemanding, patient, and does not expect reciprocation

Pragma—Practical love; lovers carefully assess compatibility in background, values, and interest to find a good match.

Anthropologists provide us with data from other cultures, indicating that love and strong feelings of attraction may almost be universal emotions. Helen Fisher (1993), a popular anthropologist and author, posits that the human animal may have evolved with feelings of attraction that are somewhat time limited. Romantic love tends to wane after a 4-year period, which she claims matches the amount of time it takes to rear a child beyond infancy. Divorce statistics, as well as her study of 62 cultures around the world, lend support to her theory that couples stay together for a period of time and then may get interested in forming new partnerships.

Researchers have found differences in love styles based on gender (Hendrick, Foote, & Slapion-Foote, 1984). In a survey of an extremely diverse group of college students, females tended to be more manic, storgic, and pragmatic than males, who seemed more ludic and erotic. Women were found to be more conservative in their views toward love and relationships, incorporating concerns over finding a mate who would be a good provider and partner. Males, on the other hand, tended to respond early on to beauty and the playful aspects of relationships, and they were less concerned with commitment.

From Theory to Practice

Most of us want to find a partner with whom we can make a relationship work. Not all relationships function in exactly the same way, yet some characteristics predict a greater likelihood of "success." The style of love may change as people age. The style of love may improve with experience. The style of love may interfere with one's getting into and sustaining the kind of relationship desired. Recognizing your values, style, and how well you "match" to your partner, therefore, becomes valuable as you seek out love and a partner.

Research and therapeutic practice have yielded insights into the variety of relationships couples create and sustain. Lonnie Barbach (2001) writes about the use of power in relationships, with each partner needing to carve out areas of control. Individuals can use "forceful power" in which needs and wants are stated, asked for, and in some cases demanded. In contrast, individuals can also use "withholding power," in which love and nurturance are withheld. For intimate relationships to be successful, neither form of power is desirable. Individuals can use their power around how money is spent, with whom the couple or each individual in the couple socializes, and even around sexual contact. Meeting one person's needs can be viewed as purposely disregarding the other's needs, and a power struggle ensues with misunderstandings, anger, and resentment. The power relationship between the couple impacts their love and commitment. Those who can successfully negotiate differing needs develop healthier and happier relationships (Barbach, 2001).

Pepper Schwartz (2001) has identified many myths about successful relationships that warrant being questioned. A few examples are "You can't be in love with two people at the same time," "Little annoying habits are unimportant in long-term relationships," and "You should always be 100 percent honest with your partner." Because human relationships are complex, she takes issues with commonly held guidelines governing behavior.

Loving more than one person can happen as we commit to a partner yet hold loving feelings for a past partner. Deciding to act on those feelings is different from having them. When couples date, they may not mind that one person is neat while the other messy; living in a home with two very different styles of where to place clothes, papers, and other items or different attitudes toward personal hygiene may prove more challenging than they had when dating. Finally, although most people feel that honesty in a relationship is fundamental to building trust and intimacy, Schwartz argues that there are times when information may need to be kept secret for the health of the relationship. Individuals are entitled to some areas of privacy, and partners may really only want to know information that they can deal with. Schwartz does caution that there are times, however, when keeping secrets can be destructive to the relationship. For example, if one person had unsafe sex outside the relationship, putting their partner's health in jeopardy, getting medical attention and discussing the situation are imperative. If real feedback is needed about behaviors such as drinking, the intimate partner is in an ideal situation to provide it. And for those for whom honesty is viewed as the key component of the relationship, keeping secrets from a partner is fundamentally incompatible with maintaining an intimate relationship.

Sexual Activity Within Relationships

We examined adult choices about sexual behaviors in greater detail in Chapter 6. In the context of relationships, individuals decide on preferences for particular behaviors, frequency of activity, and whether their behavior will occur exclusively with one partner. Research on the timing of sexual activity has often been framed with a heterosexual and marital bias. Hence, students can find reports on **premarital sex,** coitus occurring before marriage, and **extramarital sex,** coitus occurring outside of marriage. The demographics in the United States, however, indicate that there

Premarital sex Usually refers to coitus, sexual intercourse, before marriage

Extramarital sex Usually refers to coitus, sexual intercourse, outside marriage

are currently more unmarried adults than at other times in history, with an estimated three-quarters of unmarried men and two-thirds of unmarried women engaging in some form of partnered sex over the course of a year (Waite & Joyner, 2001). Consequently, making marriage as the central core from which other situations vary can be problematic.

Because of such realities, terms that are more generic and focus on the primary relationship become preferred. The term **monogamy** by strict definition refers to the practice of having one spouse at a time, but more commonly it refers to having one sexual partner. Despite much of the research on sexual behavior outside the primary relationship using the term *extramarital,* the terms **dyadic,** referring to the couple, and **extradyadic,** referring to sexual activity with someone other than the primary partner, are preferred and considered to be less biased (Wiederman, 2001a).

Christopher and Sprecher (2000) reviewed years of research focused on sexuality within relationships. As couples were together longer, whether married or in long-term gay and lesbian relationships, there was a decline in the frequency with which they engaged in lovemaking. Researchers also found that sexual satisfaction is associated with relationship satisfaction, regardless of the sexual orientation of the couple. Cohabiting couples and those dating had slightly lower levels of sexual satisfaction when compared with married couples. Factors such as race, religion, and social status were not related to the frequency of sexual activity or sexual satisfaction.

Waite and Joyner (2001), in analyzing data from the National Health and Social Life Survey, propose that couples bring different expectations about sex to their relationships depending on whether they are married, cohabiting, or dating. For married individuals, there is a long-term contract with each being able to learn what pleases the other; satisfying a spouse enhances the emotional intimacy of the relationship. Cohabiters have a lower level of commitment to each other and may not feel as compelled to develop partner-specific skills. Single individuals may be dating more than one person, aware that a long-term relationship may or may not be possible, yet the connection may be sexual regardless. Overall, viewing a relationship to be long-term, being emotionally invested in it, and being sexually exclusive were hypothesized to increase emotional satisfaction and physical pleasure from sex. As with other research, commitment becomes an important variable for both men and women when examining their emotional satisfaction with the relationship. The researchers found that physical pleasure and emotional satisfaction were higher when the sex was used to express love for the partner.

Regardless of the relationship status, the body releases the bonding chemical oxytocin and arginine vasopressin (AVP) in response to sexual intimacy. We feel closer and experience warmer feelings for the partner after sexual intercourse (Trimarchi, 2013). This is an important consequence to consider when choosing whether to be sexually intimate with a partner. Do you really want this person to feel bonded to you? Do you want this person to feel warm, fond feelings for you? And, is this a person you like enough to want to feel bonded and close to? Never-married, young adults can and do decide to remain virgins. Primarily, researchers have identified that young adults may not feel that enough love is present in the relationship, they express a fear of sexually transmitted diseases and unwanted pregnancies, their belief system supports virginity, and/or personal feelings of insecurity

Monogamy Commonly used to refer to having one sexual partner, whether married to that person or not

Dyadic sex Referring to the sexual behavior of a couple, the two people in a relationship

Extradyadic sex Referring to sexual behavior outside the primary relationship. This term replaces *extramarital sex,* which is confined to heterosexual marriages.

and inadequacy interfere with experiencing coitus (Christopher & Sprecher, 2000). What is critical is that decisions to be sexually active involve mutual consent and comfort. For some, a solid, committed relationship is key.

Americans have strong views on extradyadic and extramarital sex. When surveyed on how they viewed "married people having an affair, the majority of Americans (88%) choose the answer "morally wrong" (Pew Research. 2006). Because there are strong social sanctions against extradyadic sex, it can be difficult to assess its prevalence. Asking whether a person has been "unfaithful" or "has cheated on his or her partner" may affect research findings. Formal researchers have looked at married and cohabiting couples, and although those who cohabit have higher rates of extradyadic sex than married couples, and the rates for married couples in contemporary studies are relatively low, there are still significant numbers of people who have had sex with someone other than their spouse at least once. The variables found to be associated with more permissive extramarital attitudes are high education, low religiosity, premarital sexual permissiveness, and being male (Christopher & Sprecher, 2000). The most reliable data on extramarital sex rates comes from the earlier discussed 1992 NHSLS survey. When asked the question, " Have you ever had sex with someone other than your husband or wife while you were married?", one in four men and one in six women answer yes (Norman,1998).

Abusive Relationships

Abusive relationships are more complex than what we often imagine. It is typical to think of abuse as physically hurting another. However, the World Health Organization includes not only physical abuse but sexual, emotional and controlling behaviors abuse (WHO, 2013). Behaviors that fall into these categories are obvious markers of an unhealthy relationship. Abusive behaviors may develop slowly but tend to increase as the relationship becomes more involved. Being put down, insulted, controlled, blamed for a partner's problems ("It's your fault. . . ."), pushed, shoved, or beaten are all forms of abuse.

Abuse often begins in the dating relationship, with intimate partner violence recognized as a significant public health problem. We often assume that males are the ones who are violent. However,the Youth Risk Behavior Surveillance conducted by the Center for Disease Control(2012) found that in the junior year of high school, more males (11%) reported being "hit, slapped or physically hurt by their boy friend or girl friend than females (9%). By the senior year, males and females reported the same level of violence, one in ten.

Violence has also entered the digital realm. Teens report frequently receiving digital threats or demeaning request from their romantic partners. The website ThatsNotCool.com has tips to help set boundaries to avoid violence. It also has callout cards that can be sent by email or posted to a Facebook account that will tell someone they have crossed the line. An example of one is "Congrat! With that last text, you've achieved stalker status". (Clifford, 2009).

Lesbian, gay, bisexual, and transgendered youth when abused have the added threat of being "outed" to others who may not know of their sexual orientation. In a study of adolescents Freedner et al.(2002) found

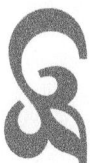

healthy sex hints 10.3

Guidelines for Healthy Relationships

Both people in a relationship have the right to

Be treated as an equal
Ask for what they want.
Be accepted for who they are.
Be treated with respect.
Express their thoughts and feelings without criticism.
Not be forced to do anything.
Feel safe when alone with each other.
Give and receive expressions of affection.
Make some mistakes and be forgiven.
Say no and not feel guilty.
Have fun.

No one in the relationship has the right to

Tell the other person where and when he or she can go out.
Act like a boss and order the other person around.
Degrade and humiliate the other person, in either public or private.
Isolate the other from friends and family.
Pressure the other to give up interests and goals.
Read the partner's personal materials without permission, search private property, or follow the other around.
Physically intimidate and harm the other person.
Use sex as a bargaining tool

that sexual orientation in general did not make a difference as to whether dating violence occurred. However, bisexual males were more than five times more likely and bisexual females more than four times more likely to be threatened with "outing" compared to their gay and lesbian peers. Lesbians had greater odds of being scared for their safety compared to heterosexual females. Cruz (2002) argues that for gay men, incidences of abuse may not even be accurately remembered, as violence is part of gendered socialization —that is, men get angry, and that anger is often expressed in violent ways.

Abuse is often a learned behavior with the abuser having experienced or witnessed abused. High conflict relationships, especially conflicting about jealousy, women's gender roles and money, are more violent than those with good conflict resolution skills. Heavy alcohol or drug use also increases the risk for violence (Jewkes, 2002). According to the American Psychological Association (2013) some other warning signs that a person may become an abusive partner include the following:

Aggressive behavior as a youth
Anger and hostility
Desire for power and control in the relationship

Belief in strict gender roles (male dominance)
Depression
Few friends and isolation from other people
Young age
Insecurity
Unemployment

Regardless, without the abusive person's getting professional help and being willing to change, the abuse will continue and the "relationship" will be between an abuser and a victim, rather than two adults in a healthy relationship. It is also likely that the violence will escalate and far too often ends in tragedy. Shelters exist across the United States for victims of intimate partner violence, with women overwhelmingly being those at greatest risk. Although those outside a violent relationship may wonder why a victim "doesn't just leave," professionals in the field know that financial dependency, children, isolation from family and friends, and fear make such flight difficult. Statistics support the fact that when a woman chooses to leave, she is at the most vulnerable point for becoming a victim of violence and possibly murder (Francese, 2001). Male and females need to be educated about the early signs of physical abuse, emotional, controlling and sexual abuse and given help to end abusive relationships in the early stage before the violence escalates to this deadly stage.

Prevention of abuse includes teaching healthy relationships skills at an early age (CDC, 2011). This would include moving from a male dominated relationship to one where partners share equal power since women who are empowered economically, educationally and socially are the most protected from violence (Jewkes, 2002). In a healthy relationship, both males and females will be empowered economically, educationally and socially thus making their commitment to the relationship a free choice.

Sexual Orientation and Relationships

Love and relationships among gay, lesbian, and bisexual adults have been subject to many myths. Perhaps one of the biggest problems lies in the secrecy involved. To be open about the relationship poses barriers that heterosexual couples seldom face. This translates into day-to-day losses such as relating stories of weekend fun with coworkers on Monday and the larger risk of losing one's job if coworkers find out about the gay or lesbian orientation. As José explains in Case Study 10.3, there can be a heavy emotional price to pay for having to keep a love relationship secret from friends and family.

Research comparing heterosexual couples and gay and lesbian couples has revealed some differences, although the similarities, such as valuing communication, sharing experiences, and laughing together, far outweigh the differences identified. The differences in values one brings to a love relationship are tied more closely to gender than sexual orientation (Peplau, 1981; Metz, Rosser, & Strapko, 1994). Similarly, gender was a more significant variable when examining differences in styles of conflict resolution. There are fewer verbal attacks, less belligerence and more of an effort to diffuse the argument when conflict occurs in same sex relationships than in heterosexual relationships (Gottman, Levenson, Swanson, Swanson, Tyson, & Yoshimoto, 2003).

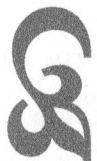

healthy sex hints 10.4

Unhealthy Behaviors After Ending a Relationship

Though some behaviors can be expected following a breakup, others become increasingly problematic if they persist. If the breakup is disrupting your life, get some help from a counselor or therapist. The following symptoms indicate a problem:

Sleeping too much or too little

Using drugs and alcohol excessively
Inability to eat
Inability to concentrate on work
Inability to study
Wanting to drop classes
Wanting to drop out of school
Driving recklessly
Making harassing phone calls to the ex-partner
Stalking or following the ex-partner around
Harassing an ex-partner's new boyfriend or girlfriend
Being violent toward the old partner or his or her property
Wanting to commit murder or suicide

Perhaps in response to the realization that gender role stereotyping is problematic when both partners are of the same sex, same-sex relationships tend to reject the traditional marriage model. Compared to heterosexual couples, gay and lesbian relationships are more egalitarian, sharing household responsibilities more evenly, share more common interest and spend more time together finances (Parker- Pope, 2010; Peplau, 1981).

Breaking Up and Ending Relationships

Just as relationships can be formed in healthy ways, they can be ended in ways that are not destructive. When feelings are mutual, both parties realize that the relationship is not working, and the breakup may not be as difficult. The experience of having a partner break up with you without your awareness of any problems, however, is quite another matter. Ending a relationship in any case is emotionally difficult and painful for most of us.

Romantic relationships end for a variety of reasons. For college students, the reasons may include being too busy with academics and sports or music commitments, transferring schools and being apart, finding someone new who excites you and with whom you want to get involved, getting pressure from family because a partner is of an "unacceptable background," and other reasons. Sometimes a crisis tests a relationship, and where one partner expected support, none was forthcoming. Whatever the reason, for at least one of the partners, the relationship wasn't working.

As discussed earlier, the end of a relationship is a perfect time to evaluate what you did and did not like in the previous relationship and your previous partner. You can use this failed relationship to refine your "must have" list for your next relationship. Take some time between relationships so you can spend time alone and with your friends. Use this period of time to reacquaint yourself with "you"-identifying what "you" think, believe and enjoy, not what "we" think, believe and enjoy. All that you learn about your wants and needs can be used to develop a better, healthier relationship when you find the person who is worthy of you.

For some college students dealing with the end of a relationship, it may be important to seek help from campus counseling centers. Whereas some students seem able to accept the end of the relationship, and move on, others find it extremely difficult to continue with their studies. College students may also need to seek counseling when their parents divorce and/or remarry. Some parents wait until their children are out of the house before initiating separation and divorce. Universities recognize the need to provide psychological health services to students.

Academic success can certainly be compromised by the energy diverted from studying to healing "a broken heart" or managing the array of emotions connected to seeing loved ones end their relationship.

✎ *Spiritual Wellness* ✎

Feelings of love and connectedness go hand in hand with spiritual wellness. To be able to be yourself and be loved for who you are contributes to our spiritual needs. The intensity of love feelings becomes apparent when we experience loss. "Loss of a loved one" is rated the highest mean measuring personal stress, and the emptiness we feel highlights how much the loved one contributed to our lives.

Depending on why a relationship ended (such as mutual change in interests, divorce, death, and the like), our emotional responses can vary. Nonetheless, it is a time to reflect on ourselves, who and what are important in our lives, and how we plan to move on. Our spiritual health is enhanced when we develop and maintain intimate relationships with family and friends as well as partners.

case study 10.3

José and Marco

José, 26, identifies as Latino American.

I'm the only son in my family and until recently was the middle child. My older sister was married, and my younger one is single. When my older sister died, my younger sister Selena and I felt increased pressure from our parents to provide grandchildren. My mother, in particular, is very religious and goes to church every day. She prays for her family, and her faith helped her deal with my sister's death. Now she prays to be blessed with a grandchild. Only one of us is going to be able answer those prayers—and Selena doesn't even have a boyfriend.

I get angry at my situation sometimes and realize that things might be easier if I would come out to my parents. On the other hand, my mother is very religious, and the church hasn't been all that welcoming. My father never gets into deep conversations, and I fear his disappointment. They've met Marco but just think he's one of my good friends. Since they live in Texas and I'm in San Francisco, it's easier to maintain the lie. Marco and I have caller ID on the phone, so we usually can tell who's calling before answering. The "right" person answers the phone.

My parents think I live alone and just have had little success dating women. I took a female friend to my senior prom, but other than her, I've never introduced my family to a girlfriend. They seem to be comfortable accepting my stories, although my mother tells me I should "settle down" and make a family.

When my sister died, it was hard to go home and not have Marco with me. And it continues to be hard to visit family without my partner. Straight people don't have to play these games. I'm getting sick of the secrets and know that I cut myself off from family because I think I am afraid they may totally reject me. I could not face the loss of my family. I may be wrong, but I'm just not ready to take the risk.

> ### Critical Thinking
>
> If you are heterosexual, compare your life to Jose's. What losses does he suffer that you do not have to experience? Imagine how your family would respond if you told them you were gay. Would they be loving and accepting? How would you feel about bringing your partner home with you and how would your family and friends react?

Personal Assessment

How Jealous Are You?

One feeling that often causes conflict between two people is jealousy, perhaps because men and women often experience and express jealousy in different ways. If partners are unable to communicate openly about an issue, a conflict may result. The following exercise is designed to help bring to light your experiences with jealousy so you may better understand yourself and your partner. If you currently do not have a partner, simply respond to the questions in terms of your last relationship or a hoped-for future one.

Directions:

Read each statement carefully, then respond yes or no in the blank following the statement.

1. You have found at times that you actually like feeling jealous. _____
2. Your spells of jealousy seem to follow a pattern, one after another. _____
3. Sometimes you get so jealous you lose your appetite or overeat. _____
4. When you hear about, or think about, your partner's former lovers, you are jealous. _____
5. You avoid close relationships with people other than your partner because such situations may cause your partner to be jealous. _____
6. You are very jealous of your partner's friends, yet you tell people you are not the jealous type. _____
7. You are apt to display fits of jealousy with no apparent cause. _____
8. You are often jealous of your partner's friends even when you know your partner has no romantic feelings toward them. _____
9. At social gatherings you are aware of every move your partner makes. _____
10. Jealousy has led you to spy on your partner. _____
11. You want to know where your partner is at all times. _____
12. It would definitely be a crisis if you were to discover that your partner had one sexual encounter with another person. _____
13. The feeling of loneliness is common to you. _____
14. You have thought of taking revenge on a person you felt was a rival. _____
15. You feel that jealousy is proof of your love for your partner. _____
16. You are jealous of your partner's hobbies. _____

Scoring:

If you have responded yes to more than five of these statements, you are allowing jealousy to control your life. To continue in this way is to leave yourself open to considerable pain and anguish. When jealousy arises, talk about it and reaffirm your commitment to your partner. You need to listen to each other.

Reactions:

Use the space provided to respond to the following questions.

1. Which statements, to which you responded yes, are of most concern to you? After discussing them with a friend or partner, explain what you plan to do differently.

2. Do you feel you are trying to control this person who is important to you? Why or why not?

Source: Your Sexuality: A Self Assessment (2nd ed.), by R. Valois and S. Kammermann, New York: McGraw-Hill, 1992, pp. 111–112.

Thought Questions

1. What is intimacy? How can a person be intimate but not have sex with a partner or have sex with someone but not be intimate?

2. What are three barriers to intimacy? Does gender role impact our ability to form intimate relationships? If so, how?

3. Explain Sternberg's model of love.

4. Give an example of a love mismatch, according to Sternberg.

5. How does romantic love differ from consummate love?

6. What are three characteristics of happy couples?

7. What are three common problems that lead to breakups and divorce?

Test Yourself!

1. Intimacy is characterized by all but which of the following qualities?
   a. Honesty
   b. Controlled emotions
   c. Openness
   d. Trust

2. Intimate friendships and intimate romantic relationships
   a. both enhance our social health.
   b. both have an erotic component.
   c. essentially induce the same emotional responses in the participants.
   d. differ substantially in their expectations of openness.

3. Which of the following statements about shyness is true?
   a. It is common for most people to feel shy at some point or other.
   b. People who are shy have low self-esteem and need professional help.
   c. Most people who are shy feel that way in all situations.
   d. Some levels of shyness help foster intimate relationships.

4. Laws and public policies have been put into place to prevent dating
   a. between two students in the same class.
   b. between supervisors and employees at work.
   c. between athletes on the same team.
   d. between two adults more than 5 years apart in age.

5. Marla met Chuck in a chat room, and they then began an online relationship. After a month, they decided that they wanted to meet face-to-face. They should follow all but which of the following pieces of advice?
   a. Let a friend know where they've gone and when they will return.
   b. Find a quiet place to be alone so that they can get to know each other.
   c. Take a cell phone.
   d. Have their own means of transportation.

6. Research on partner choice indicates that most people choose someone
   a. of a higher socioeconomic class so that there is more money to live on.
   b. regardless of the person's background, as long as there is compatibility.
   c. within a 10-year age differential, older or younger.
   d. of the same race and religion.
7. Research on attraction has revealed
   a. lesbians are only attracted to other lesbians.
   b. most men prefer large-breasted women.
   c. variations in what and who is perceived as attractive.
   d. similarities in what gay and straight men find attractive.
8. Being compatible with a partner means
   a. you share all the same values.
   b. you find each other physically attractive.
   c. you share similar values, interests, and goals.
   d. you have the same level of education.

9. John and Karen have been dating for 1 year. Prior to John, Karen dated Carlos and has remained friends with him. John is jealous. According to research, what best explains John's feelings of jealousy?
   a. Carlos is very attractive.
   b. John also likes Carlos.
   c. Karen had been sexually involved with Carlos.
   d. Karen had been in love with Carlos.
10. Theories of love are useful to couples in that they
   a. recognize different styles of love and attachment.
   b. guide couples on how to love each other.
   c. provide a framework for understanding couple behavior.
   d. teach the individual how to become a loving partner.

Journal Article

Boo, K. (2003, August 18). The marriage cure. New Yorker, 79(23), 105.

Web Resources

Go Ask Alice
www.goaskalice.columbia.edu

This site is sponsored by the Columbia University Health Service yet will answer questions mailed from anywhere.

Students will find the answers to questions about love and relationships, conflicting feelings, and other topics.

Planned Parenthood
www.teenwire.com

Sponsored by Planned Parenthood, teens and young adults can write in for information about all aspects of sexuality, including concerns about relationships.

Resource Directory for Internet Dating Sites
www.internetdating.net

The site leads the user to a variety of options from regional and international sites to religious and singles' travel sites.

Each category provides a list of links.

American Association of Sex Educators, Counselors, and Therapists
www.aasect.org

Professional certifying organization that provides links to professional help nationwide.

References

Acevedo, A. & Aron, A. (2009). Does a long term relationship kill romantic love? Review of General Psychology, 13, 1, pp59-65.

American Psychological Association. (2013). Intimate partner violence; facts and resources. Available on line: www.apa.org/topics/violence/partner.aspx?item=1

Arnst, C. (2005). Better loving through chemistry. Business Week, 3956. Hillsdale, NJ: Erlbaum.

Bailey, J., Gaulin, S., Agyei, Y., & Gladue, B. (1994). Effects of gender and sexual orientation on evolutionary relevant aspects of human mating psychology. *Journal of Personality and Social Psychology,* 66, 1091–1093.

Barbach, L. (2001). *For each other: Sharing sexual intimacy.* New York: Penguin.

Berscheid, E., & Walster, W. (1974). Physical attractiveness. In L. Berkowitz (Ed.), *Advances in experimental social psychology* (Vol. 7). New York: Academic Press.

Boostin, J. (2010, February 12). The big business of on line dating. Available on line: www.CNBC.com

Botting, D., & Botting, K. (1996). *Sex appeal.* New York: St. Martin's.

Buss, D. M., Larse, R. J., Westen, D., & Semmelroth, J. (1992). Sex differences in jealousy: Evolution, physiology, and psychology. *Psychological Science, 3,* 251–255.

Byrne, D. (1971). The attraction paradigm. New York: Academic Press.

Cann, A., Mangum, J., & Wells, M. (2001, August). Distress in response to relationship infidelity: The roles of gender and attitudes about relationships. Journal of Sex Research, 38(3), 185–190.

Carducci, B. (2000, Jan.). Shyness: the new solution. Psychology Today.

Center for Disease Control and Prevention (2012, June 8). Youth Risk Behavior Surveillance-United States 2011 [online] available: www.cdc.gov/Healthy Youth/yrbs/pdf/yrbs 12_mmwr.pdf

Center for Disease Control (2011). Understanding intimate partner violence-fact sheet. Available on line: www.cdc.gov

Christopher, F. S., & Sprecher, S. (2000, November). Sexuality in marriage, dating, and other relationships: A decade review. *Journal of Marriage and the Family,* 62, 999–1017.

Clifford, S. (2009, January 27) Teaching Teenagers about harassment. New York Times.

Corbett, S. (2001, October 14). When Debbie met Christina, who then became Chris. *New York Times Magazine,* Section 6, pp. 84–87.

DeAngelis, B. (1992). *Are you the one for me? Knowing who's right and avoiding who's wrong.* New York: Dell.

Dion, K. L., & Dion, K. K. (1987). Belief in a just world and physical attractiveness stereotyping. *Journal of Personality and Social Psychology,* 52, 775–780.

Downey, G., & Feldman, S. I. (1996). Implications of rejection sensitivity for intimate relationships. *Journal of Personality and Social Psychology,* 70(6), 1327–1343.

Egan, J. (2003, November 23). Love in the time of no time. *New York Times Magazine,* p. 66.

Fisher, H. (1993). *Anatomy of love: The national history of monogamy, adultery, and divorce.* London: Simon & Schuster.

Francese, T. (2001, November). The battered woman's experience and theories of violence. Class presentation by the Passaic County Office of Women, William Paterson University.

Freedner, N., Freed, L., Yang, Y., & Austin, S. (2002, December). Dating violence among gay, lesbian, and bisexual adolescents: Results from a community survey. *Journal of Adolescent Health,* 469–474.

Fromm, E. (1956). The Art of Loving. New York: Harper Row.

Gottman, J. Levenson, R., Swanson, C., Swanson, K., Tyson, R. & Yoshimoto, D. (2003). Observing gay, lesbian, and heterosexual couples' relationships: mathematical modeling of conflict interactions. Journal of Homosexuality, 45, pp 65-91.

Hatfield, E. (1996). *Love, sex, and intimacy: Their psychology, biology, and history.* New York: HarperCollins.

Hatfield, E., & Rapson, R. L. (1996). Love and sex: *Cross cultural perspectives.* Boston: Allyn & Bacon.

Hatfield, E., & Sprecher, S. (1986). *Mirror, mirror. . . . The importance of looks in everyday life.* Albany: State University of New York Press.

Henderson, L., Zimbardo, P., & Rodino, E. (2001). Painful shyness in children and adults [Online]. American Psychological Association. Available: http://helping.apa.org.

Hendrick, S., Foote, F. J., & Slapion-Foote, J. (1984). Do men and women love differently? *Journal of Social and Personal Relationships,* 1, 177–180, 184, 193–195.

Jewkes, R. (2002). Intimate partner violence:causes and prevention. The Lancet,vol 359, issue 9315, pp 1423-1429.

Kohl, J. V., & Francouer, R. T. (1995). *The scent of eros: Mysteries of odor in human sexuality.* New York: Continuum.

Lee, J. (1988). Love styles. In R. Sternberg & M. Barnes (Eds.), *The psychology of love.* New Haven, CT: Yale University Press.

Lewis, R. (2010). Emotional intimacy among men. Journal of Social Issues, vol 34, issue 1.

Marano, H. E.(2005, Jan/Feb.). What's a shy guy to do? Psychology Today, (38) 1.

Metz, M. E., Rosser, B. R., & Strapko, N. (1994, November). Differences in conflict-resolution styles among heterosexual, gay, and lesbian couples. *Journal of Sex Research, 31*(4), 293.

Michael, R. T., Gagnon, J. H., Laumann, E. O., & Kolata, G. (1994). *Sex in America.* New York: Little, Brown.

Nevid, J. (1984). Sex differences in factors of romantic attraction. *Sex Roles, 11,* 401–411.

Norman, M. (1998, July 4). Getting serious about adultery; who does it and why they risk it? The New York Times.

Parker-Pope, T, (2010). For Better: how the surprising science of happy couples can help your marriage succeed. New York, NY, Plume.

Peplau, L., & Cochran, S. (1988). Value orientations in the intimate relationships of gay men. In J. DeCecco (Ed.), *Gay relationships.* New York: Haworth.

Peplau, L. A. (1981, March). What homosexuals want in relationships. *Psychology Today,* 28–34, 37–38.

Pew Research Social & Demographic Trends (2006, March 28). A barometer of modern morals: sex, drugs and the 1040. Available on line: http://www.persocialtrends.org/2006/03/28/a-barometer-of-modern-morals/

Schwartz, P. (2001). *Everything you know about love and sex is wrong: 25 relationship myths redefined to achieve happiness and fulfillment in your intimate life.* New York: Perigee.

Smith, E., Becker, M., Byrne, D., & Przybyla, D. (1993). Sexual attitudes of males and females as predictors of interpersonal attraction and marital compatibility. *Journal of Applied Social Psychology, 23*(13), 1011–1034.

Sprecher, S., Sullivan, Q., & Hatfield, E. (1994). Mate selection preferences: Gender differences examined in a national sample. *Journal of Personality and Social Psychology, 66,* 1074–1080.

Sternberg, R. (1986). A triangular theory of love. *Psychological Review, 93,* 119–135.

Trimarchi, M. (2013). 10 Steps to a more intimate relationship. Available on line: http://health.howstuffworks.com

University of Florida (2013). Types of intimacy. Available on line: http//www.counseling.ufl.edu/cwc/types- of- intimacy.aspx

University of Michigan(2009, April 29). Seven-Year itch? Boredom can hurt a marriage. Available on line: http://www.sciencedaily.com/releases/2009/04/090429172241.htm

Waite, L. J., & Joyner, K. (2001). Emotional and physical satisfaction with sex in married, cohabiting, and dating sexual unions: Do men and women differ? In E. O. Laumann & R. Michael (Eds.), *Sex, love and health in America.* Chicago: University of Chicago Press.

Wiederman, M. W. (2001). Mate selection: What determines peoples' choice of particular partners? In *Understanding sexuality research.* Belmont, CA: Wadsworth/ Thomson Learning.

Wiederman, M., & Allgeier, E. (1992). Gender differences in mate selection criteria: Sociobiological or socioeconomic explanations? *Ethnology and Sociobiology, 13,* 115–124.

World Health Organization (2013). Understanding and addressing violence against women: intimate partner violence. Available on line: http//www.who.int/reproductive health/publications/violence

Zimbardo, P. G. (1977). *Shyness.* Reading, MA: Addison-Wesley. 320 Intimate Relationships

chapter
eleven

Sexual Communication

Student Learning Objectives

After reading this chapter, students will be able to

- ♥ Compare a variety of communication models.
- ♥ Describe some of the key elements that make sexual communication different and difficult.
- ♥ Assess the importance of communication in sexual relationships.
- ♥ Describe a variety of verbal sexual communication techniques.
- ♥ Describe a variety of nonverbal sexual communication techniques.
- ♥ Compare and contrast verbal and nonverbal sexual communication techniques.
- ♥ Describe some barriers to effective sexual communication.
- ♥ Describe how disabilities impact sexual communication.

activity teaser: Are you comfortable with the language of sex? Find out with the Personal Exploration Activity on page 381.

case study 11.1

Pam and Doug: Irreconcilable Differences or Poor Communication?

Pam and Doug, both 50, married. Pam identifies as an Italian American. Doug identifies as Hungarian-American.

Critical Thinking

Pam and Doug's story illustrates how important it is to communicate clearly when issues and problems in a relationship arise. How did failing to discuss other issues in their marriage influence their sexual relationship?

Pam was a non-traditional student in one of Dr. Blonna's online Human Sexuality classes. She and Doug agreed to be interviewed by Dr. Blonna for this book. After 25 years of marriage, Pam and Doug separated for six months because of "irreconcilable differences." Pam asked Doug to move out of their house so she could rethink their relationship. During that time they each began individual counseling, and after a couple of months started seeing a sex therapist together. It soon became apparent to the therapist that Doug and Pam had lost the desire to communicate effectively. After a few sessions with the therapist Doug and Pam began to realize how poor communication contributed to their marital problems. They are back together now and had this to say.

Dr. Blonna: "Could either of you please describe how communication was related to your problems?"

Doug: "I guess I'll start. I always thought Pam and I had sex problems. Our therapist showed me that the problems had as much to do with communication as sex."

Dr. Blonna: "In what ways?"

Pam: "Well, for one, he made us realize that we had just stopped talking about sex years ago."

Doug: "Not only about sex—we really stopped communicating about most things. We were both so angry most of the time that we just stopped talking and merely co-existed in the same house for over 10 years."

Dr. Blonna: "Ten years! Tell me about your sex life during this time."

Pam: "What sex life? I thought I had lost all of my sexual desire. At first I kept telling myself that it would return once the kids were older and in school. Then I told myself it would return when the kids moved out of the house and went away to college. When they left last year and I still did not feel any passion for Doug I wanted out. I needed to find out where my desire had gone."

Dr. Blonna: "So the two of you did have an enjoyable sex life in the beginning?"

Doug: "Yeah, it was good. It wasn't perfect. Pam and I were both raised in very strict households where sex wasn't discussed much and we had a lot of hang-ups about things like oral sex, but we enjoyed the physical and emotional aspects of intercourse."

Dr. Blonna: "So what happened?"

Pam: "Once the kids came and I had to stop working, our relationship changed and we never really talked about it or how we would work around it. I was angry because Doug had a low-level position in his firm and didn't earn what I expected he would. He was angry because I never lost the 20 extra pounds from the second baby, and things just escalated from there."

Doug: "Yeah, neither one of us really knew how to talk about the things that were bothering us, so they just festered and grew. Eventually our problems seemed so great that I didn't know where to start to begin addressing them."

Dr. Blonna: "So you just gave up?"

Pam: "Yeah. I just assumed that this was what happened when couples had kids and were married for more than 10 years. I just immersed myself in my children and my home and Doug spent more and more time at work and on the golf course."

Dr. Blonna: "So how did it turn around?"

Doug: "After Pam asked me to leave and I was on my own for a couple of months I realized how much I loved and respected her. I really missed her."

Pam: "I felt the same way. I guess that beneath the years of anger and holding back our feelings we really did love each other. I had never been in therapy and my therapist helped me explore all of the things I had been holding inside for so long.

Doug: "It was hard for me to talk with a therapist. I didn't want to admit that I was equally at fault for the dissolution of my marriage. He worked with me on my communication skills; asking for the things that I want and need in our relationship and it feels good."

Pam: "Yeah, after 25 years together, I feel that I can argue with Doug in a healthy way and assert myself without hurting him. It has paid off in dividends in the bedroom. I can't believe that at 50 I am enjoying sex so much. Empty nest, what empty nest?"

Communication

Communication is defined as the process by which information is exchanged between individuals through a common system of symbols, signs, or behaviors. It involves all the modes of behavior that an individual uses to affect another person. It encompasses spoken and written words as well as nonverbal messages such as gestures, facial expressions, bodily messages or signals, and artistic symbols (Watzlawick, Beaven, & Jackson, 1967).

Communicating, as Pam and Doug show us in Case Study 11.1, involves a whole range of issues from emotional comfort and security, to cultural considerations, and finally to discrete behavioral skills. Communicating about sexuality-related issues is even more complex and often

Communication The process by which information is exchanged between individuals through a common system of symbols, signs, and behaviors

more difficult because of this. Communication is the foundation of healthy sexuality. It is essential to obtaining sexual information for oneself as well as communicating information to others. Sexual communication poses unique challenges because of the difficulty of communicating in general, plus the personal nature of sexuality. Communicating effectively requires skill, patience, and commitment, as well as an understanding and mastery of sexual information. Honest and accurate sexual communication is essential in developing and maintaining good relationships and fostering healthy sexuality.

Metacommunication

Metacommunication
Communication about communication

Communication also includes the interpersonal relationship between communicators. When we are in the presence of others, it is impossible not to communicate. Activity and inactivity, speech and silence—all communicate messages. Communication occurs at two levels: the *content* level (what is actually being said) and the *relationship* level (what is going on between the communicants). This second relationship level is referred to as **metacommunication,** or communication about communication.

Pragmatics The relationship between communicators

Pragmatics refers to the relationship between communicators, and relationships are of two types—symmetrical and complementary. **Symmetrical relationships** are based on equality. Each communicator treats the other in a like fashion, minimizing differences and conflict. Symmetrical relationships are comfortable and facilitate communication. When we are involved in symmetrical relationships, we are relaxed, our conversation is not forced, and we perceive periods of silence as comfortable and not awkward (Watzlawick et al., 1967).

Symmetrical relationships
Relationships based on equality

Complementary relationships
Relationships based on differences

Complementary relationships are based on differences. Communicators maximize their differences, causing inequality and disharmony. Complementary relationships crackle with the tension in the air. Communication is forced, and periods of silence seem interminable. Complementary relationships often result in stress (Watzlawick et al., 1967).

❧ Social Wellness ❧

All interpersonal communication has a social basis. It is not just about putting thoughts and feelings into words. It also is about the relationship between you and the person with whom you are communicating. As we have seen, metacommunication proposes a framework for communicating based on symmetrical (equal) and complementary (confrontational) relationships. Symmetrical relationships foster good communication, whereas complementary ones discourage effective dialogue.

Transactional Analysis

Transactional Analysis Eric Berne's communication model based on three ego states—parent, adult, and child

Eric Berne's (1960) **transactional analysis (TA)** model examines relationships that are either symmetrical or complementary. Berne proposed that all of us have three sources of behavior, or ego states: child, adult, and parent. Each ego state manifests itself in a different communication style. Figure 11.1 illustrates the three ego states of TA.

1. *The child.* The child manifests itself through childish use of verbal and nonverbal communication. The child uses coyness, naiveté, charm and seduction, boisterousness, giggling, and whining, and is spontaneous, irresponsible, and manipulative. Our childish ego state is playful and free of restraint.
2. *The adult.* The adult is rational and objective, uses logic and analysis, and exhibits sound decision-making based on accurate perception and analysis. The adult is fair, responsible, sociable.
3. *The parent.* The parent incorporates feelings and behaviors learned from authority figures. The parent communicates the conscience of the person through words, actions, postures, behaviors, expectations, and the use of guilt or reward. The parent can be nurturing (protects, cuddles, and cares for) or critical (corrects and condemns).

According to Berne, when we communicate, our message is sent from one of our three ego states and is received by a specific ego state of another. Ideally, the ego state from which we send messages matches that of the person with whom we are talking. Thus, if we are speaking from our adult state to another person, that person should be receiving our message in his or her adult state. If this is not the case, a mismatch occurs. A mismatch is similar to the complementary message in Watzlawick et al.'s (1967) metacommunication model. Mismatches between messages sent from one state and received by another can be a source of stress and sexual miscommunication.

Figure 11.2 illustrates a mismatch that occurs when we are talking to a peer and we use our parent ego state instead of our adult state. Our friend, receiving in an adult ego state, expects us to send an adult message. Instead, we send a parent message assuming we are sending to an assumed child ego state, which creates a mismatch and is a source of stress.

Figure 11.3 illustrates another mismatch between two lovers. One is in a playful mood and communicates a sexy message from his adult state. His lover, in an adult state, receives the message, is confused, and sends back a parent message. The critical nature of the message and the condemning tone send a stressful message that resonates within the partner's child state. Mismatches like this can cool the fires of desire if they are not cleared up.

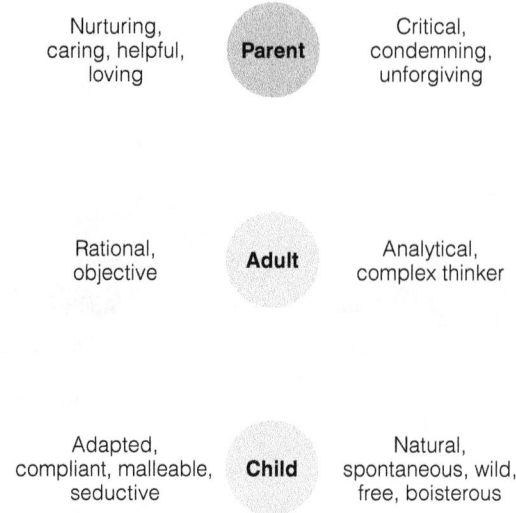

Figure 11.1 *Berne's Three Ego States* Berne identified three ego states: the parent, the adult, and the child.

Source: *Transactional Analysis in Psychotherapy,* by Eric Berne (New York: Grove Press, 1960).

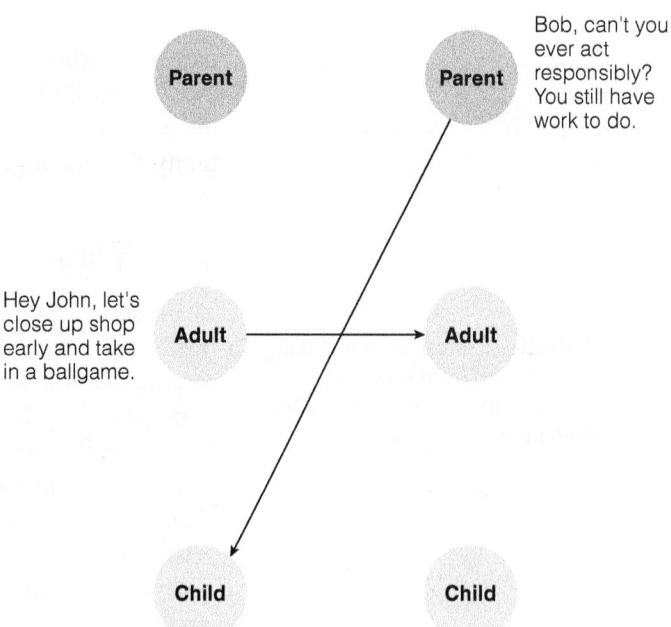

One adult addresses another adult. The second adult receives the message in an adult ego state and responds as if to a child ego state.

Figure 11.2 *Transactional Mismatch* Miscommunication occurs when people talk to each other using different ego state levels.

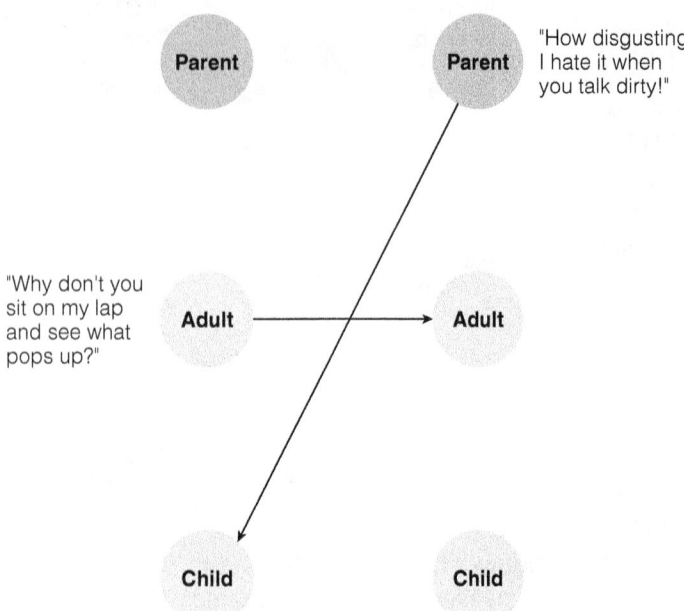

One person initiates from his adult state, using humor to signal his sexual interest. His partner responds sternly from her critical parent state, treating him like a child.

Figure 11.3 *Sexual Transactional Mismatch* Sexual transactional mismatches occur when lovers communicate about sex using different ego state levels.

Feedback A verbal or nonverbal response sent from a person receiving a message to the person sending that message

Dialogue An exchange of information in communication

Encoding Selecting the signs, symbols, emotions, and words to transmit a message

Forms of Communication

The basic forms of communication are one-way and two-way.

One-Way Communication

One-way communication is an information-giving process that does not involve or rely on feedback. Speeches, lectures, movies, TV programs, concerts, and radio broadcasts are examples of one-way communication. One-way communication is a direct and powerful way to transmit information about sexuality. Much of what we learn about sexuality in our culture is disseminated through one-way communication.

Print and broadcast media use sexual themes in their programming and to sell their products. Movies, TV programs, and music videos weave visual sexual images into their plots. Song lyrics provide auditory sexual information. We absorb most of what we learn about the cultural context of sexuality through this passive transfer of sexual information through mass media. Mass media convey messages about how our culture views sex. Mass media communicate sexual information to entertain or sell products, not to inform and educate us. Although the impact of this exposure is powerful and conveys messages about sex, the portrayal is often shallow and inaccurate, and doesn't offer the opportunity for a dialogue. It also doesn't afford the opportunity to personalize the information and explore how it relates to us as individuals.

Two-Way Communication

Two-way communication goes beyond information-giving by including **feedback.** Feedback ensures a dialogue, the key component of two-way communication. It gives us the opportunity to share information, ask questions, seek clarification, and explore ideas and feelings that go beyond those initially presented. **Dialogue** represents a true exchange of information. This is why two-way communication is essential for communicating about sexuality. Two-way communication increases the likelihood that each person will express his or her needs and wants, and will understand each other clearly. One way to explain two-way communication is through a circular model of communication.

A Circular Model of Communication

Effective communication is a circular process that involves sending and receiving coded messages, as illustrated in Figure 11.4. A sender, wishing to communicate, puts the idea and feeling of the message into a form that can be transmitted. This process of formulating a message, choosing appropriate words, symbols, tone, and expressions to represent it is called **encoding.**

case study 11.2

Susan: An Awkward Communication Circumstance

Susan, 37, single, and lesbian, is white.

Susan, a professor, is attending an out-of-town conference with some friends. She is sitting at the bar in her hotel, waiting for friends to come down and go out to dinner with her. She is nursing a drink, trying to relax.

A man seated two stools to her right tries to draw Susan into a conversation he is having with a group of his friends about the sexual differences between men and women. Susan doesn't know any of these people. She finds them not only a little drunk but also unsophisticated and shallow. Their discussion of sexual differences is childlike, and reminds Susan of a bunch of adolescents smirking and telling sex jokes in the locker room. She immediately feels uncomfortable. Susan feigns interest in what they are talking about, nodding her head while looking over their shoulders to try to spot her friends. She politely responds as if addressing a colleague and they immediately look at her as if she is from another planet. She can't relax around them as they carry on about a variety of issues she doesn't care about and trade barbs with each other. She also feels uncomfortable talking about this subject with a group of strangers who don't realize she is gay. Eventually Susan's friends arrive, and she quickly excuses herself and joins them. She is able to let down her guard, be herself, and enjoy the rest of the evening in symmetrical conversation among peers she respects and feels comfortable around.

Critical Thinking

What are the characteristics of Susan's interaction with the man at the bar that make this a complementary relationship? How does Susan being a lesbian influence the complementary nature of this interaction?

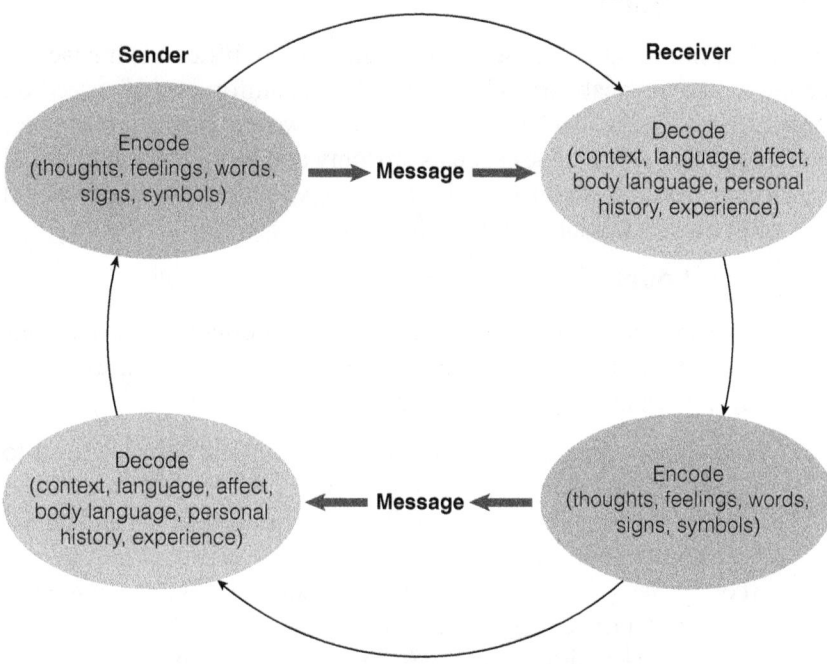

Figure 11.4 *A Circular Model of Communication* A circular model of communication assumes that senders and receivers provide feedback to each other.

Decoding The use of knowledge, memory, language, context, and personal history and experience to interpret a message

The receiver perceives and translates the message using his or her personal storehouse of knowledge and experience in a process called **decoding.**

Encoding and decoding take place within the context of the communicator's interpersonal and physical relationship. What is being said involves not only the actual message but also the physical environment of the communication as well as the relationship of the sender and receiver. A sender might alter the message depending on whether the environment is friendly or unfriendly, familiar or unfamiliar, safe or unsafe, formal or informal (Sawyer & Behnke, 2002).

In addition, a sender might send a different message in the same environment, depending on the nature of the relationship with the receiver. The message might be affected by whether the sender and receiver are friends or enemies, strangers or known to each other, peers or of unequal status (Sawyer & Behnke, 2002). Communication involves sending and receiving both verbal and nonverbal messages. Each type of message is capable of transmitting information, and is part of the encoding and decoding process.

Verbal Communication

Verbal communication is two-dimensional in that it involves transmitting both thoughts and feelings through words. The *cognitive* domain is concerned with communicating our thoughts about things. The *affective* domain involves putting our feelings into words. Many people find communicating cognitive information easier than expressing feelings.

Specificity

Specificity is crucial in effective verbal communication. The more specific the message, the more likely it is to be transmitted clearly. Vocabulary plays a big part in the specificity of our verbal communication. Having a large working vocabulary allows us to specify exactly what we want to say.

Sexual Vocabulary

One of the things that makes sexual communication difficult is the lack of a common sexual vocabulary. U.S. culture has no uniform set of agreed-on words, phrases, and sexual language level. Often we are unsure of the proper terminology for sexual topics such as anatomy and physiology and sexual behaviors. Insecurity about sexual terminology, coupled with emotional discomfort, makes talking about sex difficult.

Language Level

The level of language we use also plays a part in effective verbal communication. The four levels of language are childhood, street, everyday discourse, and scientific language (Mandel, 1980).

1. *Childhood language* is simple, cute, and fun and often is used to disguise embarrassment. Lovers have their own brand of childhood language. They may use it to describe their sexual anatomy and physiology, sexual desire, or need for pleasure. Pet names and phrases are part of this language. Lovers often use childhood language to refer to their genitalia or sexual desire. People also use childhood language when they make mistakes and seek forgiveness. "Ooops, sowwy about that," we might say in mock childhood tones.

2. *Street language* is tough, expressive, and emotional. Street language can be disarming and often is used to level the playing field when communicators do not share equal power or prestige. Tough talk can bestow power and superiority. Street language also serves to create bonds between members of subcultures by sharing a language that members of mainstream society do not understand. Rap music incorporates the power and raw sensuality of street language into a unique art form.

3. *Common discourse* is the language level of mainstream society. It is the generally accepted form of language with which most of us communicate. Most people use its words, expressions, and speech patterns in communicating information that is neither intimate nor scientific. It is the language taught in schools and used in most communications.

4. *Scientific/professional language* is the discourse of the work world and professional community. It is the language that professional peers use as they communicate about the subtleties of their chosen professions. Like street language, it usually is understood only by those who share its culture. Computer programmers, doctors, and other professionals have unique vocabularies, complete with acronyms only they understand.

When we communicate with our partners, we must use the level of language with which they are most comfortable. Miscommunication can occur when the language levels of two communicators are not the same. A language level in common is a good starting point for effective sexual communication.

Nonverbal Communication

How we say things is just as important as *what* we actually say. **Body language** describes the nonverbal messages we send through posture, gestures, movement, and physical appearance, including adornment. Our body language intentionally or unintentionally sends messages to receivers (Andersen 1999).

Body language Sending intentional or unintentional messages through body postures and movements

Lovers use nonverbal communication to express feelings, ask for things, and reinforce pleasurable activities. A moan, a hug, a seductive look—these can speak a thousand words. Placing a partner's hand in the correct spot or squeezing it when you are being touched as you want can accomplish as much as explaining these things through words.

Body Language

Positive, or open, body language is demonstrated by a relaxed posture, steady eye contact, nods of the head, and an occasional smile or happy expression. These are cues that you are an approachable sender or a receptive receiver (McGinty et al., 2003).

Negative, or closed, body language has visible signs of tension such as clenched fists or tight jaw muscles, a closed posture (arms folded, body shifted sideways, and the like), and facial expressions ranging from anger to disbelief. Negative body language can indicate either apathy or disturbance about something.

sex in society 11.1

He Said/She Said

Do men and women communicate differently? Research about this subject over the past 20 years has yielded mixed results. Men and women are socialized differently, and many researchers believe this difference emerges in the way we communicate. Women are socialized to show their feelings, whereas men have been taught to keep their feelings hidden (Michaud & Warner, 1997). Men have been taught to keep their fears and doubts disguised, because showing these is considered a sign of weakness. Men are socialized to believe that admitting weakness is unmanly (Tannen, 1990).

These beliefs can affect the way we communicate with our partners. Wives send clearer and more emotional messages than their husbands do (Noller & Fitzpatrick, 1991). Wives tend to frame their message in an emotional context, whereas husbands deemphasize affect and focus instead on issues and facts. Husbands send more neutral, less expressive messages that are harder to interpret (Tannen, 1990).

Michaud and Warner (1997) found that men and women communicate differently when dealing with problems. When dealing with "troubles talk," these researchers found that women were much more likely to offer sympathy than men were. Men were much more likely to tell a joke. Women were much more likely to be supportive, whereas men were more likely to avoid the trouble. Lastly, Tannen (1990) found that women were much more likely to listen as a way to offer support, whereas men were much more likely to try to "solve" the problem by offering advice.

McGinty, Knox, and Zusman (2003) found that female college students were more likely to engage in nonverbal feedback and were more proficient at using it than their male counterparts. Female college students in the study were also more proficient at decoding nonverbal feedback than the males who participated. McGinty et al., (2003) also found that males and females differ in how they communicate according to the nature of the relationship. There were significant differences in the communication patterns of students in "involved" versus "casual" relationships. The former group was significantly more concerned about nonverbal communication than the latter. The involved students also demonstrated greater skill in communicating nonverbally with their partners than the casual daters did (McGinty et al., 2003). Involved daters were also "less confused" about their communications than the casual daters were, and reported "working harder" on communicating (both verbally and nonverbally) clearly (McGinty et al., 2003).

Physical Appearance

Physical appearance can convey a variety of messages. A messy, sloppy, or ungroomed appearance may send encoded messages ranging from positive ("I'm comfortable enough in your presence to relax") to negative ("I don't care enough about you or myself to pay attention to my appearance"). Clothing and adornment might intentionally or unintentionally be erotic and seductive. This can affect both the encoding and the decoding process, as the sender might be trying to convey one message ("I'm trying to look my best"), while the receiver may perceive another ("This person is trying to manipulate or come on to me sexually").

Silence

Silence is a form of nonverbal communication that can be either a source of stress or a sign of comfort. Silence also can be used to hurt and control people. Silence is a stressor when wordless pauses are perceived as signs of a breakdown in communication.

Conversely, silence communicates comfort and acceptance between friends and lovers who understand that a loving bond is present despite a lack of conversation. Silence is a necessary part of effective communication that is often overlooked. We need time to listen, digest, and understand messages. Silence allows us time to reflect as we formulate our thoughts and words.

Touch

A firm handshake, a reassuring touch on the arm, a gentle squeeze of the buttocks, the placing of a partner's hand on the genitals or breast—all convey messages without speaking a single word (McBurney, 2002). Appropriately used, touch adds another dimension of communication that sometimes reaches deeper than mere words.

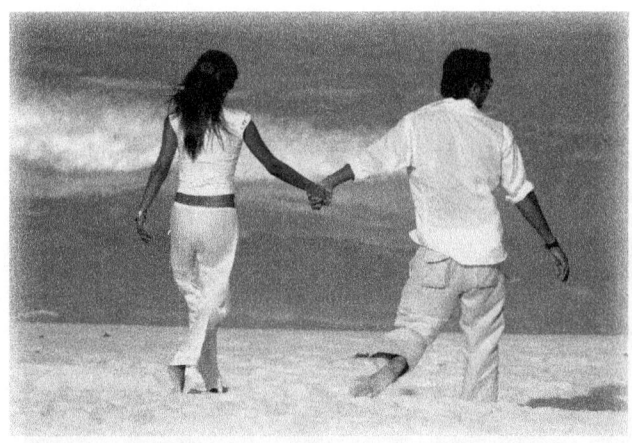

True intimacy doesn't require constant talking. Holding hands and walking silently can communicate love, trust, and a variety of other emotions.

Often we find it easier to communicate our sexual desires through touch than words. For example, a man might take his partner's hand and place it on his penis and squeeze it rather than ask, "Please squeeze my penis this hard." A woman might draw her partner's head upon her breast rather than ask, "Please suck on my nipples." A person might moan or groan rather than say, "I like it when you suck on my penis like that," or "It feels good when you rub my clitoris like that." When used inappropriately, however, the effects of touch can be devastating. A pat on the head can be a sign of endearment to a child but can embarrass or infuriate another adult. A squeeze on your friend's shoulder can show him you understand his problems and care about him. The same squeeze on your secretary's shoulder, however, can convey an entirely different meaning. A pat on a teammate's buttocks can show appreciation of a great play or an extreme effort. The same pat on a coworker's buttocks can be perceived as sexual harassment.

Space

The space between sender and receiver also affects communication. Four space zones common to communication in North America are as follows (Hall, 1973):

Intimate space (less than 18 inches)—space reserved for communication between intimate partners.

Personal space (18 inches to 4 feet)—space appropriate for close relationships that may involve touching.

Social-consultive space (4 to 12 feet) space for nontouching, less intimate relationships that may involve louder verbal communication.

Public space (more than 12 feet)—space used for formal gatherings such as addressing a large group.

Stress and sexual tension can arise when we violate these commonly accepted space parameters. For example, we find ourselves backing up to reclaim our violated space when a nonintimate person gets within the

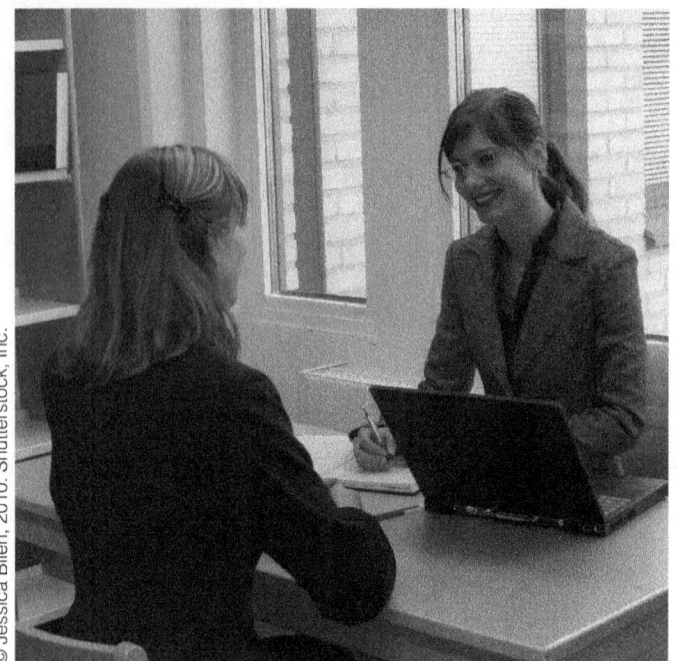

Professionals use desk and chair placements as a way to establish comfortable space requirements.

boundaries of our intimate space. Sometimes we place objects as barriers between us and other people to define our space and set allowable communication zones. Culture plays an important part in determining what is acceptable and unacceptable concerning space.

❧ *Intellectual Wellness* ❧

Intellectual wellness can facilitate communication. Effective communication, whether of a generic or sexual nature, involves three sets of skills: initiating, listening, and responding. Because these are skills, they can be developed and improved, regardless of one's current level of functioning.

Initiating Skills

Initiating sexual communication is different for new and for established relationships. Initiating skills are critical in meeting new people. Initiating skills also are important for discovering what our partners desire, as well as for communicating our own wants and needs, likes and dislikes. Partners in established relationships have a history of intimacy and trust that foster communication. The context of their communication differs greatly from that of two people who are attracted to each other but have not established an intimate relationship yet.

Despite the nature or length of the relationship, however, research shows that men and women often misread emotional cues and misinterpret nonverbal messages (Senecal, Murard, & Hess, 2003). This makes it particularly important to take responsibility for any perceived miscommunication and initiate a dialogue with one's partner to clear this up.

Nonverbal Initiating Skills

Initiating communication starts with nonverbal messages. Think about how you act when you meet for the first time someone to whom you are attracted. You make eye contact and hold it a little longer than you would if you were not interested in meeting the person. Eye contact leads to a smile, a brush of the hair, followed by another look that signals approachability.

Take the case of John and Susan. They are in the same biology lecture class of 150 students. For a couple of weeks they have noticed each other and seem mutually attracted. Today Susan decides she wants to meet John. She intentionally sits closer to him—about four seats down in the same row. She smiles at him as she takes her seat. She sees that he notices her and returns her smile.

Buoyed by this, she glances over again, tossing back a long shock of hair while reestablishing eye contact—this time for a moment longer. She decides to approach John after class and initiate a conversation with him. If John hadn't noticed Susan, returned her glance, or maintained eye contact, she might have received a different message and decided not to pursue meeting him any further.

Nonverbal communication between lovers in a long-term relationship is similar—but different because of their shared intimacy, comfort level, and experience together. Nonverbal messages are still important, however, to signal approachability and desire to communicate. They still need to establish eye contact, set the appropriate distance, and adopt a relaxed and approachable posture. Lovers can soften or strengthen their intentions with techniques such as a flirtatious look, lingering eye contact, a smile, or a serious look. Initiating nonverbal communication also can involve props for both new and established lovers. Peering over the top of a book you are reading or the drink you are nursing provides a small security blanket. The feigned dropped handkerchief is the quintessential prop that heroines in classic movies used to gain the attention of their heroes.

Leaving on the table a magazine opened to a story about sex is one way to send a message that you are interested in discussing the subject. Putting a sex manual on your coffee table or bedstand is a way to send messages of interest and approachability to your partner. Renting an erotic or romantic video is a way to introduce the topic of sex without saying a word.

Verbal Initiating Skills

Whether a person is trying to meet someone for the first time or to talk to a partner of 15 years about a sexual topic, he or she has to initiate the communication. Waiting and hoping that your partner or someone in whom you are interested will initiate is a sure way to end the communication before it begins. Take the case of Susan and John again. Clearly, from his nonverbal messages, John is at least approachable. Susan now is responsible for initiating.

Deciding what to say in first-time encounters can be excruciating. A simple rule of thumb is to be honest. Susan could simply say, "Hi, I'm Susan. I'm a little embarrassed, but I've noticed you for the past couple of weeks, and I'd like to meet you." It's now up to John either to reinforce his nonverbal display interest or to pass it up. Susan also could draw from their shared experience of the biology lecture. She might initiate by saying something like, "Hi, I'm Susan. I'm having trouble understanding something the professor just said. Can we talk?" Four common initiating techniques that can be used in both first-time and longtime relationships are open-ended questions, paraphrasing, declarative statements, and simple yes/no questions.

ᷡ *Spiritual Wellness* ᷡ

Sometimes our moral and ethical standards affect our emotions and impact negatively on our ability to communicate. We each have our own personal moral code with a unique set of values and ethics that develop over a lifetime. Taboos against behaviors ranging from masturbation to oral sex are often deep-seated and rooted in religious training. This can make it very difficult to initiate discussions and pose conflicts in communicating about some of these behaviors.

Cultural Considerations in Communication

Communicating effectively requires awareness of, and sensitivity to, various cultural influences related to verbal and nonverbal communication. The following are a few examples of common cultural considerations to keep in mind.

Verbal Communication

Cultural groups and subcultures do not necessarily share a common language. Although English is the first language spoken by most Americans, and common discourse is the level most frequently used to communicate, this is not the case for many individuals and groups. For many Americans, English is a second language, and common discourse (including slang) is often misunderstood. For these Americans, certain subjects, words, and gestures may be misunderstood or taboo.

For Americans traveling abroad for pleasure or business, this consideration is even more important. Sharing personal information, using hand gestures, squeezing an arm, and giving a peck on the cheek are all examples of communication behaviors that are common to everyday discourse among Americans. These would be considered major gaffes when used by Americans traveling in such places as China and Japan (Dou & Clark, 1999).

Perception of time and the relationship of the past, the present, and the future also vary by culture. The predominant culture in the United States is time-urgent and future-oriented. Being aware of the present and doing something now to plan for the future (such as exercising now to prevent heart disease in the future) are commonly accepted.

In daily life, people are oriented to specific times of the day and strict schedules. Some other cultures are much less interested in time and are not as oriented to specific schedules. For example, many Native American homes do not even have clocks, as people of some tribes are more concerned about the present and live one day at a time (Ivey, D'Andrea, Ivey, & Simek-Morgan, 2002).

Nonverbal Communication

A variety of nonverbal factors also vary from culture to culture. Cultures differ in their norms for territoriality and personal space. In general, people of Arabic, Southern European, and African origins sit or stand relatively close to each other when talking. People of Asian, Northern European, and North American countries are more comfortable being farther apart when they are talking (Ivey et al., 2002).

Body language varies significantly according to culture. The dominant U.S. culture places a high value on direct eye contact when speaking. In contrast, Native Americans consider continuous direct eye contact to be insulting and disrespectful. Rules about eye contact also vary by gender in certain cultures. In Islamic cultures, women are taught to avert the eyes, whereas eye contact is OK for men. The meaning and acceptability of a myriad of other nonverbal behaviors, such as pointing fingers, shaking hands, and other forms of touch, vary by culture (Ivey, D'Andrea, Ivey et al., 2002).

The following general suggestions can be helpful in verbal and nonverbal communication with people from cultures different from one's own:

- *Slow down.* People for whom English is a second language sometimes have a hard time keeping up with and understanding English when it is spoken too rapidly.
- *Minimize nonverbal distractions.* Be conservative rather than flamboyant in your use of gestures, personal space, and other nonverbal communication.
- *Look for feedback.* People who don't understand, can't keep up, or are uncomfortable with something you do or say often give nonverbal or verbal cues. These can be as overt as asking for clarification or as subtle as a turned head or lack of eye contact. Seek clarification of these cues.
- *Avoid talking louder.* Sometimes, when we are not sure we are being understood, we raise our voice, assuming that the person can't hear us. Talking too loudly, however, can be perceived as threatening or condescending, and is rarely helpful.
- *Show respect.* Being humble and respectful of cultural differences conveys the message that you care and want to understand and improve communication.
- *Use an interpreter.* If necessary, get someone to translate your message into the person's primary language.
- *Seek information.* Take advantage of opportunities to learn more about cultural differences in communication (read, travel, go to workshops, and so forth).

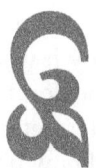

healthy sex hints 11.1

Using Open-Ended Questions to Keep a Sexual Dialogue Flowing

If you want to keep a dialogue flowing, minimize your use of closed-ended questions and maximize your use of open-ended statements. Most closed-ended questions tend to be answered with one- or two-word replies. Open-ended questions (often referred to as *open-ended statements*) cannot be answered with a simple yes or no, and require the person to elaborate.

1. Avoid the Following Types of Closed-Ended Questions:
   "Do you do like this?"
   "Did you like that?"
   "Do you still love me?"
   "Can you remember the last time we made love?"
2. Maximize Your Use of the Following Types of Open-Ended Questions and Statements:
   "Tell me what you like about this."
   "Tell me more about what you didn't like about that."
   "How do you feel about this?"
   "What are your thoughts about that?"
   "Describe that more fully."
   "What are your thoughts about. . . .?"
   "Explain that more completely."
   "What made you decide to do that?"
3. Use Open-Ended Questions and Statements To Explore Thoughts, Feelings, and Behavior. Our sexual behavior is intimately linked to both the cognitive (thoughts) and affective (feelings) domains. Take time to explore all three domains with your partner.

Open-Ended Questions

Open-ended questions are excellent for initiating a dialogue because they cannot be answered with a simple yes/no response. Imagine that you want to explore how your partner likes to be touched. You initiate, using an open-ended question such as, "Tell me more about how you like to be touched," or "What else can I do to make you feel good?" Open-ended questions require information from the other person. Your partner can't respond with a simple yes/no answer. Open-ended questions will get your partner talking and draw out additional detail and emotion.

Open-ended questions
Sentences that require information from the other person

Paraphrasing

Paraphrasing means interpreting the meaning of a message and restating it in one's own words. Paraphrasing is another way to initiate a conversation and obtain additional information by getting a person to talk. Imagine that you want to follow up on something your partner said about sex last night. You could initiate a conversation by paraphrasing your partner's comments from the previous evening.

For instance, in discussing last night's conversation about sexual technique, you might say, "I was thinking about what you said last night. What

Paraphrasing Restating a message in one's own words

I heard you say was that you like it when I squeeze your scrotum firmly," or, "So, what you were saying last night is that you really enjoy it when I bite gently on your nipples," or, "I sense from last night that you don't like it when I put my tongue in your ear." Paraphrasing requires interpretation, or reading between the lines. Your partner usually will let you know if you are on target or off base in your interpretation of the initial message.

Simple Declarative Statements

Declarative statement A verbal initiating technique that does not require a response to a message

Sometimes simple **declarative statements** about a sexual topic can initiate a dialogue. These are not as direct as the previous two techniques because they do not specifically require a response. They can be useful, however, especially to test the waters to see how someone feels or what he or she thinks about some sexual topic. Imagine you just read some sexually provocative story in a magazine and are interested in discussing it with your partner. You could simply state this as a declarative sentence: "I just read a fascinating story in this magazine about what men desire most in sexual relationships." By tossing out this simple declarative statement, you could assess whether your partner wants to pursue the discussion and gauge his or her feelings about it. You might follow up with an open-ended statement or let it pass if your partner shows no interest.

Yes/No Questions

Yes/no questions A verbal initiating technique involving a question that requires only a yes or no response

The weakest way to initiate a dialogue—and the way most of us start conversations—is to ask direct **yes/no questions.** These are questions that can be answered by a simple yes or no. They don't require explanation or embellishment in the way that open-ended statements and paraphrasing do. Although they are useful for verifying facts ("Do you like it when I touch you like this?" "Does this feel good?"), when they are overused, they can shut down a dialogue.

Listening Skills

Passive listening One-way listening; provides no feedback

There are two types of listening: passive and active. In **passive listening** the listener merely soaks in what the initiator of the message is sending. Passive listening is what we do when watching television, a movie, the radio, and so on. It is one-way communication. Although passive listening can be an effective way to receive sexual information, it is not the most effective form of listening to another person when trying to establish or maintain a dialogue.

Active listening Listening with understanding and providing feedback

Active listening is much better than passive listening for dealing with interpersonal communication because, by definition, it requires feedback. Active listeners show that they are listening by providing both nonverbal and verbal feedback. For this reason, active listening is demanding. It takes a lot of energy and concentration, and the listener can easily get distracted and lose interest.

Letting the sender know that the receiver is listening actively can be accomplished through a variety of nonverbal cues. First, the listener adopts a relaxed pose and maintains eye contact. Additional techniques include nodding the head and smiling. Simple verbal cues such as "uh huh," combined with eye contact and head nodding, are enough to let the speaker know the receiver is listening.

personal exploration activity
My Personal Sexual Dictionary

Sexual communication is made even more difficult by the lack of a comfortable vocabulary that does not offend anyone. Most of us have heard an amazing number of different words for the various parts of sexual anatomy and sexual acts. To make our own sexual communication easier, we may find it helpful to identify which words we are comfortable using and hearing used. In this activity, you will create your own personal list of sexual terms that you like and enjoy using.

For the following sexual terms, list all the words you feel comfortable using and enjoy hearing. These can be words you have made up, words from your childhood, slang, words you as a couple have made up, or technical terms. The terms for making your list are *vagina, penis, intercourse, masturbation, breast,* and *testicles.*

When you have listed all your favorites, ask your partner to do the same and then compare your list. If one of you has listed a word that the other finds offensive, discuss what about the word offends. Decide as a couple what words you want to eliminate and what words you want to use together. You may find this activity makes asking for what you want and need sexually a little easier when you have a comfortable communication tool. If you are not in a relationship now, do this exercise with a friend. You may find you are quite different in your likes and dislikes.

Responding Skills

The message receiver reacts to the initiator's message and encodes some type of feedback using verbal or nonverbal communication. If the message was understood and no further clarification is necessary, the receiver can make a simple declarative statement, acknowledging the message with agreement, disagreement, or new information. If the receiver disagrees, or has problems, he or she can use **"I" language** to express opinions. An example is "I hear what you're saying, and I understand your point, but I disagree with that position. I see it differently."

"I" language Taking responsibility for feelings by saying "I feel" versus "You make me feel"

Often, responding skills go beyond merely providing feedback and are used to get additional information needed to understand an issue or to solve a problem. Keeping the conversation going or requesting more information relies on being able to draw more information out of the initiator. Open-ended statements, paraphrasing, and simple yes/no questions, discussed earlier in the chapter, can be used to respond as well as initiate. An additional responding technique that can be powerful is mirroring.

Open-Ended Statements

The open-ended statement is an excellent responding technique because it provides feedback and also keeps the dialogue going. A response such as, "I hear what you're saying—tell me more about how you feel about masturbation," lets the sender know you are with him or her and want additional information.

Paraphrasing

Paraphrasing lets senders know you are listening but goes one step further by giving them an idea of how you interpret their message. For instance, a response such as "What I heard you say is that you can accept masturbation as a form of sexual release in general but personally don't feel good about it" lets the sender know you are listening and also provides the opportunity for the sender to know what you think he or she said. The sender usually will let you know if your interpretation is accurate or if you missed the point.

Mirroring

Mirroring Restating the message exactly, including body language

A powerful technique for providing feedback and keeping a person talking is **mirroring**—restating the person's exact words while mimicking the body posturing. This is done intentionally for impact. Mirroring is useful when someone says something that has strong emotional connotations. The message was so powerful that you do not want to risk weakening or misinterpreting it. Let's say a friend tells you she was so angry at the lewd comments a stranger made to her as she walked by him that she felt she could kill him. You would mirror it by saying, "You were so angry you felt you could kill him!" This usually prompts the person to continue and go into the greater detail you desire.

Yes/No Questions

The weakest type of response in a dialogue—and the way most of us seek additional information about something—is to ask direct yes/no questions. Although these are useful for verifying facts ("Do you like it when I touch you like this?" "Does this feel good?"), they are easy to overuse, can make people feel defensive, and can shut down a dialogue. Once the receiver encodes a response, the communication process shifts back to the sender. We have now come full circle from sender encoding, receiver decoding, receiver encoding, and providing feedback that now becomes information to be decoded by the sender. And the cycle begins all over again.

Barriers to Sexual Communication

In the next section we'll discuss overcoming barriers to effective sexual communication. Most of the barriers to effective sexual communication are related to the skills discussed previously in this chapter, and include failure to initiate, picking an inappropriate time or place, not being specific enough, lack of active listening and assertiveness, saying no when we mean yes, and failing to make requests. Although these barriers may seem insurmountable, in fact they can be overcome if you are aware of their presence, have the desire to overcome them, and are willing to work on improving your communication skills and changing them.

Failing to Initiate

One of the biggest barriers to effective sexual communication is failing to initiate. As we discussed previously in this chapter, initiating any conversation, let alone a sexual one, requires that you first realize that it is your responsibility to initiate the conversation. Whether you want to meet someone new who attracts you or discuss something with your long-term lover, you cannot wait and assume the other person will get the ball rolling for you. Failing to initiate is your problem, not the receiver's.

Using "I" language is a great way to start a dialogue, especially when discussing sexual concerns. When using "I" language, communicators take responsibility for their feelings. For example, let's say your boyfriend has made fun of your outfit in front of three other mutual friends. Rather than blame your boyfriend by saying, "You really made me feel bad," you could say, "I felt bad when you criticized my outfit in front of our friends." Rather than blame your friend for what you are feeling, express you own your feelings and state them in "I" language.

The situation and feelings about what happened should be stated in clear, simple terms. General statements like "I hate it when you treat me like a sex object" or "I hate it when you do things like that" should be avoided. Good communicators specify exactly what the other person did that they dislike. It's better to say things like "I don't like you to talk about my sexual behavior or level of desire in front of your friends," or "I really feel like a fool when you talk about my sexual needs in front of my friends." Specifying exactly *what* you dislike (talking about sexual needs) and the context (in front of your friends) clarifies the situation and leaves no room for misunderstanding.

Using "I" language when trying to meet others shows the other person that you are being responsible for your feelings and you really care: "Hi, I'm Rich. I find myself agreeing with a lot of your viewpoints about things. I really liked what you said in political science class today. Can we talk about it over a cup of coffee in the Student Center?"

❧ *Physical Wellness* ❧

Good communication takes time and energy. Often we are too tired, too stressed, and too busy to communicate effectively. Sometimes when our energy level is low, we simply don't have the energy to think clearly and communicate well. Spending our energy on talking and active listening seems beyond our ability during times of low energy. Stress also robs us of energy, puts us on edge, and contributes to our being overly defensive. It's hard to communicate effectively when we are on edge. We don't listen effectively or have empathy when we are stressed out.

Inappropriate Time and Place

Choosing the appropriate time and place to initiate a discussion about sexuality is important. To be able to relax, each person needs to feel safe and secure. This is important for establishing new relationships as well as strengthening existing ones. The best time to address issues and problems is when they occur. Taking the time to clear things up, before they are allowed to progress, can prevent problems from escalating.

Often, however, situational constraints prevent this. Other people may be around, you're in the middle of something else, or you don't have enough time right then. In these cases, you should tell the other person you need

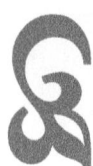

healthy sex hints 11.2

How to Initiate Sexual Conversations

The following five suggestions were designed to help you initiate sexual conversations more effectively.

1. *Take Responsibility.* Don't assume the other person will start the conversation. If you want to discuss an issue or tackle a problem, it is your responsibility to start the conversation.
2. *Don't Assume Anything.* People are not mind readers. Don't assume that other people understand how you feel or what you are thinking. Although your thoughts and feelings regarding the issue may seem obvious to you, they are often misunderstood by others until you explain them.
3. *Choose the Right Time and Place.* You may have the best intentions, but if you choose the wrong time and place to initiate your conversation it can sabotage everything. While it is best to deal with problems when they arise, it isn't always convenient (or possible) to do so. In this case, let the other person know that you have something important to discuss with them and that you will need 20–30 minutes of their time. Ask them when it would be convenient to them to talk.
4. *Use "I" Language.* Don't blame the other person for what you are feeling or thinking. Take responsibility for your thoughts and feelings by stating your concerns using "I" language.
5. *Use Open-Ended Statements.* The best way to involve the other person in the conversation once you have initiated the conversation is to finish up with an open-ended statement. This invites them to join the conversation, and minimizes the likelihood that they will respond to you with a shortened response. For example saying something like, "So what do you think about this?" or "What are your feelings about what I just said?", invite the other person to explain their position.

some time alone with him or her to discuss something important. The two of you should be in a neutral territory where you feel safe and emotionally strong, with enough time so neither of you feels rushed. In the case of meeting someone new, initiators should wait until they can speak to the person alone, away from friends.

In new relationships, talking in public in less intimate settings is sometimes better. A booth in a restaurant, a bench in the park, under a tree on campus all afford privacy yet are public enough to ensure safety and security until you get to know each other better. When dealing with problems or concerns in an established relationship, time should be sufficient to discuss the issues completely. Privacy and undisturbed time are ensured by shutting off the TV, putting the answering machine on the phone, closing the door to your room, and giving each other undivided attention. Some people prefer the privacy of their bedrooms when talking about sex. As one student explained, "I like to talk about sex in the bedroom—not when we're making love, but at other times. I like to close the door, prop up a few pillows, unplug the phone, and talk. Sometimes we'll have a glass of wine, relax, and let our feelings flow." Other people prefer discussing sex outdoors. A student described it this way: "I like to get outdoors to talk to my wife about sex. We go for a long walk somewhere in the mountains or in a local park along the canal. There's something open but private about strolling slowly, hand in hand, and discussing our feelings. It works for us."

❧ *Environmental/Occupational Wellness* ❧

Some of the barriers to effective communication are environmental in nature. Privacy, safety, and a nonthreatening, non-distracting environment are essential for effective sexual communication. Most people find that talking about intimate personal issues in public places is somewhat threatening. A walk in the woods or along the beach or in a park sometimes can create a facilitative setting and mood for communicating about sexual matters.

The workplace can be a particularly challenging place to communicate. Men and women of different cultures and ages all come together around a common work theme. The potential for miscommunication is great, so extra care must be taken to communicate effectively and to take responsibility for miscommunication.

Lack of Specificity

Being critical of a partner's behavior at times is normal in any long-term relationship. Being critical of someone's *behavior,* however, is different from being critical of the person. A sure-fire way to sabotage an attempt to discuss sexual concerns is to criticize the partner rather than the behavior. It is important to criticize the behavior, not the person. People have to understand that the other still loves them but does not like a certain behavior. The partner probably is unaware of how the behavior affects the other. The more precision in describing exactly what a person did or said, the better is the chance of clearing up the problem without hurting the person's feelings. "I really feel hurt when you reject my sexual advances" is a lot easier to deal with than "You're a jerk for rejecting me." Sexual messages are difficult to interpret clearly, even under the best of circumstances.

People in long-term relationships are no exception. Mixed messages—contradictory messages—usually are a result of nonverbal cues not matching verbal messages or people saying something they don't really mean.

For instance, if a partner asks, "Do you like it when I do this?" and the response is, "Yeah, sure," while the body is tight and the facial expression is pained, the message is mixed.

We send mixed messages for various reasons. In some cases, we are unsure where we stand or how we feel. The message is mixed because feelings are mixed. Sometimes we send mixed messages because we are unable or unwilling to be assertive and say no or tell the other person how we really feel. In the worst case, we send mixed messages because we play games and deliberately want to keep people off balance and unsure of our position. This approach may be linked to unhealthy sex role stereotyping based on positioning for power and control in relationships.

The bottom line in mixed messages is that they impair the communication process, making it difficult to understand the true meaning of what

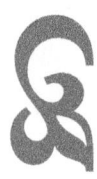

healthy sex hints 11.3

How to Be a Better Listener

1. **Keep yourself in good mental and physical shape.** We listen better when we are mentally and physically alert.
2. **Keep eye contact with the speaker whenever possible.** This will assure the speaker that what he or she is saying is being heard.
3. **Listen actively rather than passively.** In other words, exert energy and use body language to reflect what the speaker is saying. Nod in agreement, smile or laugh at the speaker's humor, and the like.
4. **Avoid distracting mannerisms.** Things such as hair twirling, fingernail inspecting, and similar behaviors convey boredom or disinterest.
5. **Ask questions** when you don't understand something the speaker is saying. Repeat what the speaker has said, in different words, to convey understanding.
6. **Resist the temptation to let your mind wander.** It's easy to do considering that a person can think much faster than he or she can speak. The best listeners make the speaker feel like he or she is the only person in the world at that moment. By following these tips, you can join the ranks of good listeners.

is going on. Healthy sexuality revolves around effective communication, based on personal knowledge and the desire to communicate honestly.

Failing to Listen Actively

Many sexual communication problems, too, revolve around failure to listen actively. Instead of giving undivided attention and providing feedback, we get caught in a variety of bad listening habits that impair our ability to listen actively.

Lack of Assertiveness

Assertiveness Pursuing one's own needs and wants without infringing on others

Aggressiveness Pursuing one's own wants and needs without regard for the rights of others

Assertiveness is a positive attribute, based on mutual respect and democracy in relationships. Assertiveness means understanding one's own wants and needs and pursuing them without infringing on others' ability to do the same. **Aggressiveness,** on the other hand, means pursuing one's needs and wants without regard to how this affects the rights of the others. Often, aggressive people get their needs met at the expense of others. Nonassertive people fail to pursue their needs and wants while allowing others to meet theirs. They fail to stick up for their rights and allow others to take advantage of them, often denying what is going on (Smith, 1993).

Assertiveness is important to effective communication. Many people are not assertive because they confuse assertiveness with aggressiveness. In an attempt to control what they perceive as aggressiveness, they act nonassertively and fail to meet their needs while allowing hostility and frustration to build up inside themselves, weakening their communication and relationships. Often, lack of assertiveness is based in religious, cultural, or gender role expectations, and transcends lack of skill or desire to assert

case study 11.3

Sirahana

Sirahana, 22, single, identifies as Iranian American.

Sirahana was a senior with a major in finance, enrolled in the human sexuality class to fulfill her free elective requirement and to learn more about herself. Normally an "A" student, Sirahana was having trouble with a couple of assignments that required her to write brief reactions about the influence of culture and religion on her sexuality.

She came to see Dr. Blonna about this matter and explained that the assignments forced her to examine things about her life and culture that were painful to her. She had been able to avoid these subjects because she had lived away from home for the past four years and was able to hide them from her parents. In a couple of months, however, school would be ending, and her parents expected her to move in with her Iranian family.

Sirahana would have to make some tough choices. She had a steady boyfriend, Sean, who was Irish Catholic. She had never told her parents about Sean because their relationship started out as a casual, lighthearted romance that neither thought would last.

Little by little, it blossomed as their attraction for each other grew. She practically lived at his off-campus apartment and wanted to move in full-time once school ended in the summer. They had talked seriously about marriage and eventually children, neither one wanting to let their religious beliefs stand in the way of their love.

Sirahana explained that she was feeling a tremendous amount of guilt over her desire to live apart from her family with Sean. Her parents, culture, and religion all expected her to follow tradition by living at home and ultimately marrying someone of her own faith. It was such a strong expectation that she felt utterly paralyzed at the thought of talking to her parents about it. She also knew that she loved Sean and wanted to start a new life with him. She didn't want to move back home.

She liked the freedom of her current life and felt less and less drawn by the covenants and traditions of her religion and culture. She also loved and respected her parents, and deeply appreciated all they had done to put her through school and rear her. She wanted to talk to them, explain exactly what she was feeling, and help them understand, but she didn't know how or where to begin.

Critical Thinking

How have your cultural beliefs and traditions influenced your relationships with current or former partners?

---

oneself. Some cultures require subjugating one's personal desires to those of the dominant partner in the relationship.

In many cultures, the male partner is the dominant member of the couple. Women are expected to put their needs behind those of their partner and behave in ways expected of them. Respecting the wishes of the partner and the culture is taught to be more important than one's own needs. The conflict between these traditional ways of behaving, and U.S. cultural values focusing on the individual and self-actualization, is a source of stress and sexual dissatisfaction for many women.

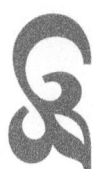

healthy sex hints 11.4

Assert Yourself With the DESC Technique

The DESC model is a powerful tool for helping you make requests, deliver criticism more effectively, and become more precise in your assertiveness. The DESC model has four steps:

1. *D—describe:* Paint a verbal picture of the situation or the other person's behavior that is a source of stress. Be as precise as possible: "Honey, when you use language like 'I'm feeling horny—let's fuck,'. . . ."
2. *E—express:* Express your feelings about the incident using "I" language: "I feel seedy and cheap" or "I feel very uncomfortable."
3. *S—specify:* Be specific in identifying alternative ways that you would prefer the person to speak or behave: "I'd like you to soften your language and say, 'I'm feeling sexy—let's make love.'"
4. *C—consequences:* Identify the consequences that will follow if the person does (pro) or doesn't (con) comply with your wishes: "In the future, if you do soften your language, I'll be much more likely to get in the mood and want to make love with you (pro)." "If you don't, and you continue to use such crude language, I can't guarantee that I won't be turned off and not feel sexy." When using this model, precision is important in describing the other person's offending behavior or actions. As mentioned previously in this chapter, focus your criticism on the offensive behavior, not the person (Bower and Bower, 1976; Greenberg, 2003).

Saying Yes When We Mean No

When people are nonassertive, they say yes to others' demands when they really want to say no. They spend an inordinate amount of time pleasing others without being reciprocated. They forsake their sexual needs and wants while granting the partner's desires. Although sharing and sacrificing are important to relationships, they become a problem when this behavior is always one-way and not reciprocated.

When people are nonassertive, they are filled with resentment and hostility toward their partner as a result. It's a vicious cycle. Originally, in an attempt to avoid conflict, discomfort, or hurting the partner's feelings, they say yes when they really mean no. This response temporarily relieves them from feeling guilty.

Unfortunately, however, when they do this, they get trapped into doing things they really don't want to do. When this result happens, they begin to feel miserable because they've lost control of their lives and lost their self-respect. Not only do they feel stressed because of this situation, but it also affects their sexual response. Desire and arousal are difficult when a person feels stressed and angry. The only way to stop the cycle is to begin to say no. This brings us full circle to the same situation as the initial one: having to say no. If people are assertive to begin with, they can avoid the aggravation and stress.

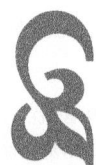

healthy sex hints 11.5

Saying No

Saying no isn't always easy, but it is essential if you are to be assertive and reduce your stress. You have the right to say no. The following are clear guidelines:

1. *Face the other person from a normal distance.* If you are too far away, you may appear timid. If you crowd the person, you border on aggressiveness.
2. *Look the person directly in the eyes.* Averting eye contact is a sure giveaway that you'll cave in.
3. *Keep your head up and your body relaxed.* Don't be a shrinking violet.
4. *Speak clearly and firmly, at a volume that can be heard clearly.*
5. *Just say no.* You don't have to clarify why.
6. *Be prepared to repeat it.* Sometimes people are persistent. Be prepared to say it again.
7. *Stick to your guns.* Don't give in. It gets easier with practice.

If you feel a need to explain why you are declining, here are a few tips for setting the stage:

1. Thank the person for the offer: "Gee, thanks, but *no.* I really can't [don't want to] . . ."
2. Express appreciation: "I really appreciate the offer, but *no.* I'm not interested/too busy/ don't want any . . ."
3. Affirm your friendship: "I enjoy your company, and I'd like to do something together, but *no.*"
4. Reject the offer, not the person: "Please don't take this personally. I like you, but *no, I don't . . .*"

Failing to Make Requests

Assertiveness is directly related to requesting things you desire and saying no to things you don't want to do. People have many reasons for not making explicit sexual requests. As we've already discussed, language poses a unique barrier. Feeling comfortable with sexual language is important, and finding a comfortable language level helps. If sex has been a taboo topic of conversation while growing up, it may be difficult to talk about openly. People enter their first relationship without having had the benefit of knowing that talking about sex is OK. Shaking this taboo is sometimes difficult. You can become more comfortable by proceeding slowly, acknowledging your fears and discomfort, and allowing yourself to take chances and grow out of your old ways of thinking and feeling.

Another barrier is not taking responsibility for one's wants, needs, and feelings. First, the individual has to find out who he or she is as a sexual person. Then the person has to accept this. The third step is to share it with the partner. The partner can't know who the other is, what he or she needs, and how to please that person without the other person's taking responsibility to communicate this.

Our sexuality is continually growing and evolving. A married student expressed it this way in class:

My wife is always saying that she shouldn't have to explain what she wants sexually. We've been together for 10 years, and I should know how to please her and what her needs are. I have a hard time with this. My own needs change from day to day and from sexual encounter to sexual encounter. One day I may want her to take the lead and initiate sex and be dominant while I lie back and let her take me. The next time we make love, I might want to initiate. I know she's the same way, but I can't tell in advance without her communicating her desires to me.

We need to take responsibility for what we're feeling and make requests accordingly, using "I" language.

✎ Emotional Wellness ✎

Emotional wellness affects the ability to communicate clearly. Communicating effectively is difficult even under the best of circumstances. Communicating about sexuality poses unique challenges because of the sensitive nature of the topic. Even though people may want to communicate more effectively, emotions sometimes get in the way. They might feel embarrassed talking about their most intimate desires, thoughts, and feelings. They also might feel guilty about some of these things. These emotions often make it difficult to think clearly and logically. A first step in sexual communication is to identify how we are feeling and to take responsibility for owning these feelings. Once we assume ownership for our feelings, we can use "I" language to communicate them to our intimate partner.

Thinking More Logically About Sex

Sometimes we fail to communicate clearly because our sexual thinking is irrational or illogical. Our sexual perspective, or belief system—as Albert Ellis (1993), the father of rational emotive behavior therapy (REBT), calls it—is disordered. Ellis believes that our *perception* of our partners and specific sexual situations (not the actual person or situation) gives them meaning and determines whether they become a source of dissatisfaction and miscommunication.

For instance, Khalid and Teri have been lovers for a year and have been happy with their sexual lifestyle. They make love about once a week and engage in a variety of sexual behaviors they find enjoyable. Last night, after they came home from the movies, Khalid wanted to make love and Teri didn't. She was tired and wanted to get to bed early. Feeling rejected, Khalid began to have doubts about their sexual relationship, wondering, "What's wrong with her? Teri should be in the mood when I am. What's wrong with our relationship?" In reality, nothing is wrong with their relationship. They are happy, enjoy each other's company, and have a satisfying sex life together. The only problem is Khalid's perception of this specific situation.

In their clinical work with neurotic patients, Albert Ellis and Robert Harper (1998) identified a group of 10 commonly held irrational or illogical beliefs about life. These beliefs form the basis of a belief system that gives one a distorted perspective for assessing potentially stressful situations. Using and understanding Ellis and Harper's theory can be simplified by grouping the 10 illogical/irrational beliefs into four categories (Walen, DiGuisseppi, & Wessler, 1980).

Awfulizing statements: These exaggerate the negative aspects/impact of a situation.

Shoulds/musts/oughts: These are beliefs that put illogical demands on oneself and others.

Evaluation-of-worth statements: These imply that some people or things are worthless or a complete waste of time.

Need statements: These are beliefs that set unrealistic, unattainable requirements for happiness.

We often blow things out of proportion, set unrealistic demands for our behavior and that of our partners, misinterpret sexual comments, or have irrational fears about discussing our wants, needs, desires, or problems with our partners. These illogical/irrational beliefs result in undesirable emotional, intellectual, physical, social, and behavioral consequences. Ellis and Harper (1998) use an ABC model to describe this interaction. In this model, the presence of an activating event, A, triggers a series of irrational/illogical beliefs, B, about A. These illogical beliefs about A (not the activating event itself) are the cause of a variety of negative consequences, C.

We'll illustrate the model again using Khalid and Teri:

A—activating event:
   Khalid wanted to make love with his girlfriend Teri when they came home from the movies, but she didn't. She said she wasn't in the mood and wanted to get to bed early.

B—irrational/illogical beliefs:
   "My girlfriend should always be in the mood." "My girlfriend should always be in the mood when I am." "Partners should always be sexually available." "People who are in love should always please their partners sexually." "She must not love me anymore." "She must be having an affair with someone else." "I'm not good enough for her."

C—Consequences
   Physical—muscle tension, upset stomach, tension headache
   Emotional—anger, depression
   Mental—irrational thoughts
   Social—retreating into isolation, breaking off all physical touching
   Behavioral—starting to drink to excess REBT uses logical thinking and positive self-talk as an aid to reducing sexual problems.

Illogical thinking Thought based on inaccurate or irrational perception of information

Ellis and Harper's (1998) ABCDE technique attempts to help us understand our illogical beliefs and self-talk and learn to substitute more rational thoughts in their place. The ABCDE technique builds upon Ellis's ABC model of **illogical thinking** by adding D (dispute) and E (evaluate). D involves disputing each illogical B and substituting a more logical belief in its place. When all of the illogical beliefs have been disputed, the effectiveness of the dispute in defusing the consequences is evaluated.

The ABCDE technique would work like this:

A—Khalid's girlfriend Teri rejecting his offer to make love

B—Khalid's irrational beliefs about A
"My girlfriend should always be in the mood."
"My girlfriend should always be in the mood when I am."
"Partners should always be sexually available."
"People who are in love should always please their partners sexually." "She must not love me anymore."
"She must be having an affair with someone else."
"I'm not good enough for her."

C—Consequences of B
Physical—muscle tension, upset stomach, tension headache
Emotional—anger, depression Mental—irrational thoughts
Social—retreating into isolation, breaking off all physical touching
Behavioral—starting to drink to excess
Illogical thinking Thought based on inaccurate or irrational perception of information

D—Dispute
Khalid decides to tackle this problem by analyzing each of these illogical beliefs and substitute more rational thoughts in their place.
1. "It's irrational for me to think that Teri should always be in the mood."
2. "It's impossible for us both to always be in sync with our sexual desire."
3. "Each partner has the right to say no when he or she is not in the mood to make love."
4. "People can be in love but on any given day not feel sexually responsive."
5. "Teri's not wanting to have sex doesn't necessarily mean she doesn't love me."
6. "Her not wanting to have sex with me doesn't necessarily mean she's doing it with someone else."
7. "I'm great for Teri. This has nothing to do with that."

E—Evaluate
As a result of working through the dispute and coming up with a more rational belief system concerning what happened, Khalid experiences the following changes: Physically, his muscles begin to relax and he can get to sleep again. His tension headache subsides. Emotionally, Khalid feels like a tremendous weight

sex in society 11.3

Ellis and Harper's 10 Illogical Beliefs

Often we are sexually dissatisfied because of illogical or irrational beliefs and expectations we have about sex and our relationships. Ellis and Harper found that when these beliefs form a belief system that is predominately irrational, we are more prone to stress and sexual dissatisfaction. Throughout the course of their clinical work, Ellis and Harper noticed recurring themes or patterns. They distilled these beliefs into 10 that form the basis of an irrational belief system or way of viewing the world. This way of viewing the world could relate to any subject. When it forms the basis of our sexual belief system, it can create sexual problems and make it difficult to communicate effectively.

The beliefs are the following:

1. You must have love or approval from all the people you find significant.
2. You must thoroughly prove adequate, competent, or achieving.
3. When people act obnoxiously or unfairly, you should blame and damn them and see them as bad, wicked, or rotten individuals.
4. You have to view things as awful, terrible, horrible, and catastrophic when you get seriously frustrated, treated unfairly, or rejected.
5. Emotional misery comes from external pressures, and you have little ability to control or change your feelings.
6. If something seems dangerous or fearsome, you must preoccupy yourself with it and make yourself anxious about it.
7. You can more easily avoid facing many life difficulties and self-responsibilities than undertake more rewarding forms of self-discipline.
8. Your past remains all-important, and, because something once strongly influenced your life, it has to keep determining your feelings and behavior today.
9. People and things should turn out better than they do, and you must view it as awful and horrible if you do not find good solutions to life's grim realities.
10. You can achieve maximum human happiness by inertia and inaction or by passively and uncommittedly enjoying yourself.

Source: *New Guide to Rational Living,* by A. Ellis and R. Harper (Hollywood, CA: Wilshire Book Company, 1998).

has been lifted from his shoulders. He feels he is thinking clearly again. Khalid stops drinking and asks Teri whether she wants to snuggle and fall asleep while he reads his book.

Communicating About Disabilities

As we have discussed, communicating sexual needs and wants is often difficult for many people because of their upbringing, the uniqueness of the subject, and the lack of a uniform language of sex. Communicating about special sexual considerations due to disabilities presents a unique challenge for the person with disabilities and his or her partner. Not only does the person have to work through personal issues surrounding sexuality in general, but he or she also has the added challenge of describing how the disability impacts sexual needs and wants (Bullard & Knight, 1981).

As we've seen, disabilities can affect sexual anatomy and physiology, sexual response, and sexual behavior. Describing these effects and the special considerations they bring to the sexual encounter can be a daunting experience for the most proficient communicator. We'll use colostomy as the disability to illustrate these challenges.

Ostomy

Ostomy is a general term used to describe an artificially created opening in the body. The prefix associated with the ostomy denotes the organ where the opening is. A *colostomy* is an opening of the colon, for example, and an *ileostomy* is an opening to the ileum (Alterescu, 1981). The actual connection of the opening to the abdominal wall is referred to as the *stoma*.

Many people are squeamish about the association of an ostomy to organs associated with human waste (urine and feces), and they have a hard time discussing the impact of the ostomy on their sexuality. A colostomy, for instance, redirects the movement of feces from the rectum and anus to the colostomy bag, which is attached to the stoma through a ring and sealed bag secured to the abdominal wall with adhesive material. The bag fills up with waste on a schedule that coincides with the person's bowel movement behavior. The consistency of the fecal material and the frequency of accumulation will vary according to the person's diet, exercise behavior, and overall health. Assuming the person with the colostomy returns to a normal lifestyle following surgery, eventually the person can expect a bowel pattern similar to what he or she experienced prior to the surgery. A person with a colostomy can learn how to clean, change, sanitize, and maintain the colostomy bag to ensure a return to a normal life and control of bowel functioning with normal hygiene.

In reality, having a colostomy does not necessarily impact sexual response and behavior. The physiological changes that occur during arousal and orgasm are, in most cases, unchanged by the procedure.

A person who has undergone a colostomy may experience nerve damage, pain, and the development of scar tissue. These can impact sexual arousal and the enjoyment of sexual activities (Alterescu, 1981). These complications can occur with any surgery, however, and are not exclusive to colostomy. A person with a colostomy can also have temporary mechanical problems associated with securing the ostomy bag to the abdominal wall and securing a leak-free attachment between the ring and the collection bag.

In most cases, sexual problems associated with colostomy are due to psychosocial factors related to the patient's self-perception, depression, and relationship concerns or problems. Desire and the frequency of sexual activity can be affected if the person with the colostomy perceives it negatively and as something that interferes with sexuality in a negative way.

Alterescu (1981) has compiled the following list of questions that many colostomy patients have:

Will my partner(s) still consider me desirable and attractive?

Will I still be capable of maintaining social usefulness as a worker and mother/ father?

Will I (male patient) be capable of achieving/maintaining an erection and ejaculating?

Will I be able to make adjustments in clothing?

Will I experience pain during intercourse?

Will my pouch interfere with my sexual activities?

How will I explain the existence of my pouch to my new partner?

Will my ostomy keep me from being the person I want to be?

Questions like these must be answered honestly and completely by the person with a colostomy and his or her partner in order to have a satisfying sex life. The communication skills discussed in this chapter will help people with a colostomy or other disabilities understand these concerns, transmit them to their partner(s), and keep the dialogue open regarding these issues so they don't lead to deeper response and relationship problems.

Foremost, this chapter has demonstrated how the responsibility for sexual communication lies with the individual. People with a colostomy or any other disability must discuss the nature of their disabilities with their intimate partners and helping professionals if necessary. They must seek to learn all they can about how their disability impacts their sexuality and take responsibility for transmitting this information to their intimate partners.

Personal Assessment

Sexual Communication Satisfaction Questionnaire

This questionnaire assesses your satisfaction with your sexual communication with your partner. Use the following scale to indicate how strongly you agree or disagree with each statement:

1 = Strongly agree   4 = Disagree

2 = Agree   5 = Strongly disagree

3 = Neither agree nor disagree

1. I tell my partner when I am especially sexually satisfied.

2. I am satisfied with my partner's ability to communicate his/her sexual desires to me.

3. I do not let my partner know things that I find pleasing during sex.

4. I am very satisfied with the quality of our sexual interactions.

5. I do not hesitate to let my partner know when I want to have sex with him/her.

6. I do not tell my partner whether or not I am sexually satisfied.

7. I am dissatisfied over the degree to which my partner and I discuss our sexual relationship.

8. I am not afraid to show my partner what kind of sexual behavior I find satisfying.

9. I would not hesitate to show my partner what is a sexual turn-on to me.

10. My partner does not show me when he/she is sexually satisfied.

11. I show my partner what pleases me during sex.

12. I am displeased with the manner in which my partner and I communicate with each other during sex.

13. My partner does not show me things he/she finds pleasing during sex.

14. I show my partner when I am sexually satisfied.

15. My partner does not let me know whether sex has been satisfying or not.

16. I do not show my partner when I am sexually satisfied.

17. I am satisfied concerning my ability to communicate about sexual matters with my partner.

18. My partner shows me by the way he/she touches me if he/she is satisfied.

19. I am dissatisfied with my partner's ability to communicate his/her sexual desire to me.

20. I have no way of knowing when my partner is sexually satisfied.

21. I am not satisfied in the majority of our sexual interactions.

22. I am pleased with the manner in which my partner and I communicate with each other after sex.

Thought Questions

1. What makes communicating about sex different from communicating about other subjects?

2. Define metacommunication. What are the parts of a metacommunication model?

3. What four sets of skills are involved in two-way communication?

4. What is "I" language? Give examples of using "I" language.

5. How do we communicate about sexuality nonverbally? Is nonverbal sexual communication accurate?

6. What is the best thing to do if miscommunication becomes apparent? Whose responsibility is it? Why?

7. Give examples of four open-ended sexual statements.

8. What is the impact of language level on sexual communication?

9. What are three barriers to effective listening?

10. What are two barriers to correcting miscommunication?

11. What should you do if you reach a communication impasse?

12. Describe the effects of a disability such as colostomy on sexual communication.

Test Yourself

1. Which statement best characterizes communicating about sex?
   a. It is easier than communicating about other topics because everyone likes sex.
   b. It is harder than communicating about other topics because of the subject and the personal nature of the material.
   c. It is easier because of the personal nature of the subject matter.
   d. It is harder because the subject is personal and immaterial.

2. Metacommunication focuses on
   a. the actual content being discussed.
   b. the content and the relationship between the communicators.
   c. the content and the metaphysical nature of human sexuality.
   d. the relationship between the communicators.

3. The key to successful communications using Berne's transactional analysis model is
   a. communicating on the same ego state as your partner.
   b. communicating on a different ego state than your partner.
   c. trying to keep your ego state out of objective communication with your partner.
   d. keeping your ego out of communications.

4. Which of the following represents a true exchange of information between two people?
   a. Selflessness
   b. Monologue
   c. Dialogue
   d. Information giving

5. Which statement best describes how men and women communicate?
   a. Research shows that men tend to focus more on wanting to solve problems, whereas women want to share emotions.
   b. Research shows that men and women are very similar in their communication patterns.
   c. Research shows that women tend to focus more on wanting to solve problems, whereas men want to share emotions.
   d. Research shows that women and men focus equally on problem solving and sharing emotions.

6. Nonverbal forms of sexual communication
   a. generally are not very useful in communicating sexual content.
   b. are often just as effective in communicating sexual needs and wants as verbal forms.
   c. should be avoided until you get to know a person better.
   d. have no place in effective sexual communication.

7. What is the relationship between language level and sexual miscommunication?
   a. Miscommunication can occur when the language levels of the two communicators differs.
   b. Miscommunication occurs because people from different countries have different words to describe things.
   c. It is easiest to avoid miscommunication by using scientific/professional language, which is the most precise language level.
   d. Miscommunication is less likely to occur if both partners use a lower language level.
8. "I" language refers to
   a. maintaining eye contact when you are communicating.
   b. being very assertive about your sexual needs and desires.
   c. taking personal responsibility for feelings.
   d. putting blame for problems on others where it belongs.
9. Using open-ended statements is effective when you want your partner to
   a. expand on how he or she feels about an issue.
   b. get a simple yes or no answer to a simple question.
   c. leave things kind of open to debate.
   d. put off closure on the subject.
10. DESC is a communication model that is useful for
   a. using verbal aggressiveness to resolve communication problems.
   b. using verbal assertiveness to resolve communication problems.
   c. describing communication problems that are descriptive in nature.
   d. expressing deep-seated sexual problems to your partner.

Web Resources

Real World University; Relationship Skills Page

http://www.rwuniversity.com/articles.cfm?id=87&action=show

Real World University's (RWU) mission is to help students succeed in college and in life by helping them identify and pursue their purpose, strengthen their character, overcome life's obstacles, and maximize their potential. This is a page from their website that is dedicated to communicating effectively in relationships.

DiscoveryHealth.Com's Love and Relationships Page

http://health.discovery.com/centers/loverelationships/loverelationships.html

This is the love and relationships page of DiscoveryHealth.Com. It offers a variety of assessments and links to other pages devoted to this subject.

References

Alterescu, V. (1981). Sexual functioning following creation of an abdominal stoma. In D. G. Bullard & S. E. Knight (Eds.), *Sexuality and physical disability.* St. Louis: Mosby.

Andersen, P. A. (1999). *Nonverbal communication: Form and function.* Mountain View, CA: Mayfield.

Berne, E. (1960). *Transactional analysis in psychotherapy.* New York: Grove.

Bower, S. A., & Bower, G. H. (1976). *Asserting yourself: A practical guide for positive change.* Reading, MA: Addison-Wesley.

Bullard, D. G., & Knight, S. E. (Eds.). (1981). *Sexuality and physical disability.* St. Louis: Mosby.

Dou, W. L., & Clark, W. (1999, Summer–Fall). Appreciating the diversity in multicultural communication styles. *Business Forum, 24*(3–4), 54–62.

Ellis, A. (1993). Reflections on rational emotive therapy. *Journal of Consulting and Clinical Psychology, 61*(2), 199–201.

Ellis, A., & Harper, R. (1998). *A new guide to rational living.* North Hollywood, CA: Wilshire.

Greenberg, J. S. (2003). *Comprehensive stress management* (8th ed.). Boston: McGraw-Hill.

Hall, E. (1973). *The silent language.* Menlo Park, CA: Cummings.

Ivey, A. E., D'Andrea, M. D., Ivey, M. B., & Simek-Morgan, L. (2002). *Theories of counseling and psychotherapy: A multicultural perspective* (5th ed.). Boston: Allyn & Bacon.

Mandel, B. (1980, Summer). Communication: A four-part process. *Hotliner, 1*(4), 6.

McBurney, L. (2002, Spring). Touch me—not there! How to be sensual without necessarily being sexual. *Marriage Partnership, 19*(1), 26–29.

McGinty, K., Knox, D., & Zusman, M. E. (2003, March).

Michaud, S. L., & Warner, R. M. (1997, October). Gender differences in self-reported troubles talk. *Sex Roles: A Journal of Research, 37* (7–8), 527–541.

Noller, P., & Fitzpatrick, M. A. (1991). Marital communication. In A. Booth (Ed.), *Contemporary families: Looking backward, looking forward.* Minneapolis: Council on Family Relations.

Nonverbal and verbal communication in "involved" and "casual" relationships among college students. *College Student Journal, 37*(1), 68–72.

Sawyer, C. R., & Behnke, R. R. (2002, Fall). Behavioral inhibition and the communication of public speaking state anxiety. *Western Journal of Communication, 66*(4), 12–23.

Senecal, S., Murard, N., & Hess, U. (2003, January). Do you know what I feel? Partners' predictions and judgements of each other's emotional reactions to emotion-eliciting situations. *Sex Roles: A Journal of Research,* 21–38.

Smith, J. C. (1993). *Creative stress management.* Englewood Cliffs, NJ: Prentice Hall.

Tannen, D. (1990). *You just don't know: Women and men in conversation.* New York: Morrow.

Walen, S., DiGuisseppi, R., & Wessler, R. (1980). *A practitioner's guide to RET.* New York: Oxford University Press.

Watzlawick, P., Beaven, J. H., & Jackson, D. D. (1967). *Pragmatics of human communication.* New York: Norton.

Wheeless, L. R., Wheeless, V. E., & Baus, R. (1984). Sexual Communication, Communication Satisfaction, and Solidarity in the Developmental Stages of Intimate Relationships, *Western Journal of Speech Communication, 48*(3), pg. 224.

chapter
twelve

Sexual Dysfunction, Sex Therapy, *and* Sexual Enhancement

Student Learning Objectives

After reading this chapter, students will be able to:

- Describe the relationship between sexual dysfunctions and the phases of the sexual response cycle.
- Describe the key components of sexual desire disorders.
- Describe the key components of sexual arousal disorders.
- Describe the main elements of orgasmic disorders.
- Describe the main elements of sexual pain disorders.
- Describe the psychological causes of sexual dysfunctions.
- Evaluate recent criticisms of the current conceptualizations of sexual disorders based on the classic sexual response cycle.
- Describe the medical and pharmacological causes of sexual dysfunctions.
- Differentiate prior learning and immediate causes of sexual dysfunctions.
- Evaluate the effects of legal and illicit psychoactive substances on sexual dysfunction.

activity teaser: How can you improve your sexual response? Find out with the Personal Exploration Activity on page 437

case study 12.1

Orgasmic Disorders: Christine

Christine, 25, single, is white.

Christine is a college senior. She has been having sex with her boyfriend, Nick, for about 3 months and has not been able to have an orgasm yet. She met with Dr. Blonna.

I'm not sure whether I have a problem, but I've been having sex with my boyfriend, Nick, since the end of the spring semester—about 3 months—and haven't had an orgasm yet.

He's a real nice guy, and I think I love him. I've been dating lots of guys since my boyfriend Tom and I broke up 3 years ago, and Nick is very special. I met him at the college gym, and we were instantly attracted to each other. He is in great shape, is very outgoing, a former athlete, and has a great sense of humor. In a way, he's a great big kid, always joking.

We started having sex from the first date and all spring made love about three to five times a week, but I never had an orgasm with him. Even though I don't come, sex with him is a lot of laughs. The only problem is that he kind of rushes through it and doesn't last very long. I haven't said anything because I kind of hoped he would get better with time.

During the summer, things cooled off because he had a summer house with a bunch of fraternity brothers and was at the shore every weekend (Friday to Sunday night) from Memorial Day to mid-September. I went down a few times but was really turned off because everyone did nothing but get drunk, act out, and sleep the days away.

Since September, we've picked up where we left off last spring, but I still can't come with him. When I masturbate by myself, I have satisfying orgasms, but not with Nick. I'm afraid that if I tell him, he'll get upset and maybe our relationship will suffer. The problem is that I like him a lot and would like the relationship to grow, but the sex is a real problem. I'm not sure what to do about the relationship.

Critical Thinking

The fact that Christine can achieve orgasm through masturbation is solid evidence that her orgasmic problems have more to do with Nick, and her relationship with him than with herself. What would you recommend Christine do in light of this?

Sexual dysfunction A disturbance or disorder in desire, excitement, orgasm, or resolution of the sexual response cycle

Sexual dysfunctions, as Christine illustrates, are complex phenomena, involving our bodies, minds, past history, relationships, and a host of other factors. According to the *Diagnostic and Statistical Manual*, **sexual dysfunction** is a disturbance or disorder in desire, excitement, orgasm, or resolution of the sexual response cycle (APA, 2000). As we discussed in detail in Chapter 7, the interaction of all five senses plays a key role in the sexual response: becoming sexually aroused, maintaining interest, having an orgasm, and feeling satisfied.

Sensory arousal combines with emotional arousal (limbic system) and conscious thought (cerebral cortex) as our sensing, feeling, thinking brain triggers and directs the organs, glands, and tissues that regulate our sexual response. Although something as common as developing and maintaining an erection seems like a fairly primitive response, in reality it is a complex result of many reactions within a complicated interdependent system. As such, sexual response isn't always an all-or-nothing phenomenon. Levels of performance and satisfaction vary.

Everyone experiences some level of dysfunction throughout the course of life. It is produced by illness, stress, fatigue, or a variety of other causes. Dysfunction is not just a heterosexual issue, either. Gay, lesbian, and bisexual people also experience sexual dysfunction (Lemonick, 2004).

Our perception, gender role, and beliefs about aging all factor into determining whether a sexual problem is or is not a dysfunction. As we'll describe, one of the mediating factors in determining dysfunction is whether the "problem" causes emotional distress or relationship difficulties. One's perception of the issue plays a big part in determining whether it even *is* a problem. If a person or partner does not perceive a sexual "problem" (premature ejaculation, for example) as troubling, is it a dysfunction or even a problem?

Gender role also factors into the mix. For years, women were taught that they were not supposed to initiate sex. Does a woman who wants sex but won't ask for it from her partner because she thinks this isn't the "proper" thing to do have a sexual dysfunction? What about our expectations of sex as we age? If we expect a decline in sexual performance and response because we view this as a normal part of aging, do these changes constitute a dysfunction? We'll address these and many other questions in this chapter.

Basson et al., (2000) carry the issue of gender-based differences a step further. They argue that emotional factors and intimacy issues are the central issues in understanding sexual response and subsequent dysfunction in women. Women, according to these researchers, are much more likely than men to have intimacy issues as the basis of low sexual desire and sexual arousal disorders. In fact, as we will examine in more detail later in this chapter, Basson et al., found that many women who have low sexual desire have no problem becoming aroused physiologically (evidence of lubrication and so forth) and achieving orgasm.

If you recall from Chapter 7, sexual functioning combines physical, intellectual, emotional, social, spiritual, and environmental well-being. We need a minimum level of physical health to ensure that all of the component body parts and systems are able to perform the myriad tasks necessary for sexual response to occur. The health of our social relationships impacts on our ability to trust our partner, relax, and let the sexual response happen. Our emotional health contributes to our self-esteem, feeling good about ourselves, and feeling comfortable with our partner. Our intellectual health contributes to being able to understand and improve our sexual technique and to make informed choices about fertility control and protecting ourselves against STDs. Our spirituality helps us connect with our inner sexuality and others in a deeper way. And a healthy environment allows us to feel safe and comfortable in our sexual space. Stevenson (2002), in an eloquent editorial, describes the interplay of the mind-body continuum in sexual response and dysfunction. He explains how the body does not exist independent of the mind and how sexual dysfunctions can never be diagnosed independently without an examination of the whole person.

Therefore, although we will use the classic diagnostic and etiologic criteria for sexual dysfunctions for practical purposes (since they are the most widely accepted), they must always be examined within the context of the whole person, not merely as just physical or psychological problems.

Physical/Medical Causes of Sexual Dysfunction

Erectile dysfunction
A disturbance or disorder related to obtaining an erection

Research findings over the past decade concerning the causes of sexual dysfunctions have created a dramatic change in our understanding of these conditions and approach to their treatment. In the past, sexual dysfunctions (particularly **erectile dysfunction,** formerly known as *impotence*) had been thought to be caused primarily by psychological factors. Most experts in the field now believe the exact opposite, especially regarding erectile disorder. Sexual dysfunction can be caused by a host of physical causes, ranging from disease and injury to the side effects of legal and illegal drugs (Goldstein, I., Auerbach, S., Palma-Nathan, H., Rajfer, J., Fitch, W., Schmitt, L. (2000). Goldstein, 2000; Johnson, Phelps, Cottler, 2004; Kloner & Padma, 2005; McCabe, 2004; Richardson, 1991).

Recent studies show that understanding sexual dysfunction may not be such a simple either-or phenomenon. It may well be that dysfunction in men is primarily related to blood flow and physical causes (therefore very amenable to pharmacological fixes such as Viagra), whereas problems in women are more related to psychosocial issues such as intimacy (Basson, 2002, Johnson, 2004, Enserink, 2005, *Drug Week*, 2001). The differences may be so great that prominent researchers in the field are calling for a reexamination of the nature of sexual response in women to shed light on how to treat sexual dysfunctions. This may ultimately change the very way dysfunctions are diagnosed and treated in men and women (Basson, 2002, Lieblum, 2000).

Cardiovascular Disease

In a study of approximately 1,300 men in the Massachusetts Male Aging Study, nearly half of the subjects (all were between 40 and 70 years of age) had experienced erectile difficulties in the previous 6 months (Heapes, 1994). Furthermore, men being treated for heart disease and high blood pressure were up to four times more likely to be completely impotent than men without these conditions. These findings implicate vascular problems (blood flow) as the major culprit in erectile problems. All forms of cardiovascular disease rob the blood and body of adequate oxygen through circulation, contributing to increased risk for sexual dysfunction (Kloner & Padma, 2005).

Behaviors that increase the risk for cardiovascular disease also can increase the likelihood of incurring erectile disorders. Smokers have been found to be four times more likely than nonsmokers to have severe erectile dysfunction (Heapes, 1994).

Other Diseases

Other physical causes of sexual dysfunction range from structural defects or changes (congenital abnormality of the penis or vagina, scar tissue, fibroids, tumors), to sexually transmitted disease, endocrine disorders, neurological

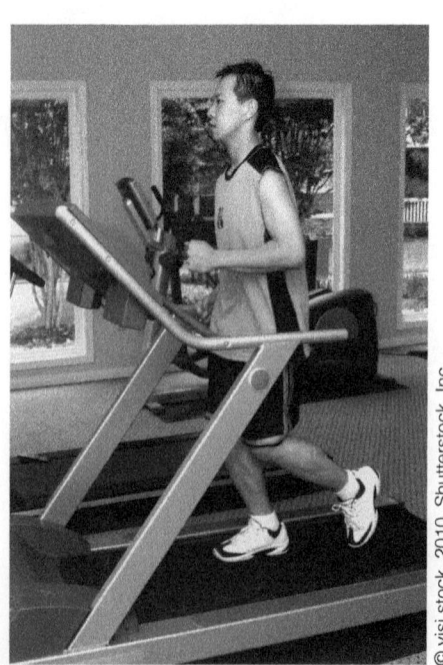

© visi.stock, 2010. Shutterstock, Inc.

Aerobic exercise can reduce the risk for developing certain sexual dysfunctions.

problems, and spinal cord injury, to deficiency diseases (insufficient hormonal production, malnutrition, vitamin deficiency), to allergic reactions (say, to spermicide). These and other medical causes can affect any or all of the phases of the sexual response cycle, resulting in a wide variety of sexual dysfunctions. Table 12.1 describes a variety of chronic diseases and disabilities and their effects on sexual functioning.

> ❧ *Physical Wellness* ❧
>
> High-level physical wellness can enhance sexual performance and satisfaction and lessen the risk for dysfunction. Physical wellness plays a crucial role in the desire and excitement phases of sexual response. Physical wellness is also linked to vasocongestion, as blood flow leading to engorgement of genital tissue and lubrication are affected adversely by obesity, arteriosclerosis, and other physical health problems. Being fit (especially attaining high levels of cardiovascular fitness) and maintaining recommended body composition promote efficient vasocongestion.

Table 12.1 Effects of Select Medical Physical Conditions on Sexual Response

Condition	Effects of Sexual Response
Cardiovascular disease	*Men and women:* sexual arousal disorder; loss of sexual desire
Spinal cord injuries	Vary according to severity and location *Men:* often lose ability to have typical erections (may have "reflex" erections); often lose ability to ejaculate *Women:* decreased vaginal lubrication; lose genital and orgasmic sensations
Complications from surgery (hysterectomy, cesarean section, tubal ligation, episiotomy)	*Women:* damage to nerves and blood vessels involved in vasocongestion; sexual arousal disorder, orgasmic disorder.
Multiple sclerosis and other neurogenic diseases	*Men:* loss of erections and ejaculation *Women:* orgasmic disorder
Diabetes	*Men:* male erectile disorder; small percentage suffers from retrograde ejaculation and less intense ejaculation *Women:* varies—some experience less lubrication and sexual arousal disorder; female orgasmic disorder

Cancer
  Breast
  Cervix
  Uterus
 	
  Prostate
  Testicles
 	
  Anorexia
  Bulimia
	
	Vary based on treatment and psychological reactions
	Minimal if treated early (bleeding; discharge)
	Vary according to amount of scarring; hysterectomy is sometimes related to sexual desire disorder in women who feel a diminished sense of femininity
	Can cause sexual arousal disorder and orgasmic disorder
	Infertility; no physiological changes but psychological stress is related to sexual desire disorder in some men who feel a diminished masculinity
	Sexual desire disorders; sexual arousal disorders
	Sexual desire disorder

Sources: McCabe 2004, Heiman, 2002a; Lewis Rosen, Goldstein, 2005; Kloner & Padma, 2005; O'Donohue and Geer (1993); Lowinson, Ruis, Millman, and Langrod (1992); Kita (2001).

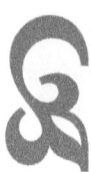

healthy sex hints 12.1

Enhancing Male Potency by Increasing Wellness

Greg Gutfield (1994) summarized findings from studies documenting the effects of a healthy lifestyle on sexual potency. These findings show that many of the roadblocks to good sex can be removed through simple lifestyle changes aimed at improving overall health status.

Three of the major culprits in sexual potency—heart disease, diabetes, and high blood pressure—often can be prevented by regular exercise and a healthy diet. Both of these also aid tremendously in weight management and controlling obesity, a major risk factor for all three conditions. The common denominator is *vascular health.* Impaired blood flow leads to poor sexual response. Increasing exercise and eating a healthy diet (low-fat, high-carbohydrate, moderate protein) enhances blood flow and vascular health.

Stress is another factor that can undermine sexual potency. Chronic stress can lower testosterone, the key hormone related to sexual desire. Less testosterone means less sexual desire. Stress also can make us angry. Men who respond to stressors by losing control and getting angry were much more likely to suffer from erectile disorder then men who were not angry. Of the men who scored highest on measures of anger, 35 percent reported moderate erectile disorder and 20 percent complete erectile disorder.

Stress management and relaxation will help moderate testosterone levels, reduce anger, and help restore potency.

Smoking increases the likelihood of erectile dysfunction and is a major risk factor in cardiovascular disease (Heapes, 1994). Smokers are four times as likely as nonsmokers to develop complete erectile disorder. The negative effects of smoking can be reversed by quitting.

Use it or lose it. "The more erections you have, the more you're likely to have" (Gutfield, 1994). Having at least three erections per week can reduce the risk for erectile disorder. Erections improve blood flow to the penis. Frequent erections help promote circulation and bring oxygen-rich blood to the area.

To improve your erectile function, make these three simple lifestyle changes:

1. Exercise regularly.
2. Eat a balanced diet.
3. Stop smoking.

Injuries and Surgery

Certain injuries also can cause erectile disorder and other forms of sexual dysfunction. An estimated 600,000 or more cases of erectile dysfunction are attributed to accidents and injuries to the underside of the penis (Parker-Pope, 2002; Kita, 2001). Athletic injuries resulting from being kicked or struck in the groin can damage the area. Extensive bicycle riding (100-mile rides) can damage the blood vessels on the underside of the penis. Falls that crush the penis against an object (such as a railing or fence) can damage the blood vessels that supply blood to the penis.

Female-centered sex therapists suggest that such injuries to women can also damage nerves and blood vessels in the pelvic region associated with sexual response in women. "Straddle" injury trauma associated with accidents such as falls from gymnastic balance beams and narrow bicycle seats can affect blood flow and nerve transmissions in women also (Parker-Pope, 2002; Kita, 2001).

Sexual dysfunction can also be traced to nerve and blood vessel damage associated with surgery. Common surgical procedures such as episiotomy, cesarean section, hysterectomy, and tubal ligations are often related to subsequent sexual dysfunctions. Cosmetic surgery involving the pelvic area (genital, cosmetic surgery, vaginal tightening, and labial reconstruction) is also associated with some forms of female sexual dysfunction (Kita, 2001).

Substance-Induced Sexual Dysfunction

Substance-induced sexual dysfunction can affect any stage of the sexual response cycle. The essential feature of this condition is the link between a clinically diagnosed sexual dysfunction and a specific substance, legal or illegal. The three diagnostic criteria of this condition are as follows:

1. The sexual dysfunction causes marked distress or interpersonal difficulty.
2. Depending on the substance involved, the condition may involve impaired desire, arousal, orgasm or sexual pain, and is fully explained by the direct effects of the substance.
3. The dysfunction is not better accounted for by a dysfunction that is not substance induced. A diagnosis of substance-induced sexual dysfunction represents a recurrent or persistent condition and should not be confused with the effects of episodic substance intoxication.

Both **psychotropic** (mind-altering) **drugs** and **somatotropic** (body-altering) **drugs** may have side effects that can produce sexual dysfunction. In some cases, the use of drugs to influence sexual response is intentional (for example, using alcohol to decrease sexual inhibitions). In other cases, the effects of drug use on sexual response are unintentional or unexpected (for example, the contributing effects of prescription antihypertensive medications on male erectile disorders) (Johnson et al., 2004; Parrish, 1997).

Psychotropic drugs Substances that are mind-altering

Somatotropic drugs Substances that are body-altering

Prescription Drug Interactions

The effects of prescribed and over-the-counter drugs are many and varied. They range from decreased vaginal lubrication associated with antihistamines (over-the-counter use by allergy sufferers) to erectile dysfunction associated with certain forms of anti-hypertensive medication. The commonly prescribed antidepressant drug Prozac (fluoxetine) has been shown to cause erectile disorder and **anorgasmia** in small numbers of male and female users, respectively (Rosen, 1991). Table 12.2 outlines common medical drugs and their associated sexual dysfunctions.

Anorgasmia An inability to achieve orgasm

Anyone who takes these drugs should have a thorough understanding of their potential sexual side effects. A potential complication associated with taking medications is the effect of combining two or more medications. The effects can range from a simple additive effect (the effect of one medication added to the effect of the other) to a **synergistic effect** (the effects of two or more drugs creating a third, enhanced, and often unpredictable effect), which can be associated with sexual dysfunction. This possibility can be especially troubling for people with chronic diseases who must take more than one medication regularly. They must guard against mixing over-the-counter medications with alcohol or illegal substances, as well as medically prescribed drugs.

Synergistic effect An enhanced, unpredictable drug effect caused by combining two or more substances

Table 12.2 The Effects of Select Medical Drugs on Sexual Response

Drug	Medical Use	Effect on Sexual Response
Hormones Estrogen and Progesterone	Replacement therapy in menopause; birth control; prostate cancer prescription	May decrease sexual desire in women; sexual arousal disorder in men
Steroids Diannabol and others	Treatment for hypogonad disorder (deficiency in gonadal function); promote growth; treatment for aplastic anemia	*Men:* atrophy of testicles; cessation of sperm production; growth of breasts; sexual desire disorder *Women:* masculination of clitoris; excessive facial and body hair
Hypertensive medications Diamox Catapres Inderal Tanormin	Control high blood pressure	Loss of sexual desire; sexual arousal disorders; orgasmic disorders
Gastrointestinal drugs Tagament Librax	Treat gastrointestinal distress and similar problems	Decreased sexual desire; sexual arousal disorders
Antihistamines	Control allergic reactions, stop runny nose, itchy eyes	Inhibit lubrication; painful intercourse
Psychiatric medications (major tranquilizers)	Control psychotic episodes	Decreased sexual desire; sexual arousal disorders; orgasmic disorders

Sources: Heiman 2002a, Enserink 2005, Witters, Venturell, and Hanson (1992); Jones and Jones (1977); Masters, Johnson & Kolodny (1996); O'Donohue and Geer (1993); Lowinson et al., (1992).

Psychotropic Drugs

Mind-altering drugs, both legal and illegal, have the potential to affect sexual response. The complexity of our vascular, neurological, and endocrine interactions during sexual response makes us particularly susceptible to the effects of psychoactive substances. The sexually-related side effects of psychoactive drugs are variable. As with all psychoactive drugs, the user's psychological well-being and environment can affect the outcome of the drug experience. A placebo effect can occur if a user has certain expectations for the drug (Johnson et al., 2004).

Depressants

Tranquilizers, barbiturates, and alcohol are all central nervous system (CNS) depressants. They reduce, depress, or slow down brain and nervous system functioning. Although they are all classified as depressants, their intended use and effects are different. Barbiturates and alcohol have a more diffuse, less targeted effect on the nervous system. Benzodiazepines (the most frequently prescribed tranquilizers selectively target neural receptors. In addition, tranquilizers and barbiturates are prescribed as medical drugs for treating psychological disorders. Their social use is illegal. Alcohol is a legal, nonmedical drug whose primary use is social.)

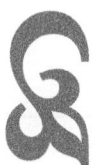 **healthy sex hints 12.2**

Dealing with Side Effects of Drugs

Drugs have many different effects. The *intended effect* is the desired outcome of taking the product. The intended effect of hypertension medication, for example, is to lower blood pressure. *Side effects* are secondary outcomes that result from taking the medication. Some side effects are beneficial, such as regulation of the menstrual cycle when taking oral contraceptives.

The drug is intended to prevent the release of an ovum, and, as a side effect, it regulates the menstrual cycle. Many side effects, however, are not beneficial for sexual response. A side effect of some hypertension medication, for instance, is a reduction in sexual desire. All drug manufacturers are required by law to provide information about side effects concerning their products. Pharmacists also are required to discuss side effects with consumers.

Ultimately, you have the responsibility for making sense of it all. Here are some tips for understanding possible adverse side effects of prescriptions:

1. Make sure you know what disease or condition you have been diagnosed as having *before* you leave your health care provider.
2. Be sure you know the name of your medication and its intended effects.
3. Understand exactly how to take it (dosage schedule, contraindications, and so forth).
4. Ask your health care provider, "What possible effects will taking this medication have on my sexual response?"
5. If the medication carries any potentially negative sexual side effects, ask, "What other medication can I take that will treat my disease [or condition] without affecting my sexual response?"
6. When you pick up your prescription, read the package insert. Ask the pharmacist to clear up any questions you have about the medication.

If you experience any negative side effects that detract from the quality of your life, go back to your health care provider.

Tranquilizers originally were divided into two categories: minor (primarily used to treat anxiety and insomnia) and major (antipsychotic drugs used to treat severe mental illness such as schizophrenia). Benzodiazepines (Valium-like drugs) are the most frequently prescribed CNS depressants. The pharmacologic effects of benzodiazepines are so different from those of the antipsychotic drugs that the terms *minor* and *major tranquilizers* are rarely used today. The primary medical use of Valium-like drugs is to reduce anxiety and treat neuroses. They work by depressing limbic functioning and thereby altering mood. Because these drugs can reduce anxiety and improve mood, they sometimes are used by people in an attempt to enhance sexual desire.

Barbiturates have a less specific, more diffuse sedative/hypnotic effect on depressing nervous system functioning. Barbiturates are used primarily as sedatives to treat insomnia. Barbiturates are rarely used to treat anxiety these days, having been replaced by safer drugs (such as the benzodiazepines). In low doses, barbiturates can induce a lazy, sleepy state. Because of this, barbiturates sometimes are used incorrectly and illegally to enhance

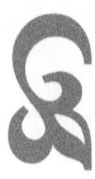

healthy sex hints 12.3

Mixing Alcohol and Medicines

Sometimes alcohol increases the effects and the risks of a medicine to potentially dangerous levels. About 100 prescription medicines can produce unwanted effects when mixed with alcohol. A few examples are presented here:

Analgesic Pain Medication
Salicylates (aspirin) Ibuprofen (Advil, Motrin)
Effects: Stomach and intestinal bleeding; bleeding ulcers

Antidiabetic Agents
Chlorpropamide (Diabinese) Tolbutamide (Orinase) Insulin
Effects: Altered control of blood sugar, most often hypoglycemia

Barbiturates
Secobarbitol (Seconal) Phenobarbital (Barbita) Pentobarbital (Nembutal)
Effects: Greater sedative effect; drowsiness; confusion

Benzodiazepines
Alprazolam (Xanax) Diazepam (Valium) Triazolam (Halcion)
Effects: Greater sedative effect; impaired motor coordination (such as driving ability)

Monamine Oxidase (MAO) Inhibitors
Isocarboxazid (Marplan) Phenelzine (Nardil) Tranylcypromine (Parnate)
Effects: Certain alcoholic beverages contain tyramine, which can cause severe high blood pressure; may be fatal.

Make sure you understand the risks associated with mixing alcohol with your prescription medications. If you have any doubts, ask your physician or pharmacist.

Source: Adapted from "Alcohol and Medications: Ask Before You Mix," publication #B–20, National Council on Patient Information and Education, 666 Eleventh St. N.W., Suite 810, Washington, DC 2001. Reprinted with permission.

Ethyl alcohol A grain alcohol that is a central nervous system depressant

sexual response by inducing a relaxed, less inhibited state of mind. In high, toxic doses, barbiturates can induce coma.

The alcohol people drink is more precisely termed ethyl alcohol, also known as ethanol. **Ethyl alcohol** is available either in its pure form, grain alcohol, or more commonly as the active ingredient in a wide variety of alcoholic beverages. Alcohol is a strong central nervous system depressant.

Unlike the other categories of depressants (tranquilizers and barbiturates), alcohol is not a prescription medical drug with specific intended effects. Alcohol creates a sedative/hypnotic effect similar to that of barbiturates. Alcohol decreases the inhibitory centers of the brain and is used primarily for its ability to reduce inhibitions (USDHHS, 2000). Therefore, people often use alcohol to enhance sexual desire. In larger doses, alcohol has effects similar to those of other depressant drugs.

When a person consumes an alcoholic beverage, about 20 percent of the alcohol enters the bloodstream immediately through the stomach lining. The remainder enters the body when the stomach's contents enter the intestines. Because the brain has a large blood supply, it absorbs a lot of

Table 12.3 Effects of Various Blood Alcohol Concentrations

BAC (%)	Effects
0.01	Mild, if any; slight changes in feeling, mood elevation
0.03	Feelings of relaxation and exhilaration; slight impairment of mental function
0.08	Diminished inhibitions; difficulty performing motor skills; impaired judgment; impaired visual and hearing acuity
0.10	Typically, little or no judgment and poor coordination
0.12	Difficulty performing gross-motor skills; impaired vision; definite impairment of mental function
0.15	Major impairment of physical and mental functions; erratic and irresponsible behavior; distorted judgment; feeling of euphoria; difficulty responding to stimuli
0.20	Confusion; decreased inhibitions; inability to move without assistance; inability to maintain upright position; may fall asleep
0.30	Severe mental confusion; difficulty in comprehension and perception; difficulty responding to stimuli; extreme distortion of sensibility; produces sleep in most people
0.40	Nearly complete anesthesia; severely depressed reflexes; possible unconsciousness or coma
0.50	Unconsciousness or deep coma; possibly death
0.60	Total depression of nerves that control heart and breathing centers; death (USDHHS, 2000).

alcohol (USDHHS, 2000). The measurement of alcohol content of blood in circulation is termed **blood alcohol concentration (BAC).** Physical and psychological effects on the body at different blood alcohol levels are shown in Table 12.3.

Small elevations in BAC are characterized by a "mellow" state, in which the body is relaxed and the person is less inhibited than usual. At this stage, sexual desire—and sexual performance—may be enhanced. With increased alcohol intake, however, the person's judgment rapidly becomes impaired, which impacts sexual decisions. Because alcohol is classified as a depressant, the initial high may be followed by a low. Some drinkers become suicidal.

Physiological responses (including sexual performance) are compromised with increasing BACs. The person may have trouble walking a straight line and maintaining balance, and the speech may become slurred. Sometimes the person vomits. At higher levels, the drinker may pass out. Chronic drinkers often have a problem with erectile dysfunction. Alcohol intoxication can even result in death. Because of the many variables—gender, weight, food consumption, simultaneous use with other medications, and so forth—the actual effects vary from person to person and cannot be predicted.

The legal drinking age is 21 in all states. Also, because of the high accident rates involving drinking and driving, laws are becoming more

Blood alcohol concentration (BAC)
A measurement of percentage of alcohol in blood; also termed *blood alcohol level* (BAL)

restrictive. A person is considered legally intoxicated at BAC levels between 0.08 and 0.10 percent, depending on the state. Sexual assault, rape, domestic violence, and crime in general are also associated with overuse of alcohol. *Moderation* is the operative word (Higher Ed. Center, 2003; Weschler, Eun, Kuo et al., 2002, Fisher, Cullen, & Turner, 2000). In Chapter 16 we talk more about alcohol-related violence.

Stimulant Drugs

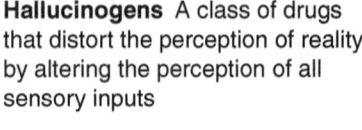

Amphetamines A central nervous system stimulant that is administered by ingestion, injection, snorting, or inhalation

Stimulants work by increasing or speeding up nervous system functioning. Three major physiological effects of stimulants are higher energy and alertness, heightened cognitive functioning, and less appetite. The major legal stimulant drugs are **amphetamines,** which come in a wide variety of brands. The major illegal stimulants are designer amphetamines (chemically synthesized variants of legal products) and cocaine (in powder and crack forms). Amphetamines are available by prescription for three intended medical purposes: treatment of narcolepsy (inadvertent falling asleep), attention deficit hyperactivity disorder (ADHD), and weight reduction.

People often use stimulants illegally in an effort to enhance sexual response. Cocaine and intravenous injection of amphetamines have been reported to create an intense burst of energy that users have described as "orgasmic." Users also report that amphetamines can help prolong sexual activity. The use of stimulants seems to interfere with the brain's ability to trigger orgasm. Although these drugs might enhance the excitement and plateau stages, some users are unable to achieve orgasm under any circumstances (Goldberg, 2006).

Hallucinogens

Hallucinogens A class of drugs that distort the perception of reality by altering the perception of all sensory inputs

Hallucinogens are a class of drugs that distort the perception of reality by altering the perception of all sensory inputs—sights, sounds, tastes, touches, and smells. Hallucinogens work by interfering with the normal function of sensory processing systems within the brain. Routine interpretation of sensory input is altered, causing hallucinations.

Some people use hallucinogens to improve their sexual response by enhancing the perception of touch and other sensations. Users also report a sense of time distortion; sexual activities seem to last longer. Three of the best-known hallucinogens are lysergic acid diethylamide (LSD), methylenedioxymethamphetamine (MDMA), and phencyclidine (PCP). Hallucinogens are illegal except as part of certain American Indian tribal ceremonies.

For many years, marijuana, or cannabis, was classified as a mild hallucinogen. Most drug authorities now place marijuana and its variants (hashish and hash oil) in its own category because of the varied effects. The effects of marijuana result in part from the varying amounts of the active ingredient, tetrahydrocannabinol (THC). High levels of THC can produce a mild hallucinogenic effect, which leads to changes in perception of sensory stimuli. Users report a heightened sensitivity to visual and auditory stimuli and an increased craving for certain kinds of foods.

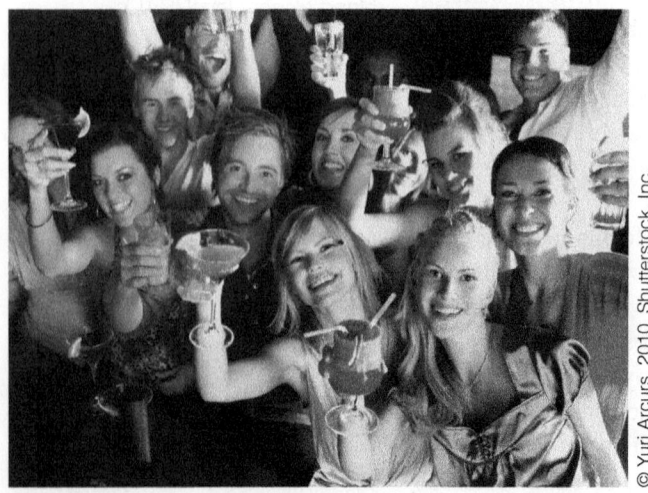

© Yuri Arcurs, 2010. Shutterstock, Inc.

Although alcohol in limited amounts can reduce inhibitions, excess consumption can make sexual arousal difficult.

The effects of marijuana on sexual response are variable. Many users report increased sexual pleasure because of enhanced sensations, as well as a distortion of space and time. This creates a "time warp" in which the sexual act seems to hang suspended.

Other users, in contrast, report that the same mildly hallucinogenic state creates a kind of paranoia that cancels out these same effects. The loss of control brought on by the distortion of perception of time and space is frightening and can diminish sexual pleasure and disorders in sexual response. Long-term marijuana use has been shown to lower testosterone (the sex hormone most related to sexual desire) and sperm levels.

Marijuana use is illegal except in two instances: (a) as an adjunct to glaucoma treatment (to relieve pressure within the eye) and (b) as a way to reduce nausea symptoms associated with chemotherapy for cancer. In both instances, strict legal regulations control its use.

Narcotics

Narcotic drugs are pain killers. They work by diminishing the transmission of pain throughout the nerve pathway. The common opium-derivative narcotics are opium, heroin, and codeine. A common myth concerning heroin addicts is that they are sexually aggressive. To the contrary, one of the side effects of heroin addiction is a diminished interest in sex.

Cautions

Any illegal drug carries the potential for toxicity, overdose, and serious physical danger because illegal substances are not regulated or controlled. Therefore, a person has no idea where or how the substance was produced, and there is no way to quantify the amount of the active ingredient in the drug or the presence of any additives. Marijuana, for instance, has varying amounts of THC and can be cured or mixed with a variety of other substances. Heroin and cocaine can be "cut" (diluting the original volume and pure form by adding ingredients to increase the volume) with anything ranging from talcum powder to rat poison.

Penalties for using illegal drugs are variable and far outweigh any perceived benefits associated with enhanced sexual response. Sexual response can be greatly diminished by spending the rest of one's life in prison. All of the four categories of drugs [depressants, stimulants, hallucinogens (including marijuana), and narcotics] have the potential to cause sexual dysfunction. Table 12.4 summarizes the effects of psychoactive drugs on sexual response.

Psychological Causes of Sexual Dysfunction

Besides being correlated with health problems ranging from cardiovascular disease to substance abuse, sexual problems and dysfunction also appears to be associated with personal psychological well-being and relationship stability (Heiman, 2002b). The two basic psychological causes of sexual dysfunction are (a) prior learning and (b) immediate causes. **Prior learning** refers to factors related to childhood development. *Immediate causes* are factors that have their origins later than childhood learning.

Prior learning Factors relating to childhood development

Table 12.4 The Effects of Select Psychoactive Substances on Sexual Response

Drug	Chronic Use or Effects of Small Doses	High Dosage
Depressants		
Benzodiazepines		
Valium	Diminished anxiety and improved social and sexual functioning	Loss of interest in sex
Librium		
Tranxene		
Barbiturates		
Amytal	Cerebral disinhibition; increased relaxation	Loss of desire; sexual arousal disorders; loss of motor control
Nembutal		
Luminal		
Seconal		
Tuinal		
Alcohol	Cerebral disinhibition; increased relaxation	After time, loss of desire; sexual arousal disorders; loss of motor control
Stimulants		
Amphetamines	Increased energy and interest in sex; ability to prolong sexual activities; "rush" similar to orgasm	After time, loss of desire and interest; loss of control; orgasmic disorders
Cocaine		
Hallucinogens		
Marijuana	Heightened awareness and sensations; time distortion (sex seems to last longer)	Decrease in testosterone; loss of desire
LSD		
MDMA		
Narcotics		
Opium	Feelings of warmth; reduction in aggression; sleepy/mellow state	Loss of desire; sexual arousal disorders; orgasmic disorders
Heroin		
Morphine		
Methadone		
Codeine		

Prior Learning

Most theorists agree that childhood learning shapes many of our fundamental attitudes, values, and beliefs about sexuality. Humans are capable of experiencing sexual and sensual pleasure from birth to death. Infants of both sexes seem to derive great pleasure from touching and rubbing their genitals against bedding and clothing. They also seem to thrive when physical bonding, breastfeeding, and other forms of intimate physical touch are established early in infancy (Montague, 1977). When this seemingly innate sexual potential is thwarted through overt or covert child-rearing practices, the seeds of subsequent sexual problems in adulthood are planted.

The messages we receive during childhood—particularly those from our parents and other primary caregivers—contribute heavily to healthy or unhealthy psychosexual development. Sex therapists widely report the relationship between severe anti-sex parenting and the development of sexual dysfunction in later life. Children who are reared in environments where nudity, masturbation, and childhood inquiry and discussion of sexuality are severely punished are more likely to develop sexual problems than their peers who are reared in more tolerant environments.

case study 12.2

Lilian's Thoughts About Her Parents' Sexuality

Lilian, 19, single, lesbian, identifies as African American.

Lilian is a freshman. She shared these feelings about her parents as sexual beings.

I never viewed my parents as sexual creatures. They never talked about sex once in my presence. My mom briefly explained menstruation to me and what to expect when I get my period, but when I interrupted and told her we had already gone over that stuff in school, she abruptly stopped and seemed relieved.

My brothers told me that my mom and dad never talked to them about sex, either. My parents are not very warm people. They never hug and kiss in public and very rarely express themselves physically.

I guess they love each other, because they seem to care about each other and respect one another's needs. It's just that they don't seem interested in sex at all. I'd never ask either of them about a sexual issue. My lover's mom kind of fills that role for me. She thinks its kind of sad that I can't talk to my own mom about it.

To tell you the truth, I can't even imagine my parents ever having sex. I guess they had to have it three times to conceive my brothers and me, but I can't even visualize it. It doesn't gross me out or anything. I just can't seem to create the picture. Funny, isn't it?

Critical Thinking

Many students can't visualize their parents having sex. As in Lilian's case this was due in part by never mentioning sex at all. How does the absence of a subject, like sex, send messages to children growing up in a household like Lilian's?

In one study, adults with the former type of childhood histories were less interested in sex, derived less pleasure from sexual relations, had more inhibitions about sexual expression, and had higher levels of shame, guilt, anxiety, and disgust than those with less rigid backgrounds (Purcell, 1985). The "sex-as-sin" message and subsequent sexual problems came from a strict or orthodox religious orientation; the more rigidly orthodox, the greater the extent of dysfunction.

Another researcher warned about associating sexual dysfunction with religious orthodoxy. Hyde (1994) notes the lack of suitable research designs and methodology associated with sex therapists' reports concerning the etiology of sexual dysfunction. Without suitable control groups, it is impossible to discern whether orthodoxy or some other factor is the problem.

Prior Learning Factors Relating to Childhood Development

Even covert practices can sabotage the development of healthy sexuality. Parents who are uneasy about sexuality may choose to deal with this subject by ignoring it. Saying nothing still sends a strong message to children about sexuality. Omitting such an integral part of life from all discussion leaves a void that children clearly perceive. They learn early that something must be wrong, shameful, or dirty about sex if it doesn't ever come up as a topic of conversation. Students often report anecdotally in class their feelings that their parents must have made love only once (for their conception) or as many times as they have siblings, because they never discussed sexuality, their desire for each other, or other sexual themes when the children were around.

Other messages about sexuality relate to gender role expectations. Males and females in U.S. culture often are reared with different sets of sexual standards and expectations. Rather than viewing sexual needs and expression as a human universal, they are reared with the belief that men and women have differing needs and wants that are gender-specific. Society also has different rules and codes of conduct concerning how to satisfy these needs. Men are expected to be more assertive in pursuing their sexual needs. Women are expected to be more demure, to rely on men to pursue them and satisfy them.

These gender role expectations can create anxiety, shame, guilt, and fear—all attributes that detract from sexual pleasure. As early as 1970, Masters and Johnson (1970) noted that rigid sex roles and a double standard concerning sexual expression were often at the root of much of their clients' sexual dysfunction.

Fifteen years later, another study found that nontraditional, less rigid gender roles were related positively to increased enjoyment with sex, greater levels of experimentation with sexual positions, oral sex, initiation of sexual encounters, and assertion of one's sexual needs and wants (Kobilinsky & Palmeter, 1984).

Male sexual dysfunction is often related to performance anxiety stemming from rigid male gender role socialization. (Zilbergeld, 1992). Many men grow up with an idealized picture of male sexuality that positions men as all-knowing, ever-ready, and being responsible for initiating sexual encounters and pleasing their partners. This view puts tremendous pressure on men to live up to those expectations.

Immediate Causes

Immediate causes of sexual dysfunction are identified as (a) failure to engage in effective sexual behavior because of either ignorance or unconscious avoidance; (b) anxiety related to performance, fear of failure, or perceived inability to please a partner; (c) perceptual and intellectual defenses against erotic feelings; (d) failure to communicate effectively with one's partner; and (e) stress and fatigue.

Ignorance/Avoidance

Failure to engage in effective sexual behavior often arises from simple ignorance. Sexual dysfunctions related to the arousal and orgasm phase often are related to lack of knowledge concerning effective techniques for achieving optimal levels of stimulation. Ignorance is often compounded by shame and guilt related to sexual experimentation, assertiveness, and admission of what is arousing. Some people unconsciously avoid exploration of the sensual and erotic and fail to take advantage of opportunities to explore sexual satisfaction.

Achieving sexual pleasure is a skill that can improve with better technique. If one perceives sexual activity as something that is learned rather than innate, and allows oneself to pursue self-improvement, many sexual problems and dysfunctions can be remedied. All five phases of sexual response can be enhanced by improving technique. People can learn how to increase desire, enhance arousal, maximize plateau, increase the likelihood of orgasm (and multiple orgasms), and enjoy resolution and the refractory period.

Good communication can enhance technique, especially when practicing with a partner and discovering what works with him or her. But, as one man said, "The way I got to become such a good lover was that I practiced a lot by myself when I was at home." Through introspection, guided readings, practice activities, and a variety of other techniques, technique and performance can be enhanced.

ᕀ *Social Wellness* ᕀ

Sex with another person is a unique social experience that cannot be separated from the emotions the two people bring to the encounter. High-level social wellness revolves around healthy relationships. And healthy relationships are based on trust, respect, commitment, love, and affection. Good sex flows out of this safe and protected context. When trust, respect, and affection are displaced by mistrust, disrespect, and fear, relationship problems ensue. Communication, which is central to good sex, often breaks down when couples are having relationship problems. When sexual needs and desires are not communicated clearly, sexual response suffers.

Performance Anxiety

Sexual anxiety resulting from fear of failure, the demand for performance, or an excessive need to please one's partner can literally shortcircuit sexual response. Any type of anxiety interferes with the ability to relax and allow vasocongestion and other sexual processes to occur. Anxiety can interfere with the level of sexual desire and ability to get aroused and to create sufficient stimulation to trigger orgasm. Anxiety interferes with the ability to become fully involved in the moment, not allowing one to be immersed in the sexual episode.

Anxiety related to a current sexual encounter is often rooted in past sexual episodes. Failure to become sufficiently aroused and maintain an erection in the past often leads to anxiety related to the present ability to perform satisfactorily. Being asked to perform sexually on demand can create resentment and anxiety related to current functioning. In a sense, anxiety fosters the anticipation of failure.

Anxiety is perhaps the greatest psychological factor associated with erectile disorder. Although **performance anxiety** is often characterized as a "male problem" because men usually are viewed as responsible for their partner's orgasm, women also suffer from this malady. The person worries over every facet of the sexual encounter: "Am I attractive enough . . . sexy enough?" "Is my penis big enough?" "Are my breasts large enough?" "Is my underwear sexy?" "Will I be able to get [sustain] an erection?" "Will my technique work?" "What if he [she] asks me to do something I'm not comfortable with or know how to do?" "Will we come together?" These and countless other thoughts and concerns set up an expectation-anxiety performance feedback loop that initiates and perpetuates sexual problems. The expectation of failure or poor performance produces anxiety ranging

Performance anxiety Fear, worry, or panic associated with one's perceived sexual behavior

from mild worry to panic. Anxiety creates physiological and psychological roadblocks that impair good performance, resulting in the kind of poor performance the person feared to begin with. In a sense, it creates a self-fulfilling prophecy. The fears are answered by "I told you so," confirming the failure. This outcome seals one's fate by making it twice as hard to correct the problem and improve performance.

Defenses

Spectatoring Becoming an outside observer of one's own sexual encounter while it is occurring

Anxiety also contributes to the perceptual and intellectual defense against erotic feelings called **spectatoring.** Spectatoring occurs when the person becomes an outside observer of his or her own sexual encounter. In a sense, the sexual encounter is reduced to an intellectual activity in which the participant steps away and critically analyzes his or her own behavior.

Whether driven by narcissistic preoccupation with self, voyeurism, or performance anxiety, spectatoring turns the participant into an observer of his or her own sexual encounter. In a sense, the spectator examines the performance of self or partner rather than becoming fully involved in the sensations and experiences. The result is a lack of enjoyment in the experience, as well as dysfunction with any phase in the response cycle.

Communication Problems

We sometimes have trouble communicating our sexual desires, needs, and wants because of feelings of shame, guilt, or fear. Maybe we have learned that sex and sexual needs are a taboo subject.

Furthermore, we may be uncomfortable with the language of sexuality. Our culture does not have a common sexual language. This makes it difficult to understand, articulate, and communicate about sexuality with our partners. Consequently, we suppress our needs and problems, anger and resentment build, and eventually this repression short-circuits the delicate balance among the neurological, vascular, and endocrine factors necessary in the sexual response.

Open communication is essential for dealing with sexual problems.

Stress and Fatigue

Finally, stress and fatigue can precipitate sexual dysfunction. When associated with other aspects of life such as work, child-rearing demands, money problems, and poor health, stress and fatigue can rob a person of vital energy and a zest for living. Stress and fatigue can affect all phases of the sexual response cycle. When men are stressed, their testosterone levels drop. Testosterone, you may recall, is the hormone most related to the level of sexual desire.

When these men participated in stress management activities, their testosterone levels and levels of sexual desire returned to normal (Singer-Kaplan, 1974). Common sense tells us that when we are tired and stressed, the last thing we seem to be interested in is sex. For the sexual response to begin and orgasm

sex in society 12.1

Cultural Considerations in Sexual Dysfunction

As we have seen, sexual dysfunction, like sexual response, is a very complex phenomenon. Basson et al., (2000) have shown that the origin of sexual desire is different for men and women. Desire disorders in women may really be related to problems associated with intimacy more than with desire.

Just as gender affects desire, response, and dysfunction, so does culture. We have seen what a big role communication plays in sexual dysfunction. The American therapeutic model emphasizes open communication between marital partners. Both partners hold equal status in the therapeutic relationship. Each is expected to take an active role and to be responsible for the therapy. How does sexual desire and dysfunction play out in cultures where this is *not* the norm?

Media coverage of Middle Eastern countries such as Iraq, Iran, and Afghanistan, where a radical version of Islam is practiced, paints an entirely different view of spousal relationships and communication between spouses. Women are clearly subservient in the marriage. They do not have equal status, power, or responsibility in the marriage. Women are routinely tortured and put to death for committing even the smallest transgression against their spouses.

In such a climate, is something like *sexual satisfaction* or *dysfunction* even in the vocabulary? Is the right to experience sexual pleasure (for the sake of pleasure itself) even a part of sexual relations between partners?

For years, organizations such as the National Organization for Women (NOW) have lobbied international organizations from the United Nations to Amnesty International to stop barbaric practices such as clitoridectomy (see Chapter 2) and various forms of torture commonly used against women in Iran, Iraq, and Afghanistan. Until women in these cultures have even the most basic human rights, healthy sexual rights will have to be put on hold.

to occur, people need to relax and let the body take over. This reaction often is not possible if a person is feeling overwhelmed or just needs a good night's sleep.

✎ *Occupational Wellness* ✎

Work-related stress is often associated with low sexual desire. Other job-related issues ranging from rotating shifts to excessive travel and long-standing separation (such as in military assignments) are also implicated in sexual dysfunction. As we have seen, injury and illness are also associated with sexual dysfunction. Some jobs and work sites are more risky than others and can indeed be hazardous to one's health.

Types of Sexual Dysfunctions

The APA (2000) classifies sexual dysfunctions as the lifelong type, acquired type, generalized type, and situational type. *Lifelong disorders* have been present since the onset of sexual functioning. *Acquired disorders* have developed after a period of normal functioning. *Generalized dysfunctions* are not limited to specific types of stimulation, situations, or partners. *Situational dysfunctions* are limited to certain types of stimulation, situations, or partners. The APA classification of sexual dysfunctions is based on traditional models of sexual response and a four-phase conceptualization of human sexual response: desire, excitement, orgasm, and resolution.

The *desire phase* originates with fantasizing and thinking about engaging in sexual activities. Sexual dysfunctions that relate to this phase are called *sexual desire disorders.*

The *excitement phase* is characterized by the buildup of sexual excitement and tension, manifested through vasocongestion. Penile tumescence and erection are physical evidence of desire in men. In women, vaginal lubrication and expansion and swelling of the vulva indicate arousal. Sexual dysfunctions related to this stage are called *sexual arousal disorders.*

In the *orgasm phase,* built-up sexual tension is released, followed immediately by psychological feelings of satisfaction and satiation. Sexual dysfunctions related to this phase are referred to as *orgasmic disorders.*

The *resolution phase* is characterized by a physiological return to the predesire stage. *Sexual pain disorders* may be present during intercourse or in the resolution phase.

As we mentioned in Chapter 7, Lieblum (2000) and Basson et al., (2000), propose a need to re-examine sexual dysfunction based in part on redefining the very nature of sexual response in women. Basson (2004) questions the presence and ordering of the traditional phases of sexual response and suggests a new model of sexual response. If such a new model of sexual response (particularly one that is more consistent with women's response patterns) becomes widely accepted, it should spur the development of a new paradigm for treating sexual dysfunctions in both men and women (Johnson, 2004).

Dysfunction Versus Disinterest

When discussing sexual dysfunctions, we must recognize the normal continuum of sexual interest and desire in all people. Some people are much more interested in sexual activity than others. The level of interest, desire, and fantasy are variable and are not the only criteria for a diagnosis of sexual dysfunction. To qualify for a diagnosis of either hypoactive sexual desire disorder or sexual aversion disorder, the condition must (a) be persistent and recurrent, (b) cause marked distress or interpersonal difficulty, and (c) not be the result of another medical or physical condition.

Little interest in sexual activity, low desire, and no fantasizing aren't necessarily dysfunctional unless they are accompanied by the three diagnostic criteria. Individuals with low levels of sexual desire still can be happy and productive, and can sustain satisfying long-term relationships as long as their partners have similar sexual traits.

Hypoactive sexual desire disorder should not be confused with voluntary celibacy or abstinence. Some people perceive celibacy as a sexual dysfunction because they believe it is "abnormal" and abstinence is "unnatural." Celibacy is not a sexual dysfunction. Not all celibate people lack sexual interest and desire. Most of us choose to be celibate and abstain from sexual activity at times in our lives, for a variety of reasons.

Sexual Desire Disorders

Sexual desire disorders include hypoactive sexual desire disorder and sexual aversion disorder.

Hypoactive Sexual Desire Disorder

Hypoactive sexual desire disorder is a dysfunction characterized by very low levels (or complete absence) of sexual desire. Individuals with this condition do not initiate sexual activity and may engage in sexual relations only begrudgingly at the insistence of their partner. They have little or no motivation to seek sexual stimulation and are increasingly undisturbed by this lack of opportunity.

Three APA (2000) criteria are necessary to diagnose hypoactive sexual desire disorder: (a) persistent or recurrent deficiency or absence of sexual fantasy or desire for sexual activity; (b) marked psychological or interpersonal distress attributable to the disorder; and (c) no other psychological disorder (such as major depression or posttraumatic stress disorder), medical condition, or direct physiological effects of a drug or medication.

The onset of hypoactive sexual desire disorder can be as early as puberty but usually begins in adulthood, after a period of adequate sexual interest. This dysfunction often is associated with chronic stress, interpersonal difficulties, and problems related to intimacy and commitment.

Although loss of sexual desire can be chronic or episodic, depending on the underlying relationship and psychological problems, hypoactive sexual desire disorder is a chronic condition. Temporary loss of sexual desire is a common byproduct of recovery from depressive disorders (Warnock, 2005; Sceifo, 2002).

Hypoactive sexual desire disorder A dysfunction characterized by very low or complete absence of sexual desire

Sexual Aversion Disorder

Sexual aversion disorder is characterized by disgust and active avoidance of any genital sexual contact with a sexual partner. People who have sexual aversion disorder report anxiety, fear, disgust, or revulsion when confronted with a sexual opportunity with a partner. The aversion may be to a specific aspect of sexual contact (such as genital secretions or vaginal penetration) or to all sexual stimuli, including kissing and touching (APA, 2000).

People with this disorder may have extreme psychological distress, panic attacks, and physical symptoms such as dizziness, nausea, and breathing difficulties. These symptoms often are accompanied by impaired relationship functioning and unusual "covert" strategies to avoid sexual contact (immersion in work, going to sleep early, neglecting personal appearance, abusing substances, and so forth).

Sexual aversion disorder A disorder characterized by disgust and active avoidance of any genital sexual contact

Sexual Arousal Disorders

Sexual arousal disorders differ from sexual desire disorders in that the latter are related to lack of desire and the former to the inability to achieve sufficient levels of arousal. The arousal phase of sexual response depends on vasocongestion, which affects erection in men and vaginal lubrication and expansion and swelling of the external genitalia in women. Vasocongestion involves a complex interplay between psychological variables (desire, trust, affection) and physiological variables (unrestricted blood vessels, a healthy endocrine system). Similarly, the causes of sexual dysfunction related to vasocongestion can be psychological, physiological, or both (Fisher, 2004; Munarriz, Kim, Goldstein et al., 2002).

case study 12.3

Hypoactive Sexual Disorder: The Case of Rhonda

Rhonda, 45, married, is white.

Rhonda is a part-time evening student. She has been married for 20 years and has three children, ages 19, 17, and 14. A homemaker for the past two decades, Rhonda has returned to school to earn a second degree in computer science (she already has a bachelor's degree in English). Rhonda met with one of the authors for counseling.

I'm not even sure why I came to see you. I've never discussed this with anyone before. We were discussing hypoactive sexual disorder in class today, and I think I have it. I've been married to Ed over 20 years. We met in college in the seventies, fell in love, and were married in 1976. Our sex life was great for the first 10 years of our marriage. Even with the pregnancies, the kids, staying home, and all, sex was always a strong part of our relationship. It all changed about 10 years ago.

Ed and I had been drifting apart a little. His career had taken off, and I was home with the kids. He felt we didn't have as much in common any more, and I was getting boring. It's hard when you're raising three kids almost by yourself. Ed is on the road almost 40 percent of the time, traveling all over the world for his job. One day he's in Japan, the next in Indianapolis. Meanwhile, I'm schlepping one kid off to soccer, another to band practice, and the third to the mall to work.

Anyway, we began to pull back from each other sexually. Sex became such a hassle. Half of the time Ed claimed he was too tired or busy with work. Other times he'd pop in, fresh from some exciting business trip to Europe or somewhere exotic, and expect me to be Miss Bubbly, drop everything, and jump in the sack with him. I really resented that and just withdrew.

Our sex life slipped from two or three times a week, when he was home, to two or three times a month. There were even some months when we didn't have sex at all.

It seems as though for the past 2 years I don't even care if we don't have sex at all. I'm not even sure if I miss it, but I know something is terribly wrong. I guess I thought these kinds of feelings were inevitable after being together for 20 years.

Female Sexual Arousal Disorder

The major characteristic of this female dysfunction is the persistent or recurrent inability to attain or maintain sufficient vaginal lubrication and swelling to complete the sexual activity. Vasocongestion is impaired, and the vagina and external genitalia do not become fully engorged with blood. As a result, penetration is restricted, which may result in painful intercourse, avoidance of sexual relations, and a disturbance of the relationship. Female

case study 12.4

Sexual Aversion Disorder: The Case of Josh

Josh, 25, single, is African American; Suzanne, 30, is divorced and white.

Josh, a senior, is an excellent student; he works for a large investment firm. He is finishing his degree in finance. He grew up in a strict, conservative family and remembers being severely punished for masturbating when he was a child. He came to the office of one of the authors to seek guidance concerning a sexual problem he had. Josh began by saying, "I feel really strange talking to you about this, but you seem very understanding and I need to talk to someone." After receiving some reassurances and permission, he began his story.

I met this wonderful woman, Suzanne, at work this semester. She is 30 years old, divorced with no kids, and is one of the stock traders for the company. She is gorgeous, funny, and bright. We hit it off immediately. I'm not a virgin, and I've been engaged in the past, but I'm hardly what you'd call sexually experienced. I like sex and all that, but I'm kind of conservative and not into any kinky stuff. Intercourse is okay, but oral sex repulses me. I start to get nauseous just thinking about it.

Anyway, Suzanne and I began dating, and from the start she was very passionate. She wanted to have sex on our first date, but I held off, told her I was tired and needed to get up early the next day. I wasn't ready for her and needed time to get to know her. I was surprised she wanted to see me again, but she did, and we talked about my need to get to know her better before we began to have sex. She said she really liked me and it was OK—we wouldn't rush into a sexual relationship.

After about a month, we finally had sex. We went back to her place after dinner and a movie, and she had a glass of wine. We started to kiss and undress, and everything was great until she started to kiss me on the chest and stomach. I felt her head begin to go lower, and as she reached my penis, I began to stiffen up and push her away. I guess she thought I was teasing, because she persisted and even laughed. When I began to lose my erection, she knew something was wrong and stopped. I was so embarrassed I didn't know what to say.

She told me it was OK, that we'd try to work it out, but I just couldn't perform that night. I told her we'd have intercourse the next time, but I just couldn't enjoy oral sex. I really like her and want to make this relationship work. My fiancée broke our engagement because of this same issue three years ago, and I don't want to lose Suzanne.

Critical Thinking

It is not uncommon for couples to differ in terms of what they need or want to be sexually satisfied. What advice would you give Josh and Suzanne for dealing with the issue of oral sex?

---

sexual arousal disorder is often accompanied by a sexual desire disorder and female orgasmic disorder.

The three APA diagnostic criteria for female sexual arousal disorder are (a) persistent or recurrent inability to attain or maintain an adequate lubrication/ swelling response; (b) marked psychological distress; and

(c) not caused by another psychological condition (such as major depression), the effects of a medication or drug, or a general medical condition (APA, 2000).

Women who have sexual arousal disorder simply do not become sufficiently aroused to have or enjoy sexual relations. Sexual arousal disorder often is accompanied by sexual desire disorders and female orgasmic disorder (Fass, 2004, Basson, 2002).

Male Erectile Disorder

Often called *impotence,* male erectile disorder is the persistent or recurring inability to attain or maintain an adequate erection for the completion of sexual activity. Erectile disorder is related to a complex interplay of physiological and interpersonal issues and has different patterns. Some men with the disorder are unable to attain an erection at all. Others are able to get an erection but lose it upon penetration. A third group of males are able to attain an erection and complete penetration but lose their erection during thrusting. Some men with this condition report having morning erections or being able to attain erection during masturbation. Others are unable to attain an erection through masturbation (Swindle, Cameron, Lockhart, 2004). About 40 percent of men over the age of 40 and up to 70 percent of men 70 years old or older suffer from erectile disorder (Goldstein, 2000).

The three APA diagnostic criteria for male erectile disorder are (a) marked distress or interpersonal difficulty, (b) no other coexisting psychological condition, and (c) no direct physiological effects of a substance or preexisting medical condition. Men who have male erectile disorder often are anxious, fear failure, and doubt their sexual performance. These psychological concerns often result in lack of sexual excitement and pleasure, avoidance of sexual intercourse, and disturbance in sexual and marital relationships (APA, 2000).

Isolated episodes of inability to obtain an erection are almost universal among men. The reasons include, among others, stress, fatigue, depression, and anxiety (Goldstein, 2000).

Orgasmic Disorders

Orgasmic disorders
Dysfunctions related to the orgasm phase of sexual response

Orgasmic disorders are dysfunctions related to the orgasm phase of sexual response. These disorders center on the inability of men and women to release pent-up sexual tension through orgasm. These people are interested in sexual relations and are able to become sexually aroused. Their problems relate to their inability to move to the next stage of sexual response, orgasm.

Female Orgasmic Disorder

Formerly known as *inhibited female orgasm,* female orgasmic disorder is a persistent or recurring delay in or absence of orgasm following a typical excitement phase. Three specific APA criteria must be met to diagnose this condition: (a) the absence of orgasm following a "normal" excitement phase, (b) accompanying marked distress or interpersonal difficulty, and (c) not the result of another medical or psychological condition or direct physiological effects of a substance.

The "normal" excitement phase is highly variable. The clinician has to assess what is a normal excitement phase for any given patient. This assessment takes into account the woman's sexual experience, history, and the level and adequacy of stimulation she receives. A normal excitement phase for one woman may be markedly different from that of another woman (Basson, 2002).

Because the female capacity for orgasm increases with age, female orgasmic disorder is more prevalent in younger women. As women experience more variety of sexual stimulation, become more knowledgeable about their bodies, and better communicate their needs to their partner, they tend to gain orgasmic facility. Most female orgasmic disorder is lifelong rather than acquired, as women who learn to be orgasmic rarely lose this capacity.

When orgasmic disorders are situational, they often are related to issues such as stress, fatigue, overindulgence of food or drink, or relationship problems such as poor communication and poor technique. Many, if not most, women do not receive enough direct clitoral stimulation through back-and-forth vaginal thrusting. Vaginal intercourse alone does not always provide enough clitoral stimulation for orgasm (Johnson, 2004; Hite, 1977).

Emphasis on intercourse (especially the man-on-top position) as the only acceptable sexual outlet for women can be the root of the problem. Often, women who are unable to achieve an orgasm through vaginal intercourse find that they can achieve it during cunnilingus or masturbation or with additional manual clitoral stimulation during coitus. Some educators and therapists call women who never have had an orgasm "preorgasmic," implying that all women are inherently capable of achieving orgasm. These professionals prefer to view the inability to orgasm as a developmental learning issue versus a dysfunction (Barbach, 1982; Dodson, 1974).

❧ *Emotional Wellness* ❧

Emotions are related intimately to sexual response. All phases of the sexual response cycle are subject to the effects of emotions. Sexual interest and desire are fueled by positive emotions such as happiness, love, joy, respect, and trust. Negative emotions (especially directed at a partner), such as anxiety, anger, hate, fear, disgust, and mistrust, make interest and desire difficult at best and impossible for most. For the body to respond properly, the mind must let go and relax. Arousal and orgasm also are affected by our emotions. The ability to prolong and enjoy sex is affected in part by emotions. Relaxing and becoming immersed in the sensuality of the plateau stage are difficult if we are feeling anxious, rushed, fearful, or angry. We just want to hurry up and get it over with. When we can relax, let down our guard, and allow our senses free rein, we can enjoy the plateau.

Orgasm is contingent on the buildup of tension through adequate stimulation. It is triggered when we give up mental control and allow our body to be swept along in the ecstasy of physical pleasuring. This is difficult if we are on guard, tense, angry, or resentful.

Resolution might be considered a thankful end to a resentful experience in which partners uncouple, roll over, and fall asleep. Or the resolution phase can be a special time. Lovers who are emotionally healthy can bask in the afterglow of loving time spent pleasuring each other.

Male Orgasmic Disorder

Inhibited male orgasm A persistent or recurrent delay in or absence of orgasm following a normal excitement phase

Formerly known as **inhibited male orgasm,** this disorder is a persistent or recurrent delay in or absence of orgasm following a normal excitement phase. As for female orgasmic disorder, the three APA diagnostic criteria that must be met in making this diagnosis are (a) absence of orgasm following a "normal" excitement phase, (b) marked distress or interpersonal difficulty, and (c) not the result of a preexisting medical or psychological condition or physiological effects of a medication or other drug.

Men who have this condition most commonly cannot reach orgasm during intercourse. They usually are able to reach orgasm if intercourse is accompanied by manual or oral stimulation of the penis. In less common manifestations, the men are able to experience orgasm only after a substantial amount of noncoital stimulation. A smaller group of men with male orgasmic disorder are able to ejaculate only through masturbation or upon waking from an erotic dream.

Men who have male orgasmic disorder are able to experience pleasure during the excitement phase of sexual activity and enjoy the beginnings of a sexual encounter but rapidly lose interest. For these men, thrusting and prolonging sexual activity are a chore rather than a pleasure. Many men with male orgasmic disorder have a pattern of paraphiliac sexual arousal and are unable to experience orgasm without the object of their desire.

Premature ejaculation The persistent or recurring early onset of orgasm and ejaculation

Another male orgasmic disorder is **premature ejaculation,** the persistent or recurring onset of orgasm and ejaculation shortly after penetration or before the man wishes it. The condition is diagnosed after the following three APA criteria have been met: (a) the clinician must take into account factors that affect the duration of the excitement phase such as age, novelty of the partner or scenario, and the frequency of activity; (b) accompanying marked distress and interpersonal difficulty; and (c) not a result of the effects of a substance.

Sometimes premature ejaculation is related to the level of desire and excitement. An extremely high level of sexual arousal can trigger orgasm prematurely and does not represent the true disorder. Occasional episodes are common and are not a problem if they do not cause marked distress and interpersonal difficulty. Also, specific exercises can be practiced to delay orgasm.

With sexual experience and aging, most men learn to delay orgasm. As with women, this technique is related to learning from experience and better sexual communication. Some men continue to have premature ejaculation under all circumstances. Others incur this disorder only when they are with a new partner. Premature ejaculation can create tension and discord in sexual relationships and deter single men from dating and initiating new relationships because of fear and performance anxiety.

Sexual Pain Disorders

The most common sexual pain disorders are dyspareunia and vaginismus. Medical conditions also can result in pain during sexual intercourse.

Dyspareunia

Dyspareunia Genital pain associated with sexual intercourse (such as STDs or scar tissue) or substance use

Dyspareunia is genital pain associated with sexual intercourse. It may be present before, during, or after sexual intercourse and can affect both men and women. Symptoms range from mild discomfort to sharp pain (Phillips, 2000).

Three APA diagnostic criteria must be met to diagnose this condition: (a) recurrent or persistent pain associated with sexual intercourse; (b) marked accompanying psychological distress or interpersonal difficulty; and (c) not caused exclusively by vaginismus or lack of lubrication, a preexisting psychological or medical condition, or the direct effects of a substance.

Sexual pain disorders are not the result of insufficient excitement (which can account for insufficient lubrication and erection and tense muscles) or poor technique. Nor are they a result of medical conditions that affect sexual functioning (APA, 2000). Sexual pain disorder is diagnosed when these other conditions are ruled out and the pain has no clear-cut physiological or medical basis (Phillips, 2000).

Vaginismus

Vaginismus is the recurrent or persistent involuntary contraction of the perineal muscles surrounding the outer third of the vagina during attempted penetration with a penis, finger, tampon, or speculum. In some cases, even the anticipation of vaginal penetration can cause muscle spasms. Symptoms range from mild discomfort and tightness to severe contractions and cramping.

Vaginismus Painful, involuntary contractions of the outer third of the vagina during attempted penetration

The three APA diagnostic criteria that must be met to diagnose this condition are (a) recurrent or persistent involuntary spasm of the musculature of the outer third of the vagina upon insertion, (b) accompanying psychological distress or interpersonal difficulty, and (c) not caused by a preexisting psychological or medical condition (APA, 2000).

Vaginismus usually is discovered upon first gynecological examination or the onset of sexual intercourse. It is more common in young women than older women but can become chronic if it is not treated. It is a primary contributing factor to unconsummated marriages and can limit the development of relationships. Vaginismus is more common in women who have negative attitudes about sex, as well as females who have a history of sexual abuse or trauma (Phillips, 2000, Basson, 2002).

Sexual Dysfunction Caused by a General Medical Condition

The essential features of this disorder are pain, hypoactive sexual desire, male erectile dysfunction, or other types of sexual dysfunction that are direct physiological effects of an established medical condition. Medical conditions range from obvious sexual disorders such as sexually transmitted diseases to inapparent conditions such as arteriosclerosis.

The three diagnostic criteria that must be met to establish the presence of this disorder are (a) clinically significant sexual dysfunction resulting in marked distress or interpersonal difficulty; (b) medical history, physical examination, or laboratory findings fully explaining the dysfunction as the direct physiological effect of a general medical condition; and (c) not better accounted for by another mental disorder.

A Survey of Sexual Dysfunction

At a meeting of the Office of Research on Women's Health, National Institutes of Health, the director of the Partnership for Women's Health at Columbia, Marianne Legato (1999), reported that 43 percent of women and 30 percent of men have some sexual dysfunction. Figure 12.1 presents the various problems by gender. Many of these problems respond well to various treatments.

A New Paradigm for Understanding Sexual Dysfunction

As we mentioned in Chapter 7, Basson's theory of sexual response sheds new light on the importance of intimacy in understanding sexual interest, desire, arousal, and satisfaction. It also can be used as the basis for understanding sexual dysfunction and how to treat it (Lieblum, 2000). According to this new paradigm, understanding sexual desire disorders, for example, requires a deeper emphasis on examining the role of intimacy in relationships.

Since Basson et al., (2000) found that intimacy seeking is often the motivation for sexual desire in women, sexual desire disorders may in fact be more related to lack of intimacy than lack of desire. Desire in women often springs out of intimacy with a partner. Women diagnosed with "low sexual desire" may in fact have normal levels of desire for sexual activity but inadequate intimacy in their relationships. Insufficient intimacy can manifest itself as "low sexual desire" because the two are interrelated. For these women, sexual desire (physical sexual release) is not the starting point in their sexual response; the desire for intimacy is (Lieblum, 2000).

For example, if someone asked his or her female partner, "Do you want to have sex?" the answer might be "No, let's snuggle." The person initiating might interpret this as his or her partner not wanting to have sex, while the female partner might view this as a prelude to sexual activity or as a *big* part of her sexual activity. Additionally, Basson et al., (2000) found that women with reported low internal feelings of sexual desire might seek to initiate sexual activity with their partners out of a desire to generate intimacy.

Similar issues arise when examining sexual arousal disorders. In men, erection is a clear-cut indicator of arousal. The classic physical manifestation of sexual arousal in women, vaginal lubrication, has been found to be a much less reliable indicator of arousal than previously believed. Lieblum (2000) reports that some victims of sexual assault report lubricating during an assault, whereas some women who have an absence of lubrication due to estrogen deficiency report being "psychologically" aroused. Furthermore, most women are unaware of whether they are lubricating and experiencing genital swelling associated with vasocongestion (Lieblum, 2000).

Female orgasmic disorder relies on a very male-oriented view that orgasm is something easily documented and observable. Whereas orgasm in men is distinguished by contractions and ejaculation, the experience in women is much less clear. Little is known regarding female ejaculation and the emission of fluid other than urine. As Basson et al., (2000) note, many women report that they need not experience orgasm to feel sexually satisfied. This leads one to wonder whether the absence of orgasm should be the basis for a dysfunction.

Lief (1985) argued that a major problem with models of sexual response (and consequently sexual dysfunction) is that they fail to recognize any end point to the phenomenon. Lief believes that measures of "satisfac-

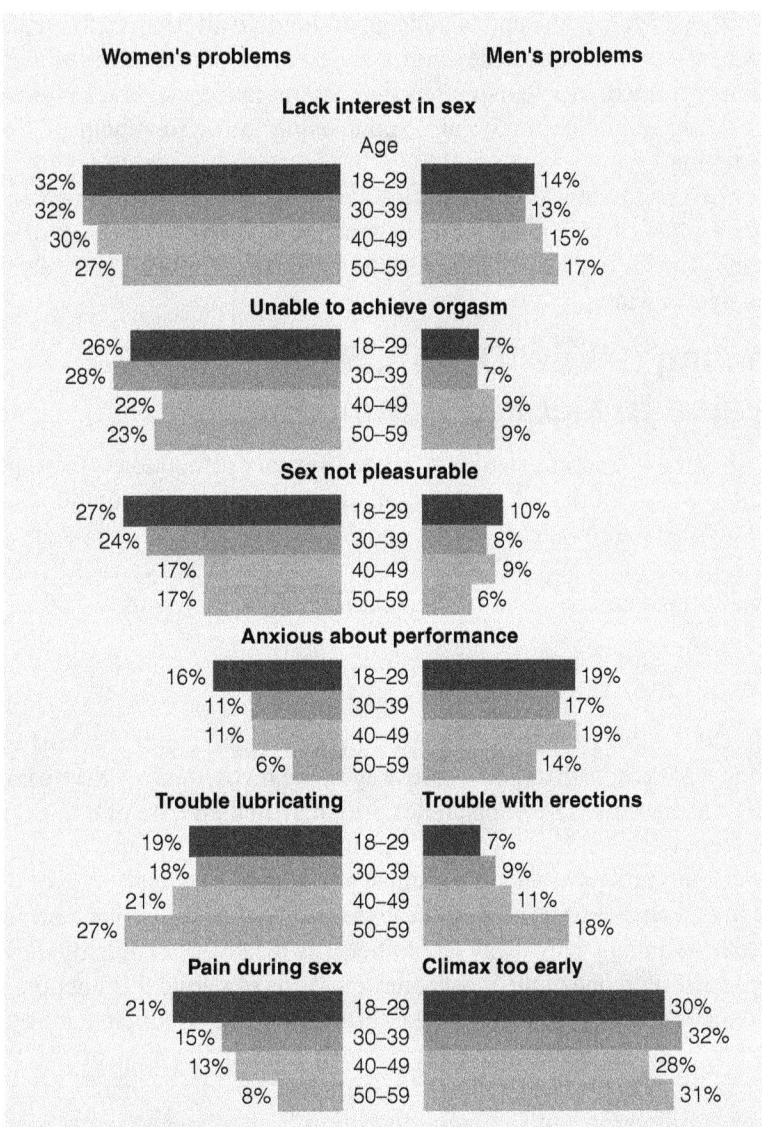

Figure 12.1 *Sexual Dysfunction by Gender and Age*

Source: National Health and Life Survey, 1992.

tion" with the experience should be part of any model. This approach would help us understand sexual response in a more subjective way, similar to how real people define it.

Treating Sexual Dysfunctions

Because the origin and nature of sexual dysfunction are multifaceted, diagnosis and treatment are also usually multifaceted. Treating impaired sexual functioning is complex, with many interdependent components. Sexual dysfunction can be caused by physical problems (for example, arteriosclerosis, which impairs vasocongestion), emotional disorders (excessive stress or negative emotions), spiritual distress (no longer being in love with a partner, lack of self-love), or simple ignorance (poor technique, inadequate stimulation).

Often, sex therapy and enhancement involve all four components. In 1959, Masters and Johnson developed a systematic approach to sex therapy that incorporated an extensive physical examination (to root out organic causes) and individual and couple counseling in the treatment of sexual dysfunction.

Most sex therapists take an extensive medical history, and many incorporate a physical examination as part of the diagnostic work-up of their patients. The individual and couple approaches to counseling and treatment have many variations.

Treating Sexual Dysfunction Related to Medical Conditions

The first step in treating medically related sexual dysfunction is to properly diagnose the condition. A thorough medical examination, combined with a detailed sexual/medical history, guides the therapist in diagnosis. The overwhelming majority of cases of erectile disorder are caused by medical conditions and respond to medical treatment (Lewis et al., 2005; De Tejada, 2002).

Viagra, Levitra, and Cialis

Since 1998, three drugs have been introduced in the United States for the treatment of erectile disorder. These drugs have revolutionized the treatment of erectile disorder. Their appeal lies primarily in their ease of use. Prior to the advent of these drugs, erectile disorder was treated primarily through drug injection therapy, vacuum pumps, and surgical implants. As we'll see later in this chapter, all three of these treatments were invasive, and interrupted lovemaking in one way or another. The discovery of drug therapy for erectile disorder, one of the most common forms of sexual dysfunction, will go down as one of the medical breakthroughs of the twentieth century.

Viagra The drug sildenafil, prescribed for the treatment of erectile disorder

Viagra, the trade name for Sildenafil, was the first of the three drugs to go in the United States in April 1998. The recommended dose of Sidenafil/pill varies but following ingestion Viagra goes to work in about 30 minutes. The effects last for 3–5 hours with a 4-hour average duration (Wooten, 2004).

Viagra immediately became one of the best-selling drugs ever to hit the marketplace. The response to the drug by men who have erectile disorder was staggering. After 3 weeks on the market, Viagra was being prescribed at a rate of at least 10,000 prescriptions a day (Handy, 1998). By the year 2000 over 20 million prescriptions for the drug were being filled worldwide (Rosen & McKenna, 2002).

Unlike injectable drugs, pumps, and implants that produce an erection regardless of a man's level of desire, Viagra enables the production of an erection if desire is present. In other words, Viagra does not produce desire. It is a sexual arousal drug. Viagra works in consort with sexual desire to produce erections. Once a man feels the desire for intercourse, Viagra allows arousal and erections to proceed (Wooten, 2004). If a man is not interested in sex or has little sexual desire, Viagra will not work effectively. Viagra is effective only if a man is sexually aroused and NOS has been released (Wooten, 2004).

As we discussed in Chapter 7, the muscular and vascular changes of erection are controlled by a complex chemical reaction involving nitric oxide synthase (NOS) and the conversion of **guanosine triphosphate** (GTP) into guanosine monophasphate (GMP). This starts a chain reaction resulting in the relaxation of smooth muscle tissue in the penile tissue, allowing it to engorge with blood (Rosen & McKenna, 2002; Wooten, 2004).

Guanosine triphosphate
A chemical that controls the muscular and vascular changes of erection

During sexual arousal, if the man feels sexual desire, GMP is released from cells in the penis that are stimulated by the brain and nervous system. The GMP triggers receptor cells in the spongy erectile tissue, allowing muscles there to relax and penile arteries to dilate. As the erectile tissue expands, it squeezes shut the veins responsible for removing the blood to the area. After orgasm, GMP is broken down by a normally occurring enzyme called *phosphodiesterase 5* (PDE5) (Rosen & McKenna, 2002; Wooten, 2004).

Most men with erectile disorder don't produce enough GMP to override the ever-present PDE5. Their erectile tissue doesn't expand enough to squeeze the veins shut, and consequently the penis does not attain complete erection. Viagra works by suppressing the effects of PDE5, allowing even a limited amount of GMP to cause erections (Rosen & McKenna, 2002).

Another important thing to know about Viagra is that "more" is not better. Viagra is generally prescribed in either 50- or 100-milligram tablets but can be effective in as small as 25 mg. doses (Wooten, 2004). The correct dose is the smallest needed to create the desired effect. The penis has a limited number of receptors for GMP, and the body can process only so much of it. Taking a bigger dose of Viagra will not allow more GMP to be processed than the body can handle. Men who are not having problems with GMP production will not obtain any enhanced erectile effects from taking the drug, because the body is already processing as much GMP as it can handle. Any enhanced erectile response reported probably is placebo effect rather than an effect of Viagra (Handy, 1998).

Levitra (Vardenafil) and Cialis (Tadalafil)

Levitra (Vardenafil) and Cialis (Tadalafil) work basically the same way as Viagra but differ primarily in their specificity, absorption, and potency. The specificity of these three drugs relates primarily to their ability to target the PDE 5 enzyme while not affecting other PDE enzymes. A side effect of Viagra is to influence other PDE enzymes while targeting PDE 5. For example, the PDE 6 enzyme is involved in retinal function and color recognition. A common side effect of Viagra is mild abnormal vision due to it influencing PDE 6 as well as PDE 5. Both Levitra and Cialis are more specific in their ability to target PDE 5. Neither is associated with the mild vision disturbances associated with Viagra. Of the three drugs, Cialis is the only one whose absorption is unaffected by food. Food definitely influences the absorption of Viagra and because of this it should be taken on an empty stomach. While Levitra can be taken with or without food, studies have shown that high-fat meals can delay its absorption (Rosen & McKenna, 2002; Wooten, 2004). The last variable, potency, refers to the duration of effectiveness of the medication. As we mentioned, Viagra takes about 30 minutes to work and the effects last about 4 hours. Levitra becomes

sex in society 12.2

Why No Viagra for Women ?

If Viagra and other drugs have been so effective in reversing the effects of PDE-5 in men, thereby enhancing sexual arousal, why don't they work similar magic in women? There are two main reasons for Viagra's limited effectiveness in treating women's sexual dysfunction; (1) Viagra is a drug to enhance sexual arousal, not sexual desire, (2) most women with a diagnosed sexual dysfunction do not have problems with vasocongestion.

In Chapter 7 we clearly established the link between nitric oxide synthase (NOS) and sexual response in men and women. In men, NOS is released in the spongy erectile tissue of the penis. In women, it is produced in the erectile tissue of the vestibular bulbs, the body and crura of the clitoris and in the tissue of the walls of the vagina (O'Connell, Sanjeevan, Hutson (2005). In both men and women NOS converts guanosine triphosphate (GTP) to guanosine monophosphate (GMP) and starts a chain reaction initiating vasocongestion and sexual arousal (Rosen & McKenna, 2002). In this chapter we discussed how PDE-5, a normally-occurring enzyme, is responsible for degrading GMP and reversing vasocongestion once we either reach orgasm or cease stimulation. As we've seen in this chapter, most problems related to male sexual arousal are not related to lack of desire; they are linked to the breakdown of GMP by PDE-5. Viagra works wonders in correcting this.

The main reason that Viagra seems to be less of a breakthrough for women than for men is that for most women with a sexual dysfunction, vasocongestion is already occurring. For the majority of women seeking sex therapy, vasocongestion is not the issue (Basson et al., 2000). As we mentioned earlier in this chapter, Viagra does not enhance sexual desire. As we've seen in Basson et al's (2000) work in studying sexual response in women, sexual interest, sexual desire, and sexual arousal are all very interrelated and thrive on intimacy. Because Viagra doesn't influence intimacy directly, its utility as anything other than a placebo is limited to those women with problems related to blood flow and engorgement of genital tissue (Boschert, 2000). In these women Viagra has been shown to increase blood flow and enhance sexual arousal (Berman, Berman, Lin et al., 2001; Laan et al., 2002).

Clearly, additional research is needed to more thoroughly understand the physiological and psychosocial mechanisms at work during female sexual arousal. Great strides have been made in the last five years. There is a huge potential market for drugs that can treat female sexual dysfunction. Some advocates see a $3-billion-a-year market on the horizon (Fass, 2004). Others. However, doubt the market for women will ever equal that for men, and question whether female sexual dysfunction is even a disease that warrants the risk of side effects that new medicines pose (Fass, 2004).

effective about 25 minutes after ingestion and lasts up to about 24 hours. In one clinical study of Levitra, some subjects were able to obtain erections that were suitable for intercourse as early as 16 minutes after dosing (Padma-Nathan, Kaufman, & Taylor, 2003). Cialis is the most long-lasting of the three drugs. Cialis begins to work after 30 minutes and is effective between 24–36 hours (Wooten, 2004). During this time a user can achieve additional erections without having to take another does of the medication.

The most common side effects of these drugs are headache and facial flushing. As mentioned, Viagra use has been associated with altered vision. The dosages for all three drugs vary. Consult your physician for the appropriate dose, schedule, and use of these and any drugs (Wooten, 2004).

Drug Injections

Prior to Viagra, most medically caused erectile disorders were treated with self-injections of a drug (alprostadil, a synthetic prostaglandin, is a common one) directly into the penis. The drug works by relaxing the muscles of the spongy erectile tissue, allowing the arteries to dilate and engorgement to occur. Men (and often their partners) were taught how to administer the injections using tiny needles similar to the ones diabetics use to inject insulin. The injections produce a pinprick sensation that patients usually tolerate well.

Unlike Viagra, injection treatment produces an erection without requiring the brain to initiate it through sexual desire. The injections lead to erections in approximately 15 minutes. The medication is premeasured in doses that will produce erections that last for approximately an hour (Goldstein et al., 2000).

Another method of delivering alprostadil involves inserting tiny pellets of the drug directly into the urethra. A small plastic tube containing a plunger product is inserted about 1 inch into the urethra. When the plunger is pushed, it releases the drug, which resembles tiny rabbit food pellets, into the urethra. Within 10 minutes the drug begins to take effect (Goldstein et al., 2000).

Vacuum Pumps

Prior to Viagra and injectable drug therapy, vacuum pumps and surgical implants were used to treat erectile disorder. The vacuum pump is a flexible plastic sleeve that is placed over the penis and secured at the base of the lubricated penis with an elastic band. Suction is applied to the sleeve, by mouth or a small hand pump, through a tube that connects at the other end. The pump draws blood into the penis, filling the erectile tissue and thereby causing an erection. Once the man achieves a sufficient erection, the sleeve is removed and the band is kept in place to trap the blood for about half an hour (Raina, Agawarl, Ausmundson, et al., 2005).

Implants and Other Surgery

Implant treatment involves the surgical implantation of an inflatable penile prosthesis. The device consists of two hollow cylinders connected to a fluid-filled reservoir and a pump. The cylinders are implanted in the shaft of the penis, the reservoir in the abdomen, and the pump in the scrotum. When the man desires an erection, he activates the pump, which fills the cylinders and causes erection. After intercourse, he turns a valve, which empties the cylinders back into the reservoir. Figure 12.2 depicts a penis pump. Implant surgery is considered radical treatment and should be considered only if other forms of treatment fail (Montague, 2000). It can lead to permanent damage that could make a natural erection impossible.

Finally, some structural problems in sexual anatomy may have to be corrected with surgery. Examples are removing scar tissue and freeing adhesions that cause pain during intercourse.

Hormone Treatments

Certain medical conditions, particularly those of the endocrine system, respond to medication or hormone replacement therapy. Correcting a hormonal imbalance

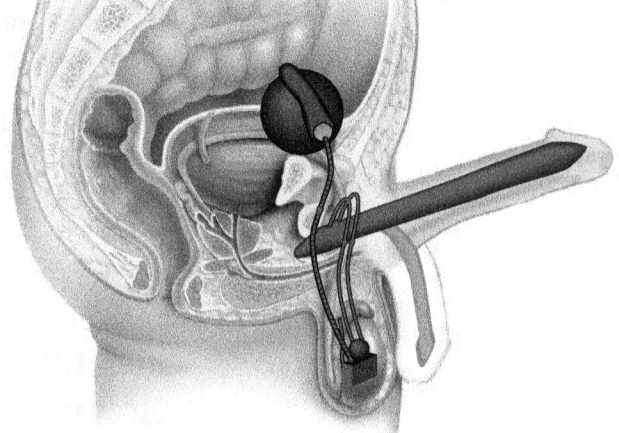

Figure 12.2 *Penis Pump* The penis pump uses a closed system consisting of a hydraulic pump (hidden in the testes), a fluid reservoir (concealed in the abdominal cavity), and expandable chambers (hidden in the penis). To produce an erection, fluid is pumped from the reservoir to the chambers.

that might affect disorders of sexual arousal might best be treated through the oral administration of hormone replacement therapy. Sometimes endocrine glands need help in being stimulated to begin producing adequate amounts of sex hormones.

Medications are available that activate endocrine glands to release their hormones. Although testosterone is often considered a male hormone, both men and women have testosterone, and it is believed to play an important role in libido. As levels of this hormone decline with age, sexual interest may wane. Many women are helped by taking testosterone, in low enough doses to prevent any male secondary characteristics to develop. Also, estrogen improves vaginal lubrication in postmenopausal women.

Other Medical Treatments

Still other sexual dysfunctions are related to a disease that can be treated or cured with medication. Sexual pain disorders associated with sexually transmitted infection, for instance, respond quite well to treatment or cure of the underlying disease condition. Sexual arousal disorders related to cardiovascular problems such as arteriosclerosis often can be improved through medication designed to change blood biochemistry and improve the flow of blood and blood pressure.

Treating Drug-Induced Sexual Dysfunction

Similar to treating organic-based sexual dysfunction, the treatment of drug-induced sexual dysfunction begins with a thorough sexual/medical history and medical examination. The assessment includes current drug use (licit and illicit). The specific drugs are analyzed for possible side effects and interactions to assess their role in the sexual dysfunction. The therapist examines the onset of the sexual dysfunction in relation to the onset of drug use.

Many commonly prescribed medications, alone or in combination with other prescription or over-the-counter medications or psychoactive substances, have potential negative side effects related to sexual response. Sometimes treatment is as simple as changing the dosage of the medication or switching to a similar drug with different side effects. An example is provided by medication for controlling high blood pressure.

A common side effect of certain hypertension medications is erectile dysfunction. Changing the medication often relieves the erectile problem and still controls the patient's high blood pressure. In other cases, treatment consists of avoiding additional medications or substances that, when taken with the prescribed drug, result in sexual dysfunction. Patients often are unaware of the potentially troubling side effects of combining substances.

Treating Psychosocially Based Sexual Dysfunction

Several different sex therapy approaches can be applied when the origin of the dysfunction is psychosocial in nature. The therapeutic approach has four main variables:

- The therapist's theoretical framework
- Duration and schedule of treatment

- Individual versus couple or group approach
- Use of surrogates

Sex therapists come from a variety of backgrounds. Some are physicians with advanced training in psychiatry, sex therapy, psychoanalysis, or counseling. Others are psychologists, psychoanalysts, counselors, and social workers. No uniform credentials are required for sex therapists across the United States; credentialing requirements vary from state to state. Each of these professionals has a philosophical and theoretical framework regarding sex therapy that guides his or her work.

Psychoanalysts, for example, take a psychodynamic approach to treatment that is grounded in the work of Freud. A basic element in their approach is helping the client gain insight into the origin of his or her problem (Kring, 2000). Counselors using a behaviorist approach, in contrast, do not believe it is necessary to delve deeply into their clients' past to help them gain insight into the origin of their problem. Rather, the behaviorist focuses on the here and now and examines the nature of the problem, how the client perceives it, and how it directly affects the person's quality of life.

The therapist's theoretical framework is intimately related to the duration and schedule of therapy. A psychoanalyst might spend several sessions just getting to know the client and establishing trust while beginning to look back into his or her past. A Masters and Johnson–trained therapist team would be finished with therapy by that time because the approach is to get right down to the business of treating the presenting problem in an intensive 2-week program.

Some sex therapists work only with individuals. Most however, believe that sexual dysfunction can be understood and treated only within the context of the relationship. Couples are seen together and individually, and treatment involves treating the couple as well as the individual. Others incorporate group therapy to help couples view their problems in a broader context (Corliss & Steptoe, 2004).

Finally, some sex therapists provide explicit help by using trained **sex surrogate** partners. Although these surrogates are sexually responsive trained professionals who serve as partners for clients, the American Association of Sex Educators, Counselors, and Therapists (AASECT, 1998), one of the leading professional groups charged with certifying sex therapists, does not recommend their use in the treatment of sexual dysfunctions.

Sex surrogate A person who acts as a substitute sex partner during therapy

Most sex therapy is eclectic, combining elements from various forms of psychotherapy, education, and medicine (Bach, Barlow, Wincze, 2004, Rosen, Seidman, Menza et al., 2004). Six common threads that seem to underlie the practice of sex therapy, regardless of the therapist's theoretical framework, are (a) permission-giving, (b) limited information, (c) specific suggestions, (d) selfawareness, (e) communication training, and (f) use of masturbation.

Permission-Giving

Permission-giving is the unconditional support the therapist offers for becoming a fully self-actualized sexual being. Clients are given permission to explore any thoughts, feelings, desires, fantasies, and behaviors that might enhance their sexual pleasure. They also are given permission not to engage in behaviors and relationships that undermine their sexual and other well-being.

Information-Giving

Information-giving or education is a key element in all forms of sex therapy. Because most people receive little or no formal sex education, they often are misinformed about simple issues that can undermine their sexual enjoyment, such as penis size, level of sexual activity, and effects of aging. Often, providing information, along with permission giving, is liberating enough to help people work their way out of some sexual dysfunctions.

Information-giving can include didactic sessions with the therapist related to the individual's specific concerns, guided reading (reading a prescribed set of materials), and viewing instructional videotapes. Providing limited information helps change negative attitudes, open lines of communication, and develop sexual skills necessary for enhancing performance and pleasure.

Specific Suggestions

Each person or couple has unique problems and needs that can be addressed through specific suggestions. The main technique in this regard is "homework assignments" with one's partner. The range of specific suggestions varies depending on the nature of the problem and the specific individual or couple involved. Usually these homework assignments require the couple to practice activities and techniques that the therapist has discussed with them. These often are coupled with communication activities designed to help couples open up and share their feelings with each other.

> ### ❧ *Intellectual Wellness* ❧
>
> Many sexual problems are based on ignorance, illogical thinking, irrational expectations, and poor technique. Intellectual wellness is fostered through knowledge, logical thinking, rational expectations, and improved sexual technique. Much of sex therapy revolves around relearning what good sex is and what being a good lover means. These things can be taught. You can learn about sexual response and what to expect during lovemaking. You can learn to understand the factors that influence interest, desire, plateau, orgasm, and resolution and begin to set more realistic and logical expectations about lovemaking. You can learn techniques and practice your skills (by yourself or with your partner) and become a better lover.

Self-Awareness

Increased self-awareness is a natural outgrowth of permission- and information-giving. Many of the specific suggestions prescribed as homework help individuals and couples focus on their sensual/sexual response. This is the first time many clients have spent focusing on their sexual response and specific techniques related to sensual and sexual arousal.

Sensate focus Nongenital pleasuring used to heighten sensuality without sexual activity

One commonly used activity is called **sensate focus.** In the early stages of sex therapy, the couple is instructed to refrain from sexual activity involving genital contact. This approach is designed to relieve performance anxiety and other forms of anxiety and to allow the couple to focus on nongenital pleasuring.

personal exploration activity
A Great Sex Life

Unfortunately, many of us have just a few sexual issues and hang-ups that may cause our sex life to be less than great. However, there are many things we can do to increase our enjoyment and physical response so that we can have a better sex life. Your task is to find one or more methods to incorporate that would improve your sexual response.

While reading this chapter, compare your sexual response to various sexual disorders. Your goal is to find one that is similar to an issue that you may have experienced. Then choose a sexual therapy that you can try to see whether it improves the way you respond. You may choose one to do alone or with a partner. If you cannot find anything you need to improve, try one of the therapies just for fun. You may find something like sensate focus increases the enjoyment you already experience and may decide to incorporate it in your routine sexual activities. Look for some therapy that would increase pleasure or skill, and give it a try. Hopefully, you will find the results worth the work.

During the first phase of sensate focus (Figure 12.3), each partner is given a turn to explore the other's body. The breasts and genitals are off-limits. The intent is not to give sexual pleasure but instead to establish awareness of touch by paying attention to the textures, contours, and temperature of the partner and to attend to what it feels like to touch and be touched.

The partner doing the touching is in control and is not driven by the needs of the person being touched. The initial stage is supposed to be conducted as silently as possible. The person being touched is allowed to convey (either verbally or nonverbally) when the partner's touch makes him or her uncomfortable.

During the second phase of sensate focus, touch is extended to include the breasts and genitals. The couple receive instructions similar to those in the first phase and are advised to gradually expand the touch to include the genitals. The purpose is still to experience the sensation of touch and to discover what types of touch are most pleasurable.

A simple technique called *handriding* is used during this phase. This involves having one partner place his or her hand over the partner's and to guide it on an exploration of the other's body. The guiding hand non-verbally communicates by increasing or decreasing the pressure, changing the speed or type of motion, and holding the hand to linger. The idea is to help the partner who is doing the touching understand the preferences of the partner being touched without controlling the action. The partner doing the touching is still in control but is guided along.

In the third phase of sensate focus, the couple is asked to explore each other at the same time. Rather than take turns, the couple doubles the amount of sensory input by mutual exploration. This simulates real-life touching and allows the couple the opportunity to get lost in the sensations of touch without the pressure to have intercourse.

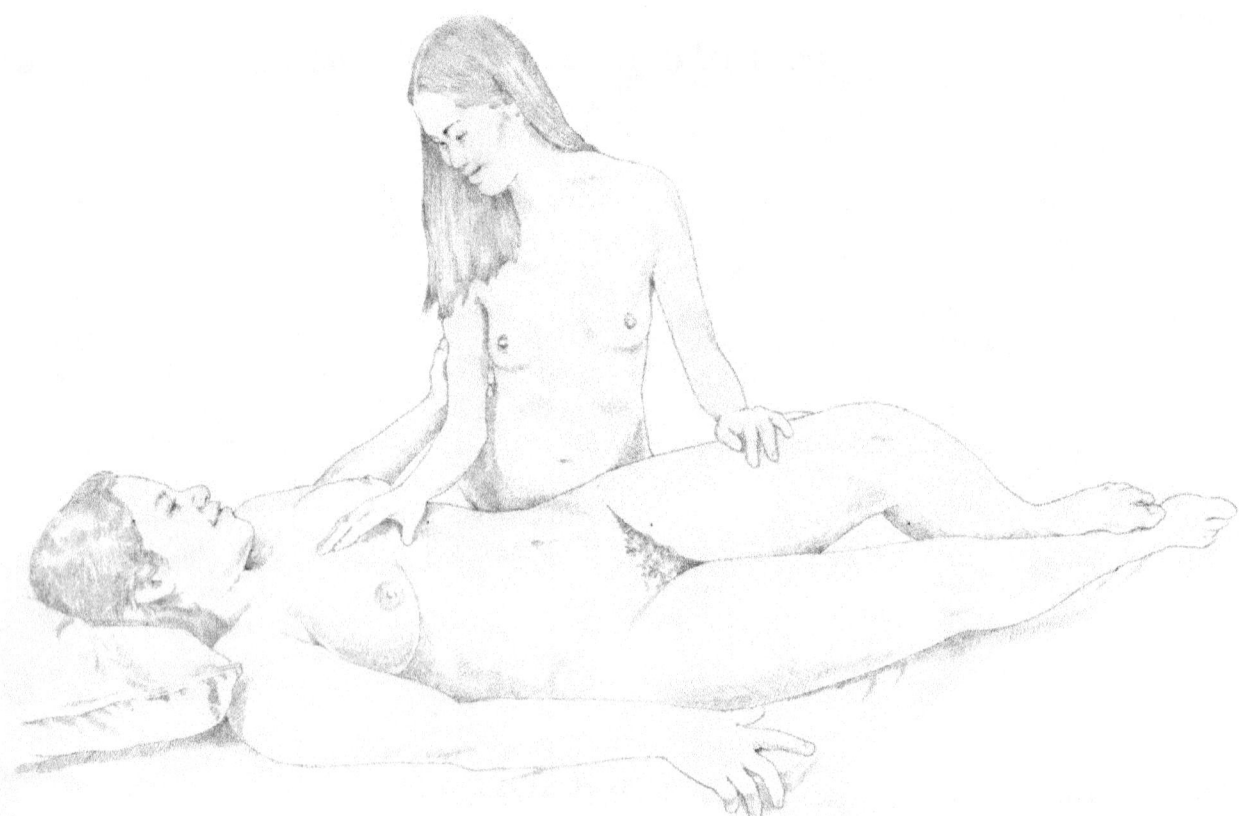

Figure 12.3 *Couple Practicing Sensate Focus* During the first stage of sensate focus, couples practice nongenital pleasuring.

In the last stage of sensate focus, the couple shifts to the female-on-top position without attempting full penetration of the penis. In this position, the woman can rub her clitoris directly against her partner and stimulate his penis with her vulva and vaginal opening. This position may or may not result in arousal and full erection in her partner. The purpose is not to cause full arousal and intercourse, but if an erection occurs, she can put the tip of the penis into her vaginal opening. The couple are instructed to continue to explore each other, using full body contact to explore the sensations of touch and arousal. After the couple has worked through the stages of sensate focus successfully and is comfortable with it, the two of them usually are ready to experience full intercourse without difficulty.

Communication Training

Couples can learn how to communicate nonverbally through sensate focus and other awareness-building activities. Often, nonverbal communication—such as placing a hand or other body part in a certain position or holding a partner to linger at what he or she is doing—can transmit information that will help treat sexual problems. Improving verbal communication —in particular, expressing needs and desires and communicating using "I" language instead of blaming one's partner—is integral to all forms of sex therapy. Communication building can occur during sessions with the therapist and as homework assignments.

Use of Masturbation

Sex therapy commonly includes masturbation, both individual and mutual. It can be used in sexual arousal disorders to help both partners explore the types, intensity, and duration of stimulation necessary for full arousal. It also can help the couple learn how to delay orgasm in cases of premature ejaculation.

A variation of masturbation used to treat premature ejaculation is the squeeze technique, illustrated in Figure 12.4. During manual stimulation of her partner, the woman is instructed to stop periodically and apply firm pressure for a few seconds to the frenulum and coronal ridge with her thumb and first and second fingers, respectively. This squeezing reduces her partner's urgency to ejaculate. She can continue to masturbate her partner, stopping periodically to squeeze. Through this technique her partner can learn to delay ejaculation.

Masturbation also can be used to treat female and male orgasmic disorder. Often these conditions are related to inadequate sexual stimulation. Through permission giving, sensate focus, and masturbation, men and women can learn the type, intensity, and duration of stimulation necessary for orgasm.

Treatment progresses from individual masturbation, to masturbation in the presence of the partner, to being masturbated by the partner, to using masturbation as a prelude to intercourse.

Masturbation, coupled with the use of increasingly larger dilators can be used to treat some cases of vaginismus. Women are taught to use permission giving, self-awareness, and masturbation to initiate sexual arousal and to use the varying sizes of dilators for 10 to 15 minutes at a time to introduce objects into her vagina. The goal is to work up to a penis-size dilator and then make the transition to a real penis.

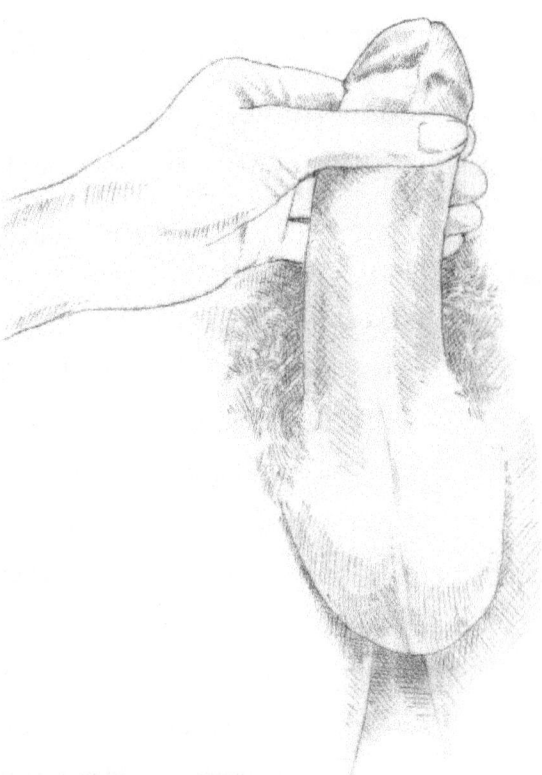

Figure 12.4 *Squeeze Technique* During the squeeze technique, the partner's erect penis is periodically squeezed to inhibit ejaculation.

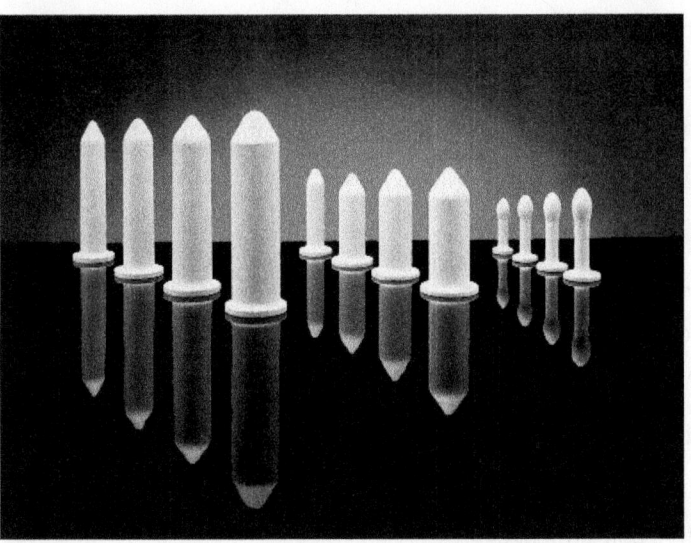

Image courtesy of CooperSurgical Milex Pessaries.

Vaginal dilators come in varying sizes and colors.

Personal Assessment

Are You an Addict?

Substance abuse is not only a risk factor for sexual dysfunction; it can destroy your life. This assessment is designed to help you assess whether your current drug use is considered addictive. The following questions were written by recovering addicts in Narcotics Anonymous.

Please answer yes or no.

1. Do you ever use alone?

2. Have you ever substituted one drug for another, thinking that one particular drug was the problem?

3. Have you ever manipulated or lied to a doctor to obtain prescription drugs?

4. Have you ever stolen drugs or stolen to obtain drugs?

5. Do you regularly use a drug when you wake up or when you go to bed?

6. Have you ever taken one drug to overcome the effects of another?

7. Do you avoid people or places that do not approve of you using drugs?

8. Have you ever used a drug without knowing what it was or what it would do to you?

9. Has your job or school performance ever suffered from the effects of your drug use?

10. Have you ever been arrested as a result of using drugs?

11. Have you ever lied about what or how much you use?

12. Do you put the purchase of drugs ahead of your financial responsibilities?

13. Have you ever tried to stop or control your using?

14. Have you ever been in a jail, hospital, or drug rehabilitation center because of your using?

15. Does using interfere with your sleeping or eating?

16. Does the thought of running out of drugs terrify you?

17. Do you feel it is impossible for you to live without drugs?

18. Do you ever question your own sanity?

19. Is your drug use making life at home unhappy?

20. Have you ever thought you couldn't fit in or have a good time without using drugs?

21. Have you ever felt defensive, guilty, or ashamed about your using?

22. Do you think a lot about drugs?

23. Have you had irrational or indefinable fears?

24. Has using affected your sexual relationships?

25. Have you ever taken drugs you didn't prefer?

26. Have you ever used drugs because of emotional pain or stress?

27. Have you ever overdosed on any drugs?

28. Do you continue to use despite negative consequences?

29. Do you think you might have a drug problem?

Are you an addict? This is a question only you can answer. Members of Narcotics Anonymous found that they all answered different numbers of these questions yes. The actual number of yes responses isn't as important as how you feel inside and how addiction has affected your life. If you are an addict, you must first admit that you have a problem with drugs before any progress can be made toward recovery.

Do You Suffer from Erectile Disorder?

Take the Viagra erectile disorder self-assessment at http://www.viagra.com/rate-your-sexual-health.aspx and calculate your score. If the results indicate that you may be suffering from erectile disorder, consult your physician for further assessments.

Thought Questions

1. How do the categories of dysfunctions mesh with the stages of the sexual response cycle? Why are they set up this way?

2. What are two dysfunctions related to sexual desire?

3. When does low interest in sexual activity become a desire disorder?

4. What is the relationship between cardiovascular health and sexual arousal disorders?

5. What does the term *preorgasmic* mean?

6. What are three illness-related causes of sexual dysfunction?

7. What are three medication-related causes of sexual dysfunction?

8. Are isolated episodes of sexual dysfunction normal? If so, why?

Test Yourself

1. Which of the following best characterizes the relationship between cardiovascular disease and sexual dysfunction?
   a. There is very little relationship between cardiovascular disease and any form of sexual dysfunction.
   b. All forms of high blood pressure medication causes impotence in most men and women.
   c. The majority of cases of erectile dysfunction are related to cardiovascular disease.
   d. A small percentage of cases of erectile dysfunction are related to cardiovascular disease.

2. Damage to the blood vessels of the underside of the penis causing erectile dysfunction
   a. can be minimized by using protective athletic cups and contoured bicycle seats.
   b. cannot be minimized by using protective athletic cups and contoured bicycle seats.
   c. is unrelated to sports and other athletic activities.
   d. is grossly overstated.

3. The negative effects of alcohol and other depressant drugs on sexual response begin when
   a. their depressant effects impair good judgment.
   b. their depressant effects move beyond inducing relaxation and reducing anxiety to create paranoia.
   c. their depressant effects move beyond inducing relaxation and reducing anxiety to inhibiting blood flow and other metabolic functions.
   d. their depressant effects put users to sleep.

4. Although stimulant drugs such as cocaine and amphetamines seem to provide energy and increased sexual interest,
   a. they can inhibit orgasm and result in diminished desire.
   b. they do not last long.
   c. their long-term use is misunderstood.
   d. they can cause death due to the strain of orgasm.

5. The use of narcotics such as heroin is associated with
   a. increased sexual interest.
   b. no change in sexual interest.
   c. decreased sexual interest.
   d. distorted sexual interest.
6. Which of the following best describes the relationship between the types of sexual dysfunction categorized by the American Psychiatric Association (APA) and the sexual response cycle?
   a. They are the same thing.
   b. The types of sexual dysfunction correspond to the sexual response cycle.
   c. They are very different from the APA, which takes a very psychiatric approach to this problem.
   d. They are similar but different.
7. What is the difference between sexual disinterest and sexual aversion disorder?
   a. They are the same thing.
   b. People with sexual aversion disorder are anxious about, fear, or are disgusted with sexual activity, whereas those with sexual disinterest are just not very interested in sex.
   c. People with sexual disinterest disorder are anxious about, fear, or are disgusted with sexual activity, whereas those with sexual aversion disorder merely avoid sex.
   d. People with sexual disinterest usually progress to sexual aversion.

8. Which statement best characterizes the use of Viagra in women?
   a. Viagra is an effective treatment for women with female sexual arousal disorder.
   b. Viagra is not an effective treatment for women with female sexual arousal disorder because the condition in women is usually not associated with vascular problems.
   c. Viagra is more effective in women than in men.
   d. Viagra is a very effective treatment for women with female sexual arousal disorder because the condition in women is usually associated with vascular problems.
9. Viagra works in the treatment of male erectile disorder by
   a. increasing sexual desire.
   b. increasing testosterone levels.
   c. relaxing stress associated with performance.
   d. relaxing erectile tissue, allowing penile arteries to dilate.
10. Which of the following is not commonly used in eclectic sex therapy?
   a. Surrogate sex partners
   b. Communication training
   c. Specific suggestions
   d. Masturbation

Web Resources

Viagra Home Page
www.viagra.com

This site is a comprehensive resource for the drug and has had nearly 10 million visits.

National Foundation for Sexual Health Medicine (NFSHM)
http://www.internet-web-directory.com/Detailed/L946077/

A nonprofit organization dedicated to educating the medical community and the public about sexual health. NFSHM addresses the growing need for current information on sexual health by offering information and training to clinicians and the general public. Click the "Resources" link on the top of their page for access to their journals and other resources.

Mental Health Net
http://mentalhelp.net

Net guide to mental health, psychology, and psychiatry; addresses the symptoms, online resources, and organizations concerning sexual problems of dyspareunia, exhibitionism, female and male orgasmic disorders, female sexual arousal disorder, fetishism, frotteurism, gender identity disorder, male erectile disorder, premature ejaculation, sexual masochism and sadism, transvestic fetishism, vaginismus, and voyeurism.

References

American Association of Sex Educators, Counselors, and Therapists. (1998). *Ethical guidelines for sex therapists.* Washington, DC.

American Psychiatric Association (APA). (2000). *Diagnostic and statistical manual of mental illness* (4th ed., text revision). Washington, DC.

Bach, A. K., Barlow, D. H., Wincze, J. P. (2004). The Enhancing Effects of Manualized Treatment for Erectile Dysfunction Among Men Using Sildenafil: A Preliminary Investigation. *Behavior Therapy*, Winter 2004, 35 (1) pg. 55–73.

Barbach, L. (1982). *For each other: Sharing sexual intimacy.* Garden City, NY: Doubleday.

Basson, R., Berman, J., Burnett, A., Derogatis, L., Ferguson, D., Fourcoy, J., Goldstein, L., Graziotto, A., Heiman, J., Laan, E., Lieblum, S., Padma-Nathan, H., Rosen, R., Seagraves, K., Shabsigh, R., Sipsk, M., Wagner, G., & Whipple, B. (2000). Report of the International Consensus Development Conference on Female Sexual Dysfunction: Definitions and classifications. *Journal of Urology, 163,* 888–893.

Basson, R. (2004). Recent advances in women's sexual function and dysfunction. *Menopause.* 2004 Nov–Dec11(6):714–25.

Basson, R. (2002). Are our definitions of women's desire, arousal and sexual pain disorders too broad and our definition of orgasmic disorder too narrow? *J Sex Marital Ther.* 2002 July–Sept.28(4):289–300.

Berman, J. R., Berman, L. A., Lin, H., Flaherty, E., Leahy, N., Goldstein, I., Cantey-Kiser, J. (2001). Effect of sidenafil on subjective and physiologic parameters of the female sexual response in women and sexual arousal disorder. *Journal of Sex and Marital Therapy*, 27 pages 411–420.

Boschert, S. (2000, July). Women don't get a rise out of taking Viagra. *Ob Gyn News, 35*(13), 23–24.

Corliss, R., Steptoe, S. (2004). The Marriage Savers. *Time*, vol. 163, no. 3, Jan 19th 2004, pp. 88–92.

DeTejada, I. S. (2002). Molecular mechanisms for the regulation of penile smooth muscle contractility. *International Journal of Impotence Research* 2002 (14) Supplement 1, pp. 6–10.

Dodson, B. (1974). *Liberating masturbation.* New York: Dodson. *Drug Week.* (2001, August 24). Viagra-type drugs unlikely to solve many women's sexual response problems [Online]. Article A78895438. Available: NewsRX.net.

Enserink, M. (2005). Let's Talk About Sex—and Drugs. *Science* 308, June 10, 2005. pgs. 1578–1580.

Fass, A. (2004). Quest for Desire. *Forbes*, Vol. 174, Issue 11, Nov., 29, 2004. pp. 115–116.

Fisher, B. S., Cullen, F. T., & Turner, M. G. (2000). *The sexual victimization of college women.* Washington DC: U.S. Department of Justice.

Fisher, H. (2004). *Why we love; the nature and chemistry of romantic love.* New York: Henry Holt and Company.

Goldstein, I., Auerbach, S., Palma-Nathan, H., Rajfer, J., Fitch, W., Schmitt, L. (2000). Axial penile rigidity as primary efficacy outcome during multi-institutional in-office dose titration clinical trials with alprostadil alfadex in patients with erectile dysfunction. *Int J Impot Res.* 2000 Aug 12; (4):205–11.

Goldstein, I. (2000). Male sexual circuitry. *Scientific American* August 2000, Vol. 283, Issue 2, pp. 70–75.

Goldberg, R. (2006). *Drugs across the spectrum.* Englewood, CO: Morton.

Gutfield, G. (1994). The prescription for male potency. *Prevention, 46*(11), 78–82.

Handy, B. (1998). The Viagra craze. *Time, 151*(17), 50–53.

Heapes, T. (1994). Smoking your sex life away. *Muscle & Fitness, 55*(4), 42.

Heiman, J,R. (2002a). Sexual Dysfunction: Overview of Prevalence, Etiological Factors, and Treatments. *The Journal of Sex Research* v. 39 no. 1 (February 2002) p. 73–78.

Heiman, J. R. (2002b). Psychologic Treatments for Female Sexual Dysfunction: Are They Effective and Do We Need Them? *Archives of Sexual Behavior* Vol. 31 number 5, Oct. 2002, pp. 445–450.

Higher Education Center. (2003). *Sexual assault: Alcohol and other drugs.* http://www. Edc.org/ hec/pubs/factsheets/fact_sheet1.html.

Hite, S. (1977). *The Hite report.* New York: Dell.

Hyde, J. S. (1994). *Understanding human sexuality* (5th ed.). New York: McGraw-Hill.

Johnson, S. D., Phelps, D. L., Cottler, L. B. (2004). The Association of Sexual Dysfunction and Substance Use Among a Community Epidemiological Sample. *Archives of Sexual Behavior*, Feb. 2004, 33 (1) pp. 55–63.

Johnson, J. (2004). Exposed at last; the truth about your clitoris. In Worcester N.

Jones, H. B., & Jones, H. (1977). *Sensual drugs: Deprivation and rehabilitation of the mind.* London: Cambridge University Press, pp. 387–389.

Kita, J. (2001). The sex crusaders. *Men's Health, 16*(9), 98–106.

Kloner, R., Padma, N. H. (2005). Erectile Dysfunction in patients with coronary artery disease. *International Journal of Impotence Research*, Jun 2005, Vol. 17 Issue 3, p. 209–215.

Kobilinsky, S., & Palmeter, J. (1984). Sex role orientation, mother's expression of affection toward spouse and college women's attitudes towards sexual behaviors. *Journal of Sex Research, 20,* 32–43.

Kring, B. (2000). Psychotherapy of sexual dysfunction. *American Journal of Psychotherapy*, Vol 54 no. 1, Winter 2000, pp. 97–101.

Laan, E., Van Lunsen, R. H., Everaerd, W., Riley, A., Scott, E., Bodell, M. (2002). The enhancement of vaginal vasocongestion by sidenafil in healthy premenopausal women. *Journal of Women's Health and Gender-Based Medicine*, pp. 357–365.

Legato, M. (1999). *Summary: U.S. Department of Health and Human Services, Public Health Service, National Institutes of Health: A report of the task force on the NIH Women's Health Research Agenda for the 21st century. Vol. 1: Executive summary* [Online]. Available: www:4.od.nih.gov/orwh/report.pdf.

Lemonick, M. (2004). The Chemistry of Desire. *Time*, Jan 19th, 2004, pp. 62–68.

Lewis, J. H., Rosen, R., Goldstein, I. (2005). Erectile dysfunction. *Nursing*, February, 2005, 35(2) p. 64.

Lieblum, S. R. (2000, November). Redefining female sexual response. *Contemporary ObGyn, 45* (11), 120–131.

Lief, H. (1985). Evaluation of inhibited sexual desire: Relationship aspects. In H. S. Kaplan (Ed.), *Comprehensive evaluation of disorders of sexual desire* (pp. 59–76). Washington, DC: American Psychiatric Press.

Lowinson, J. H., Ruiz, P., Millman, R. B., & Langrod, J. G. (1992). *Substance abuse: A comprehensive textbook* (2nd ed.). Baltimore: Williams & Wilkinson.

Masters, W. H, & Johnson, V. E. (1970). *Human sexual inadequacy.* Boston: Little, Brown.

Masters, W. H., Johnson, V. E., & Kolodny, R. (1996). *Human sexuality* (5th ed.). New York: HarperCollins.

McCabe, M. P. (2004). Exacerbation of Symptoms Among People With Multiple Sclerosis: Impact on Sexuality and Relationships Over Time. *Archives of Sexual Behavior*, December, 2004, 33 (6) pp. 593–601.

Montague, D. K. (2000). How to implant a three-piece inflatable penile prosthesis. *Urology Times*, Jul 2000, Vol. 28 Issue 7, pp. 32–34.

Montague, A. (1977). *Touching: The human significance of the skin.* New York: Harper & Row.

Munarriz, R., Kim, N. N., Goldstein, I., Traish, A. M. (2002). Biology of female sexual function. *Urol Clin North Am.* 2002 Aug; 29(3):685–693.

National Council on Patient Information and Education (2001). Alcohol and Medications: Ask Before You Mix, publication #B-20, Washington, DC: National Council on Patient Information and Education.

O'Donohue, W., & Geer, J. H. (1993). *Handbook of sexual dysfunctions: Assessment and treatment.* Needham Heights, MA: Allyn & Bacon.

O'Connell, H. E., Sanjeevan, K, V., Hutson, J. M. (2005). Anatomy of the clitoris. *J Urol.* 2005 Oct; 174(4 Pt 1):1189–95.

Padma-Nathan, H., Kaufman, J., & Taylor, T. (2003, June 28–July 1). *Earliest time of onset of erections with vardenafil determined in an at-home setting.* Paper presented at the Second International Consultation on Erectile and Sexual Dysfunctions, Paris.

Parker-Pope, T. (2002). Studies link bicycling to impotence. *Wall Street Journal*, Oct 15th, 2002, p. D1.

Parrish, M. (1997). Up, up, and away. *Playboy,* *44*(6), 92–99.

Phillips, N. A. (2000). Female sexual dysfunction: evaluation and treatment. *American Family Physician*, Vol 62, number 1, July 2000, pp. 127–142.

Purcell, S. (1985, August 25). *The relationship between religious orthodoxy and marital sexual functioning.* Paper presented at annual meeting of American Psychological Association.

Raina, R., Agawarl, A., Ausmundson, S., Lakin, M., Nandipati, K. C., Montague, D. K., Mansour D., Zippe, C. D. (2005). Early use of vacuum constriction device following radical prostatectomy facilitates early sexual activity and potentially earlier return of erectile function. *International Journal of Impotence Res*. 2005 Aug 18, pp. 57–87.

Richardson, J. D.(1991). Medical causes of sexual dysfunction. *Medical Journal of Australia,155,* 29–33.

Rosen, R. C., McKenna, K. E. (2002). PDE-5 Inhibition and sexual response; pharmacological mechanisms and clinical outcomes. *Annual Review of Sex Research.* Volume 13 pages, 36–88.

Rosen, R. C., Seidman, S. N., Menza, M.A., Shabsigh, R., Roose, S. P., Tseng, L. J., Orazem, J., Siegel, R. I. (2004). Quality of life, mood, and sexual function; a path analytic model of treatment effects in men with erectile dysfunction.. *International Journal of Impotence Research*, Aug 2004, Vol 16 Issue 4, pp. 334–340.

Scelfo, J. (2002). Bored with sleeping? Sleep and Sex. *Newsweek* v. 140 no.3 (July 15, 2002) p. 45.

Singer-Kaplan, H. (1974). *The new sex therapy.* New York: Brunner/Mazel.

Stevenson, R. W. D. (2002, January). Sexual dysfunction: Attending to the mind–body continuum. *Medical Aspects of Human Sexuality, 2,* 7–9.

Swindle, R. W., Cameron, A. E., Lockhart, D. C. (2004). The Psychological and Interpersonal Relationship Scales: Assessing Psychological and Relationship Outcomes Associated With Erectile Dysfunction and Its Treatment. *Archives of Sexual Behavior* Vol. 33, Issue 1, Feb. 2004, pp. 19–30.

United States Department of Health and Human Services USDHHS (2000). Alcohol and health: Tenth special report to the US Congress. *NIH Publication* 00-1583. Washington DC: US Government Printing Office.

Warnock, J. (2005). Acquired, Generalized, Female Hypoactive Sexual Desire Disorder: I Had It, I Lost It, I Want It Back. *Psychiatric Times*, August, 2005, Vol. 22, Issue 9, pp. 45–52.

Weschler, H., Eun, L. J., Kuo, M., Sebring, M., Nelson, T. F., & Lee, H. (2002). Trends in college binge drinking during a period of increased prevention efforts: Findings from four Harvard School of Public Health college alcohol study surveys: 1993–2001. *Journal of AmericanCollege Health,* 50(5), pp. 203–217.

Witters, W., Venturelli, P., & Hanson, P. (1992). *Drugs and society.*3rd ed. Boston: Jones & Bartlett.

Wooten, J. M. (2004). Erectile Dysfunction. *RN,* October, 2004, No. 67 (10), pp. 40–45.

Zilbergeld, B. (1992). *The new male sexuality.* New York: Bantam.

thirteen

Human Reproduction

Student Learning Objectives

After reading this chapter, students will be able to

- Describe the dynamics of conception.
- Describe normal developmental characteristics during the three trimesters of pregnancy.
- Assess the influence of a variety of negative personal behaviors (such as alcohol use) on prenatal development.
- Describe personal health behaviors that enhance pregnancy outcomes.
- Identify a variety of alternatives to traditional conception and parenting.
- Describe a variety of factors related to infertility.
- Identify options available to enhance fertility.
- Describe the process of childbirth.
- Evaluate options for labor and delivery.
- Identify areas where health policies affect individual choices.

activity teaser: Are you ready to be a parent? Find out with the Personal Exploration Activity on page 391.

case study 13.1

Ana, Then and Now

Ana, 24, identifies as Dominican American.

One day in class, Ana shared with her peers that she had had a child at the age of 15. Her boyfriend at the time was a senior in high school. They seldom used any method of birth control; he told her not to worry, and she figured that since she had been a virgin up until then, there really was not much to worry about. He knew what he was doing.

Ana was not particularly aware of when she got her period, didn't understand fertility too well, and when she hadn't had her period for 3 months, realized that she may be pregnant. She was able to do a pregnancy test, and when it came up positive, she felt so confused. Eventually, she told her mother, who was upset yet very supportive. They went to the local hospital that had a teen clinic, and from that point of 16 weeks' pregnant forward, she received the prenatal care she needed. The birth was hard, but the baby was healthy.

Finishing high school and going on to college was always a part of Ana's dreams. And she followed that dream. What she didn't do then, she admits, was be a very good mother. Her mother "mothered" her son, and they all continued living at her home. The father of the baby hasn't had too much to do with them, although occasionally he visits or sends some money.

Today, Ana is a 24-year-old college senior, married and pregnant again. She laughs as she recounts how the baby's due date is 2 weeks after graduation. She planned this pregnancy, has been receiving prenatal care all along, and knows what to expect during delivery. Her sonogram let her know that she is having another boy, and from all reports he is developing normally. She feels so lucky that her husband is an active father to her older son and has been so involved with her pregnancy. He actively participates at the birthing classes and has his camera ready for the delivery. This time around, Ana knows she can be the parent she needs to be.

Critical Thinking

If Ana's family had not been supportive at the time of her first pregnancy, what kinds of decisions may she have had to make at that time?

What impact might those decisions have had in contrast to how she is living now?

In the not so distant past, when a child asked his or her parents "Where did I come from?", the answer was usually not very complicated. There may have been discussion about the sperm meeting the egg, the baby developing and then childbirth. However, children asking this question today may receive answers that are far more complicated, as the ways in which babies are "made" and "born" have become more varied.

Imagine that a child asks her parents, "Where did I come from?" and gets the following answer:

> Mom and Dad weren't able to have a child in the typical way, but we very much wanted to become parents. Because Mom's ovaries didn't work quite right, we went to the fertility bank, where we found an ova donor who was a lot like Mom. Her skin and hair color were like mine, and we seemed to like to do the same things. She seemed a good match for me.

418

personal exploration activity
The World's Greatest Parent

Taking care of a baby before it is born is essential to the well-being of the child. However, the hard work has just begun. Parenting is complex and challenging, and often we are totally unprepared for the job. The following interview activity will help you begin the process of determining what you will need to do to be an effective, loving parent.

It is time to put your friends to work again to help you gather some ideas about healthy and unhealthy parenting. Interview five of your friends or acquaintances using the following questions, recording all of their answers in a journal.

1. What are the characteristics of a good parent?
2. What are the characteristics of a poor parent?
3. What are some things your parents or friend's parents did that you would like to do with your children?
4. What are some things your parents or friend's parents did that you will not do with your children?
5. How did your parents or friends' parents handle sexuality that you will also do with your children?
6. How did your parents or friends' parents handle sexuality that you will not do with your children?
7. In what activities will you encourage your children to participate?
8. What activities will you discourage your children from participating in?

When you have finished interviewing, review your list and add ideas you have about each question. Can you incorporate the ideas you gathered so you can be "the world's greatest parent"?

> *Dad found out that his body didn't make enough sperm, so he used the sperm directory and also found a good match. The laboratory was able to join the donated ova with the donated sperm, and then a very kind lady carried you as you grew inside her uterus. Nine months later we watched your birth and took you home!*

Even though one couple would not likely utilize all of this technology, each facet is possible today. Not even the U.S. legal system has been able to keep up with the rapid changes in reproductive technologies, with some very modern and difficult questions posed to the courts.

To date, individuals and couples alike have turned to the legal system for what sometimes seem Solomonesque decisions concerning their fertility and reproductive rights. For example, in one divorce case, the couple even fought over the ova that had been taken from the wife's body. The wife wanted control over the embryos she believed to be her only chance at a pregnancy, and the husband wanted them destroyed. The court found that the frozen embryos were part of the property to be split in a divorce. The wife was awarded custody of the embryos. On appeal, the husband got "custody" of the embryos—and he destroyed them. Other cases have focused on unhealthy babies born from donors and large amounts of money having exchanged hands, leaving the "buyer" unhappy with his or her "purchase." Indeed, having babies has moved from the bedroom and out into the medical, technological, legal, and business worlds.

To Parent or Not to Parent

The decision about whether or not to have children may be the most life changing and important decisions one will ever make. While most people think very carefully about who and when to marry, many never closely examine whether they really want to take on the awesome responsibility of having and raising a child. However, unlike marriage where divorce is an option, a child is a lifelong responsibility. Some individuals and/or couples care for a friends' child for the weekend or get a dog to help assess how well they work individually and as a couple with the responsibilities of caring for a dependent. If after careful examination, they decide to become parents, they then face the decisions of how many children to have, when to have them, and how far apart to space them, all aspects of **family planning.** With reproductive technologies becoming more familiar and accessible, prenatal screenings more widespread, and better prenatal care more available, prospective parents have the opportunity to improve the health and welfare of their babies. In addition, if biological parenthood is not possible, adoption opportunities—albeit at great personal, emotional, and financial expense—exist both within and outside the United States.

Family planning The conscious effort of deciding to have a family, including when to have children, how many, and how far apart to space them

❧ *Intellectual and Emotional Wellness* ❧

Becoming a parent has many intellectual challenges. Individuals find themselves thinking about their values, what is important, and how best to rear a child. College students may find that the challenges of college preclude time to take care of children. Particularly with young children, little time may be available to attend classes, read, study, and prepare papers. More and more colleges and universities are providing child care facilities, yet comprehensive care, including infant care, is limited.

Becoming a parent requires emotional readiness. Some individuals know "I'm just not ready to do this now." The role of mother or father has been so idealized that reality comes as a major shock to many new parents. Finding no time for oneself, with another person so totally dependent on the parent, is a new experience. The lack of sleep that accompanies new parenthood also takes its toll. When babies have colic and cry for what seems like months, can you be the patient, adoring parent that you envisioned being? How well are you able to put another's needs above your own?

The emotional/mental illnesses of the parents certainly have an impact on the welfare of the children. Parenthood and the care of a baby are not always "natural," positive experiences for which everyone is ready. The ideal for a child is to live with parents who are emotionally healthy, parents who love themselves and are able to fully love their child or children. Perhaps we all need to work on learning to love ourselves and live positively before we contemplate having children.

sex in society 13.1

Who Makes Appropriate Parents?

Society makes judgments about who would make appropriate parents, with the ideal not matching up well to the diverse realities of American families. Income, age, marital status, and sexual orientation become a few of the focal points for commentary and public policy.

Young teens who become parents are part of the "teen pregnancy problem" in the United States. School dropout rates and teen parenthood often intersect with poverty, lack of academic achievement, and a focus biased in the direction of the girl (Cassell, 2002). Compared to living with two parents, research indicates that a child growing up in a household headed by a young, poor teen mother is twice as likely to drop out of high school, 2.5 times as likely to become a teen mother, and 1.4 times as likely to be out of school and unemployed (Cassell, 2002). There is a growing and perhaps long overdue need to address the sexual and reproductive rights of males. For males, age at first intercourse, early fatherhood and living apart from their biological children, higher rates of infection, and marriage and divorce rates all seem to be exacerbated by poverty (Alan Guttmacher Institute, 2002). The development of policies to promote healthier families requires addressing the experiences of both males and females.

In 1997, a woman who had "tricked" a fertility program by claiming to be in her early 50s when she actually was in her early 60s subsequently gave birth to her first child at age 62. This prompted numerous editorials and angry letters to editors in newspapers across the country. How selfish for a woman to become a mother at that age! In contrast, when actor Tony Randall fathered his first child in his mid-70s, he was not subject to as much ridicule or outrage.

Nonetheless, waiting until older to become a parent has its drawbacks. Although it is no longer unusual to see "gray-haired parents "at PTA meetings of elementary- aged children, women in particular still struggle with their "biological clocks." Sylvia Ann Hewlett (2002), in the book *Creating a Life: Professional Women and the Quest for Children,* reported on a national survey of high achieving women. She found

that 42 percent of these women working in corporate America still did not have children at age 40. Although admittedly some women in the group chose a professional career with no thoughts of having children, others found themselves childless by circumstance. The decision to become a parent after age 35 for women can mean greater reliance on infertility programs, with or without success, not to mention great financial expense. The concept of a "ticking biological clock" does not affect men in the same way. At the same time, being close to two generations older than a child can impact family dynamics.

When lesbian and gay couples choose to parent, they often find themselves being judged by a culture that traditionally has defined parenthood as a heterosexual right. Psychological studies have shown that good parenting is the key ingredient to raising healthy children, not the sexual orientation of the parents. The concern that having gay or lesbian parents will deprive a child of the opposite sex's influence is common yet without a scientific basis. Apart from the realities that children are exposed to many individuals throughout their schooling, play, neighborhoods, and media, the key to good development is to have a caring, consistent adult with good parenting skills. A comprehensive report conducted by the American Psychological Association concluded that there is no evidence to suggest that gay and lesbian parents are unfit to parent or that their children's healthy development is compromised in any way (Patterson, 1995).

The American Academy of Pediatrics issued a statement in 2002 supporting co-parent and second-parent adoptions by same-sex couples: "There is a considerable body of professional literature that suggest children with parents who are homosexual have the same advantages and the same expectations for health, adjustment, and development as children whose parents are heterosexual." In addition to adoption, lesbian couples may choose to use artificial insemination with donor sperm to create their families. As described in Case Study 13.2, lesbian couples today have more options for bearing children and sharing in the joys of parenthood.

case study 13.2

The Joy of Matthew

Elizabeth, 30, is white.

I remember when I came out as a lesbian to my family and friends—it took a little while to live openly and share my life with those closest to me. I also thought that as a lesbian I had to give up my dreams of owning a home, getting married, and having kids. Then I met Maria, and everything changed. Maria and I have been together for 6 years now and have built a really fulfilling life together. We have a home. We had a commitment ceremony and would have married if that had been an option. And we have our wonderful son, Matthew.

Maria and I were together 3 years before we decided to begin building our family. We know gay and lesbian couples who have adopted children, others who have children from previous marriages, and those who had a child biologically together. After a lot of discussions, we decided to have our own biological child. There we were with all those eggs, but no sperm. We needed a donor.

After even more discussion—and I mean lots of talking and soul searching—we decided that Maria would be the biological mother. I know that many couples "plan" their children, but for two prospective parents of the same gender, the planning is more complicated and takes on a lot of the same issues faced by infertile heterosexual couples. We had to know when Maria was fertile and then inseminate her at the right time. And as with all couples trying to create a pregnancy, success does not necessarily happen right away. It took nearly 9 months before Maria became pregnant. Believe me, this baby was planned and so very wanted!

Luckily, we had found our way to a gay-friendly health clinic that referred us to a helpful physician. With donor sperm, insemination took place at home. We're not quite sure yet what we're going to tell Matthew about how he was conceived, but since he's a baby, we have time to figure out how best to explain things. Even though friends may be curious about the donor, they've been really understanding and respect our privacy.

For now we're just basking in the joys (and challenges!) of parenthood. Maria is breastfeeding Matthew, but all other parenting roles we share. Our son has a hyphenated last name representing both of us, and I have legally adopted him to ensure I have the same parental rights as Maria. Maria is "Mama" to Matthew, and I'm "E-Mom" for "Elizabeth Mom." But the other night, he pointed at Maria and said, "Mama," then pointed at me and said, "Mama." He gets it. Smart kid.

Almost as wonderful as Matthew himself has been the growing awareness that people see and accept us as the loving family we are. While there is certainly much more that needs to happen when it comes to lesbian and gay rights, we feel very lucky to live at a time where there is so much more acceptance and understanding. We have a great support network of family and friends. We always had great support from our doctor, and the birth-

ing experience at the hospital was totally positive. We haven't experienced any homophobia as we meet other families, and we have families with all different structures in our life. All we hear over and over again is what a great kid Matthew is. People could care less that he's got two moms instead of a mom and a dad. That's pretty neat.

Matthew is safe, secure, and totally loved by his two moms and the wonderful people we're lucky enough to have in our lives.

Not everyone wants to be a parent. The number of those choosing not to have children appears to be increasing. Today nearly one- in- five American women reaches the end of her childbearing years never bearing children, compared to one in ten in 1970. The explanations for this increase include a decrease in social pressure for women to have children, better economic opportunities for women and better contraception choices. Among women in their forties, an equal number are childless either by choice or because they cannot have children. In 2002, among those 40-44, six percent were childless by choice, six percent wanted children but were infertile and 2% were hoping to have them in the future (Livingston & Cohen, 2010). These numbers do not even include all of the males who do not choose to have children. The overall birth rate in the U.S. declined eight percent between 2007 and 2010. The birth rate for those 15-44 was the lowest since 1920, perhaps currently due to the great recession (Livingston & Cohen, 2012). And, certainly, plenty of evidence shows that not everyone is able to be a good parent. Too often, individuals are asked, "When are you going to get married?" and once in a committed relationship, "When are you two going to have children?" If individuals or couples respond that they don't want children, some people are taken aback, as if an offense has been committed. Only recently has the language changed to become less judgmental. Couples without children are now often referred to as *childfree* rather than *childless.* In any case, planning to become a parent rather than stumbling on impending parenthood has clear advantages. The wellness model at the end of the chapter provides a useful framework for assessing your readiness for parenting.

The Menstrual Cycle and Ovulation

A pregnancy begins with the union of an ovum (or ova) and a sperm, a process called **fertilization** or **conception.** For conception to take place, the sperm must get to the ovum within a 24-hour period after its release from the ovary, a process known as **ovulation.** Ovulation occurs about 14 days before a woman's next menstrual cycle. Consequently, it is often difficult if not impossible to predict when ovulation will occur. The timing depends on the length of the cycle itself—a piece of information not available until the cycle is over. Stress, poor nutrition, and other issues may cause a woman's menstrual cycle to be early or late thus making the prediction very unreliable.

Couples who want to conceive try to predict when fertility is most likely. Women who have cycles that are 25 days long will ovulate closer to the first day of menstruation (the first day of the cycle). Women whose

Fertilization/conception Union of the sperm and ovum

Ovulation The release of an egg from the ovary

cycles are 31 days in duration will ovulate farther from the first date of the cycle. (See Chapter 2, Figure 2.9, which illustrates the menstrual cycle and timing of ovulation.) Understanding when a woman is fertile allows us to know when conception can take place.

Women who pay close attention to their body changes throughout the menstrual cycle may be more successful at predicting ovulation. The cervical mucus goes through changes: At ovulation it is clear and thin like egg white. Sometimes a discharge signals ovulation.

Changes in body temperature can be used to monitor ovulation. Women use a basal body temperature thermometer to determine slight fluctuations in temperature. Ovulation is marked by a few tenths of a degree drop, followed by an increase, in which the body temperature remains slightly elevated until the next menstrual cycle. The temperature must be taken first thing in the morning, before any activity, tooth brushing, or drinking of hot or cold beverages. Careful charting over a period of months is necessary to see individual patterns (see Figure 14.1, the basal body temperature chart, in Chapter 14).

In recent years, the pharmaceutical industry has been producing ovulation kits, which purport to detect critical hormonal changes signaling that ovulation will occur within 1 to 2 days. The kits can be helpful, although frequent use could become costly.

Conception

Fallopian tubes Conduits connected to the uterus through which the egg passes into the uterus during ovulation. Fertilization usually takes place at the outer third of the tube

Conception results from the successful journey of a group of sperm to the outer third of the **fallopian tube.** After being deposited in the vagina, ideally close to the cervix, sperm must make their way into the uterus, over to and up the fallopian tube where the ovum is waiting. Some argue that conception is enhanced when sperm arrive "early" and wait for the ova to be released.

A normal ejaculation usually contains between 250 and 500 million sperm. Although only one sperm penetrates the membrane of the ovum at conception, millions are needed for conception. For a male to be considered fertile, the sperm count must be 15 million/milliliter of semen, there must be a high number of sperm with normal shaped oval heads and long tails and at least 40% of sperm are moving- wriggling and swimming (Mayo Clinic, 2012). Sperm survive best in an alkaline environment, and many die when confronting the acidity of the male urethra and female vagina. Continued losses result from sperm not heading toward the correct tube (the two tubes alternate in egg production each month). Finally, the much smaller group reaches the ovum. Consequently, though the sperm count starts at millions, only a few thousand make it to the fallopian tube, and a couple hundred get close to the ovum.

Descriptions of conception have often left mental images of the valiant, strong, surviving sperm successfully attacking and breaking through the membrane of the ovum. Research has demonstrated that the process is more complicated. A mature ovum will release the chemical **allurin,** which attracts the sperm. The sperm that ultimately penetrates the outer membrane of the ovum is able to do so because of **fertilin,** a protein on its plasma membrane (Sherwood, 2004). The ovum extends microvilli up from its surface, which hold down the sperm and push other sperm away. Finally, the egg pulls the sperm inside toward its nucleus. This process and its aftermath are depicted in Figure 13.1.

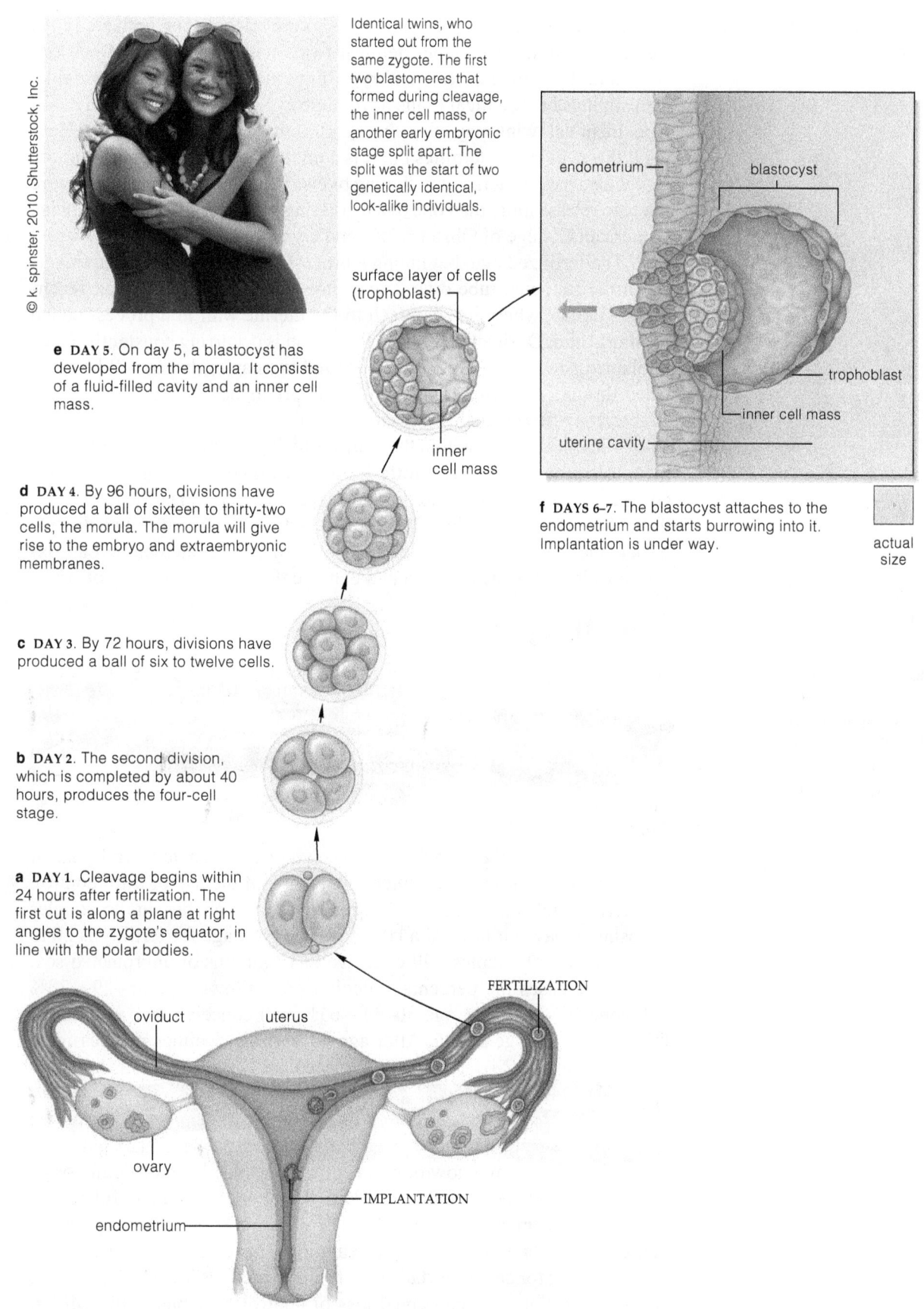

© k. spinster, 2010. Shutterstock, Inc.

Identical twins, who started out from the same zygote. The first two blastomeres that formed during cleavage, the inner cell mass, or another early embryonic stage split apart. The split was the start of two genetically identical, look-alike individuals.

e DAY 5. On day 5, a blastocyst has developed from the morula. It consists of a fluid-filled cavity and an inner cell mass.

surface layer of cells (trophoblast)

inner cell mass

d DAY 4. By 96 hours, divisions have produced a ball of sixteen to thirty-two cells, the morula. The morula will give rise to the embryo and extraembryonic membranes.

c DAY 3. By 72 hours, divisions have produced a ball of six to twelve cells.

b DAY 2. The second division, which is completed by about 40 hours, produces the four-cell stage.

a DAY 1. Cleavage begins within 24 hours after fertilization. The first cut is along a plane at right angles to the zygote's equator, in line with the polar bodies.

endometrium

blastocyst

trophoblast

inner cell mass

uterine cavity

f DAYS 6–7. The blastocyst attaches to the endometrium and starts burrowing into it. Implantation is under way.

actual size

oviduct   uterus   FERTILIZATION

ovary

IMPLANTATION

endometrium

Figure 13.1 *Fertilization in the Fallopian Tube*

Sterility The permanent inability to reproduce

Vasectomy The surgical sterilization of the male that involves cutting and tying off the vas deferens

Fraternal twins will result if two eggs are released and both are fertilized by different sperm, and identical twins will be produced if one egg splits and develops into two embryos. Fraternal twins are no more alike than siblings but identical twins have same eye color, hair color and blood type. Identical twins may even share a placenta during development. Having twins does run in families but it is a myth that twins skip a generation. Age is a contributing factor to having twins. Women older than 30 are more likely to release more than one ova increasing the chance for fraternal twins (American College of Obstetricians and Gynecologist, 2012).

The fertilized egg, beginning a process of rapid cell division, travels down the fallopian tube over 3 to 4 days and sometimes longer, reaching the uterus, where it will attach to the uterine wall in a process called **implantation.** During this time, cell division is occurring constantly. Once implanted, the fertilized egg, now referred to as an **embryo,** will be nourished through the remaining term of the pregnancy. After 8 weeks, the structure is referred to as a **fetus.**

The environment within the uterus is highly protected. The fetus floats in, and is protected by, **amniotic fluid.** The **placenta,** an organ of interchange that attaches to the uterine wall, passes oxygen and nutrients through the umbilical cord to the fetus and passes waste products and carbon dioxide back to the mother. Unfortunately, as will be discussed later, numerous toxins may also cross the placenta and damage the fetus in a variety of ways.

Infertility

Although pregnancy and childbirth are "natural" occurrences, they don't occur easily for all couples. Infertility affects 10% of all couples in the United States (Lentz, 2012). Based on surveys conducted by the National Center for Health Statistics (NCHS) in 2010, 6.7 million women between ages 15 and 44 had an impaired ability to have children; the number of infertile married couples was reported to be 1.5 million (Centers for Disease Control [CDC], 2010).

Infertility is the inability to conceive or impregnate after 1 year of regularly engaging in sexual intercourse without the use of birth control. The fertility rates have declined in recent years probably due to couples choosing to have children at a later age. The peak age for fertility is 20 to 24 when 86% of couples will conceive in 12 months of unprotected sex. As age increases the percentage declines as follows: age 25–29—78% will conceive in 1 year, age 30–34—63% will conceive in 1 year and it falls to 52% for age 35–39. After age 40, fertility declines progressively and more rapidly (MD Consult, 2007, Medical Clinics of North America, 2008). Approximately one third of cases are related to female factors, one third of cases relate to male factors, one tenth to problems in both partners and in the remaining cases no cause can be found (Miller 2012). On occasion, individuals may know or suspect that they may have difficulty or be unable to reproduce. For others the knowledge comes as a painful reality. Over half of women described infertility as the most upsetting experience of their lives. Many will experience emotions similar to those experienced when grieving for any important loss. Typical reactions include depression, anger, frustration, and perceived loss of control over one's life (Miller, 2012). In recent years, reproductive technologies have greatly expanded to enable couples to biologically become parents. The pregnancies that result,

sex in society 13.2

Ethical Issues and Reproductive Technologies

Among attempts to have a child, surrogate motherhood remains an option—albeit a controversial one. The case of Mary Beth Whitehead in 1986 brought the complicated issues of surrogacy to national attention. Whitehead had signed a contract with a New Jersey couple and was artificially inseminated with the husband's sperm. After giving birth to a baby girl, Whitehead decided that she didn't want to give up the child for adoption. The courts became involved, and the story spread across the popular media. For a while the baby girl even had two names. The outcome of the court case was that the child was given to the adoptive parents, with Whitehead being granted visitation rights.

As a result of this case, a number of legal and ethical issues were brought to national attention. To some people, the use of surrogate mothers extends the array of reproductive options for infertile couples. It represents a choice that is both private and not much different from traditional adoption. To others, it represents exploitation of women's bodies. Those who are able to pay hire women whose need of income may be paramount. The contractual elements, fees involved, and possible legal challenges all contribute to the debate over surrogate mothering.

Another public case had to do with John and Luanne Buzzanca. After 6 years of infertility treatments, the couple turned to a laboratory that supplied donor sperm and ova, paid a surrogate, and finally became parents in San Francisco in April 1995. Shortly after the birth, John filed for divorce and refused to make child support payments on the grounds that he wasn't the baby's father in any true legal sense, despite having earlier signed a contract agreeing to the child's birth. The Superior Court agreed, claiming that baby Jaycee had been conceived in a petri dish, from anonymous donors, and carried and delivered by a surrogate mother with no genetic ties to her. Consequently, according to California law, not only was John not the father, but Luanne was not the legal mother. By California law, the child had no parents.

A petition filed with the California Court of Appeals for the Fourth Circuit (March 1998), however, resulted in the determination that both John and Luanne Buzzanca were the legal parents of Jaycee (Vorzimer, O'Hara, & Shafton, 1998). As a result of that ruling, individuals who use assisted reproductive technologies and intend to be considered the parents can finalize their parental rights before the child is born, regardless of whether they use a traditional or a gestational surrogate. Specific to this case, because John Buzzanca initially had consented to using donor sperm and a surrogate to produce a child, he was viewed as the father and, therefore, has financial responsibilities to Jaycee.

In January, 2009, Nadya Suleman, a single mother of 6 gave birth to an additional 8 children conceived through invitro fertilization. These births ignited a controversy over the ethics of implanting multiple ova when the guidelines recommend implanting only 2 embryos in young women. This prompted the California Medical Board to investigate the fertility doctor to determine if the standards of medical practice had been violated. These births also created much debate over the issue of a single mom with no source of income choosing have so many children through invitro fertilization.

---

though, come at great physical, emotional, and financial cost and do not always result in a successful birth.

Prevention of infertility has become an important focus in educating future parents. Behavioral changes prior to attempting to become parents can have very positive impacts on decreasing the risk of infertility. Reducing the risk of STD's by minimizing the number of sexual partners, using barrier contraception and screening regularly for STD's can greatly decrease the female's risk for scarring the fallopian tubes. Maintaining a healthy weight (body mass index 18-25) all throughout life increases the probability of normal ovulation. Being overweight (body mass index over 25) or

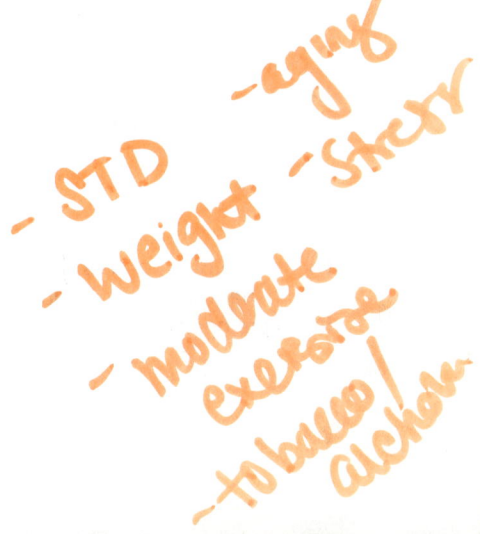

underweight (body mass index of 17 or less) is associated with infertility due to lack of ovulation

Moderate exercise and responsible alcohol use are also important health habits. Those who exercise heavily more than 7 hours a week and consume high intakes of alcohol delay conception (Hornstein & Gibbons, 2008). Tobacco use by females and males increases risk of infertility. Individuals are urged to take control and practice healthy behaviors to maintain their reproductive ability thus giving themselves the choice of whether to have children or not.

Infertility in women is most often caused by problems with ovulation. As discussed earlier, simple lifestyle factors such as stress, body, weight, poor diet, and strenuous athletic training can affect hormonal balance and ovulation. The most important contributor to problems with ovulation is aging. One third of couples are infertile when the female is 35 or over. The ovaries' ability to ovulate declines with age, especially after 35. Female infertility can also be caused by blocked fallopian tubes resulting from pelvic inflammatory disease, endometriosis, or surgery for an ectopic pregnancy. The most preventable causes of infertility are gonorrhea and chlamydia. Up to 15% of women infected with chlamydiawill develop pelvic inflammatory disease which may cause infertility or an ectopic pregnancy (CDC, 2013).

Male infertility is often a result of problems with manufacturing of the sperm or the ability of the sperm to reach the egg. As with the female, life style can influence fertility with alcohol and drugs temporarily reducing sperm quality. In addition, environmental toxins and lead may cause male infertility. Sperm production problems can develop as a result of mumps, some sexually transmitted diseases, severe testicular injury and tumors. If a male is unable to ejaculate due to diabetes, prostate or urethral surgery, antihypertensive medication or lack of erection, this will of course not allow the sperm to reach the egg. (MD Consult, 2005) Age is also a factor for male infertility with a key risk factor for infertility being the father's age of 40 or greater (deLaRochebrochard & Thonneau, 2003). The assessment of male infertility is often frustrating because it is quite difficult to determine the specific cause of male infertility or best treatment for his infertility (Swerdloff, R. & Wang, C., 2008).

Numerous tests, with varying degrees of invasiveness, have been developed to determine the cause(s) of infertility. Males and females alike initially will have complete physical assessments, including a detailed medical and lifestyle history. The man will be asked to ejaculate into a sterile cup, after which his sperm will be tested for viability and motility. If problems are found with the sperm, correct diagnosis and treatment follow. These might consist of lifestyle changes, hormone treatment, treatment for a **varicocele** (an enlarged vein in the scrotum impairing blood flow), and artificial insemination with his sperm.

Tests for the female typically begin after months of first charting her menstrual cycle by taking her basal body temperature to assess ovulatory status. A medical history and physical will be part of the evaluation. **Hysterosalpingograms** are tests that determine whether the fallopian tubes are open. Diagnostic Laparoscopy is used for couples with unexplained infertility, endometriosis and pelvic adhesions (Kuohung, W. & Hounstein, 2008).

Varicocele An enlarged vein in the scrotum impairing blood flow

Hysterosalpingograms Tests that determine whether the fallopian tubes are open

If the infertility is suspected to result from absence of ovulation, treatment will depend on the age of the female. For young females under 30, the focus will be on timing intercourse to correspond with ovulation. Normal sperm can live at least 3 days but the ova can only be fertilized in the first 12-24 hours following ovulation. The focus will also be on lifestyle changes such as weight loss/ gain and decreasing exercise, smoking cessation, and decreasing alcohol intake. (Kuohung & Hounstein, 2008). In addition, women can be treated hormonally. One problem with hormonal treatment is the increased possibility of multiple births—some of which receive a lot of media coverage and attention. Multiple-birth babies, however, are almost always premature and frequently have health problems. Whereas normal gestation takes place over a 40-week period, multiple births usually do not go to term. Each additional fetus shortens the gestation period. When babies are born around the 32nd week of a pregnancy, for example, they weigh little more than 2 pounds and require weeks of treatment in a neonatal intensive care unit. Decades ago, these babies would not have survived. Today, more drugs and technology are available to keep these infants alive. The costs on many levels—physical, social, emotional, and financial—can be staggering. In 2000, it was estimated to cost over $58,000 to deliver twins and close to $282,000 for quadruplets (Wright, Schieve, Reynolds, & Jeng, 2003). Case Study 13.3 describes some of the emotions and experiences typically associated with infertility.

Some women first undergo pelvic surgery to conceive and carry a pregnancy. Endometriosis, a condition in which endometrial tissue grows outside the uterus and in some cases literally wraps around and blocks off the fallopian tubes, can be treated with surgery. Myomectomy, a surgical procedure used to remove fibroid growths but preserve the uterus, can help women as well.

When a woman's fallopian tubes remain blocked, **in vitro fertilization (IVF)** becomes an option. Her ovaries are first stimulated using hormones, so that more than one ovum matures each month. After surgically removing the eggs, they are joined with sperm in a laboratory. Often three or four **blastocysts** (preembryos) then will be placed directly into the woman's uterus if the woman is over 35. for those under 35, the recommendation is that no more than 2 be place in the uterus. Generally, the more embryos that are transplanted, the higher the rate of success. Researchers are also finding that the age of the woman impacts the success of the procedure. Nationally, live-birth rates ranged from 37 percent for women under 35, 29 percent for those 35-37, 20 percent for those 38-40 and only 4 percent for women over 42 (Paulson, 2008). As women age, it can become more difficult for them to become pregnant for a variety of reasons, including quality of the ova and blockage of the fallopian tubes.

Some couples confront the reality that a pregnancy will result only from the use of donor sperm or donor ova. Fertility clinics can provide information to couples that allow them to choose donors who match them in physical appearance, background, and interests. Because college students are considered young and healthy, they may be approached as possible donors. You may find advertisements in your college newspaper seeking sperm and ova donors. For women in particular, the money offered is enticing and intended to compensate for the health risks involved. High doses of hormones are prescribed, which stimulate multiple ovulations. The ova

In vitro fertilization (IVF) A procedure in which ova are removed from the woman's body and fertilized with sperm in a laboratory; the embryo is surgically implanted into her uterus.

Blastocysts Spherical clusters of cells, also known as preembryos, that form shortly after conception

case study 13.3

Anthony's Story of Infertility

Anthony, 40, identifies as Italian American.

Looking back on it now, it all seems so distant. My wife and I married in September of 1989. We planned a perfect life together, filled with love and joy. We thought that most of this joy would come from the children we planned on having.

I don't know whether it was the combination of my going back to college full-time and the pressures of conceiving or whether it just wasn't "God's time" (a phrase we held to that kept our faith), but getting pregnant just wasn't happening. At first we kidded about it. Then we decided to pay more attention to having sex around my wife's ovulation date. Purchasing and using the special thermometer that allowed us to take her basal body temperature was the beginning of a host of infertility treatments. We came to hate that word infertility as much as the constant advice to "relax."

One year passed, and no pregnancy. I thought about how my brother's infertility was remedied by an operation to remove a varicocele. Six months after his surgery, his wife became pregnant. The operation had helped his sperm count, which had been both low and with slow-motility sperm.

Now it was my turn. I delivered more sperm samples to a variety of medical centers than I care to remember! I had such anxiety as I tried to ejaculate into cups, being in public medical facilities with what seemed to be everyone knowing what I was doing. It was determined that I was a candidate for varicocele surgery. Finally our problems would be solved! I had the surgery and hoped to become a father soon. No such luck.

My wife was given two fertility drugs to improve our chances of children. Clomid didn't work. Serephene didn't work. She was then scheduled for a laparoscopy to allow the doctors to see what was going on. It turned out that she had endometriosis, cysts on her ovaries, and one of her fallopian tubes was smaller than the other. All these problems were described as "fixable" and, paired with my problem, could have explained why we weren't getting pregnant. After the necessary surgery, we regained our hope.

Months and months of trying came and went. Negative pregnancy tests . . . trying again . . . waiting and hoping that she wouldn't get her period. Anger and sadness when her period came. And trying again. Lovemaking

Critical Thinking

Anthony's case highlights the lengths couples may go to in their attempts to reproduce.

With health care so costly, should limits be placed on what options individuals and couples can exercise? How far would you be willing to go to have a baby when the time is right for you?

Assisted reproductive technology (ART) Infertility interventions in which a laboratory is involved with the union of the sperm and egg

are harvested and then retrieved surgically. Both hormone ingestion and surgery carry some risk to the woman's health.

The **assisted reproductive technology (ART)** refers to fertility treatments in which both eggs and sperm are handled by a laboratory. The federal government requires all medical centers in the United States that use

became a job. We were so upset that we were often no-shows at family christenings and children's birthday parties.

After a period of time, the doctor suggested artificial insemination with my sperm. My wife would be put on fertility drugs to increase her chances of ovulation. I would provide a sample—legal masturbation, as I called it—and the sperm would be injected into my wife using a long syringe. We agreed to the procedures. Each time we prayed and prayed yet continued to get negative results.

Not being ready to consider adoption—people were kindly suggesting that to us—we enrolled at the reproductive clinic at a local hospital, known for its successes with infertile couples. I was now 33 years old, finished with college, and fortunately employed at a place with good health benefits. The doctors there suggested in vitro fertilization. We agreed. I had to inject fertility drugs into my wife's buttocks for 21 straight days prior to "the day." Prayer got me through that. Retrieval of the eggs was successful, and we were told that there were seven excellent embryos. The doctors would put three back into my wife's uterus.

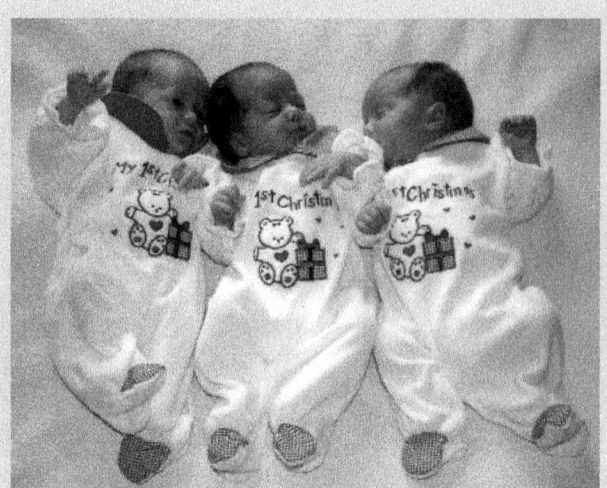

Anthony's triplet girls.

Picture Courtesy of the authors

My wife had to be monitored daily at the hospital, giving blood and having ultrasounds. The egg retrieval was done on March 17, Saint Patrick's Day. The embryos were put back on March 20, the first day of spring. We would have to wait 14 days for the results. Those were the longest 14 days of our lives.

On Easter Sunday we received the exciting news that she was pregnant! Tests conducted 2 weeks later confirmed that she was carrying triplets. We were grateful . . . scared . . . overwhelmed. There was never a question that, despite the high risks associated with multiple births, we would keep all three babies.

After 20 weeks of bed rest and daily monitoring, my wife gave birth, with me at her side, to three beautiful girls. The road was long and bumpy. It took almost 6 years of trying. Although we had been angry, sad, and frustrated, we never lost our faith. We supported each other from start to finish. And now I live with the four most beautiful women in the world, all coming in "God's time."

ART to report data to the CDC on an annual basis. Assisted reproduction can stem from a couple's fresh eggs and sperm, donor eggs and sperm, "thawed" embryos, and so forth. For 2011, there were 163,038 ART procedures attempted, with 47,849 live-birth deliveries and 61,610 infants born (CDC, 2011). Overall, about half of all couples who go through the rigors of these procedures are able to take a baby home. The success decreases as the woman ages. This is not the information most people hear when the discussion of assisted reproductive technology takes place. Infertile couples come to learn that attempts do not mean automatic success and that multiple births with their concomitant issues are a risk. In addition, there is an increased risk of several birth defects for the infant conceived by ART (Van Voorhis, 2007).

Couples spend varying amounts of time, money, and certainly emotional energy being tested and evaluated for the causes of the infertility. Those who consider IVF can expect to pay $15,000 for each attempt. Each cycle has a 25% chance of resulting in a live birth leading the average cost per baby to be $62, 000 (Henderson, 2006, Guzick, 2002). Class differences become readily apparent, as those with financial resources and better health insurance plans clearly have an advantage. In addition to the cost consideration, assisted reproductive technology appears to double the risk of having a child with low birth weight or a child with a major birth defect (Mitchell, 2002).

After examining the issues of assisted reproductive technology, it becomes evident that it is not a simple fix for infertility. Those who know that they really want children should take steps to insure that they remain fertile. As discussed earlier, avoiding sexually transmitted diseases or having them treated promptly helps maintain a healthy reproductive tract. In addition, those who really want children should consider having them between the ages of 25 and 35. During those years fertility is high and pregnancy is safest (Heffner, 2004). Because fertility declines for the female by 35 and for the male by 40, delaying the decision to have children until later in one's life and career may result in dependence on ART or not being able to have children.

Preconception

Preconception care is an essential element for optimizing both the health of the fetus and the mother. The goal of preconception care is to identify issues that could affect the pregnancy and to make changes prior to becoming pregnant (American College of Obstetrics and Gynecology, 2013). The most critical development for the fetus is in the early days after conception, days 17-56, when the mother may not know she is pregnant and before the first prenatal visit. A preconception visit to the health care provider includes education on the topics of nutrition, drug use before and during pregnancy, healthy body weight,smoking and alcohol education, and medical and family history. If a woman is obese she will be advised to lose weight prior to conception. Folic acid supplements will be recommended to reduce this risk of neural tube defects. (ACOG, 2013). The CDC now actually recommends folic acid supplement of 0.4 mg for all women who have a chance of conceiving even if they are not attempting to get pregnant (Gabbe, 2012). All of this preconception education helps the woman understand that once she decides to attempt conception, she needs to care for herself as if she is already pregnant. Preconception care gives her the tools to create the healthiest environment possible for conception and development of her baby.

Pregnancy

Confirming a pregnancy in years past meant that a woman had to see her physician, have a urine test, and wait for days for the results. Today, determining whether a woman is pregnant is as simple as purchasing a home pregnancy kit at the local pharmacy. Home pregnancy kits are designed to detect the presence of **human chorionic gonadotropin (hCG),** a hormone present in the urine of pregnant women. Because this hormone is secreted as the fertilized egg implants in the uterus, early testing can confirm a pregnancy. Many kits can be used reliably within a day or two of a missed period, although reliability improves if used a week after a period is missed (Consumers Union, 2003b). Overall, a woman must be aware that her period was due to have early feedback that she is pregnant.

Human chorionic gonadotropin (hCG) A hormone secreted during pregnancy that shows up in the urine of pregnant women; the basis for determining pregnancy using home kits

Although home pregnancy tests are 85 to 95 percent accurate, medical laboratory tests are the most accurate. Two types of blood test for pregnancy detection are available from a caregiver. One of the test, the quantitative test, can detect pregnancy as quickly as 6-8 days after ovulation (MD Consult, 2012). False positives can happen. When a woman has given birth recently, had a miscarriage, or is taking certain fertility drugs, a test may show that she is pregnant when she is not. In all cases, the woman should follow up with a visit to a physician. A pelvic exam will indicate an enlarged uterus associated with pregnancy and also will allow the physician to estimate the duration of the pregnancy and project a birth date.

Many women never realize they are pregnant since fifty percent of pregnancies are unplanned and of these fertilized eggs, almost half die and are aborted spontaneously (miscarry) before the woman even suspects she is pregnant. Of the women who know they are pregnant, the miscarriage rate is 15-20% with most occurring before the seventh week. The majority of miscarriages are caused by chromosome issues that prevent the fetus from developing. Other factors that can cause a miscarriage include heavy smoking and alcohol use, illegal drug use and environmental toxins (Storch, 2012).

Gestation

A pregnancy is measured from the first day of a woman's last menstrual period, with the expected period of **gestation** averaging 40 weeks. A normal birth will take place between the 38th and 42nd week. Deliveries before 38 weeks are considered premature, and after 42 weeks, the extended time may threaten the health of the baby, so labor may be induced. A mathematical calculation called the *Naegele's rule* is used by obstetricians, nurse midwives, and other health care providers to help estimate the expected date of birth (McCloskey & Bulecheck, 1996). When a woman's menstrual cycle is regular and she hasn't been on oral contraceptives, the measurement is useful; nonetheless, many babies are actually born before or after their "due date." To calculate the estimated due date, take the first day of the last menstrual period, subtract 3 months, and then add 7 days. (Women need to keep track of their menstrual cycles

Gestation The period of time representing pregnancy and development of fetus from conception to birth

Tubal ligation The surgical sterilization of the female that involves cutting and tying off the fallopian tubes

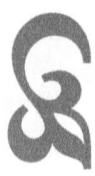

healthy sex hints 13.1

Ratings of Home Pregnancy Tests

The Consumers Union tested 18 pregnancy test kits for their performance, including average cost, ease of use, and sensitivity. The most highly recommended kit is listed first, down to the worst performer listed at the bottom of the chart.

Notes: Except as noted, all the tests came packaged in pairs. Overall score is based on the test's hCG sensitivity, both at the recommended reading time and after 10 minutes; and on the ease of reading the result. hCG *sensitivity* was measured by adding progressively higher concentrations of hCG to female urine, then conducting the test according to package instructions. The higher the level of hCG it took to produce a positive result, the lower the sensitivity score. *Ease of reading* was based on the intensity of the line signifying a positive result; the more intense the line, the higher the score. None of the products tested had consistently intense lines at all the hCG concentration levels they detected. *10-minute hCG sensitivity* was evaluated by reading the results at the maximum allowable reading time of 10 minutes. Price is a national average based on a survey of prices paid in supermarkets and drugstores.

Overall Ratings — In performance order

Rating key: Excellent ● · Very good ◕ · Good ○ · Fair ◔ · Poor ●

BRAND & MODEL	PRICE/ NO. TESTS	OVERALL SCORE (0–100)	HCG SENSITIVITY	EASE OF READING	10-MINUTE HCG SENSITIVITY	RECOMMENDATIONS & NOTES
First Response Early Result Pregnancy Test	$18.09/2		Excellent	Good	Excellent	Wick-type stick. Best combination of sensitivity and reliability.
Answer Quick & Simple One-Step Pregnancy Test	$15.22/2		Very good	Good	Very good	Wick-type stick. No wick protection; possibly messy to use.
Answer Pregnancy Test	8.14/1		Very good	Fair	Excellent	Wick-type stick must be dipped in a cup. No wick protection; possibly messy to use.
Clear Blue Easy One Minute Pregnancy Test[1]	16.02/2		Good	Good	Very good	Wick-type stick. Easier to read than most.
Clear Choice At Home Pregnancy Test	9.11/1		Excellent	Fair	Excellent	Jar. Some samples failed to work.
e.p.t. Pregnancy Test	16.72/2		Good	Poor	Excellent	Wick-type stick.
ClearPlan Easy Pregnancy Test Pack	17.617/3		Good	Fair	Very good	Wick-type stick.
Inverness Medical Early Pregnancy Test[2]	10.77/2		Fair	Fair	Excellent	Cassette type.
American Fare (Kmart) Easy to Read Pregnancy Test[1]	9.35/2		Fair	Poor	Excellent	Wick-type stick.
CVS Pregnancy Test	10.86/2		Fair	Poor	Good	Wick-type stick.
Target Brand One Step Pregnancy Test	7.99/2		Fair	Poor	Good	Wick-type stick.
Walgreens One Step Pregnancy Tests	12.99/2		Fair	Poor	Very good	Wick-type stick.
Sav-On Osco (Albertson's) One Step Pregnancy Test	12.99/2		Fair	Poor	Good	Wick-type stick.
Inverness Medical Early Pregnancy Test[2]	12.56/2		Fair	Poor	Good	Wick-type stick.
Rite Aid One Step Pregnancy Test	7.23/1		Fair	Poor	Good	Wick-type stick.
Eckerd One Step Pregnancy Test	12.67/2		Fair	Poor	Fair	Wick-type stick.
Equate (Wal-Mart) Pregnancy Test[1]	7.92/2		Fair	Poor	Excellent	Wick-type stick. Some samples failed to work.
Confirm Pregnancy Test	11.19/2		Fair	Poor	Fair	Wick-type stick. Some samples failed to work.

[1] Reformulation in progress.

[2] Renamed Accu-Clear Early Pregnancy in March 2003.

Notes: Except as noted, all the tests came packaged in pairs. *Overall* score is based on the test's hCG sensitivity, both at the recommended reading time and after 10 minutes; and on the ease of reading the result. hCG *sensitivity* was measured by adding progressively higher concentrations of hCG to female urine, then conducting the test according to package instructions. The higher the level of hCG it took to produce a positive result, the lower the sensitivity score. *Ease of reading* was based on the intensity of the line signifying a positive result; the more intense the line, the higher the score. None of the products tested had consistently intense lines at all the hCG concentration levels they detected. *10-minutes hCG sensitivity* was evaluated by reading the results at the maximum allowable reading time of 10 minutes. *Price* is national average based on a survey of prices paid in supermarkets and drugstores.

Source: Consumers Union (2003b, p. 47).

as a general health practice, but especially around pregnancy.) For example: Jessica's last period began on February 2. Subtracting 3 months brings her to November 2, and adding 7 days makes her estimated due date November 9.

Pregnancies are divided into trimesters, each having unique characteristics. Figure 13.2 is a time line showing features of each.

First Trimester

During the first trimester of the pregnancy, all structures and systems develop in rudimentary form. At the end of 3 months, the fetus has arms, legs, feet, toes, fingers, and the vital organs and body systems are functioning. The mother's taking drugs during the first trimester can have a particularly damaging effect on the fetus. One overpowering argument for planning a pregnancy lies in the fact that without planning, the mother unintentionally may be taking medications with **teratogenic effects,** causing fetal malformations. As suggested earlier, women who are trying to get pregnant should take care of themselves as if they are already pregnant. This will help protect the developing embryo during that time between conception and when pregnancy is determined. For example, women need to take folic acid supplements prior to getting pregnant and during the pregnancy to prevent neural tube defects. Neural tube development is complete within 28 days after conception and this is often before the woman knows she is pregnant. Taking preconception folic acid supplements would reduce neural tube defects by 50%. (MD Consult, 2007). At the end of the first trimester, the fetus is approximately 4 inches in length and weighs approximately 1 ounce. At this point, the hands are more developed than the feet and the arms are longer than the legs. The bones and muscles are beginning to grow and the skin is almost transparent (ACOG, 2011).

Second Trimester

The second trimester is marked by growth and maturation of all the fetal systems. As the fetus grows in size and the uterus stretches, the mother's pregnancy becomes evident. During the fifth month of pregnancy, fetal movement is usually active enough for the mother to feel and the fetus sleeps and wakes regularly. In females, the eggs have formed in the ovaries and in males the testicles begin to descend from the abdomen into the scrotal sac. By the end of the second trimester, the fetus is close to 12 inches long and weighs between 1 and 1.5 pounds. The sex organs are apparent, as is body hair, including eyebrows and eyelashes. The eyes begin to open and the lungs are fully formed but not functioning. Neonatal intensive care units, equipped with the proper medications and

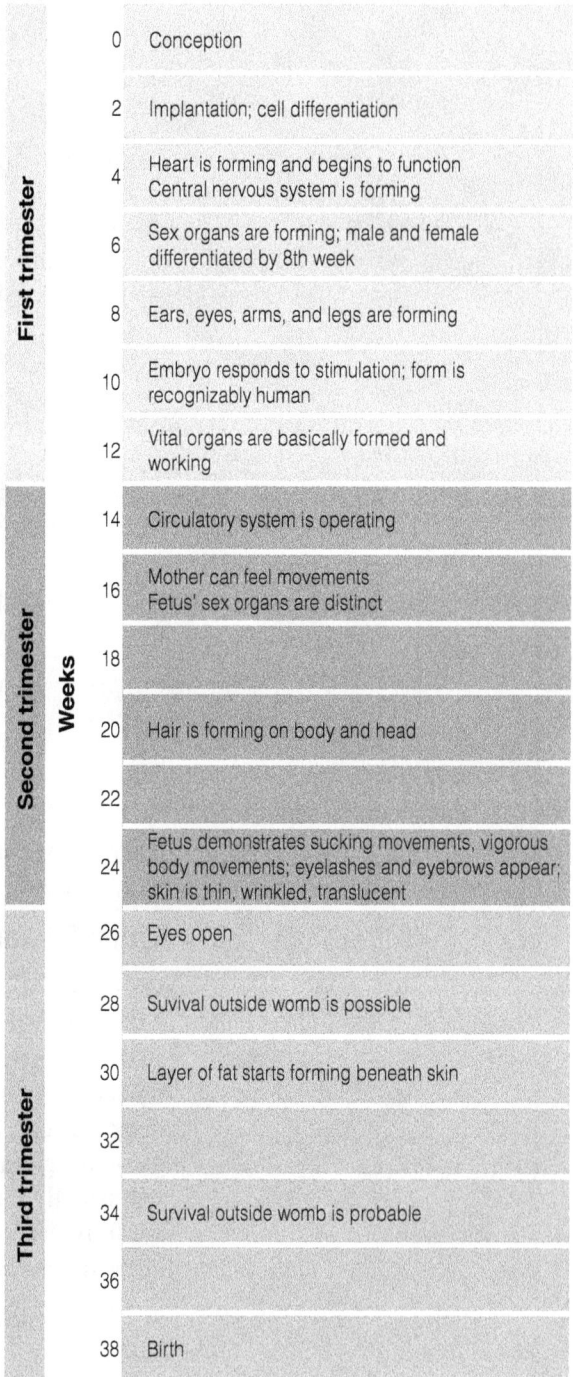

Fetal development

Weeks	
First trimester	
0	Conception
2	Implantation; cell differentiation
4	Heart is forming and begins to function. Central nervous system is forming
6	Sex organs are forming; male and female differentiated by 8th week
8	Ears, eyes, arms, and legs are forming
10	Embryo responds to stimulation; form is recognizably human
12	Vital organs are basically formed and working
Second trimester	
14	Circulatory system is operating
16	Mother can feel movements. Fetus' sex organs are distinct
18	
20	Hair is forming on body and head
22	
24	Fetus demonstrates sucking movements, vigorous body movements; eyelashes and eyebrows appear; skin is thin, wrinkled, translucent
26	Eyes open
Third trimester	
28	Suvival outside womb is possible
30	Layer of fat starts forming beneath skin
32	
34	Survival outside womb is probable
36	
38	Birth

Figure 13.2 *Fetal Development*

Teratogenic effects Side effects of drugs and other substances that cause birth defects

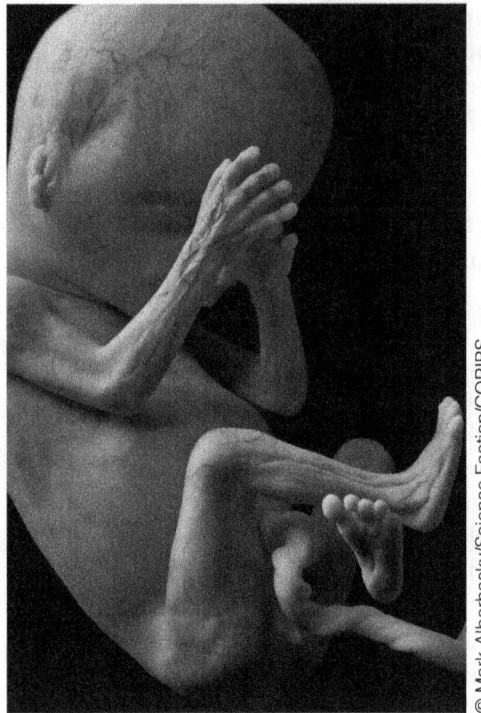

Fetal development at 20 weeks

technology, can help some babies born prematurely at the end of the sixth month of pregnancy to survive (ACOG, 2011).

Third Trimester

During the third trimester, the fetal systems continue to grow and mature. Early in this trimester, the fetus kicks and stretches and responds to sound. The eyes open and close and react to light. The taste buds develop and the fetus can distinguish sweet and sour taste. The mother may even feel the baby hiccup. With all the major development finished, the fetus rapidly gains weight and in the ninth month gains ½ pound per week. The fetus will usually turn and settle into a head down position for birth. The lungs are fully developed and ready to function on their own (ACOG, 2011). At birth, the average baby weighs 8 pounds and is approximately 20 inches in length.

Physical, Psychological, and Social Effects of Pregnancy

Clearly, pregnancy has a powerful impact on health. The woman experiences a number of physical changes as her body responds to the physical demands of the pregnancy. Carrying an ever larger baby in the front of one's body puts demands on all the systems. Pregnancy and childbirth may well be the greatest physical challenges in a woman's life.

✎ *Physical Wellness* ✎

Pregnancy and childbirth clearly have an impact on a woman's health, and parenting affects the health of all caregivers. The mere fact that pregnant women are advised to gain between 25 and 35 pounds to have a healthy baby can put a strain on many body systems. Blood pressure may increase. Respiration becomes more labored. Muscles and ligaments must stretch. Throughout pregnancy, women report varying degrees of fatigue, shortness of breath, heartburn, indigestion, nausea, gas, constipation, headaches, leg cramps, backaches, water retention, varicose veins, and difficulty sleeping. Nerves may be impinged upon by the developing fetus; sciatica is a common complaint. Maintaining a healthy pregnancy requires good prenatal care, focusing on nutrition, exercise, and monitored use of medication. Any problems that develop can then hopefully be managed without harm to the developing fetus.

Emotionally, fathers and mothers both respond to pregnancy in various ways. A planned pregnancy should connect to positive feelings—happiness, joy, excitement. Even so, periods of anxiety and fear about pending parenthood are normal. The high hormone levels in pregnancy affect women's moods and may result in being weepy, irritable, and upset but for many women, pregnancy is a wonderful and amazing period in their lives. As the projected date of birth gets closer and closer, pending parenthood, or the addition of another child to the family, becomes all the more real. Couples might have difficulty concentrating on anything but the soon-to-arrive baby.

Pregnancy may affect social relationships as well. Because the birth of a child, and having children, changes our lives in so many ways, some people report feeling awkward around those who have not had the experience of pregnancy. Once children are born, relationships may go through periods of additional strain. Couples with children are talking about their baby's smallest accomplishment or where to buy diapers at the lowest expense, whereas childfree couples may be discussing their latest vacation. Continuing to be able to relate to each other's lifestyle can test the bounds of friendship.

Relationships with family members also may change. Excited grandparents can be a tremendous source of support. Relations between adult children and their parents may improve as the new parents come to better understand the roles of mother and father. In some situations, however, grandparents offer unsolicited advice and become controlling. Something as basic as naming a child and honoring relatives can be a source of tension.

Couples can manage the stresses associated with pregnancy, and later child rearing itself, by communicating openly. Private time to share what can be an intensely spiritual event becomes important. Couples also need time away from the baby to help maintain their bond and the strength of their relationship.

Sexual Activity During Pregnancy

Sexual activity, harmless in a normal pregnancy, can continue throughout the pregnancy. Changing hormones may cause an increase in some women's level of desire and a decrease for others. Beginning in the 4th month of pregnancy some women experience dizziness while lying on their backs, therefore positions for intercourse may need to change. For many couples, intercourse continues until the birth of the child but not for all. However, sharing intimacy is always important and pregnancy is no exception. Couples can achieve non sexual intimacy by romancing one another with long walks and candle light dinners. Physical intimacy can be achieved in ways other than intercourse such as erotic kisses, hugging, massage and oral sex. One caution with oral sex is for the male to avoid blowing into the vagina during pregnancy.

If a pregnancy has been determined to be high-risk, a physician may advise modifications in lovemaking patterns. Sexual activity causes increased uterine activity, perhaps due to orgasm, nipple stimulation, or prostaglandins in semen. Women who are at risk for preterm labor or who have previously lost a pregnancy are often advised to either use condoms or avoid intercourse (Gabbe, 2012).

Prenatal Care

As discussed earlier, care should begin with preconception care when a woman considers getting pregnant, even before she stops using effective birth control. This allows her to make some lifestyle changes such as eating nutritious foods, exercising, losing weight, avoiding drugs and alcohol, to create a healthy environment in which the embryo can implant. This is the one time during the life of this future child that the mother can take total control over the child's food intake and environment. There may be no better gift the mother can give the child than this healthy environment in which to grow and develop. Creating a healthy environment for both the mother and developing fetus is the focus of both preconception and prenatal care. Good prenatal care enhances the health of the mother and developing baby and reduces the possibility of congenital birth defects. The basic components of prenatal care are healthy nutrition, exercise, medical monitoring, and, when medications are necessary for the mother's health, careful monitoring of those medications.

Getting good prenatal care is tied to making an early connection with a health care provider. Traditionally, women have relied on physicians who specialize in obstetrics and gynecology (ob-gyn) for care and delivery. Gynecologists specialize in reproductive health, yet not all will also provide obstetrical care, which focuses on pregnancy and childbirth. Family practitioners, nurse midwives, and lay midwives may also provide care.

Nutrition

Healthy eating should begin before the woman tries to become pregnant and continue during pregnancy and breast-feeding. Making these important changes in food intake will optimize the mother's health, reduce the risk of complications during pregnancy, and reduce birth defects and chronic diseases for the child in early and later life (American Dietetic Association (ADA), 2008). Poor nutrition results in low birth weight and impaired development of the central nervous system, another strong argument for healthy eating. Large quantities of calcium are needed for bone and tissue development and women who do not tolerate milk can be counseled to eat yogurt or cheese to help reach the needed amounts (Gabbe, 2012). Making the healthiest food choices can be a challenge for many women. A helpful tool for simplifying food choices is the U.S. Department of Agriculture "ChooseMyPlate" site. Pregnant women are encouraged to use the "Super Tracker-Daily Food Plan for Moms" section of the site to help them select a healthy intake of nutrient dense foods. Pregnant women enter their age, height, weight, physical activity and stage of pregnancy and this is used to make recommendations tailored to meet individual needs. A pregnant woman is not eating for two as is so often suggested. She actually only needs about 300 extra calories a day so she must choose her foods carefully to ensure adequate nutrition for the baby. She needs to pay attention to her intake of all nutrients—protein, carbohydrates, fats, vitamins, minerals, fiber, and water. Because pregnant women also require more folic acid, iron, and calcium, a prenatal vitamin is usually recommended. In addition to making smart food choices, women need to eliminate foods that may negatively affect fetal development. Caffeine in moderation, 2 cups of brewed coffee, is fine but excess should be avoided. Caffeine is found in many foods so she needs to become a careful consumer. Pregnant women should also avoid raw fish, fish high in mercury, and undercooked meat, poultry or seafood (American College of Obstetrics &Gynecology (ACOG), 2011).

Appropriate weight gain for the mother depends upon her pre-pregnancy weight. The general recommendation is that women who begin at a normal weight should gain between 25 and 35 pounds over the course of their pregnancy. This can be accomplished by eating an extra 300 calories a day. Women who are overweight should gain 15 to 25 pounds; those who are underweight should gain between 28 and 40 pounds. (Gabbe, 2012). Researchers have been examining the type of weight gained rather than the precise amount; weight from fat and weight from fluid can have a different impact on the health of the baby. Other researchers are looking at the time within the pregnancy when the weight is gained, rather than the actual amount gained.

Weight gains during pregnancy can range from less than 15 pounds to 50 pounds or more and still produce a healthy baby. What is certain is that women should gain weight and should not engage in a weight loss diet during a pregnancy. Figure 13.3 shows the breakdown of weight for a 30-pound weight gain. Actual weight gain will be reflected in the weight of the baby and the other variables cited. By the end of the pregnancy, the mother needs to have gained 4-6 pounds in fat and protein which are important for successful breast-feeding (Gabbe, 2002).

Exercise

Daily exercise is important for all of us and pregnancy is no exception. Pregnant women are encouraged to include moderate exercise for 30 minutes or more each day. The primary concern in choosing the type of exercise is loss of balance, especially late in the pregnancy when the center of balance changes. Swimming, cycling, walking and yoga are all excellent choices of exercise during pregnancy. One caution is that women need to avoid getting overheated enough to raise the core temperature to 100 degrees. In most situations this can be avoided by not exercising when it is hot and humid, and by drinking plenty of fluids. Daily exercise may help prevent gestational diabetes. (ACOG, 2011).

That too much exercise may cause miscarriage or harm the fetus is a myth (Sizer & Whitney, 1997). Moderate exercise during pregnancy has the benefits of improving muscle tone and alleviating pregnancy-related discomforts such as backache, bloating, constipation, and swollen hands and feet. Whether pregnant or not, exercise relieves stress, improves mood, gives the woman a sense of control of her body, and promotes relaxation and better sleep (ACOG, 2011).

Substances to Avoid During Pregnancy

Because so many substances can cross the placenta, pregnant women are advised not to take any drug without first consulting a physician. Table 13.2 highlights safety concerns related to various drugs as categorized by the Food and Drug Administration. In practical terms, however, that may not be possible, particularly given inadequate health care services for many women. Public health messages have been created to make women aware of the dangers of consuming alcohol and smoking during pregnancy. Increasing awareness is the first strategy. Actually getting women to stop drinking and smoking is more difficult.

It is estimated that getting women to stop smoking during pregnancy would reduce infant deaths by five percent and reduce the number of low birth weight infants by 10 percent. (Rayburn & Phelan, 2008). Smoking cigarettes and inhaling secondhand smoke both affect the health of the fetus negatively. Cigarette smoke reduces the amount of oxygen in the bloodstream, adversely affecting fetal growth and nicotine decreases uterine blood flow. These effects contribute to the increase in risk of low birth weight, premature birth, still birth, sudden infant death syndrome and respiratory illness for the infant (Gabbe, 2012).

According to the Centers for Disease Control and Prevention, Fetal Alcohol Syndrome cost the United States more than $4 billion dollars per year (CDC, 2012). Because no level of drinking is known to be safe, pregnant women are encouraged to abstain totally. Women who are trying to become pregnant or who use poor birth control also should not drink since they may be pregnant for a few weeks before they know it (Gabbe, 2012). The blood alcohol concentration (BAC) of the mother is the same as that of the fetus, so the impact to the fetus is greater. The higher the alcohol intake the greater the impact and the greater the lifelong problems associated with this intake. An occasional glass of wine or a beer has not been shown to have this impact. Yet, there is a risk and it may not be worth taking.

Fetal alcohol syndrome (FAS) is a cluster of effects found in babies as a result of their mother's drinking. Heavy drinking is a major risk to the fetus and a reduction, even in mid pregnancy can have a beneficial effect (Gabbe, 2012). Children born with FAS have a small head, abnormal facial features, sleep disorders, short stature, a wide space between the eyes and between the nose and upper lip, hyperactivity, and mental retardation.

Women who abuse cocaine, heroin, and other opiates risk having babies addicted to the abused substance. What is less well known is that many other drugs can have damaging effects.

Fetal alcohol syndrome Effects on embryo and fetus of pregnant woman's alcohol consumption; symptoms include facial abnormalities, mental retardation, and nervous system damage

Baby	7.5	pounds
Placenta	1.5	pounds
Amniotic fluid	2	pounds
Uterine enlargement	2	pounds
Maternal breast tissue	2	pounds
Maternal blood volume	4	pounds
Fluids in maternal tissue	4	pounds
Maternal fat	7	pounds
Average total:	30	pounds

Note: Based on a 30-pound weight gain

Figure 13.3 *Breakdown of Weight Gain During Pregnancy*

Source: What to Expect When You're Expecting, Murkoff, H., Eisenberg, A., and Hathaway, S.

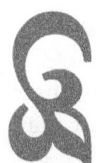

healthy sex hints 13.2

For Pregnant Women

To reduce complications during pregnancy, at delivery, and after delivery:

1. Begin preconception care when you decide you want to become pregnant and prenatal care as soon as you know you are pregnant. If you cannot afford prenatal care from a private physician, it is available through your local public health department. Prenatal care is important for a. consistent monitoring of the status of the mother and fetus; b. consistent monitoring of the mother's weight gain; c. consistent monitoring of the mother's nutritional needs.
2. Do not use any psychoactive substances, including tobacco and alcohol, during pregnancy. Drug use may cause problems in the pregnancy and damage the unborn baby.
3. Do not become pregnant without being certain that you have been immunized against German measles.
4. Schedule any of the fetal tests suggested by your health provider.

Table 13.1 Food Intake for Pregancy

Food Group	Serving Size	Servings/day
Breads, cereal, rice, and pasta group	1 slice bread 1/2 cup of cooked cereal, rice, or pasta 1 cup ready-to-eat cereal	6–9
Vegetable group	1 cup raw leafy vegetables 1/2 cup of other vegetables, raw or cooked; ¾ cup vegetable juice	4
Fruit group	1 medium apple, banana 1/2 cup chopped fruit 3/4 cup of fruit juice	3
Milk, yogurt, and cheese group	1 cup of milk or yogurt 1 1/2 oz. natural cheese 2 oz. processed cheese	4 or more
Meat, poultry, fish, dry beans, eggs, and nuts group	2–3 oz. of cooked lean meat, poultry, or fish 1 oz. meat = 1/2 cup cooked dried beans, 1 egg, 1/2 cup tofu, 1/3 cup nuts, 2 T. peanut butter	2 or more 2–3 ounce servings

Source: Journal of the American Dietetic Association, 2002; Cox, & Phelan, 2008.;
US Dept of Health and Human Services, 2008.

∽　*Environmental/Occupational Wellness*　∽

When women become pregnant, they need to determine whether their work surroundings are free of toxins and other pollutants that may affect the fetus. For example, exposure to radiation can damage the fetus. Some women who were smokers stop during their pregnancies but unfortunately return to smoking once the baby is born. Not only are they then harming themselves, but the quality of the air is unhealthy for the baby.

Ideally, new parents should be given support by their employers. Some companies are considered "family-friendly" and provide leave to new parents, birth parents, and adoptive parents. On-site day care is available at some private and public institutions. Flexible work schedules are recognized as valuable to the ever increasing number of working parents. Overall, however, the United States is not in the forefront of providing quality day care and family support compared to other industrialized nations.

Prenatal Screening

Various screening procedures are available to help determine the health of the fetus. The American College of Obstetricians and Gynecologist recommends that all pregnant women be offered genetic screening. Carrier tests determine if one parent is a genetic carrier of a disease. Certain diseases are hereditary—thalassemia and cystic fibrosis, among many others—and some prospective parents want to know whether they are carriers of a disease and their specific risks for having a baby with the disease. The cystic fibrosis carrier testing is available for all pregnant women and a family history of other diseases will trigger a recommendation for other genetic testing (ACOG, 2011).

For example, Jews of Eastern European descent are at risk for passing on the gene for Tay Sach's disease, an incurable neurological disorder that results in the degeneration of what appears to be a healthy baby and death by age 5. Knowledge that the parents are carriers may influence their decision to reproduce or terminate a pregnancy that bears the fatal illness. *Typical tests all during the pregnancy include blood tests* at varying points throughout pregnancy. Blood testing has been encouraged especially to detect HIV, STD's, blood type, past rubella (German measles) infection and other potential health issues. During the first trimester, screening tests for the pregnant mother include blood tests and ultrasound performed between 11 and 14 weeks to test for Down syndrome and trisomy 18. During the second trimester women will have a blood test called "multiple marker screening" that will test for Down syndrome, trisomy 18 and neural tube defect (ACOG, 2011).

If any of the above routine tests indicate that a woman is at increased risk for having a baby with birth defects, diagnostic tests can provide more information. These tests include the following:

1. *Chorionic villus sampling (CVS)*. CVS is conducted between the 10th and 12th week of gestation. A small sample of cells are taken from the placenta usually through the cervix, to screen for genetic abnormalities. Because of the early timing of the test, neural tube defects and

structural deformities—to legs, arms, and so on—cannot be detected. (An ultrasound can be conducted during the second trimester to identify structural anomalies.)

2. *Detailed Ultrasound Exam.* Ultrasound uses high-frequency sound waves to create a **sonogram,** a picture of the fetus. The sonogram outlines all structures in the fetus, showing the heart, kidneys, and liver as well as the full skeleton. At 18 to 20 weeks of pregnancy, the ultrasound can detect structural abnormalities in the skull, brain, spine, heart and other organs as well as cleft lip, incomplete development of the diaphragm, and so forth (Marks & Miller, 2002). For the couple receiving such feedback, there is emotional upset and difficult questions to be answered. Sometimes surgical corrections can be made during pregnancy or shortly thereafter. Other couples choose to terminate the pregnancy, which would be a second-trimester procedure.

Sonogram The picture of the fetus produced by an ultrasound screening

3. *Amniocentesis.* **Amniocentesis** involves removing a small amount of the amniotic fluid and culturing the fetal cells that have sloughed off and are in the fluid. A complete genetic analysis then can be performed, identifying a number of potential diseases and conditions. The genetic analysis also yields the sex of the offspring, but couples are not given that information unless they want it. The test usually is conducted between the 15th and 20th week of gestation. Because an ultrasound is conducted prior to doing an amniocentesis, couples learn of the structural health of the fetus as well.

Amniocentesis Removal of the amniotic fluid

Amniocentesis is recommended particularly for women who become pregnant after age 35, because the rate of birth defects related to chromosomal abnormalities rises as women get older. Particular attention has been given to babies born with Down syndrome. Although the rate of Down syndrome increases with age, eighty percent of affected babies are born to mothers under 35 (Heinzman & Khan, 2010). Rates associated with other chromosomal abnormalities also increase when the mother is 35 or older and the father is older than 55. Increased age of the father has been associated with autism and schizophrenia (Gabbe, 2012).

4. *Alpha-fetoprotein (AFP) screening.* The AFP test involves taking a blood sample from the pregnant woman between the 15th and 18th week of pregnancy. The fetal liver produces alpha-fetoprotein, and high levels in the mother's blood indicate neural tube defects. These defects include anencephaly, in which the upper portion of the brain and head is missing or underdeveloped, and spina bifida, in which the spinal cord is pushing through the spine. Most babies with anencephaly are stillborn or die shortly after birth, whereas babies with spina bifida, depending on the extent of the disability, can live fairly functional lives.

5. *Other tests.* Women with good prenatal care visit their obstetrician or nurse midwife on the recommended schedule to ensure that the pregnancy is progressing normally and that no health problems are developing. During the last weeks of the pregnancy, weeks 38-41, she will make weekly visits.

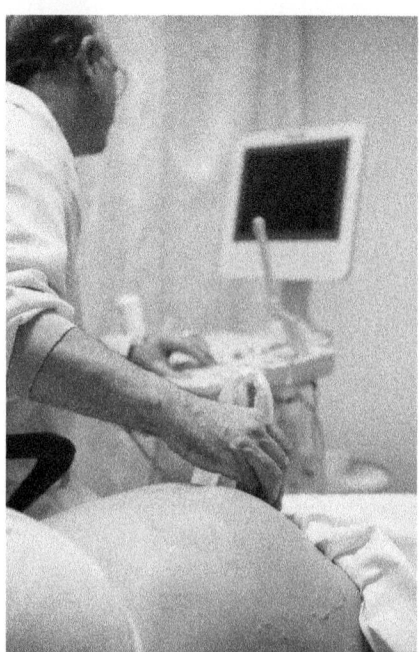

Ultrasound testing can determine position of the baby, abnormalities, and often the sex.

At each visit, the uterus is measured to ensure that the organ is expanding according to average measurements. The obstetrician or nurse midwife estimates growth of the fetus partly by measuring expansion of the uterus. Also, the woman's blood pressure is taken to watch for signs of hypertension. Each visit includes a weight measurement.

Childbirth

Childbirth encompasses labor and delivery. Although the baby is born from the mother's body, the experience is increasingly viewed as one to be shared by the couple. Stories of experiences with childbirth vary from couple to couple, woman to woman, and birth to birth, even for the same woman.

For much of history, women helped women birth their babies. With the advent of "modern medicine," obstetricians began to deliver babies. Mothers left their other children at home, went to a hospital, and gave birth, while the fathers waited in the expectant fathers' waiting room. By the end of the 20th century, birthing became an extended family event with much greater support and participation from partners, family, and friends.

Depending to some extent on geography and the availability of health care providers, couples do have choices as to where and how their baby is born. Most babies in the United States are born in hospitals. Establishing a relationship with a private gynecologist/obstetrician, hospital clinic, or birthing center will determine where the baby is born. Although facilities share some fundamental aspects of delivery, they can have philosophical differences in practice and procedures. Being informed about the staff, facilities, and philosophy will enhance the birth experience. The type of health insurance, if any, that the couple has may be the driving force in making a choice.

The Childbirth Process

Childbirth is a three-phase process, shown in Figure 13.4, occurring over a 12- to 14-hour period on average. Some women have a rapid labor, delivering even before they can make it to the hospital. Others report long labors of 30 or more hours. The length of labor is affected by many factors including fetal size, fetal position, epidural use and the mother's body mass index (Gabbe, 2012). The first stage of labor is the longest; it also tends to be longer for a first delivery than subsequent births. A number of signs indicate that labor is beginning:

- The uterus begins to contract. As labor progresses, these contractions become more regular, closer together in time, and more intense.
- The thick mucous plug that has been covering the cervix, protecting the pregnancy, is dislodged. Because this mucus can be stained with blood, it sometimes is referred to as a "bloody show."
- Rupture of the amniotic membranes releases much of the amniotic fluid in the uterus that has protected the baby, and it trickles or gushes from the vagina. Not all women experience loss of amniotic fluid early in labor; it may happen later in the process. Other women may think their membranes have ruptured but actually may be experiencing urinary incontinence from all the pressure. Because the risk of infection increases after the rupture of membranes, women who think their "water has broken" should get in touch with their health care provider.

First Stage

The first stage of labor is the longest of the three stages and is divided into early and active labor. In early labor the cervix begins to dilate and mild to moderate contractions begin. This part of the labor can last hours or even days. This is followed by active labor where the cervix dilates to 10 centimeters (4 inches), the diameter needed for safe passage of the baby's head. During active labor, which often lasts eight hours, the contractions get stronger and closer together. **Effacement,** the thinning of the cervix, also takes place during this phase. The end of the first stage of labor, called transition, is marked by the most intense contractions, and the woman now often feels the urge to push (Mayo Clinic, 2011).

Effacement Thinning of the cervix during first stage of labor

Second Stage

The second stage of labor involves the actual birth. This is a short stage for some women—one to three pushes and the baby is out and for others it may last several hours. An **episiotomy,** once performed routinely, is now performed only when absolutely necessary because the procedure increases the mothers risk for perineal and vaginal trauma and anal sphincter disruption. Based on the evidence showing a lack of maternal benefits of having an episiotomy, currently only 10-17% of births involves an episiotomy compared to 87% in 1976. (Gabbe, 2012). Once the head is out of the vagina, the baby's airway will be cleared and the umbilical cord will be checked to make sure it is free. The rest of the baby will then emerge into the world.

Episiotomy The surgical cutting of the perineum to facilitate childbirth now considered medically unnecessary

Third Stage

The third stage of labor consists of delivery of the the placenta, which had been attached to the uterine wall, and the umbilical cord, which has been cut at the baby's abdomen but remains attached to the placenta at the other end. Delivery of the placenta, sometime called **afterbirth,** takes about 5-10 minutes. During the third stage, women may experience the rush of emotions associated with the birth itself and holding their newborn. The mother can breast-feed her infant during the delivery of the placenta. The first moments and hours after the birth of the child are very important in the maternal-infant attachment process. There should be as many opportunities as possible for the new parents to be with their newborn immediately after birth and as often as possible in the next few days. This bonding process is characterized by fondling, kissing, cuddling and gazing at the infant. Modern hospitals can encourage this bonding by having flexible hours for fathers, infant rooming with the mother and supporting breast-feeding (Gabbe, 2002).

Afterbirth The placenta, umbilical cord, which has been cut at the baby's abdomen but attached to the placenta, and membranes expelled after the birth of a child

Delivery Options

Couples now have a variety of delivery options that include not only the traditional method but also birthing centers, home births, and cesarean deliveries.

Traditional Delivery

What has come to be viewed as traditional today is different from the traditional delivery of years ago. Both mother and father are typically present at the delivery, which takes place in a hospital. Some fathers videotape and

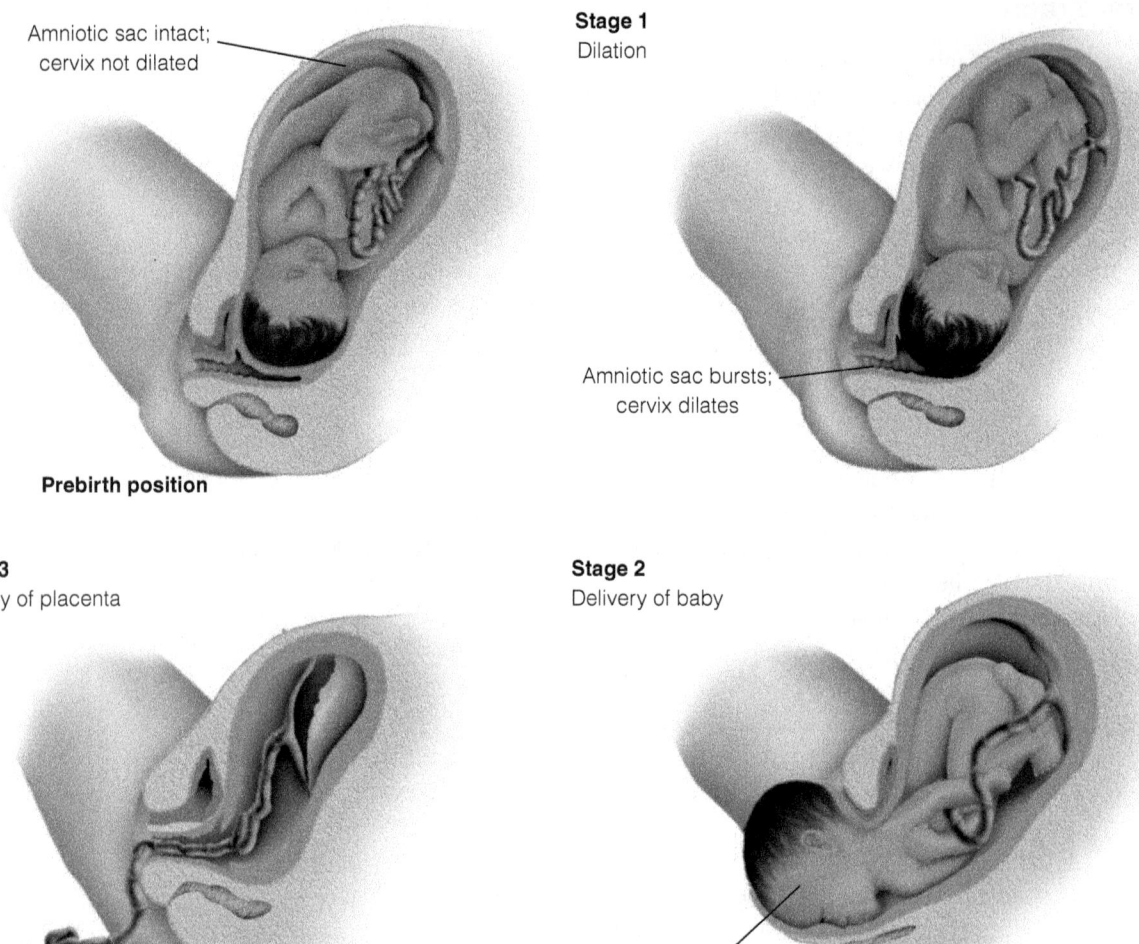

Amniotic sac intact;
cervix not dilated

Stage 1
Dilation

Amniotic sac bursts;
cervix dilates

Prebirth position

Stage 3
Delivery of placenta

Stage 2
Delivery of baby

Placenta separates from
uterus and is delivered

Fetus's head turns,
crowns, and is delivered

Figure 13.4 *Stages of Childbirth*

photograph their child's first minutes. Prior to that, couples attend prepared childbirth classes that teach about pregnancy and childbirth. Taking childbirth education classes such as Lamaze helps a woman reduce the fear and pain often associated with labor. Childbirth education gives the woman and her partner/coach the tools to help her relax, improve her labor and delivery and perhaps even decrease the need for pain medication.

Some women come to their deliveries with a "coach," who may not necessarily be the father of the child. For lesbian couples, the partner helps with the birth. Some women want their own mothers or sisters to be present. Whatever the circumstance, most hospitals have modified their obstetrical practices to allow for one or more family members or designated friends to participate in the birth.

Many hospitals offer family centered care where the woman goes through labor, delivery and recovery all in the same room. Often it is a very home like setting where the partner stays with the woman and after the birth, the baby sleeps in the room. There is also often the option of the "in hospital birthing center" that is either in or next to the hospital. These also offer a home like atmosphere with the advantage of being close to medical help if needed (Conaway, 2012).

Hospital births afford both mother and baby the availability of technology and monitoring. Some facilities also are known for their neonatal intensive care units, which become particularly important if the baby is at high risk—premature, physical deformities, infant in other than head-first position, blood incompatibility between mother and fetus, **toxemia,** multiple births, and so on.

Toxemia A highly dangerous condition during pregnancy when high blood pressure occurs

Hospitals are set up to give women a lot of attention, with specialized nurses to care for the mother and the baby. Hospital births give women more options for managing pain. Although individuals may have decided beforehand what their philosophy of birth is, the true test comes during labor. Some women manage their pain well and find that the breathing techniques they learned in their childbirth classes prepared them well. Relaxation techniques and hypnosis also can be helpful in managing the discomfort associated with labor.

The most popular pain relief is the **epidural anesthetic** used by 60% of women (Camann, 2005). The epidural which relieves pain in 10-20 minutes can be administered once a woman has dilated to 5 centimeters. This numbs her abdominal area, removing pain and discomfort while allowing labor to progress. Women who have an epidural must remain in bed. Its advantage is that the dosage of the drug is monitored in such a way so that the woman regains the capacity to push the baby out at the time of delivery. However, an epidural may decrease her ability to push effectively. Of concern is the strong association shown in retrospective studies between the use of epidural analgesia and the increased rate of cesarean delivery (Camann, 2005). There is also concern that it increases the risk of use of forceps or vacuum extraction and may prolong labor in vaginal birth (Eltzschig et al, 2003).

Epidural anesthetic An injection of a drug into the spinal cord during labor to dull pain

Even though hospitals maintain nurseries, the baby spends most of the time in the room with the mother. Hospitals have greatly eased visitation restrictions. Fathers have few limitations on the amount of time they can spend in the room, and some choose to sleep at the hospital. Siblings, too, can visit their newborn brother or sister. Gone are the days when the family looked at the new addition briefly behind glass windows.

Birthing Centers

Birthing centers gained in popularity with the growth of the women's movement in the 1970s. Women were taking an increased role in the birth of their own babies and asking for changes to traditional delivery. Birthing centers were operated by nurse midwives who worked under the supervision of obstetricians, in close physical proximity to hospitals.

The unique feature of birthing centers is the belief that the woman, with the support of her partner, should have as much control over the birthing process as possible. They were the first places where the space for deliveries was "homey," incorporating birthing beds, wallpapered rooms, and rocking chairs. They also cut back on the use of fetal heart monitors so the woman could move around more easily during the first stage of labor. Women could take showers, eat lightly, and have family, including their other children, with them.

Women who deliver at birthing centers usually are screened to rule out high risk cases. Multiple births, health conditions that warrant close medical monitoring —for example, diabetes and heart conditions—and being over 40 years of age are situations in which a hospital birth is encouraged or required.

As hospitals have increasingly embraced some of the offerings of birthing centers—leaving women to labor and deliver in one room, making those rooms more attractive and less stereotypically hospital-like, having nurse midwives on staff—free-standing birthing centers away from hospitals may be a less attractive option now.

Home Births

Delivering babies at home may be a personal choice or may result from rapid labor. Lay midwives have delivered many babies at home. Today, the attitude toward home birth is that it puts the life and welfare of both the baby and mother at risk. Because of the risk of charges of medical malpractice, obstetricians do not conduct home births, and only a select number of licensed nurse midwives will do so. In contrast, the majority of the world's babies are born at home, particularly in non-industrialized countries.

Cesarean Deliveries

Cesarean delivery (c-section) The surgical form of childbirth in which an incision is made through the abdomen and uterus to deliver the baby, placenta and umbilical cord

Breech position A birth position in which the buttocks or foot rather than the baby's head presents at the cervix

Cesarean delivery, or **c-section,** is a surgical procedure done for a variety of reasons related to the health and survival of either the mother or the baby, or both. In 2010, nearly 1 in 3 live births in the US was a cesarean birth, the highest rate ever reported. This rate is high by contrast to that of other industrialized nations. Since 1996, the total rate has increased 71%, due in part to the increase in maternal age, maternal choice and legal pressures (Menacker & Hamilton, 2010). C-sections are generally done when the baby is in a **breech position**—feet or buttocks presenting first. Other indications for cesarean delivery are incompatibility between the baby's head size and size of the mother's pelvis, a large baby, signs of fetal distress picked up by fetal heart monitors, weak contractions of the uterus and prolonged labor, or problems with the placenta and identified bleeding. If the surgery is performed under emergency conditions, such as a detached placenta, general anesthesia is administered. In other situations, where time allows, anesthesia can be given with an epidural, which allows the mother to remain awake and, in many hospitals, her partner to be present. A mother who has a cesarean for one birth will not necessarily need to have the next baby by cesarean birth.

Postpartum

The *postpartum* period represents the time after the birth, with all its various dimensions of change. First-time mothers and fathers are "new" to parenthood and sometimes overly anxious. Parents having a second, third, or fourth child, by contrast, will find themselves focused on the needs of the baby along with those of their other children. If the baby has health problems and has to stay in the hospital longer than the mother, the emotional feelings at the time are intensified.

Women, whether breastfeeding or bottle feeding, will experience marked changes in their hormone levels, which in turn affect emotions. Levels of estrogen and progesterone drop rapidly within 24 hours and then continue dropping until the body reaches its pre-pregnancy levels. It is normal to experience unexplained sadness, often termed "baby blues," after birth. For some, the blues last a few hours; for others, they can last for 1 to 2 weeks. Postpartum depression (PPD) can start after the birth and affects up to 15 percent of mothers. Women may have feelings of anxiety and deep sadness. Some may not have any interest in their babies, whereas others become overly worried. There appears to be an association between depression prior to pregnancy or during pregnancy and experiencing post partum depression (Informed Health Online, 2012).

One of the major adjustments postpartum is the effect of lack of sleep on the body. Some newborns wake to eat every 2 to 3 hours, and for those women who breastfeed, the burden of being available and awake cannot be equally divided. Anthony, in Case Study 13.2, later shared that for the 1st year with his triplets, there was never 1 hour when all three were asleep at the same time! Prolonged sleep deprivation affects mood, energy, interest in socializing, and ability to concentrate.

One very positive change for most women is the loss of some of the weight they gained during pregnancy. Immediately after birth, a woman will lose 10-13 pounds from the combination of the weight of the baby, placenta, amniotic fluid, and blood loss. By the six week milestone, 28% of women will be at their pre-pregnant weight (Gabbe, 2002).

Adjustment in this period also includes a reassessing of roles—parent, partner, individual. Who comes first? Fatigue for the parents, with the simultaneous constancy of attending to a baby, may interfere with any desire to resume lovemaking. After birth, the uterus produces a bloody discharge called **lochia,** which can be on again/off again for weeks. If a woman has an episiotomy or cesarean section, the incision will also need to heal. As a result, physicians will often advise women to wait until their first postpartum medical appointment before resuming sexual intercourse. Overall, any sexual activity can be reintroduced into a couple's lifestyle once the woman and her partner feel comfortable.

Lochia The uterine discharge that is released over a period of weeks after childbirth

Breastfeeding

Worldwide four in five mothers breast-feed their babies for one year yet only one in five American mothers do so. Women today are strongly being encouraged to breastfeed their babies, even for a short period of time. The American Academy of Pediatrics recommend babies be exclusively breast-fed for 6 months while the World Health Organization recommends breast-feeding for two years (American Dietetic Association, 2009). Even women who have a career can continue to breast feed once they return to work. Techniques such as decreasing the amount of times they nurse and pumping breast milk to leave for caretakers can give women the option to continue breast-feeding (Gabbe, 2002).

Breast milk is tailored to meet the nutritional needs of the infant and brings numerous health benefits. Perhaps one of the greatest benefits of breast feeding is that it reduces the risk for sudden infant death syndrome and death from other causes. Breast feeding improves an infant's immune response, reduces the risk for a variety of chronic diseases, contributes to better cognitive skills, stimulates bonding between mother and child and promotes better health in premature infants. Additional benefits include allergy prevention, lower asthma risk, and better mouth and tooth development in the baby. Breast-feeding is thought to give the baby better control of its intake, thereby reducing later obesity (American Dietetic Association, 2009). Breast-feeding also benefits the mother in a variety of ways. Post partum depression risks are lower and bone density increases. The breast-feeding mother will also burn extra calories helping her return more quickly to her pre-pregnancy weight. In addition, her uterus will also shrink faster (American Dietetic Association, 2009). Women who breast-feed lower their risks for ovarian cancer and breast cancer. Breast-feeding may also have a calming effect on mothers, allowing an easier transition into motherhood. Oxytocin spikes during breast-feeding and this may have an anti-anxiety effect and help promote bonding with the baby. Breast-feeding may even be a mood elevator (Rabin, 2006). In addition to all of the health benefits, breast-feeding is convenient and is less expensive than formula. In our "Go Green" world, breast-feeding is the environmentally friendly choice (Leung & Sauve, 2005).

Not all women want to breast-feed, and they need to know that improved formulas do provide the essential nutrients needed by the newborn. Mothers have many choices in types of formulas that are available for infants who are less than twelve months old. These formulas vary in nutritional and calorie content, taste and cost.

❧ *Social and Spiritual Wellness* ❧

Once children become a fact of life, notions of family expand and change. Relationships with parents, employers, and friends take on new dimensions and demands.

Caring for children is a 24-hour job, not easily filled by one person. Will parenting responsibilities be shared? Will we work well as a team to care for and raise our child ? What networks of support are in place? Will the mother work? Is child care available? Play groups? Recognizing what is required helps promote social health.

Parenthood can convey a sense of purpose and add meaning to life. Parents often discover new meaning in life/death issues as they become responsible for another human being. Parenthood brings with it an ongoing assessment of the relationship to one's child. Is the child like me? Does that matter? Can I love this child? Can I help him/her grow and be free to live his/her own life? What happens when parents die? If children die?

Although answering some of these questions may be uncomfortable and difficult, doing so is essential to plan for responsible parenthood. Parents need to have a will and designate guardians. Some children know of adults who became their godparents, yet those individuals may or may not assume an active role throughout their lives.

Personal Assessment

Assessing Readiness for Parenting

Using the wellness model, assess your readiness on each dimension. Issues that focus specifically on the pregnancy itself are weighted more toward the female parent. Nonetheless, for both males and females, parenthood touches on all dimensions of health and wellness.

Physical Wellness

Are you physically healthy? Is your weight, blood pressure, and respiration within a normal range?

Do you have any chronic illnesses that may impact your ability to conceive? Maintain a pregnancy? Experience childbirth?

Are you taking any medications that may affect the normal growth and development of the fetus?

Do you regularly use any drugs recreationally? Are you addicted to any substance? Could you stop using caffeine, alcohol, or other recreational drugs?

What are your sleep patterns? How well do you function with interrupted sleep?

Are you physically fit? Do you exercise regularly?

Do you have any physical disabilities that may affect your ability to maintain a pregnancy? Go through childbirth? Take care of a child? If so, do you have the resources to make pregnancy, childbirth, and caregiving manageable?

Intellectual Wellness

Have you thought about the roles and responsibilities of being a parent?

Have you thought about why you want to become a parent? Do they seem sound?

Have you read any educational material on pregnancy, childbirth, and parenting skills?

Have you assessed your financial readiness for parenthood?

Do you have the financial resources to provide for a child—food, clothing, medical expenses?

Emotional Wellness

Are you excited about becoming a parent?

Are you comfortable with the person you are? Do you love yourself? Are you able to offer love to another?

Do you handle frustration well? Anger?

Are you currently struggling with any emotional problems that could interfere with your becoming a parent?

Have you been diagnosed with any problems or mental conditions for which you take medication? If so, would a pregnancy aggravate your condition? Would parenthood affect your condition in any way?

Thought Questions

Social Wellness

Is the quality of your relationship with your partner healthy?

Are you considering being a single parent?

What is the quality of your relationship with your family of origin? Will family members be involved as grandparents, aunts, cousins, uncles? Is that important to you?

What is the quality of your relationship with the family of your partner? Will any of them be involved as grandparents, aunts, cousins, uncles? Is that important to you?

Do you have other social support networks? Neighbors? Friends?

Spiritual Wellness

Have you thought about the impact of parenthood on your life?

Do you feel ready to be responsible for another? Nurture and love another? Put someone else's needs above your own?

Do you and your partner share similar beliefs about religion? Would having a child bring to the surface any tensions and differences?

Environmental/Occupational Wellness

Are you currently living in a place where you can stay?

What kind of living space will you provide for a baby? Is it safe, smoke-free?

What kind of a community will you live in? Is the area safe? Can you easily get around (say, with a stroller)?

Do you have access to medical care? For you? For a baby?

Do you have access to a supermarket or other store for items such as baby food and diapers?

Do you have access to transportation?

Are you currently employed? If so, is your workplace "family-friendly"?

Does your employer have child care facilities?

Do you have family health care coverage through your work?

The answers to these questions can give you a sense of whether or not you are ready for parenthood. Keep in mind that no one is totally prepared for parenthood. It has too many unknowns, and the personal experience far exceeds your imagination and descriptions provided in books. Thinking about the issues, preparing for the possibilities, and being ready on many levels is part of good decision making and planning.

Thought Questions

1. When is the "right" time to have a baby? What are some of the considerations that go into this?

2. What happens in the process of fertilization and conception?

3. What major changes in the fetus are associated with each trimester?

4. What are the basic wellness guidelines to ensure a healthy pregnancy?

5. What tests and other technological advances are available to aid with pregnancy, labor, and delivery? How do these contribute to political debate?

6. What are the differences in hospital versus home (or birth center) births?

7. What is the role of the midwife?

8. What is cesarean birth? What is the rate of c-sections in the United States? What factors contribute to the high rate in the United States?

Test Yourself

1. Which would be the least helpful to a woman trying to determine whether or not she was fertile?
   a. Using a home pregnancy kit
   b. Looking for the presence of cervical mucous
   c. Taking her morning temperature
   d. Keeping track of her menstrual cycle on the calendar

2. Fertilization of the ovum takes place
   a. at the cervix.
   b. in the vagina.
   c. in the fallopian tube.
   d. in the uterus.

3. Home pregnancy tests look for the presence of _____ in a woman's urine.
   a. increased levels of estrogen
   b. human chorionic gonadotropin (hCG)
   c. increased levels of progesterone
   d. increased levels of testosterone

4. A normal period of gestation takes how long?
   a. 28 weeks
   b. 40 weeks
   c. 36 weeks
   d. 45 weeks

5. Good prenatal care requires that a health care provider monitor all but which of the following?
   a. A woman's nutritional intake
   b. Fetal size and growth
   c. A woman's medication use
   d. A woman's sexual interest

6. Guidelines for recreational alcohol use during pregnancy include which of the following?
   a. Women should only drink beer.
   b. No more than three glasses of wine per week.
   c. No safe limits for alcohol consumption have been established.
   d. No alcohol use until the third trimester of pregnancy.

7. Prenatal screening tests, such as amniocentesis, are primarily designed to
   a. determine whether labor will be normal.
   b. determine whether the fetus is developing normally.
   c. determine health risks to the mother because of pregnancy.
   d. determine whether the fetus is male or female.

8. A woman should suspect that labor is beginning if
   a. she experiences nausea.
   b. she feels some intermittent cramping.
   c. she is 40 weeks pregnant.
   d. she passes a bloody, mucous plug.

9. A cesarean delivery may be performed because
   a. the baby is in a breech position.
   b. the mother is overweight.
   c. the parents have requested it.
   d. the first stage of labor is too short.

10. A baby is born during the _____ stage of labor.
    a. first
    b. second
    c. third
    d. fourth

Web Resources

SuperTracker for Moms
www.choosemyplate.gov

The U.S.D.A education site that tailors the pregnant woman's food recommendations according to her individual needs and stage of pregnancy. Nutritionist and health care providers are recommending this as the primary source of nutrition information. It can also be used as a food intake guide for breast-feeding women.

International Council on Infertility Information Dissemination (INCIID)
www.inciid.org

A nonprofit organization committed to providing information about diagnosis, treatment, and prevention of infertility and pregnancy loss. The site accesses fact sheets and transcripts of auditoriums with renowned experts, more than 150 referrals and links to nonprofit organizations providing quality, sound infertility information, such as the American Society of Reproductive Medicine and the International Federation of Fertility Societies.

Infertility Resources
www.ihr.com/fertililty

Offers extensive information about infertility organizations and clinics, IVF, egg donor, financial issues, subject matter experts, sperm banks, Internet newsgroups and mailing lists, research, journals, medications, infertility medical supplies, and adoption. The infertility educational articles offer diagnosis, male factors, treatment, drugs/medication, psychological and social issues, plus financial and legal information.

March of Dimes
www.modimes.org

A nonprofit organization providing information on birth defects, prenatal screening tests, prenatal care guidelines, and other research related to pregnancy.

National SHARE Office
www.nationalshareoffice.com

A national organization with affiliates that provide resources and support for parents who have experienced miscarriage, stillbirth, or death of a baby.

Planned Parenthood Federation of America
www.plannedparenthood.org

Provides information and resources related to a full range of reproductive health issues.

References

Alan Guttmacher Institute. (2002, February/March). In their own right is new report addressing the sexual reproductive health needs of American men. *SIECUS Report, 30*(3).

American Academy of Pediatrics. (2002). *Policy on same sex adoption* [Online]. Available: www.aap.org/policy/ 02008t.htm.

American College of Obstetricians and Gynecologists(2011, August). Routine tests in pregnancy. Frequently Asked Questions (FAQ 133), available: http://www.acog.org

American College of Obstetricians and Gynecologists (2011, August). Nutrition during pregnancy. Frequently Asked Questions (FAQ 001), available: http://www.acog.org

American College of Obstetricians and Gynecologists (2011, August). Exercise during pregnancy. Frequently Asked Questions (FAQ 119), available: http://www.acog.org

American College of Obstetricians and Gynecologists(2011, August). Routine tests in pregnancy. Frequently Asked Questions (FAQ 133), available: http://www.acog.org

American College of Obstetricians and Gynecologists(2011, August).Screening for birth defects. Frequently Asked Questions (FAQ 165), available: http://www.acog.org

American College of Obstetricians and Gynecologists(2011, August).How your baby grows during pregnancy. Frequently Asked Questions (FAQ 156), available: http://www.acog.org

American College of Obstetricians and Gynecologists (2012, June). Evaluating Infertility. Frequently Asked Questions (FAQ 136), available: http://www.acog.org

American College of Obstetricians and Gynecologists (2012, June). Having Twins. Frequently Asked Questions (FAQ092), available: http://www.acog.org

American Dietetic Association (2009). Position of the American dietetic association: promoting and supporting breast-feeding. Journal of the American Dietetic Association. 109 (11). Pp 1926–1941.

American Dietetic Association (2008). Position of the American dietetic association:Nutrition and lifestyle for a healthy pregnancy outcome. Journal of the American Dietetic Association. 108 (3). pp 1926–1941.

Carson, M. & Ehrenthal, D. (2008). Medical Issues from Preconception Through Delivery: A Roadmap fro the Internist. Medical Clinics of North America. Vol. 92 Issue 5.

Camann, W. (2005). Pain relief during labor. New England Journal of Medicine. 352, (7). 718–719.

Cassell, C. (2002, February/March). Let it shine: Promoting school success, life aspirations to prevent school-age parenthood. *SIECUS Report,* 30(3).

Center for Disease Control and Prevention (April, 2007). Morbidity and Mortality Weekly Report. [online] Available: www.cdc.gov.

Center for Disease Control and Prevention (2010). Infertility. [online] Available: http://www.cdc.gov/nchs/fastats/fertile.htm

Center for Disease Control and Prevention (2011). Assisted reproductive technology[online] Available: www.cdc.gov.

Center for Disease Control and Prevention (2012). Fetal alcohol spectrum disordersSyndrome. [online] Available: www.cdc.gov.

Center for Disease Control and Prevention (2013). Chlamydia. [online] Available: www.cdc.gov.

Conaway, B. (2012, December 2). How do you want to deliver your baby? WebMD. Available: http://www.webmd.com/baby/features/childbirth-options-whats-best?print=true

Consumers Union. (2003b, February). When the test really counts. *Consumer Reports,* 68, 45–47.

Eltzschig, H, Lieberman, E., & Camann, W. (2003). Regional anesthesia for labor and delivery. New England Journal of Medicine, 348, (4), 319–332.

First Consult (2013). Pregnancy: medical topics;first consult. Available: http://www.mdconsult.com

Gabbe (2002). Gabbe:Obstretrics-normal and problem pregnancies, 4th edition. Churchill Livingston, Inc.

Gabbe (2007). Gabbe: Obstretrics- normal and problem pregnancies. 5th edition. Churchill Livingston, Inc.

Gabbe(2012). Gabbe:OBstretrics-normal and problem pregnancies. 6th edition. Churchill Livingston, Inc.

Guzick, D (2002). Should insurance for in vitro fertilization be mandated? Editorial. New England Journal of Medicine, 347, (9) 686–688.

Haffner, L. (2004). Advanced maternal age—how old is too old? New England Journal of Medicine, 351 (19), 1927–1929.

Heinzman, D., &Khan, S., (2010). Down Syndrome. MDConsult Resources.available: http://www.mdconsult.com

Henderson, J. (2006). Gonadotropin therapy prior to in vitro fertilization was more cost-effective than immediate in vitro fertilization. Evidence-based Obstetrics and Gynecology. Vol 8 issue 9.

Hewlett, S. A. (2002). *Creating a life: Professional women and the quest for children.* New York: Hyperion.

Hornstein, M. & Gibbons, W. (2008). Initial Infertility consultation in couples planning pregnacy: Lifestyle factors. [online] www.utdol.com

Informed Health Online (2012). Postpartum depression. Available: http://www.ncbi.nlm.nih.gov

Kuohung, W. & Hornstein, M. (2008). Evaluation of female infertility. Up to Date. [online] www.utdol.com

deLaRochebrochard, E. & Thonneau, P. (2003). Paternal age > or =40 years: an important risk factor for infertility. American Journal of Obstetrics and Gynecology. 189 (40), 901–905.

Lentz (2012). Lentz: comprehensive Gynecology. Sixth Edition. Mosby.

Leung, A. & Sauve, R. (2005). Breast is Best For Babies. Journal of the National Medical Association. 1010–1019.

Livingston, G. & Cohn, D. (2010).More women without children. Pew Research Center Publications Available: http://pewresearch.org/pubs/1642/more—women-without-children

Livingston, G. & Cohn, D. (2012). Immigrant women lead recent drop in U.S. births and birth rates. Pew Research Social &Demographic Trends. Available: http://www.pewsocialtrends.org/2012/11/29/immigrant- women- lead- recent- drop- in- U.S.- births- and- birth- rates

Marks, J., & Miller, M. (2002). Reproductive health technology and genetic counseling. In G. Wingood & R.DiClemente (Eds.), *Handbook of reproductive health.* New York: Kluwer Academic/Plenum.

Mayo Clinic (2011). Stages of labor. Baby its time. Available: http://mayoclinic.com/health/stages-of-labor

Mayo Clinic (2012).Healthy sperm: Improving your fertility. Available: http://mayoclinic.com/health/stages-of-labor

MD Consult (2005). Clinical Topic Tours- Infertility. [online] Available: www. Mdconsult.com

MD Consult (2007).Evaluation of the infertile couple. [Online]. Available: www. MDConsult.com

MD Consult (2007). Pregancy. [Online]. Available: www. MDConsult.com

MD Consult (2012). Pregancy tests-how do pregnancy test work? [Online]. Available: www. MDConsult.com

Medical Clinics of North America (2008, September) Infertility. Volume 92, Issue 5.

Menacker, F. & Hamiltion, B. (2010). Recent trends in cesarean delivery in the United States. NCHS Data Brief (35) available: http://www.cdc.gov

Miller, C.(2012). The emotional strain of infertility. Available: www.intelhealth.com

Murkoff, H., Eisenberg, A., & Hathaway, S. (2002). *What to expect when you're expecting.* New York: Workman.

Office on Women's Health, Department of Health and Human Services. (2002, November). Pregnancy and medication [Online]. Available: www.4woman.gov/faq/ pregmed.htm Ostrea, E., Late, M. (2004, September). Education campaign takes on lagging breast-feeding rates. The Nations Health.

Lukacz, E.,Hull, A.,Scherger, J., Danakas, G., & Jones, K. (2010). Pregnancy. MD Consult Resources. Available: http://www.mdconsult.com

Rabin, R. (2006, June 13) Breast-Feed or Else. The New York Times.

Rayburn, W. & Phelan, S. (2008). Promoting Healthy Habits in Pregnancy. Obstestrics and Gynecology Clinics. Vol 35 Issue 3.

Storch, S. (2012). Miscarriage. MedlinePlus. Available: http://www.nlm.nih.gov/medlineplus/ency/article/001488.htm

Sullivan, D. L. (2001). The expectant mother's guide to prescription and nonprescription drugs, vitamins, home remedies, and herbal products. New York: St. Martin's Griffin.

Swerdloff, R. & Wang, C. (2008). Evaluation of Male infertility. Up to Date. [online] www.utdol.com

U.S. National Center for Health Statistics. (2001). Vital statistics of the United States annual 2001, No. 76. In *Statistical Abstracts of the United States: 2001.* Washington, DC: U.S. Government Printing Office.

Van Voorhis, B. (2007). In vitro fertilization. New England Journal of Medicine. 356 (4). pp. 379–385.

Wright, V., Schieve, L., Reynolds, M., & Jeng, G. (2003, August 29). Assisted reproductive technology surveillance—United States, 2000. *Morbidity and Mortality Weekly Report, 52* (SS-9).

US Preventive Services (2008). Primary Care Interventions to Promote Breast-feeding: US Preventive Services Task Force Recommendation Statement. Annals of Internal Medicine.149: 560–564.

chapter

fourteen

Fertility Control

Student Learning Objectives

After reading this chapter, students will be able to:

- ♥ Differentiate the following terms: fertility control, contraception, birth control, and family planning.
- ♥ Compare the theoretical effectiveness and the effectiveness of actual use.
- ♥ Determine personal level of risk for unintended pregnancy.
- ♥ Develop a personal plan for controlling fertility.
- ♥ Explain the different mechanisms of fertility control.
- ♥ Evaluate a variety of fertility control methods.
- ♥ Determine which methods work best for different types of users.
- ♥ Describe how fertility control requires change over the life cycle.
- ♥ Identify which methods work best in reducing the risks for STD and HIV infection.
- ♥ Evaluate the health aspects of various fertility control methods.

activity teaser: How do you really feel about abortion? Find out in the Personal Exploration Activity on page 458.

case study 14.1

Joe's Vasectomy

Joe, 34, is white.

The best present I ever gave myself was my vasectomy. I belong to an HMO, and it cost me a dollar to have it done. I'll always feel it was the best dollar I ever spent. I guess I've used almost every method available with my wife and my girlfriends before I got married. All these methods had one problem or another, so I promised myself that after the kids were born, I'd take responsibility and get a vasectomy.

The week after my second son was born, I told my wife I wanted to have it done. She was glad that we could stop using condoms and fertility awareness and supported my decision. The procedure was uneventful. I was in and out in 1 hour. The only glitch was that the anesthesiologist had to give me three shots of painkiller before they could make the incision.

After about 2 weeks, my follow-up tests were negative, and we had sex for the first time without worry of my wife getting pregnant. The first time was in the shower. It was great. I can't remember the last time we made love in the shower. Getting the vasectomy was the biggest boost to our sex life in the past 10 years!

Critical Thinking

Sterilization is often something college students can't envision, yet it remains a very popular form of birth control worldwide. Could you imagine either you or your partner being sterilized after having had the children you wanted?

Many people use the terms *birth control, contraception,* and *family planning* interchangeably when referring to controlling fertility. Although the three terms are similar because they refer to strategies for preventing unintended pregnancy, they are vastly different in terms of their nature and scope. Although most people probably agree that avoiding unintended pregnancy is a good idea, how to accomplish this goal generates tremendous disagreement.

Family planning implies the desire to have children at some point in time. Planning a family involves postponing childbearing until it is desired, spacing subsequent births and avoiding pregnancy at other times. As discussed in Chapter 13, family planning may also include all the reproductive technologies available to facilitate a pregnancy as well as adoption. Family planning does not refer to specific methods or techniques to avoid unintended pregnancy.

Contraception refers to all methods designed to prevent conception or fertilization. Contraceptive methods work by preventing the sperm and egg from uniting to cause fertilization. These methods include noninsertive sexual activity, barrier methods, hormonal contraception, withdrawal, fertility awareness, and sterilization. How effective these methods are ranges from "not very" to "almost complete" at the other end of the spectrum.

Birth control is a broad term encompassing all methods designed to prevent pregnancy and birth. It includes all contraceptive methods, what may be considered postconceptive methods, and abortion, which is designed to interrupt an established pregnancy. At its most literal, birth control also includes infanticide, although such a practice is generally viewed with repugnance and considered a crime.

Family planning Postponing children until the optimal point in one's life

Contraception Methods designed to prevent conception

Birth control The broadest term covering all methods designed to prevent the birth of a child

Effectiveness: Theoretical and Actual Use

One of the most important questions regarding any method of fertility control is "How effective is it?" Effectiveness is measured in two ways: theoretical use and actual use.

The **theoretical effectiveness (also called perfect use)** of any fertility control method estimates how it should work if it is used consistently and correctly. It is the ideal effectiveness of the method, determined through laboratory research and experimental studies. Theoretical effectiveness research designs attempt to control for as many variables as possible that may interfere with correct and consistent use. Failure of the method accounts for most of the ineffectiveness. Theoretical effectiveness is the lowest expected percentage of women who will get pregnant while using the method.

The **actual-use effectiveness (also called typical use)** of any fertility control method is how it actually works when real people use it under normal circumstances. This is the observed effectiveness of the method, determined by following a group of actual users for 1 year to see how many get pregnant. Actual-use studies are not subject to the same rigorous controls as most theoretical effectiveness studies. Consequently, user failure (failure to use the method consistently and correctly each time a couple has intercourse) largely accounts for the lack of effectiveness. Actual-use effectiveness is a combination of method and user failure, expressed as the percentage of women who get pregnant after 1 year of using the method. Comparison of methods is also done describing *typical-use failure rates* and *perfect-use failure rates*. Current studies base lowest and typical failure rates on the first year of observation. First-year data more accurately represent the risk of getting pregnant for someone using the method for the first time. Here, we will report data from studies that use first-year failure rates.

Theoretical effectiveness or perfect use effectiveness The lowest expected percentage of women who will get pregnant while using a given contraceptive method

Actual-use effectiveness or typical use effectiveness The percentage of women who get pregnant while using a contraceptive method for 1 year

Choosing a Method

When contemplating which fertility control method to use, people pose questions ranging from "Which method am I most likely to be committed to using? Which method am I more likely to use consistently?" "Is it safe and effective?" Would I be comfortable using a method? A couple's religious and cultural background may also play a role in decisions about fertility control. No contraceptive method is 100 percent perfect and without risk. Some methods might offer the level of effectiveness you want but lack aesthetic appeal. You may like a method, but your partner hates it. A health care provider might recommend a method that looks ideal on paper, but you might feel squeamish about using it. The self-assessment at the end of the chapter will help you examine your feelings about the various methods.

Given this confusing array of things to consider, what is the best method of fertility control? The best method is the one the person or couple uses consistently and correctly. It is the one that those involved are happy with, that offers the level of protection desired, and that fits the needs of those involved at this point in life. For college students today, choices about fertility control overlap with concerns about STD/HIV risk reduction. Some methods are highly effective in their ability to prevent pregnancy yet offer no protection against infection.

From a public health standpoint, overall costs become a factor in providing services to those least able to pay. Title X of the Public Health Service Act was designed to make comprehensive voluntary family planning services available. Today clinics that are funded through Title X provide services to 25% of women who obtain contraceptives services (Alan Guttmacher Institute, 2011.) As women seek newer, more expensive methods and clinics and programs struggle with smaller budgets, the issue of "choice" and making methods available becomes ever more challenging.

It is important to realize that needs will change over time. Therefore, people would do well to review their fertility control needs periodically and make changes accordingly. Table 14.1 provides a summary of contraceptive methods.

Table 14.1 Comparison of Contraceptives

Method	Typical-Use Effectiveness	Perfect-Use Effectiveness	Protection Against STDs	Accessibility*
Continuous abstinence	0.00	0.00	Complete	Couple communication
Outercourse	N/A	N/A	Good against HIV; reduces risk of others	Couple communication
Sterilization				
Men (vasectomy)	0.15	0.1	None	Requires physician and/or hospital access
Women (tubal ligation)	0.5	0.5	None	
Implanon	0.02	0.01		Requires physician for insertion
IUD				
ParaGard (Copper T 380A)	0.8	0.6	None	Requires physician for insertion
Mirena (Copper T)	0.1	0.1	None	
Lunelle (injection); taken off the market	N/A	0.05	None	Requires physician for injection
Continuous breastfeeding	2.0	0.5	None	Only useful at early stages of infant feeding
Depo-Provera (injection)	3.0	0.3	None	Requires physician for injection
Progestin-only pill	8.0	0.3	None	Requires physician for prescription
NuvaRing (ring)	N/A	0.3	None	Requires physician for prescription
Ortho Evra Patch	N/A	0.3	None	Requires physician for prescription
Male condom	15.0	2.0	Good against HIV; reduces risk of other STDs	Over-the-counter
Female condom— Reality	21.0	5.0	Reduces risk of vaginal and cervical infection	Over-the-counter
Diaphragm	16.0	6.0	Limited	Requires physician for fitting. Spermicide is purchased independently.
Cervical cap				Requires physician for prescription
Women who have not given birth	16.0	9.0	Limited	
Women who have given birth	32.0	26.0	Limited	

Table 14.1 (*continued*)

Method	Typical-Use Effectiveness	Perfect-Use Effectiveness	Protection Against STDs	Accessibility*
Fertility awareness/Periodic abstinence	25.0		None	Requires woman to fully chart menstrual cycle, be aware of probable timing of ovulation, and then abstain from coitus.
Postovulation method		1.0		
Symptothermal method		2.0		
Cervical mucus (ovulation method)		3.0		
Calendar method		9.0		
Withdrawal	27.0	4.0	None	Requires the male to control timing of ejaculation
Spermicide	29.0	15.0	None	Over-the-counter
No method	85.0	85.0	None	
Emergency contraception— Plan B	Reduces risk of pregnancy by 75–89 percent		None	Over-the-counter

*Reproductive health care services can be provided by private physicians, clinics, nurse practitioners, nurse midwives, and physician's assistants. Costs for methods vary depending on whether the individual has medical insurance, has prescription drug coverage, or must pay out of pocket. For methods bought over the counter, there is some variability in pricing, and overall costs relate to the frequency of using the method.

Sources: Based on information from www.plannedparenthood.org (2003); Nelson, Hatcher, Zieman et al. (2003); S. Bernard, personal communication (November 29, 2003).

✏ *Physical and Intellectual Wellness* ✏

Making good decisions about controlling fertility is a multifaceted process. It is essential that you learn how you and your partner's bodies function. So much information is now accessible on the Internet, making learning about anatomy, physiology, and the biochemistry of the human body and health less of a mystery. Learning about birth control at the time of Margaret Sanger's pioneering efforts in the early 1900s was viewed as obscene, landing her in jail. Today a variety of sources of information are available to help you decide what is available and appropriate.

Fertility control, first, is affected by one's level of physical wellbeing. Overall physical health influences the fertility methods available to you. For example, physical conditions such as hypertension and diabetes are contraindications for oral contraceptives. Having a history of pelvic inflammatory disease precludes using an IUD. Health status also affects how you use certain methods. For instance, gaining weight necessitates refitting of a diaphragm.

Consistent and proper use of fertility control methods can enhance physical wellbeing. Practicing fertility control carries less risk to a woman than getting pregnant and having a child. The risk of dying associated with pregnancy and childbirth is much greater than that for using fertility control.

Certain methods impart specific health-enhancing benefits. Hormonal contraception offers protective effects against a variety of diseases including ovarian cancer and endometrial, along with possible improvement for acne and menstrual cramps. Barrier contraceptives reduce the risk of cervical cancer, as well as some STDs. Fertility awareness can give women a greater understanding of vaginal health and how their bodies work.

Mechanisms of Action

Although birth control methods can be grouped in a variety of ways, we've chosen the following seven categories according to their mechanisms of action.

1. *Provide nonpenetrative sexual pleasure.* This group of methods, sometimes called *outercourse,* provides options for the satisfaction of sexual desire and orgasm that do not involve the penis penetrating the vagina. Methods in this category include kissing, hugging/rubbing, massage, masturbation, use of sex toys, and oral-genital sexual contact.

2. *Prevent sperm from meeting egg.* These methods work either by withdrawing the penis prior to ejaculation or by predicting ovulation and avoiding unprotected intercourse during fertile times. The r IUD is also included in this category.

3. *Provide barrier between sperm and egg.* This group of methods is characterized by putting a mechanical or chemical device between the sperm and the egg (hence the term barrier). In either case, these methods prevent the sperm and egg from uniting in the fertilization process. Methods in this group include male condom, female condom, diaphragm, contraceptive sponge, cervical cap, and spermicides.

4. *Prevent release of egg.* Ovulation is suppressed by altering the hormonal balance in the body. This prevents the pituitary gland from stimulating the release of hormones necessary to trigger the release of an egg from the ovary. Methods in this group include oral contraceptives, NuvaRing, Implanon, emergency contraception and the Evra patch.

5. *Surgically block passage of sperm or egg.* Methods in this category work by sealing off the main egg and sperm transport routes (fallopian tubes and vas deferens, respectively). Female and male sterilization comprise this group.

6. *Prevent implantation.* Methods in this group work by preventing the implantation of a possibly fertilized egg in the uterine lining. These methods encompass the Mirena intrauterine device (IUDs) and emergency contraception. As discussed later, however, evidence seems to suggest that the IUD may prevent sperm from fertilizing the egg.

7. *Terminate an established pregnancy.* This group consists of methods that end an established pregnancy. Methods include abortion, both medical and surgical.

Nonpenetrative Sexual Release

Outercourse Nonpenetrative sexual activities such as massage and masturbation

Nonpenetrative activities are sometimes referred to as **outercourse** and include massage, masturbation, manual stimulation of one's partner, and the like. These activities provide sexual release but do not involve vaginal penetration (McDonough, 1995). It is important to understand that there are lots of ways to be sexual without risking pregnancy.

The actual-use effectiveness of sexual activities that do not involve vaginal penetration has not been established. If vaginal penetration doesn't occur, no mechanism is available for live sperm to reach a mature ovum. Theoretical effectiveness, therefore, should approach 100 percent.

Unprotected anal intercourse is not included in this group because, although it doesn't involve vaginal penetration, the close proximity of the anus could allow migration of fluids across the perineum and into the vagina. Ejaculating near the vagina is discouraged for this reason.

Celibacy/Abstinence

The first category of nonpenetrative methods is celibacy and abstinence. These two terms are often used interchangeably, yet their meanings are distinct. Although the definition of celibacy means to avoid sexual relations, the term is often most associated with a religious decision not to marry. Abstinence refers to practicing self-restraint and, in the area of fertility control, not having sexual intercourse. People often assume that celibacy and abstinence mean total avoidance of all forms of sexual release. This is not true. A person can be celibate or abstain from sexual intercourse but still masturbate or use other forms of nonpenetrative behaviors to release sexual tension (Norris, 1996).

Many researchers have addressed the issue of failure rates of abstinence, partially in an attempt to counter the rhetoric that only abstinence is 100 percent effective. As with any method, theoretical effectiveness rates differ from actual-use effectiveness rates. User failure rates are connected to how correctly and consistently the method is used. If an individual practices abstinence at a particular point in time, that person will never become pregnant or get a partner pregnant. When abstinence as a method fails, it is because of user failure (Pinkerton, 2001).

Outercourse Activities

Couples may choose to touch each other in a variety of ways that do not risk pregnancy. For example, the sucking, licking and rubbing, and tongue probing associated with kissing are pleasurable while imposing no risk for pregnancy. Kissing usually is associated with hugging and rubbing. Once commonly referred to as petting, these activities can take on new meaning when visualized as a viable form of fertility control. Hugging and rubbing, even with the clothes on, can be intensely pleasurable and can be carried to the point of orgasm with no risk of pregnancy. With a little imagination, these safe sex activities can be erotic and provide a satisfying outlet for sexual desire by themselves or when other fertility control methods are unavailable.

Somewhat riskier are activities in which partners are partially clothed or naked. The risk is that it puts the participants in a very tempting situation that may be difficult to control. Nongenital massage is a great sensual delight and can be a stand-alone sensual activity or part of activities culminating with orgasm. Partners can manually stimulate each other to orgasm without worrying about conception. Sex toys also offer a safe, low-pregnancy-risk sexual option

The various forms of oral-genital sexual contact (fellatio, cunnilingus, anilingus) offer a sexual option with low risk for pregnancy. Unlike abstinence and nonpenetrative sexual behavior, however, oral-genital sexual contact can pose risks of disease transmission. We will discuss these risks in detail in Chapter 15.

Preventing Sperm from Reaching Egg (Nonsurgical)

Sperm can be prevented from reaching the ova through coitus interruptus and fertility awareness methods.

Coitus Interruptus (Withdrawal; Pulling Out)

Coitus interruptus is one of the most commonly used and least understood of all the fertility control strategies. *Coitus interruptus* is a Latin term, literally meaning interrupting intercourse by withdrawing the penis prior to ejaculation.

For a typical, user the probability of pregnancy is about 22% during the first year of use (Hatcher et al, 2011). Two factors seem to contribute to the relatively low typical use effectiveness: human error (not withdrawing the penis in time) and use of the method during peak fertility (midcycle versus other times during a woman's menstrual cycle). There is some controversy over whether the pre-ejaculate contains sperm. In two studies no sperm were found in the preejaculate and in two other studies small amounts of sperm were found. Though the number of sperm found were low, there were enough to possibly cause a pregnancy even if the male withdraws his penis before ejaculating (Hatcher et al, 2011).

The number of couples having ever used coitus interruptus as their method is increasing. In 2008,over half of women surveyed answered that they had ever used this method compared to only one in four in 1992 (Hatcher et al, 2011). For women who cannot risk getting pregnant, this is not a reliable choice since it is at the bottom of list of contraceptives in effectiveness. Some users argue that coitus interruptus is free, readily available, and a "natural," "effective" method of fertility control. In a sense, this belief is true. Coitus interruptus is free, it is always available, and it is relatively effective (78 percent versus 5 percent for "hope and a prayer"). Nonetheless, couples would be much wiser to choose a method with higher reliability and STD protection.

You'll remember from Chapter 3 that orgasm in men is a two-step process. The first step, ejaculatory inevitability, begins with the man feeling the contractions initiating the expulsion of semen that occurs during the next step, emission. Many couples, especially sexually inexperienced ones, overestimate the man's ability to withdraw his penis in time if he waits for ejaculatory inevitability. Timing the removal of the penis so closely sets the stage for method failure. This is difficult for sexually inexperienced men to do. Simultaneously, a woman worried about whether her partner will "pull out" in time cannot fully relax and enjoy the lovemaking. (It is possible for couples to practice the timing of withdrawal by having the female use a backup method of birth control.)

Another way to do coitus interruptus is to withdraw prior to any sense of ejaculatory inevitability and finish with a nonpenetrative sexual method (such as masturbation) or oral-genital sex. This offers more variety in your sexual experience and reduces the risk of unintended pregnancy. You are able to enjoy vaginal intercourse while reducing the risk of pregnancy.

We suggest that all men who intend to use coitus interruptus urinate before they initiate any sexual activity. Also, we recommend that during sexual arousal and plateau, the couple remove any existing preejaculatory fluid (with a tissue or orally) before intromission of the penis. This will remove some of the fluid. These precautions should also be repeated if more than one act of intercourse occurs.

The last thing to consider with coitus interruptus is your fertility status. One way to increase the effectiveness of coitus interruptus is to limit its use to less fertile times of the menstrual cycle. Avoiding intercourse during peak fertility times will increase its effectiveness.

With an typical use effectiveness of 78 percent (Hatcher, 2011), 22 in 100 women using this method in their first year will get pregnant. This effectiveness compares poorly with other contraceptives that are available and offers no protection against transmission of STDs and HIV. This method usually is recommended for couples in disease-free, monogamous relationships for whom a pregnancy would perhaps not be ideal but would be acceptable.

Fertility Awareness

Fertility awareness, also known as *natural family planning* and the *rhythm method,* is a strategy based on avoiding unprotected intercourse during peak fertility. Peak fertility can be estimated by combining knowledge about an individual woman's menstrual cycle with the latest scientific findings about egg and sperm viability. The four fertility awareness methods are calendar, basal body temperature, cervical mucus, and combined. Each of these methods requires understanding of the specific woman's menstrual cycle and her fertile periods, discussed in Chapter 13. Perfect-use effectiveness data for individual fertility awareness methods are shown in Table 14.1.

Calendar Method. The calendar method of fertility awareness uses the menstrual cycle history to estimate future ovulation. Once a woman can estimate the day she is likely to ovulate, she can build a **safe zone** around this day by factoring in how long an egg (24 hours) and sperm (5 days) can live. This safe zone represents days prior to and after ovulation when the presence of live sperm could result in fertilization.

Steps involved in the calendar method are as follows:

1. Keep a log of your menstrual cycle for 8 months. The first day of your cycle is the first day of menstrual bleeding. The last day of the cycle is the last day prior to the onset of bleeding.
2. Subtract 18 from your shortest cycle. This represents your first unsafe day.
3. Subtract 11 from your longest cycle. This represents your last unsafe day.
4. Avoid unprotected vaginal intercourse during your unsafe days.

Example:
Mary charted her menstrual cycles for 9 months. Her longest cycle was 31 days. Her shortest cycle was 28 days. Thus:

28 + 18 = 10 (Day 10 is her first unsafe day.)
31 + 11 = 20 (Day 20 is her last unsafe day.)

During days 10 to 20, Mary should avoid unprotected vaginal intercourse.

Fertility awareness Natural family planning

Safe zone A fertility awareness concept that factors ovulation and length of time sperm and eggs can live as a time to avoid intercourse

Cervical Mucus Method. The cervical mucus method works by checking changes in cervical mucus during the menstrual cycle to predict ovulation. Mucus present in the cervix and vagina cause changes described as "wet" or "dry." In general, wet conditions represent fertile, unsafe days, and dry conditions designate infertile, safe days.

Menstruation masks mucus changes. Immediately following menstruation the cycle moves from infertile (dry) to fertile (wet), back to infertile (dry), and into menstruation. During infertile times of the cycle, cervical mucus is scanty, and the vagina and vulva feel dry (some women report an absence of totally dry days). During fertile periods, cervical mucus is abundant, clear, and stringy (it resembles the consistency of egg whites and will stretch if you try to pull it apart), and the vagina and vulva feel wet. Vaginal mucus should be checked a few times a day for a few months to observe how it changes. This can be done by inserting a finger and gathering mucus from the cervix and vaginal walls.

Once you are comfortable with interpreting these changes, you can monitor yourself as follows:

1. Check your cervical/vaginal mucus each time you urinate. Insert a finger and obtain a specimen or wipe a small amount from the vulva and examine it.
2. Record the changes.
3. Once you note the initial wetness, consider yourself fertile. The vagina should feel moist but not distinctly wet. Mucus should be thick, cloudy, and whitish.
4. Notice, a few days later, that your vagina and vulva feel distinctly wet. The mucus becomes more profuse and is stringy and slippery. See if you can stretch a specimen between your thumb and forefinger. If you can do this, you are fertile.
5. Continue checking your mucus. About 4 days after your wettest day, the mucus decreases and is no longer detectable. You should return to a drier state, indicating that ovulation has occurred. It is now safe to resume unprotected intercourse.

As a caution, production of mucus and vaginal/vulval wetness can be altered by antihistamines and other medications, douching, vaginal infection, contraceptive foam, jelly, and lubricants. For maximum effectiveness, this method should be combined with the calendar method to cross-validate the conclusion. For instance, if your calendar indicates that you are approaching midcycle and you don't feel the characteristic wetness, something may have altered your production of mucus. When in doubt, use a backup method.

Basal Body Temperature. To practice this method, you will need a basal body thermometer. This method relies on recognizing the slight, but measurable, change in basal **body temperature (BBT)** associated with ovulation (Hatcher et al., 1998).

The procedure is as follows:

1. Each morning, immediately upon rising, take your temperature using the basal body thermometer. Do not eat, shower, smoke, or do anything else before taking your temperature. Do this every day for 3 months.

Basal body temperature (BBT) The lowest body temperature of a healthy person during waking hours

2. Record your temperature on a special grid, as illustrated in Figure 14.1.
3. After 3 months, note the changes in your cycle. Normally, between 12 to 24 hours prior to ovulation, a woman's basal body temperature will drop (the decrease varies from none to about 0.3 of 1 degree).
4. Note the subsequent rise in temperature, indicating that ovulation has occurred. The preovulatory drop in temperature is followed by a rise in temperature 0.4 to 0.8 degrees Fahrenheit above your readings for about 6 days preceding the rise.
5. Assume that unprotected intercourse is safe after 3 days of sustained temperature rise.

Because this method does not predict ovulation (it notes when ovulation occurs), sexual activity prior to temperature changes may result in unintended pregnancy. Therefore, this method is best used in combination with either the calendar or the cervical mucus method, which help predict ovulation. The temperature charts should match the calendar charting of safe and unsafe days and the characteristics of wet and dry mucus.

Symptothermal Method. The symptothermal method designates the combination of BBT and mucus methods. It also incorporates some signs indicating that ovulation is imminent or has occurred.

Providing a Barrier Between Sperm and Egg

Barrier methods are among the oldest and most well known of all methods used to control fertility. They are so named because they work by literally placing a barrier (mechanical, chemical, or a combination) between the sperm and the egg. Although these methods share the same mechanism of action, they differ in terms of how they are applied or inserted.

Barrier methods Nonsurgical contraceptive measures that prevent the sperm and egg from uniting

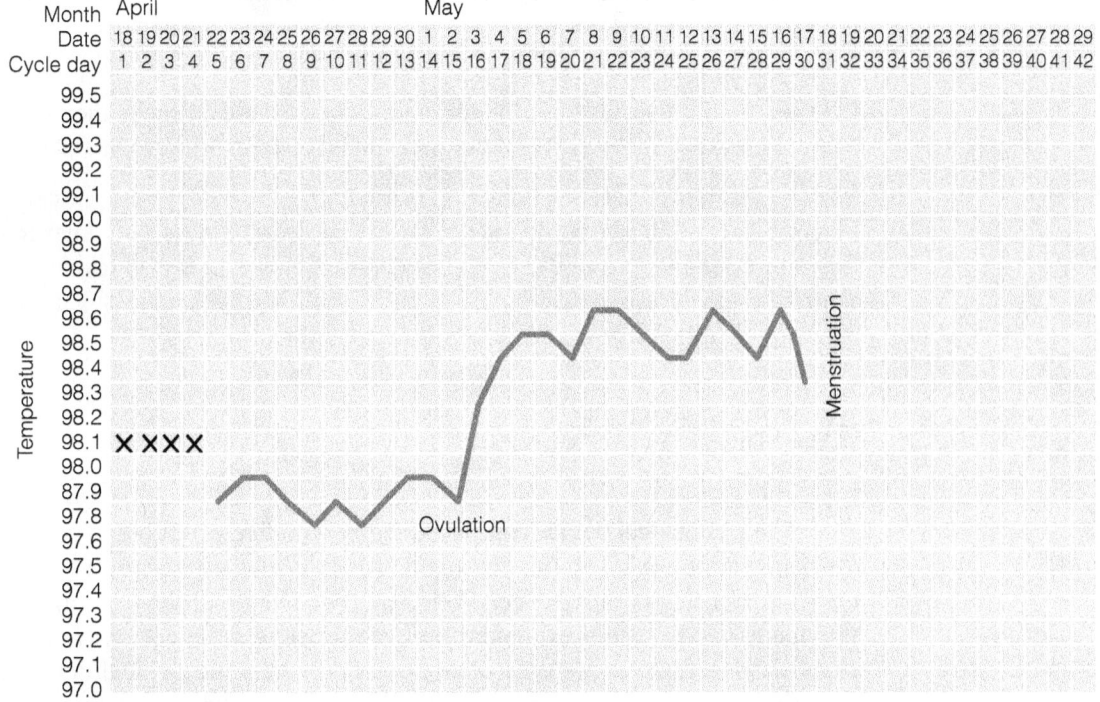

Figure 14.1 *Basal Body Temperature (BBT) Chart*

case study 14.2

Lester and Sophia: Making Choices

Lester, 20, identifies as biracial; Sophia, 20, identifies as Latina.

Lester and Sophia are both juniors who have been in a monogamous relationship for 6 months. Lester had two girlfriends in high school and, before Sophia, dated casually at college. Sophia dated casually in high school, and then as a freshman dated a man from her job for a year. The two have been having sex for the past 3 months and sometimes even use nonpenetrative forms of sexual activity as a way to prevent unintended pregnancy.

LESTER: Sophia and I take turns as far as who is responsible for birth control. When we first had sex, I took out a condom . . . my father taught me that the man should always carry a condom. Sophia also had a condom with her! It was impressive meeting a female who also had them. We both are comfortable buying condoms, but also like to do other things that don't involve using birth control.

SOPHIA: Right. When I first met Lester, I didn't know how much to trust him and didn't want to rush into a heavy sexual relationship. I had taken the pill when I was a freshman but went off of it when the relationship ended. I have a box of condoms in my dorm room "just in case." As Lester and I got more romantic, we did the "safer sex" things—massages and masturbating each other. And we had fun.

LESTER: Sophia will give me a long massage and then bring me off using her hand. There are times I like that more than having intercourse.

SOPHIA: I feel the same way. Sometimes I'm not in the mood to have sex, but I like to relax and get a massage. Or, I just want to please Lester and don't worry about who's giving and who's getting.

LESTER: Sophia also has this vibrator or massager we use on each other. It's a little kinky, but she uses it and her hand and the sensations are intense.

SOPHIA: It's funny because I bought the vibrator for me before I met Lester. I found that I could have really intense orgasms masturbating with it. I never figured Lester and I would have such a good time with it. It also takes off some of the pressure to always use birth control. Maybe someday I'll go back on the pill. For now switching off suits us fine!

Critical Thinking

How would you react if your female or male partner showed they were ready for intercourse by having a condom available? Would you enjoy trying some of the other ways of enjoying each other's body's that Lester and Sophia include?

The mechanical devices use latex and polyurethane barriers to cover the penis (male condom), line the vagina (female condom), or protect the cervix (diaphragm, sponge, cervical cap). The chemical devices either provide a stand alone spermicidal barrier that covers the cervix (foam, suppositories, film) or are used in combination with a mechanical device (gel/diaphragm or cap, spermicide impregnated in sponge, spermicidal lubricant for condoms.

Male Condom

The male condom is one of the oldest known fertility devices. Three types of condoms are currently available in the United States: latex, polyurethane, and natural lamb membrane. As more aggressive efforts were made to reduce the incidence of HIV/AIDS, condom promotion around the world has increased. Along with that has come more creative marketing, packaging, and choices, including shapes, colors, thickness and sizes. Each type is manufactured under stringent quality control and tested electronically before being sold (Hatcher et al, 2011). Almost all tested condoms meet the stringent standards with no differences found based on price, thickness or manufacturing country (Consumers Union, 2009).

The male condom works by covering the penis and trapping the ejaculate, thereby preventing it from being deposited in the vagina. Condoms reduce the risk of transmitting STD organisms that might be present in the ejaculate, vaginal fluids, vagina or in lesions on the penis. If a couple plans to use condoms as a primary birth control, they are advised to buy emergency contraceptive pills in advance to have in case the condom slips or breaks. The condom slipping or breaking happens in approximately 2 percent of all acts of intercourse using a condom (Hatcher et al, 2011).

Latex Condoms. Latex condoms come in a variety of shapes, colors, and sizes. Latex condoms come individually wrapped in foil or other sealed packets. They are rolled up to the size of a half-dollar or are folded.

Latex condoms can be lubricated (with either a spermicide or a nonspermicidal lubricant) or nonlubricated. Most nonlubricated latex condoms are dusted with powder or cornstarch to facilitate putting them on an erect penis. Latex condoms come in a variety of shapes. The traditional shape is a long, uniform sheath, with a rounded end and now, condomes that are tapered toward the closed end are also available. Each of these shapes comes with the choice of a reservoir tip, a a small nipple that protrudes about 3/4 inch at the sealed end, to catch the ejaculate. Latex condoms also can be scented or unscented, flavored or unflavored, colored or transparent, and ribbed or smooth.

Form-fitting condoms generally mimic the shape of the penis. They are wider at the opening and taper to their narrowest dimension close to the end, where they flare out again in the shape of the glans of the penis. They tend to fit more snuggly than traditionally shaped condoms.

The theoretical effectiveness of condoms is 98 percent. Stringent manufacturing standards ensure uniformly high quality. Typical use effectiveness is 82 percent. The most common reason for condom failure is that couples do not use a condom during every act of intercourse. Two other contributors to failure are slippage and breakage of condom. To help prevent these, use proper technique when putting the condom on the penis (Hatcher, et al, 2011). Figure 14.2 describes the steps involved in using a male condom properly.

Some men and women are allergic to latex and itch, become dry, burn, and develop a rash when exposed to it. These people may not be able to use latex condoms (or diaphragms). They are good candidates for natural membrane condoms or the female condom. These condoms may not provide the same level of STD protection as latex and polyurethane condoms. Condoms are also available with a spermicidal lubricant. However, spermi-

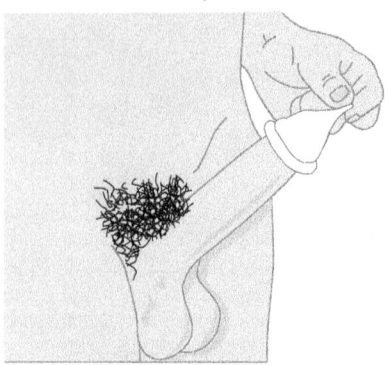

Pinch or twist the tip of the condom, leaving one-half inch at the tip to catch the semen.

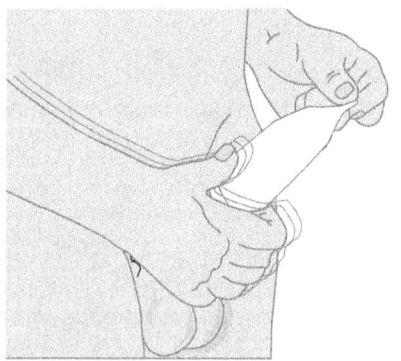

Holding the tip, unroll the condom.

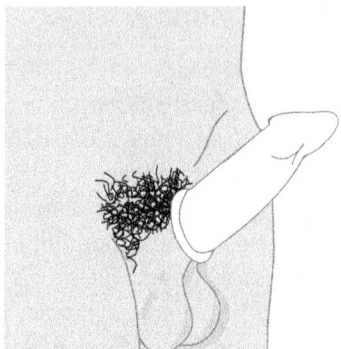

Unroll the condom until it reaches the pubic hairs.

Figure 14.2 *How to Use a Condom*

cide is no longer recommended because it does not improve effectiveness. Most manufacturers have stopped making spermicidal condoms (Hatcher et al, 2011).

The marketing of condoms has become creative and diversified over the years. Durex's Performa and Trojan's Extended Pleasure are marketed to help males prolong excitement and delay ejaculation. By placing benzocaine, a mild anesthetic, inside the tip of the condom, the medication can numb the head of the penis yet not be transferred externally to one's partner. Condoms are also produced in flavors such as chocolate and mint, to encourage their usage during oral sex. Other condoms are marketed to the gay community along with messages about their value as part of safer sex practices.

Natural Lamb Membrane Condoms. Unlike their latex cousins, natural lamb membrane condoms are not uniformly manufactured from scratch. They are made from the intestines of commercially slaughtered lambs. They are shipped to the condom manufacturer, where they are cleaned and inspected prior to being cut and sealed at one end. Even though each condom is slightly different from the next, they all must pass safety inspections and are held to the same standards as latex condoms.

Natural membrane condoms tend to fit more loosely than latex condoms. Some secure themselves to the penis with the help of a small elastic band sewn into the base. Others are snugger and grip the penis much like a latex condom. Natural lamb condoms are wet. They are sealed in a foil or other pouch with more liquid than latex condoms to keep them from deteriorating.

Natural lamb condoms offer an entirely different feel than their latex cousins. They simulate human tissue as closely as is possible. The combination of the material (lamb membrane), its wetness, and the loose fit makes natural lamb condoms feel almost like the lining of the vagina or mouth.

As a cautionary note, studies have shown that the surface of natural skin condoms contains small pores that permit the passage of viruses, including the hepatitis B

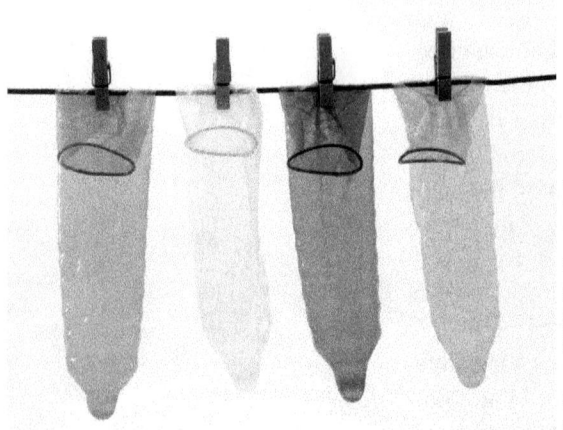

© dino o, 2010. Shutterstock, Inc.

Condoms come in different colors and styles.

virus, herpes simplex virus, and HIV (Cary, 1999). Sperm, however, are not able to penetrate these pores because sperm are much larger than viruses.

Female Condom

The female condom is a loose-fitting polyurethane pouch that is inserted into the vagina, covering its walls and protruding over the vulva. The female condom works by containing a man's semen after he ejaculates into his partner's vagina. It also offers protection against STD bacteria or viruses that might be in the man's semen or emanating from penile lesions.

Female condoms are made from a polyurethane material that is similar to latex but is less penetrable. The female condom is lubricated with a silicon based lubricant. Unlike the male condom, it does not come in different shapes, sizes, colors, or flavors. Female condoms are uniform in size and have a ring at both ends. The rings help with insertion and ensure a proper fit. The ring at the closed end loops around the cervix, anchoring it in place in a way that is similar to a diaphragm (discussed next), although the female condom does not require a prescription. The female condom is inserted like a diaphragm. You first fold the ring in half, then insert it similar to the way a tampon is inserted and feel the inner ring notch against the cervix (see Figure 14.3).

A major advantage of the female condom is that it provides women a reliable source of nonprescription protection against both pregnancy and STDs. A woman does not have to rely on her partner for this protection; she can control the method. It can also be inserted up to 8 hours prior to intercourse adding convenience as an advantage. A disadvantage of the female condom is that it costs more than a male condom. Some women have reported that there may be noise during thrusting, which can be distracting, embarrassing, and/or humorous depending on one's comfort with one's partner. Like the male condom, it can be used only once. It is considered at least as effective as the male condom in preventing transmission of STDs, including HIV.

The theoretical effectiveness of female condoms is 95 percent; typical use effectiveness is 79 percent; (Hatcher et al., 2011). Researchers found that the female condom rarely breaks, although slippage occurs in approximately 1 in 10 uses, and women may be exposed to semen in up to 1 in 5 uses. Furthermore, a woman is most likely to be exposed to semen if she and her partner experience mechanical problems with the condom, if there is a large disparity between the size of the penis and the size of the woman's vagina, and if intercourse is very active (Alan Guttmacher Institute, 2003b). As with the male condoms, couples should have emergency contraception available in case the condom slips, breaks or the female is exposed to semen.

Diaphragm

The diaphragm is a spring-loaded rubber or plastic dome that is inserted into the vagina and anchored between the wall of the vagina and the cervix (see Figure 14.4). It is nonlubricated, so before insertion, spermicidal jelly must be placed around the rim and on the inside of the dome for it to work properly. It is not designed to form an impenetrable barrier against the cervix. It works by covering the cervix and thereby blocking access of most sperm

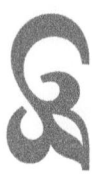

healthy sex hints 14.1

Eroticizing Condom Use

Condoms have been making a steady resurgence as a contraceptive method, yet many couples still find condom use unacceptable or not as desirable as making love without one. The following tips on eroticizing condom use might change your thinking about them.

1. It's all in your head (the one on your shoulders).
   - Start to examine your thoughts about condoms.
   - Don't buy into the myth that you can't have great sex if you use a condom.
2. Be prepared.
   - Keep a supply of condoms handy.
   - Distribute packets in the bedroom chest, living room end table, downstairs and upstairs bathrooms, and other places where you might have intercourse.
3. Practice condom use by yourself.
   - Men: Masturbate using a condom (this will help you get used to the feel); practice putting one on under a variety of conditions (in the dark, with lights, one-handed, and so forth)
   - Women: Practice putting a condom on a simulated penis (such as a vibrator); practice putting one on with your mouth.
4. Try several styles/brands.
   - Find a brand and style that feels right for you.
5. Use extra lubrication.
   - Smear some water-soluble lubricating jelly (not petroleum-based products) on the head of your penis before putting on the condom.
   - Smear extra jelly on the outside before penetration. This will help prevent the condom from breaking.
6. Make condom use (and penetration) just one part of lovemaking.
   - Read Chapter 8 about viewing lovemaking as a gourmet meal (you can enjoy a lot of erotic delights before even putting on the condom).
7. Don't rush to remove the condom.
   - Enjoy the afterglow of orgasm. After a while, hold the condom firmly against the base of your penis and pull out.
8. Take turns with birth control.
   - Trade off responsibility every month (condoms this month, spermicides or oral sex the next month, and so on), and you might find using a condom less objectionable.

to the egg. Any sperm that are able to get around the edge of the diaphragm are immobilized by the spermicide contained in the dome.

A diaphragm must be fitted by an experienced health care professional. This person can determine the proper size to fit into the vagina so the diaphragm will rest comfortably between the cervix and the top portion of the vagina. Diaphragms should be refitted if the woman gains or loses more than 10 pounds, has an abortion, or has a full-term pregnancy (Hatcher et al., 2011).

The theoretical effectiveness of diaphragms is 94 percent. Typical use effectiveness is 88 percent—higher than the male condom. As with condoms, the drop off in effectiveness is primarily a result of human error

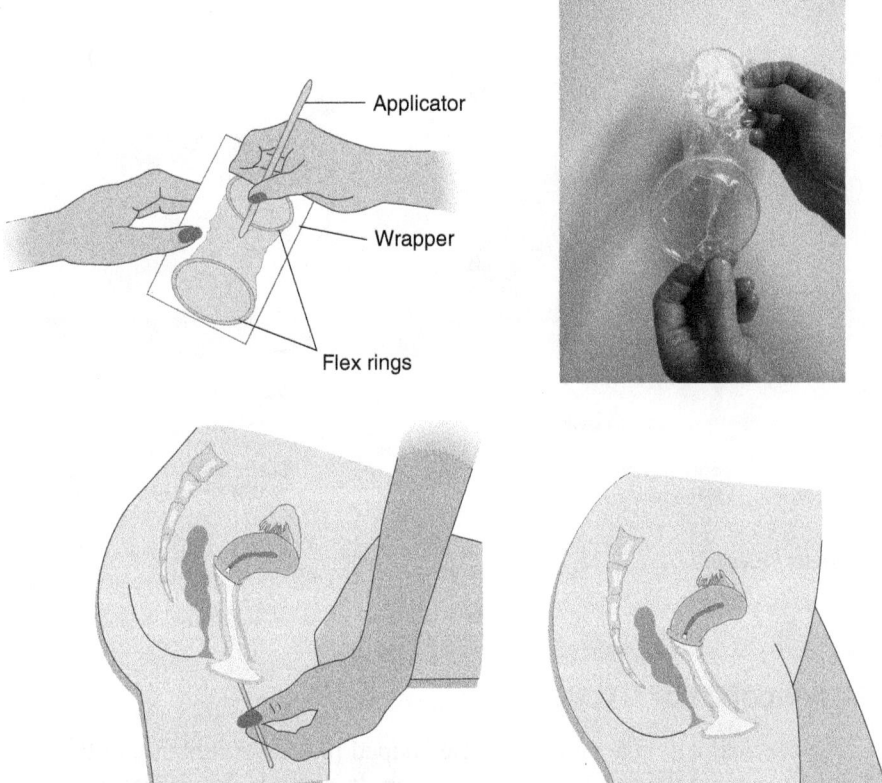

Figure 14.3 *Inserting a Female Condom*

associated with incorrect and inconsistent use. It is recommended that women be given emergency contraception as a backup in advance (Hatcher et al., 2004).

The steps in inserting a diaphragm are as follows:

1. Insert the diaphragm up to 6 hours before intercourse.
2. First smear spermicidal jelly (see later discussion for more detail) around the rim, and put about 2 teaspoons inside the dome.
3. Stand with one leg raised, supported on a chair or similar object.
4. Bend the diaphragm in half by moving it with the spring action, and insert it as far into the vagina as possible.
5. Push it the remaining distance with your finger until you feel the rim notch behind your cervix.
6. Leave it in place at least 6 hours (but no more than 24 hours) after intercourse.
7. Use a condom or added spermicide for additional protection for each additional act of intercourse.
8. After at least 6 hours from the last ejaculation, remove the diaphragm by pulling it out with a finger.
9. Wash it off with clean, soapy water; dry it; dust it with corn starch; and put it into its case.
10. If you are uncomfortable touching yourself or want to get your partner involved, have your lover remove (or insert) the diaphragm.

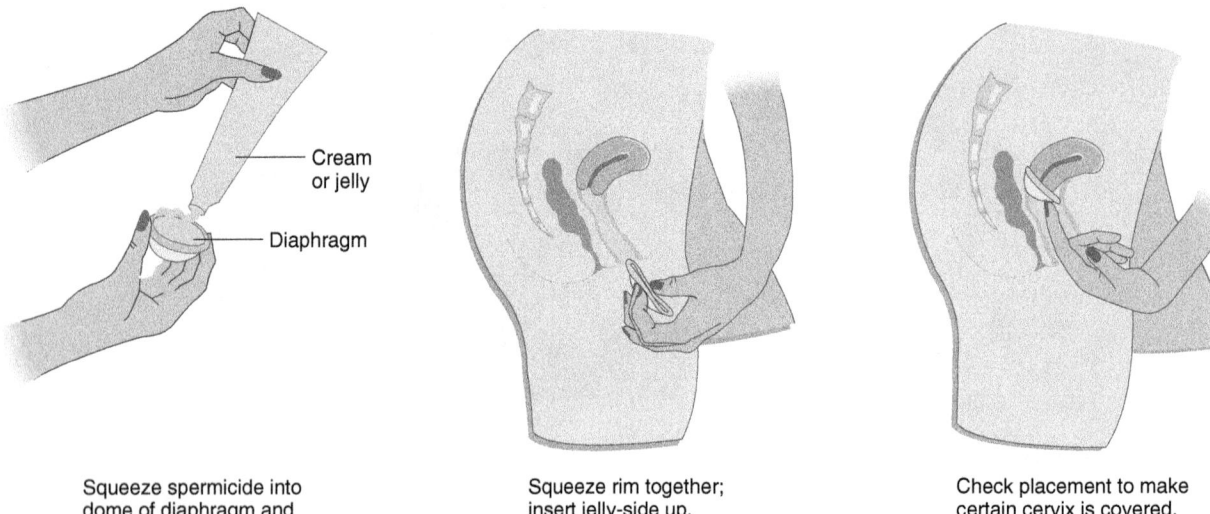

Squeeze spermicide into dome of diaphragm and around the rim.

Squeeze rim together; insert jelly-side up.

Check placement to make certain cervix is covered.

Figure 14.4 *The Diaphragm and How to Insert It*

Cervical Cap

The cervical cap is a small, thimble-shaped plastic or rubber cap that fits snugly against the cervix through suction. It is available in three sizes and must be fitted by a health care professional. It works in a fashion similar to the diaphragm, blocking the passage of sperm while utilizing spermicidal jelly as a backup to immobilize sperm that may enter around its rim.

The cervical cap differs from the diaphragm in these ways:

- The cervical cap anchors to the cervix through suction rather than by pressing against the walls of the vagina and the cervix the way the diaphragm does.
- The cap is much smaller and less conspicuous than the diaphragm.
- The cap requires less spermicide (because of its smaller size).
- The cap does not require additional spermicide with additional episodes of intercourse.

Theoretical effectiveness of the cervical cap is comparable to that of other vaginal barrier methods, those being the female condom, diaphragm, and sponge. However, the cervical cap does not work as well for women who have given birth compared to those who have not. The perfect-use failure rate in the first year for parous women (those who have given birth) is 26 percent compared to 9 percent for nulliparous women (those who have not given birth). The typical-use failure rate, by comparison, for parous women is 40 percent in the first year of use, compared to 20 percent for nulliparous women (Nelson et al., 2000). It is advised, therefore, that emergency contraception be kept as a backup at times of possible failure.

The cervical cap may be inserted up to 6 hours prior to intercourse. It must remain in place at least 6 hours but no more than 48 hours after the male ejaculates. To use the cervical cap:

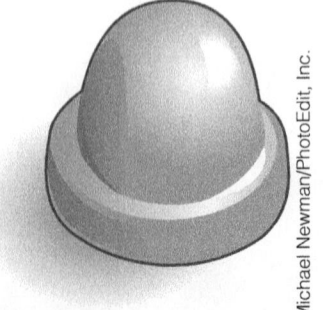

Michael Newman/PhotoEdit, Inc.

The cervical cap fits snugly against the cervix.

1. Fill the cap with spermicidal jelly.
2. Using the thumb and forefinger, squeeze the cap and push it into the vagina all the way to the cervix. Once it reaches the cervix, release it with a small twist, notching it in place.
3. If multiple acts of intercourse take place, additional spermicide is not needed, but the woman should check that the cap is in place.
4. To remove, insert a finger up the vagina, catch the strap on the outside of the cap, and pull it sideways out of the vagina.
5. Wash it out, and store in a dry, cool place.

Vaginal Contraceptive Sponge

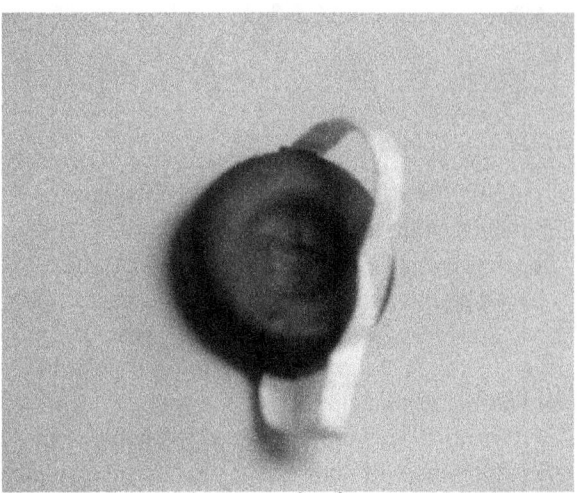

The vaginal sponge is a soft, white, polyurethane sponge filled with spermicide. It works the same way

The sponge provides protection for up to 24 hours.

as the diaphragm and cervical cap: It creates a double barrier (absorbent polyurethane sponge and spermicide) that blocks and absorbs sperm while chemically deactivating them.

The sponge works for 24 hours even with multiple acts of intercourse. Women who use the sponge need to wait for 6 hours after intercourse to remove the sponge and should avoid leaving it in for over 24 hours due to the risk of toxic shock syndrome (Hatcher et al, 2011). With the sponge, no additional applications of spermicide are needed if additional ejaculations occur within that time period. This feature allows greater flexibility in sexual activity without the need for using additional spermicides.

Sex in Society 14.1, "Update on the Sponge," traces the history of this once-popular method. A major advantage of the sponge is that it is a nonprescription device. Sponges typically cost approximately $3 to $5. Like the diaphragm and the cervical cap, the vaginal contraceptive sponge provides a protective barrier against the cervix. If used many times a day the nonoxynol- 9 in the sponge may irritate the vaginal lining and make users more at risk for STD and HIV transmission (Planned Parenthood, 2013).

For women who have never had children, the vaginal contraceptive sponge is similar in effectiveness to the diaphragm and the cervical cap. Its theoretical effectiveness is 91 percent, and actual-use effectiveness is 88 percent. It is less effective in women who have previously had a child (Hatcher, 2011). It is advised, therefore, that emergency contraception be kept as a backup at times of possible failure.

To use the contraceptive sponge:

1. Moisten the sponge with 1 to 2 tablespoons of water.
2. Insert it deep into the vagina up to 24 hours prior to intercourse. Its smaller size makes insertion easier than the diaphragm.
3. Leave the sponge in place for at least 6 hours after the last ejaculation. (Once in place, a woman can have multiple episodes of intercourse without the need for additional spermicides.)
4. Remove the sponge by slipping a finger through the sewn-in loop and pulling out of the vagina.
5. Dispose with regular trash. (Do not flush down toilet.)

sex in society 14.1

Update on the Sponge

In March, 1994, Whitehall-Robbins Healthcare in Hammontown, New Jersey, stopped manufacturing the Today Sponge. At that time, Whitehall-Robbins was the only company producing contraceptive sponges. The company stopped production of the sponge after being cited by the Food and Drug Administration (FDA) for unacceptable manufacturing standards. At no point did the FDA cite any problems associated with the sponge itself.

Ironically, many average women learned that the sponge would no longer be available from a now-famous episode of *Seinfeld*. In this storyline, Elaine learns that her chosen method of birth control is being taken off the market. In response, she runs around New York City buying up whatever sponges remain on store shelves. Her need to carefully monitor her supply leads her to wonder whether each prospective date is "sponge-worthy."

Allendale Pharmaceuticals in New Jersey bought the rights to make Today, and it has been distributing it via the Internet with Canada as its distribution base. The sponge is now again available over the counter without a prescription.

Another sponge, Protectaid, was developed in Canada in 1996 by Axcan Limited, a division of Axcan Pharmaceuticals. It is similar to the Today Sponge in size, shape, use, and instructions. Its manufacturers claim that it offers a major advantage over the Today Sponge in that it has three active spermicidal ingredients: nonoxynol-9, benzalkonium chloride, and sodium cholate. One significant difference, however, is that Protectaid does not have an attached string for easy removal.

World travelers learn that countries have differing laws about what drugs and medical products are available either by prescription or over the counter. The Internet has become a useful resource for information as well as marketing; Allendale Pharmaceuticals has been able to make their product available to women who can order the sponge online. Because neighboring Canada has approved the method, women in the United States can purchase the Today Sponge online and get questions answered at a 24- hour hotline service based in Canada.

Chemical Spermicides

A wide variety of chemical spermicides are available as stand-alone fertility control methods or to be used in conjunction with mechanical barriers as previously discussed. They all work by immobilizing and killing sperm, though they vary in form and method of application. They are available as nonprescription fertility control devices at most drug stores. It was previously thought that nonoxynol-9 was also effective in killing the organisms that cause syphilis, gonorrhea, and genital herpes, HIV/AIDS, and other STDs. To the contrary, the frequent use (more than two times a day) of nonoxynol-9 may actually increase the prospects of infection transmission due to irritating the skin (Hatcher et al., 2011).

The best-known spermicides are foams, gels, and creams. These work by creating a chemical barrier suspended in a shaving-cream-like foam, clear gel, or smooth cream. All three are inserted into the vagina, near the cervix, using a cylindrical applicator (see Figure 14.5). They create an immediate, effective chemical barrier against sperm. These spermicides may be inserted no more than 1 hour prior to intercourse.

Spermicidal film is different, however, because it is not immediately effective. It takes about 15 minutes to transform from its original shape into an effervescent liquid once inserted into the vagina (VCF Contraceptive. com, 2012).

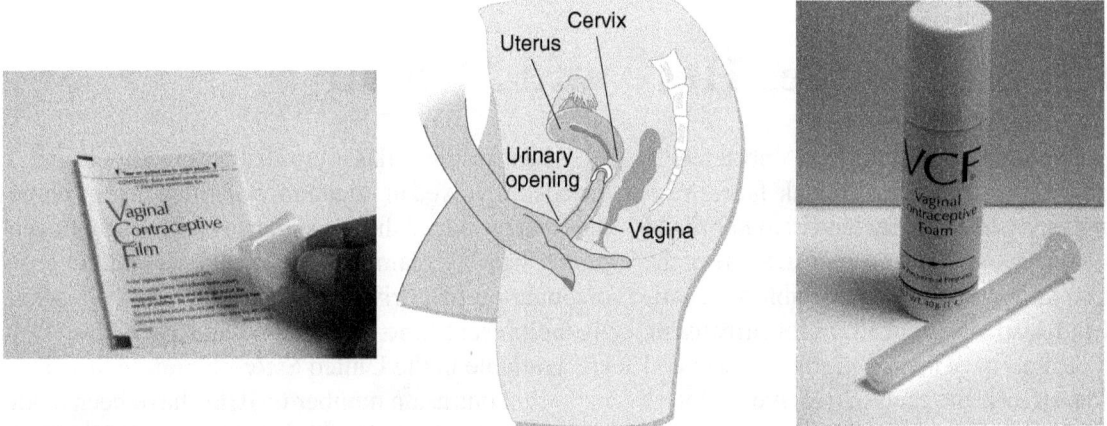

Figure 14.5 *Selected Spermicides and How to Insert Them*

Spermicidal suppositories are waxlike cylinders about the size of earplugs. They are applied in the same way as rectal suppositories, except into the vagina. Like film, the suppository requires about 15 minutes to liquefy after insertion into the vagina.

General instructions for using spermicides are as follows:

1. Fill the applicator with the product.
2. While lying down, insert the applicator deep into the vagina, near the cervix.
3. Push the plunger until the contents are completely released against the cervix.
4. If intercourse proceeds longer than one hour, stop and insert another applicator full of spermicide.
5. Insert a new application for each episode of intercourse.

The effectiveness of vaginal spermicides is similar regardless of the specific type. Foam, gel, cream, film, and suppositories are much the same in outcome. The theoretical effectiveness of spermicides is 82 percent. Typical use effectiveness is much lower, at 72 percent.

Women who are at high risk for HIV should not use spermicides because these products may actually increase the risk of transmission. Spermicides should also be avoided by women who are not willing to accept the high risk of failure. To improve effectiveness, spermicides can be combined with condoms.

Preventing Implantation of Fertilized Egg

Intrauterine Devices

The intrauterine device (IUD), is the most commonly used reversible contraception in the world and is among the safest and most effective methods of contraception available today. The IUD works primarily by preventing the sperm from fertilizing the egg. IUDs are not abortifacients, meaning they do not function by ending a pregnancy. They combine a foreign body and the effect of either copper or the hormone levonorgestrel to prevent pregnancy. The foreign body causes an inflammation in the uterus that is deadly to the sperm and ova, and prevents implantation. In addition, the inflammation harms sperm motility leading to decreased functioning of the

sex in society 14.2

Intrauterine Devices Here and Abroad

When teaching undergraduates about intrauterine devices, faculty may get met with blank faces from those who have never heard of such an item nor could imagine having one inserted into the uterus. Some of the original IUDs on the market were responsible for a variety of painful and deadly complications for early users. Although new designs have improved effectiveness and minimized side effects, the method received a lot of "bad press," and lost favor among many women.

In the 1970s, the Dalkon Shield was a commonly prescribed IUD. A significant number of users did not tolerate it. Because of its irregular shape and large size, the Dalkon Shield triggered strong uterine contractions as the body attempted to expel it from the uterus. The contractions often resulted in the shield penetrating the uterus and creating other problems, including severe infection that resulted in pain, hemorrhage, and sometimes death. The company that made the Dalkon Shield lost a civil lawsuit brought by users and their families and subsequently took the product off the market and went out of business. In practice, health care providers would advise this method for women who had been pregnant and had children. It also gave no protection against STDs, and HIV in particular, making it even less popular in the late 20th century.

Many safe IUDs were discontinued because of the costs involved in litigation, even though the companies that produced these products were found innocent of any liability claims. Consumer fears and the costs of litigation had driven most IUDs from the market. At the present time, the Mirena and ParaGard IUDs are available in the United States.

By contrast, a number of IUDs have been available abroad. Family Health International (FHI; 1996) reports that the IUD is the most widely used reversible contraceptive used worldwide, with approximately 100 million users. Rates of IUD use vary from country to country, with the highest rates reported to be in China. FHI reports that obstacles to greater use involve better training of health care professionals and educational efforts needed to overcome misinformation. A study in Kenya found resistance to the copper in IUDs, which may have tarnished in the package; women were afraid of the greenish color. Professional training in the Philippines had to focus on the myth that the IUD was too big for Filipino women and their accompanying fears that it traveled around the body (FHI, 1996). Overall, the IUD is a cost-effective method of birth control, particularly in nations with large populations of people without large numbers of health care providers.

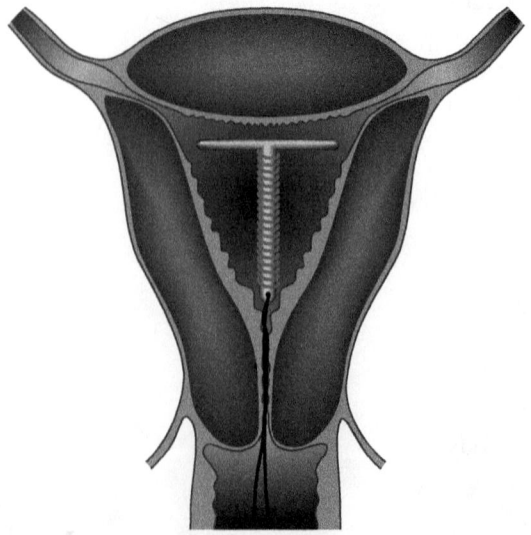

Figure 14.6 *An Inserted IUD*

sperm and to sperm death. The two models currently available for use in the United States are ParaGard T which is wrapped in copper and the Mirena, also T shaped and wrapped in progesterone. ParaGard, the copper IUD, uses copper to change uterine and tubal fluids thus decreasing sperm function and impairing implantation. The progestin released by the Mirena IUD thickens the cervical mucous, impairs the endometrial growth, and harms the sperm function. The progestin may also prevent ovulation due to systemic absorption from the uterus (Hatcher et al.,2011). Figure 14.6 shows an inserted IUD.

Once inserted, the IUD provides continuous protection with no further need for the user to do anything except to check the string monthly to be sure it is in place. The user can insert one or two fingers into the vagina and feel for the string. If she feels the string, the IUD is in place. If she doesn't, she should see her health care provider immediately and consider herself fertile.

Intrauterine devices have the advantage of providing long-term effectiveness. Once inserted, the ParaGard, also known as the Copper T, can be worn for up to 10 years. The Mirena, the newest IUD on the market, releases the hormone levonorgestrel, a synthetic progestin. It has the advantage of preventing ectopic pregnancy, lessens menstrual cramping, and decreases the amount of menstrual blood (Planned Parenthood, 2013). Mirena can be worn for up to 5 years. The 5-10 years of contraception costing typically $500-$1000 makes both methods cost effective.

The IUD is an excellent contraceptive for most women, including teens, who cannot or do not want to take hormones and for women who have and have not had children.

The IUDs are safe, very effective, and long lasting but easily reversible contraception. In addition, the IUD is convenient and allows spontaneous sexual activity. The IUD's effects on menstruation depend on which IUD one chooses. For those using the copper IUD, menstrual blood loss and cramping may increase. For those using Mirena, amenorrhea (not menstruating) occurs in 20 percent of women. IUD's do not protect against STD's so condoms will need to be used if the woman has multiple partners or non monogamous relationships (Hatcher et al, 2011).

The IUD is so effective that it can be thought of as nonpermanent sterilization. Theoretical effectiveness and actual-use effectiveness of IUDs are similar. Theoretical- use effectiveness of the copper IUD is 99.4 and actual effectiveness is 99.2. For the Mirena the theoretical and actual effectiveness rates are the same, 99.8 percent (Hatcher et al, 2011).

Women who are considering using an IUD should visit a health care provider experienced in inserting IUDs. The provider will measure the size and depth of the uterus by dilating the cervix and using special probes to measure it. This procedure, called sounding, is necessary for the safe insertion of any IUD.

If the woman decides to use the IUD, the provider will insert the IUD using an insertion device. Once inserted, the provider pushes the IUD into place in the uterus and removes the device. The provider locates the string attached to the end of the IUD and trims it to a shorter length. The string will pass from the uterus through the cervix and hang into the vagina. The woman has to demonstrate that she can find the strings, as they let her know whether the IUD is still in place. Although the woman can find the string with her finger, her sexual partner will not feel the string during intercourse. If the woman experiences bleeding or extreme cramping or cannot find the strings, she must go back to the provider immediately.

Preventing Release of Ova

The methods that prevent the release of an egg are hormonal. Focusing on managing a woman's ovulation has been extremely popular over the years, with the newest methods of birth control emerging in that area. Hormones can be taken orally, implanted under the skin, by injection, by vaginal insertion, and via a patch. Newer, varied, and hopefully less problematic methods of hormone distribution have been developed, tried, and, in some cases, removed from the market.

Fertility control does not take place within a vacuum. On a national level, personal fertility control is influenced by legislation that ensures the availability of safe, tested contraceptive methods and unrestricted access to these methods for all users. In December 2000, the U.S. Equal Employment Opportunity Commission (EEOC) argued that for employers' prescription plans to deny coverage for contraception was a violation of Title VII of the Civil Rights Act of 1964, as amended by the Pregnancy Discrimination Act (National Abortion and Reproductive Rights Action League [NARAL] & NARAL Foundation, 2001). By contrast, prescription plans had been covering the costs to men of Viagra, the drug developed to treat erectile dysfunction. In 2002, when a female student at George Washington University complained, the university revised the student health insurance plan to include prescription contraceptives. Since 1998, 26 states have some legislation that gives women financial support from their insurance companies. (NARAL, 2003).

At the local level, users must feel safe in procuring medical care and fertility control. Medical and health care providers, clinics, drug stores, schools, and other outlets for fertility control information and services should be safe and accessible for all, yet in practice they are not.

Oral Contraceptives

Oral contraceptives are formulated as combination pills of synthetic estrogen and progesterone, or progestin-only pills (POPs), commonly referred to as minipills. Combination pills are the most commonly used oral contraceptives. The combinations and levels of hormones contained in birth control pills have been changing constantly since their introduction in the early 1960s. Pills that are currently available contain the minimum levels of hormones necessary to carry out their intended functions and are much lower than the original formulations. This has resulted in a safer pill with fewer side effects (Hatcher et al,2011). In fact, using the birth control pill is safer than carrying a pregnancy to term.

Combination birth control pills work in several ways. The progestins in the combination oral contraception provide most of the contraceptive effect by suppressing ovulation and causing the cervical mucus to thicken. The progestins stop the pituitary gland from secreting leutinizing hormone (LH), the hormone that induces ovulation. Estrogen also contributes to stopping ovulation by suppressing the release of follicle stimulating hormone (FSH), which is necessary for the release of a mature ovum (Hatcher et al, 2011).

Normally, levels of estrogen, FSH, and leutinizing hormone (LH) are low during the initial phases of the menstrual cycle. The hypothalamus senses this and triggers the pituitary gland to secrete estrogen, FSH, and LH just prior to midcycle. If there is no surge of these substances, there is no release of a mature ovum.

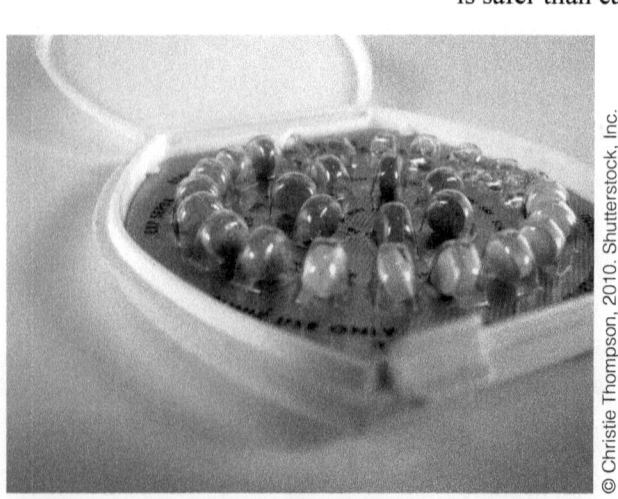

© Christie Thompson, 2010. Shutterstock, Inc.

Birth control pills come in containers that are easy to use and allow you to see if you've missed any.

Oral contraceptives are highly effective in controlling fertility. The theoretical effectiveness is over 99 percent. Typical use effectiveness is 91 percent. The drop off is associated with human error in failing to take pills consistently and correctly. For women who correctly and consistently use the pill, even the first year failure rate is less than 1% (Hatcher et al, 2011). The key to success is highly motivated pill users.

Traditionally, birth control pills were packaged in 28- pill packages, that included seven hormone free placebo pills designed to help keep the woman on schedule. Women now have many more choices with varying numbers of active pills and hormone free pills. Seasonal has 84 consecutive hormone pills with 7 placebo pills. This allows the woman to have only 4 periods of menstrual bleeding per year. Yaz and Loestrin-24 have 24 days of hormone pills and only 4 days of placebo. Lybrel, has no hormone free days allowing users to avoid having a menstrual period for a full year.

Women are instructed to use a quick start method when prescribed the pill. Using quick start, the woman takes her first pill immediately in the health care provider's office. This appears to improve the likelihood that she will continue taking the pill (Plastino & Sulak, 2008). The woman will then take a pill each day until she has consumed them all. The length of time will depend on what type of hormone regimen she has chosen.

Consistent use is crucial for maximum effectiveness. The woman should try to take the pill at the same time each day. This will help develop the habit of taking one pill each day, keep the same amount of hormones in the blood level, and ensure consistent use. Some women prefer to take the pill each morning as part of their ritual for getting ready for school or work. Others take it at night as part of a night-time sleep ritual. The time is up to her. Taking the birth control pill should become part of the lifestyle, just like brushing the teeth. It becomes so routine that she doesn't even have to think about it.

If a pill is missed, the woman should take two the next day. Missing one pill will not compromise the effectiveness of the method. Missing two pills, however, does reduce the effectiveness of oral contraceptives, and a backup fertility control method such as condoms will be necessary. If she misses two pills, she should take two immediately and two the next day. After that, she should continue to take one each day until they are all gone.

Long-Acting Combination Pills. In 2003, the FDA approved an oral contraceptive called Seasonale. Women take tablets with combination hormones for 84 days, followed by 1 week of placebo tablets, making a 91-day regimen. Women using Seasonale will get their periods four times per year, rather than the monthly periods associated with traditional birth control pills. Both rates of effectiveness as well as risks and side effects match those of traditional birth control pills. Similarly, there is no protection against sexually transmitted infections (FDA, 2003).

Progestin-Only Pills. Also it referred to as *minipills,* progestin-only pills are to be taken every day. The same precautions and instructions for missed combination pills apply to the minipill. Progestin, the same artificial progesterone used in combination pills, is taken by itself. It works by inhibiting ovulation in some cycles, thickening the cervical mucus, altering the composition of the endometrium, and reducing the activity of the cilia in the fallopian tubes. Combined these work to reduce the likelihood of fertilization and implantation.

Positive Side Effects. Birth control pills offer many advantages for women. They are frequently prescribed for women with irregular periods to regulate the menstrual cycle as well as to provide fertility control protection. Other menstrual advantages include lessening of cramps, decreasing the amount of bleeding and decreasing symptoms of PMS. While taking hormonal contraception females have what is referred to as withdrawal bleeding instead of a true menstrual period. Other benefits are the decrease in the risks of both ovarian and endometrial cancer. Hormonal contraceptives decrease a female's risk of dying from colon cancer and decreases benign breast conditions such as cysts. The pill is also beneficial in the treatment of acne and will decrease menstrual migraine headaches and iron deficiency anemia (Hatcher et al, 2011).

Negative Side Effects. Some women experience negative side effects when taking oral contraceptives. The most common side effects mimic symptoms attributed to pregnancy: nausea, vomiting, breast tenderness, and headaches. Although hormonal contraceptives can have some side effects, there are also myths about side effects of the pill. Three common myths are: that the pill can decrease sex drive: the pill can affect long term fertility; and the pill can harm a pregnancy if taken while pregnant. None has been shown to be true. One major worry for many women is that the pill may make her gain weight. This is also not true as shown in studies comparing pill users and non pill users. There is also no increase risk of breast cancer among pill users, another scary myth. (Hatcher et al, 2011).

Many of the side effects of the pill can be minimized or eliminated by changing the formula or brand of pill. Combination pills differ slightly by manufacturer in the amounts of estrogen and progesterone. If the combination of these hormones in the present pill is causing unacceptable side effects, the health care provider can change the prescription and the woman can try a different formulation. The birth control pill also can interact with other medications. In some cases, oral contraceptives lessen the effectiveness of the other medications. Or other medications can lessen the effectiveness of the pill. Table 14.2 details some of these interactions.

Although, as with any medication, the risks associated with oral contraceptives have to be considered, most of them can be reduced through proper screening of the woman by a health care professional. The benefits far outweigh the risks.

Another way to view the risks associated with use of the pill is to put them into a broader perspective. Most of us assume many risks in the course of a day without even thinking about them. A taken-for-granted activity such as driving a car puts us at a much higher risk of dying than does using the pill or other fertility control techniques. We accept the risk because it is worth assuming. The activity (driving a car, for instance) adds so much to our daily quality of life that we accept the risk it entails. We also do whatever we can to decrease the risks associated with driving. We use seat belts, obey speed limits and other traffic laws, don't drink and drive, and so on. Nonetheless, high blood pressure, migraine headaches, blood

Table 14.2 Effects of Common Medications on the Pill

Interacting Drugs	Adverse Effects (Probable Mechanism)	Comments and Recommendations
Acetaminophen (Tylenol and others)	Possible decreased pain-relieving effect (increased metabolism)	Monitor pain-relieving response.
Alcohol	Possible increased effect of alcohol	Use with caution.
Anticoagulants (oral)	Decreased anticoagulant effect	Use alternative contraceptive.
Antidepressants (Elavil, Norpramin, Tofranil, others)	Possible increased antidepressant effect	Monitor antidepressant effect.
Barbiturates (Phenobarbital and others)	Decreased contraceptive effect	Avoid simultaneous use; use alternative contraceptive for epileptics.
Benzodiazepine tranquilizers (Ativan, Librium, Serax, Tranxene, Valium, Xanax, and others)	Possible increased or decreased tranquilizer effects including psychomotor impairments	Use with caution. Greatest impairment occurs during menstrual pause in oral contraceptive dosage.
Beta-blockers (Corgard, Inderal, Lopressor, Tenormin)	Possible increased blocker effect	Monitor cardiovascular status.
Carbamazepine (Tegretol)	Possible decreased contraceptive effect	Use alternative contraceptive.
Corticosteroids (cortisone)	Possible increased corticosteroid toxicity	Clinical significance not established.
Griseofulvin (Fulvicin, GrifulvinV, and others)	Decreased contraceptive effect	Use alternative contraceptive.
Guanethidine (Esimil, Ismelin)	Decreased guanethidine effect (mechanism not established)	Avoid simultaneous use.
Hypoglycemics (Tolbutamide, Diabinese, Orinase, Tolinase)	Possible decreased hypoglycemic effect	Monitor blood glucose.
Methyldopa (Aldoclor, Aldoment, and others)	Decreased hypertensive effect	Avoid simultaneous use.
Penicillin	Decreased contraceptive effect with ampicillin	Low but unpredictable incidence; use alternative contraceptive.
Phenytoin (Dilantin)	Decreased contraceptive effect; possible increased phenytoin effect	Use alternative contraceptive. Monitor phenytoin concentration.
Primidone (Mysoline)	Decreased contraceptive effect	Use alternative contraceptive.
Rifampin	Decreased contraceptive effect	Use alternative contraceptive.
Tetracycline	Decreased contraceptive effect	Use alternative contraceptive.
Theophylline (Bronkotabs, Marax, Primatene, Quibron Tedral, TheorDur, and others)	Increased theophylline effect	Monitor theophylline concentration.
Troleandomycin (TAO)	Jaundice (additive)	Avoid simultaneous use.
Vitamin C	Increased serum concentration and possible increased adverse effects of estrogens with 1 gram or more per day of vitamin C	Decrease vitamin C to 100 milligrams per day.

Source: *Contraceptive Technology* (16th ed.) by Hatcher, Trussel, Stewart, et al. (New York: Irvington, 1998). Used with permission.

clots, and stroke have been associated with the use of birth control pills by select groups of women.

Oral contraceptives are not recommended for women who have a history of high blood pressure or stroke; blood clots or a history of blood clots; have or had breast cancer; and women who smoke, especially if they are over 35 and/or heavy smokers. Women who smoke should quit smoking to allow them to safely use hormonal contraceptives. It is important to remember that the majority of young healthy women are good candidates for hormone based contraception.

Ortho Evra Patch

The Ortho Evra Patch administers hormones through the skin, and has effectiveness rates similar to birth control pills. The patch is thin, beige in color, and measures 1.75 inches on each side. A woman wears a patch for 1 week, replaces it on the same day for 3 consecutive weeks, and is "patch-free" during the fourth week (Planned Parenthood, 2013). Like birth control pills, Evra may increase the risk for blood clots. Side effects are similar to those of the pill with the addition of breast tenderness and skin irritation at the site of application. As with all the forms of hormonal contraception, the effectiveness for pregnancy prevention is high (99 percent theoretical effectiveness and 91% typical use), but there is no protection against STDs (Hatcher et al, 2011).

Women have two options for the first cycle of using the patch; start on the first Sunday after the menstrual period or start the first day of the menstrual period. For the Sunday start she will also need to use 7 days of additional protection. Women can apply the patch to the buttocks, lower abdomen, upper torso, or upper arm. *The patch may not be applied to the breasts.* The manufacturer advises that the patch not be put where makeup, lotions, or creams are applied. The adhesive on the patch is designed to last the week, regardless of showering or bathing, swimming, exercise, or humidity.

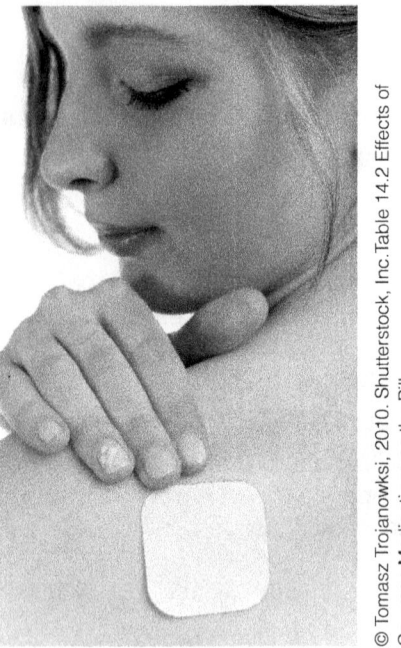

The patch can be placed on the shoulder, arm, or abdomen, but never on the breast.

© Tomasz Trojanowksi, 2010. Shutterstock, Inc.Table 14.2 Effects of Common Medications on the Pill

Vaginal Contraceptive Ring (NuvaRing)

The NuvaRing works on the principle of a woman having a 28-day cycle: 3 weeks of hormonal control followed by 1 week of no hormones thus allowing withdrawal bleeding. The NuvaRing appears similar to the plastic ring at the end of the female condom, and it is inserted by the woman deep into the vagina, where it remains for 3 weeks. Although insertion is relatively simple, involving folding the ring and pushing it up the vagina, a woman must be comfortable touching that part of her body in order for this method to work. At the end of the 3-week period, the ring is removed by hooking the index finger under the ring and pulling it out. Kits come with a timer, yet a woman needs to remember to take out the ring, wait a week, and put in a new one. If the ring is left in longer than 4 weeks, a woman may lose her birth control protection. Couples do not feel the ring, and it rarely falls out.

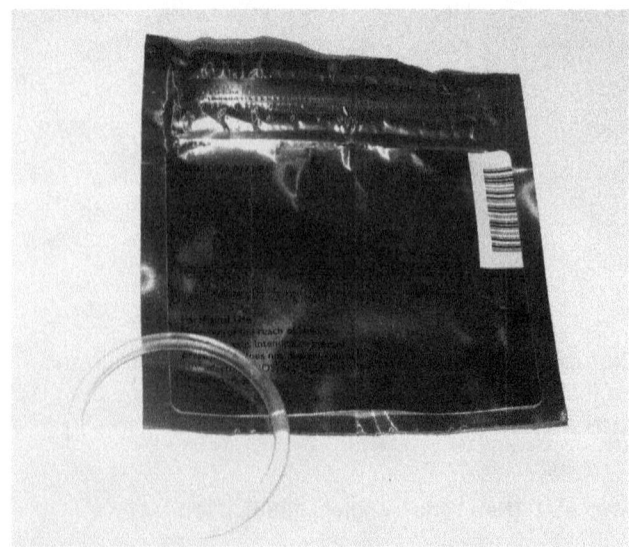

The NuvaRing dispenses hormones through the vagina.

Again, as with other hormonal methods of birth control, NuvaRing's risks include increased risk of blood clots. Some women report experiencing headaches and vaginal wetness. Some of the advantages of the vaginal contraceptive ring include that it does not cause weight gain, it is convenient, and hormone levels needed for contraception are reached within 1-3 days of insertion (Hatcher et al, 2011).

Emergency Contraception Pill

Three Emergency contraceptive pills are available in the US and include ella, Plan B One-Step and Next Choice (the generic of Plan B). Plan B and Next Choice are available over the counter to women and men 15 and older. A prescription is needed for ella and for those under 15 who choose Plan B or Next Choice. It is wise for all sexually active women to buy a supply in advance in case it is needed. Plan B is progestin only and designed to be administered as soon as possible after unprotected intercourse. It can be used up to 5 days after unprotected sex but the sooner it is used, the more effective it will be. The early administration of the pills works to delay or prevent ovulation, inhibit fertilization or may at times prevent implantation of a fertilized egg. It never works to disrupt an implanted pregnancy and therefore is not an abortion. Nausea and vomiting are side effects experienced by 13-29% of women. Taking emergency contraception, even for multiple times, has no effect on future pregnancies or fertility nor does it cause birth defects if the woman is pregnant when she takes it. However, emergency contraceptiton is not recommended for routine use since it is less effective than many contraceptives. If a woman does not get her menstrual period within 3 weeks, it is recommended that she take a pregnancy test (Hatcher et al., 2011). Overall, the rate of effectiveness is between 75 and 89 percent, although research conducted by the World Health Organization found only 1.1 percent of women who used progestin-only emergency contraception went on to become pregnant (Nelson et al., 2000).

Injectable Contraceptive

Depo-Provera, the most commonly used injectable contraceptive, is a progestin-only hormonal contraceptive. Its action is the same as the minipill. A major advantage of Depo-Provera over these other methods is the way in which it is administered: by injection every 3 months. The injections can be administered in either the arm or the buttocks. A single injection provides 3 months' worth of protection.

Depo-Provera has one of the highest typical use effectiveness rates of all fertility control methods, at 94% and a theoretical use of 99 percent. This rate can be attributed mostly to the nature of administering the product. There is no room for actual-use error. Once the shot is administered, the user doesn't have to remember to do anything.

Because Depo-Provera does not contain estrogen, it does not produce many of the side effects associated with combination pills. Nevertheless, it does produce two noticeable side effects: weight gain and infrequent but prolonged periods. Many women discontinue Depo-Provera because of predictable weight gain (5.4 pounds average during the first year; some women gain three times that). It also produces scanty menstrual flow and **amenorrhea** in some women and irregular but long periods in others. A third side effect of Depo-Provera is that prolonged use may result in temporary

Amenorrhea Absence of menstruation at some time after a female has reached menses

Table 14.3 Comparison of Newer Contraceptive Methods

	Monthly Injectable	Implant	Intrauterine System	Ring	Patch
Office visits	Once/month	Insertion/ removal	Insertion/ removal	Prescription	Prescription
Easily reversible	Yes	Yes	Yes	Yes	Yes
Dosing frequency*	Once/month	3–5 years	1–10 years	Every 4 weeks	Weekly
User controlled	No	No	No	Yes	Yes
Discreet	Yes	Sometimes	Yes	Yes	Sometimes

*The type of hormonal implant and intrauterine device/system will determine the dosing frequency.
Sources: Adapted from Baylor College of Medicine (2002) and Planned Parenthood Federation of America (2003).

and usually reversible loss of bone density. Some women also experience an increase in depression when using Depo-Provera (Hatcher et al., 2011)

Contraceptive Implants

Contraceptive implants are among the most effective contraceptive available with a typical user failure of only .05 % making them equal to the IUD and sterilzation. Implanon and Nexplanon, the contraceptive implants available in the US, consist of a single rod approximately 4 centimeters long and 2 millimeters in diameter, which is designed to provide hormonally controlled protection for up to 3 years (Planned Parenthood, 2013). The implant releases progestin and within 24 hours of insertion is thought to be reliable. Similar to birth control pills, it works by inhibiting ovulation, thickening cervical mucus so that sperm are inhibited in their travel, and altering the endometrium so that it wouldn't support a fertilized egg (Hatcher, 2011). User satisfaction is high for this method perhaps due to the ease of use, relief of dysmenorrhea and discreetness of method. Like other hormonal forms of birth control, it offers no protection against sexually transmitted infection. Irregular bleeding and headaches are the most reported side effects.

Table 14.3 compares some of the newer contraceptive methods.

Future Methods for Males

It should be obvious that the hormonal discussion so far focuses solely on the female body. Over the years, the research question has been posited as to whether hormonal control of male sperm production would be possible. Giving synthetic androgens to men, whether orally, by injection, or by implant, could theoretically reduce sperm production. Finding the right reduction in testosterone without affecting a man's sex drive and causing other side effects is the challenge. Gossypol, made from cottonseed oil, has been shown in large studies to stop sperm production without changing testosterone levels. Another promising option for further research is anticancer drugs that reduce normal sperm production. This challenging research is continuing but it does not appear that any new options for male contraception will be available any time soon (Hatcher, 2011).

Preventing Sperm from Reaching Egg (Surgical)

Sterilization is the most common form of contraception used today in the United States and in the rest of the world (Hatcher, 2011). The sterilization methods that prevent sperm from reaching the ova consist of vasectomy and tubal sterilization. Sterilization does not prevent sperm and ova from being released. It works by blocking the path of either the sperm or the egg as a result of surgical removal of a small section of the vas deferens (vasectomy) in the male or fallopian tubes (minilaparotomy, laproscopic and hysteroscopic) in the female The ends of the vas deferens and fallopian tubes are closed in a variety of ways including sealing with heat, using rings or clips or stitching shut.

All sterilization procedures should be viewed as permanent, because once these structures have been surgically altered, there is no guarantee that they can be rejoined. Ova or sperm that are produced after sterilization cannot continue their journey, so they die, break down, and are excreted from the body as waste products.

Both male and female sterilization have a typical and perfect use effectiveness rates of higher than 99 percent.

Of the two procedures, vasectomy is the simplest and less costly, costing half that of female sterilization. Vasectomies are performed as outpatient visits and last no longer than 30 minutes. Female sterilization is also relatively simple and usually takes under an hour to perform.

Both procedures require a conference with the person desiring sterilization to ensure that he or she understands the permanence of the procedure. The majority of women and men do not regret their decision to have the sterilization procedures. However, for both sexes regret was more common in those who chose to have the procedure before age 30. A change in life circumstances during the rest of the reproductive years may contribute to this regret and caution is advised (Hatcher et al, 2011).

Vasectomy

No major preoperative testing procedures are done for a **vasectomy.** During the initial consultation, patients are advised to bring an athletic supporter to wear home after the procedure.

The patient disrobes and lies on his back on the examination table. He is given a local anesthetic in the scrotal skin, not the vas deferens and remains awake throughout the entire procedure (see Figure 14.7). The physician locates the vas deferens and makes a small incision in the scrotal sac. The physician isolates the vas deferens and cuts out a small piece. The two surfaces are then clipped, treated with heat or tied off and the scrotal incisions closed. (Cutie & Dorgara, 2012). The same procedure is repeated on the other vas deferens. The patient is instructed to rest for a short time and is then free to leave. The entire outpatient stay is usually no more than an hour.

It is recommended that patients rest for 2-3 days and wait a week before having intercourse or exercising strenuously. Sperm will remain in the body of many men for as long as 3 months requiring use of a condom or other back up method of birth

Sterilization Techniques (vasectomy and tubal ligation) that prevent sperm from reaching ova

Vasectomy A male sterilization procedure in which the vas deferens are cut and tied, clipped or heated to block the transport of sperm

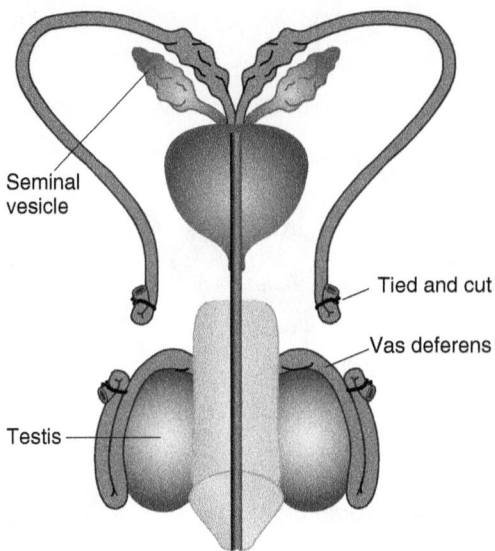

Figure 14.7 *Vasectomy*

control. Men are instructed to bring a semen specimen in for analysis after 3 months and a minimum of 20 ejaculations. This is the most reliable way to make sure there are no remaining sperm in the body and if the test is negative, intercourse is safe without a backup method (Cutie & Dorgara, 2012).

Side effects of a vasectomy are relatively mild; the most common are pain and tenderness. These can be minimized or controlled by wearing scrotal support (brief style underwear) and keeping an icepack on the scrotum for 4 hours to reduce the chances of swelling, bleeding or pain. Analgesics can also help reduce discomfort (Hatcher et al, 2011).

Female Sterilization

The two sterilization procedures used most often with women are interval tubal sterilization called laparoscopy and tubal sterilization after childbirth called **mini-laparotomy.** This surgical procedure occurs 1-2 days after childbirth and requires either general or local anesthesia. A small incision is made in the abdomen to remove a section of the each fallopian tube. The woman will not have to extend her hospital stay after birth so it is a convenient time for many women. The procedure only takes 20-30 minutes and women usually recover within 1-2 days.

Laparoscopic Sterilization

This is an outpatient procedure using either general or spinal anesthesia. A small incision is made near the navel, and a **laparoscope** is inserted to locate the fallopian tubes. The surgeon then uses rings or clips or heat to close the fallopian tube and then repeats this procedure on the other fallopian tube (see Figure 14.8). Women go home the day of the procedure. This method results in an almost invisible scar and allows women to return to normal activity quickly, within 1-2 days.

In 2002, Essure received FDA approval as a new method of sterilization for women. The advantage to the method is that it can be performed as an outpatient procedure without the use of general anesthesia or incision since the path for insertion is through the vagina, cervix, and uterus. A physician inserts a small metal spring into each fallopian tube. The coils lead to the development of scar tissue in the tube, which effectively blocks the passageway. Because it takes approximately 3 months for the fallopian tubes to become blocked, women are advised to use a backup method of birth control until their health care provider confirms that the tubes are blocked with scar tissue. (Planned Parenthood, 2013).

Side Effects. Both procedures require several days to a week to heal. Mild abdominal pain or tenderness is common. Intercourse may be resumed after one to two weeks.

As with a vasectomy, side effects are relatively rare. Minor complications may include infection and healing of the incision. As with any surgery, women confront risks related to anesthesia (Hatcher et al., 2011).

Mini-laparotomy A female sterilization procedure performed following the birth of a child in which the fallopian tubes are cut to block transport of the egg

Laparoscopic Sterilization A female sterilization procedure done at a time other than childbirth in which a surgical instrument is used to cut and tie back the fallopian tubes to block passage of the ova and thereby prevent fertilization

Laparoscope A flexible surgical instrument with a cameralike attachment that can be inserted into the abdomen to view the fallopian tubes and other organs

Seminal vesicle Testis Tied and cut Vas deferens

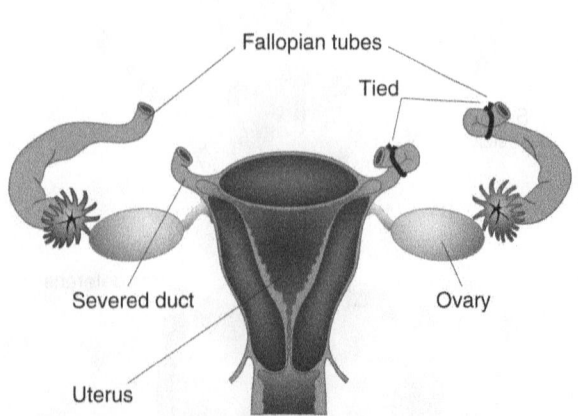

Figure 14.8 *Tubal Ligation*

case study 14.3

Mindy's Experience with Abortion

Mindy, 29, is white.

Mindy is a successful small business owner, she has been married to Bob about 5 years, and they have a 2-year-old daughter. This is the account of her decision to have an abortion.

I grew up in a small town and was raised to think that abortion was killing. I remember seeing those films about little babies being tossed out in the garbage after their mothers had abortions and all the posters and billboards with pictures of fully developed fetuses and the headings "Abortion is murder." I couldn't imagine anyone ever having an abortion. But then I got pregnant and began to look at things differently.

I was away at college. I was a 19-year-old sophomore and had been having sex with my boyfriend, Michael, for about 6 months. We were using my diaphragm for birth control, and, to tell you the truth, I don't ever remember having any problems with it. I used it faithfully, every time we had sex.

I couldn't believe I was pregnant. I was frantic. I must have had five pregnancy tests until I finally accepted the fact. I couldn't have this baby! I cried for 2 days, and Michael was very supportive. Sometimes we cried together as we tried to figure out what to do. I knew in my heart that I wasn't ready to be a mother. I still had 3 years of school left, plus graduate school. I had no job, no time, and psychologically just couldn't handle it.

I went to a local abortion clinic. The people were great. They gave me all the information I needed, I took tests, and they assured me that because I was only 6 weeks pregnant, the procedure they would use was safe and relatively simple. I scheduled an appointment and went home to think about it.

It wasn't an easy decision, but I felt I had no acceptable choice. I didn't think I could handle being pregnant, having a baby, and then give it up for adoption or foster care. I didn't want to tell my parents. I wasn't sure how they'd react and didn't want to jeopardize my being away at school.

They were paying for everything, and I wasn't sure if they'd force me to drop out.

I felt sad for a few weeks after my abortion. I wished I hadn't gotten pregnant and didn't have to make the decision, but sometimes life doesn't always work out the way you plan. I got over it gradually, finished out the school year, and graduated on time 2 years later. Now, 10 years later and the mother of a 2-year-old girl, I know I never could have been the mom I am now. Although it was a tough decision, it was the right one for me.

Critical Thinking

How do you feel about the decision that Mindy and Michael made about the pregnancy? What if they hadn't agreed to the same resolution to the unplanned pregnancy? How do you think you would have handled the same situation?

Terminating an Established Pregnancy

Established pregnancies can be terminated through surgical and medical means. **Abortion** is defined as the termination, spontaneous or induced, of an established pregnancy and relates to **viability.** A viable fetus, if born, has a reasonable chance of living. In the United States the time definition for viability is 24 weeks (gestational age starting at conception).

About one-third of all abortions are *spontaneous abortions,* or miscarriages. They result from a variety of conditions ranging from physical trauma to a breakdown of the uterine lining. *Induced abortions* account for the remaining two-thirds. Induced abortions involve purposely ending an established pregnancy, (Guttmacher, 2007). Currently, 43% of unintended pregnancies end in abortion. At this rate, by age 45 more than one third of all American women will have had an abortion (Guttmacher, 2013). In an abortion, the endometrium, placenta, and embryo or fetus are removed from the uterus. Abortion procedures are of several types, related to the length of the pregnancy and other extenuating circumstances.

Induced abortions have been legal in the United States since 1973, when two U.S. Supreme Court decisions, *Roe v. Wade* and *Doe v. Bolton,* determined that the decision to have a first-trimester abortion need concern only a woman and her physician. States could not use legislation to deny a woman's choice of first trimester abortions. The ruling did allow states the ability to set standards for second- and third-trimester abortions. The overwhelming majority of women (90 percent) who terminate their pregnancies do so in the first trimester and more than 60% take place at or before eight weeks (Hatcher, 2011). For women who have had prenatal screenings and receive information about serious health problems in the fetus, a second-trimester abortion becomes an option, particularly since amniocentesis results are not returned until the 18th week of gestation or later.

Third-trimester abortions remain very rare yet are extremely controversial and have been the focus of much legal wrangling and debate. The term *late-term* abortion is applied to cases where the viability of the fetus is not possible, and an attempted birth will leave serious health problems for the mother, resulting in termination during the third trimester. Opponents of the procedure refer to it as "partial birth abortion," a term that has worked its way into media and legislative discussions. In 2003, President George W. Bush signed the Partial Birth Abortion Ban Act, yet three federal courts issued temporary restraining orders against its enactment, claiming the language was vague and did not include preserving the mother's life.

Surgical Methods

Surgical methods include vacuum aspiration, dilation and curettage (D&C), dilation and evacuation (D&E)

Vacuum Aspiration

Vacuum aspiration is the most widely used procedure for early abortions. It can be performed in a medical office or clinic for pregnancies less than 14 weeks gestation (Hatcher et al.,2011). This is an outpatient procedure

Abortion Termination of an established pregnancy through surgical or nonsurgical techniques

Viability Fetus has a reasonable chance of living outside of the uterus usually at age of 24 weeks

Vacuum aspiration An induced abortion procedure in which uterine contents are removed by suction; used for early abortions

using local anesthesia and cost between $300-$950. Aspiration is done with either a hand held suction device or a suction machine. The contents of the uterus are gently removed with this suction. A curette, a narrow metal loop, is sometimes used after the suction to remove any remaining contents of the uterus. When the curette is used, some call the procedure a D & C, dilation and curettage (Planned Parenthood, 2013).

A vacuum aspiration abortion usually can be performed in approximately 5-10 minutes. It is safe and usually causes few side effects. The cervix is dilated, and a vacuum tube is inserted into the cervix. At the end of the tube is a **cannula,** which is attached to a vacuum pump (aspirator) used to suction off the contents of the wall of the uterus (endometrium, fetus/embryo, and placenta). Figure 14.9 (see page 458) shows this procedure.

Cannula A tapered, strawlike tube used in the vacuum aspiration method of abortion

❦ *Emotional and Spiritual Wellness* ❦

Spirituality plays a big role in how people evaluate fertility control methods and which ones they ultimately choose. Religions have various beliefs regarding fertility control, with variations from division to division, and sometimes region to region. From a broad perspective, all decisions about pregnancy relate to the underlying theme of interconnectedness. The decision to create a new life or to prevent the unintended creation of life is fundamentally a spiritual issue.

The decision to end a pregnancy is not made lightly. Some women don't even tell the male involved, choosing only to seek support from close friends. Deciding to have an abortion may be kept secret from parents and siblings as well. Both males and females may need counseling to deal with the emotional aspects of the decisions they've made.

When couples confront second-trimester abortions, they may find privacy not an option. Family, friends, and coworkers may have been aware of a planned pregnancy. Explanations about deciding to have a second-trimester abortion can be very difficult to share. Again, counseling and support groups can be very helpful.

Dilation and Evacuation (D&E)

Dilation and evacuation (D&E), usually performed later than 14 weeks, combines vacuum aspiration and medical instruments to gently remove the contents of the uterus. In preparation for the procedure, practitioners may insert a laminaria several hours to days prior to the procedure. The laminaria is made of dried seaweed that expands and gently dilates the woman's cervix. (Hatcher et al.,2011).

Dilation and evacuation (D&E) A second-trimester abortion procedure in which the cervix is first dilated, and then the fetus removed by suction and medical instruments

Like first-trimester abortions, women seek to terminate pregnancies in the second trimester for a variety of reasons. As discussed in Chapter 13, couples do not get the results of prenatal screening tests such as amniocentesis or chorionic villus sampling until the second trimester.

Surgical abortions are very safe procedures. The risk of death from childbirth is 11 times higher than that of abortions performed before 20 weeks (Planned Parenthood, 2013). Since the legalization of abortion in 1973, the death rate for the procedure has dropped steadily.

Medical Abortions

Medical abortions account for 17% of all non hospital abortions and have a high acceptability rate among women who have experienced them. Of those who had a medical abortion, eighty-four percent said they would choose a medical abortion over a surgical abortion if they faced the choice again (Christen-Maitre, Bouchard, & Spitz, 2000; Guttmacher, 2011). Medical abortions are most effective if woman is less than 8-9 weeks pregnant. These abortions do not involve surgical intervention but rather the use of medications to terminate a pregnancy. Figure 14.9 illustrates this method. Abortions can be induced by administering agents that work two ways: (a) by initiating the breakdown of the endometrium, making it impossible to sustain the pregnancy and (b) by causing the uterus to contract and expel its contents.

RU-486 is the drug mifepristone and was marketed in 2000 as Mifeprex. It is an antiprogesterone drug that works by blocking the absorption of progesterone, the hormone necessary for continued viability of the endometrium. If progesterone is blocked, the uterine lining will no longer support fetal development. A second drug, misoprostol (a type of prostaglandin), is administered at home a few hours to 3 days later, causing uterine contractions. These contractions cause the uterine lining and products of conception to be sloughed off within 4-5 hours for over half of women and the remaining usually abort within a few days (Planned Parenthood, 2013).

RU-486 Known as the "abortion pill"; mifepristone, a drug used to induce menstruation by blocking the absorption of progesterone and thereby preventing the uterine lining from supporting an embryo

Medical abortion

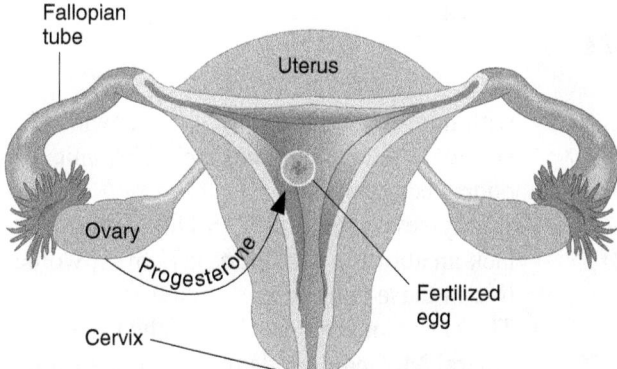

Progesterone, a hormone produced by the ovaries, is necessary for the implantation and development of a fertilized egg.

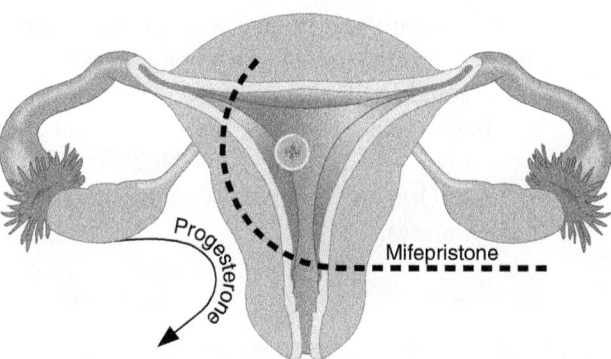

Taken early in pregnancy mifepristone blocks the action of progesterone and makes the body react as if it isn't pregnant.

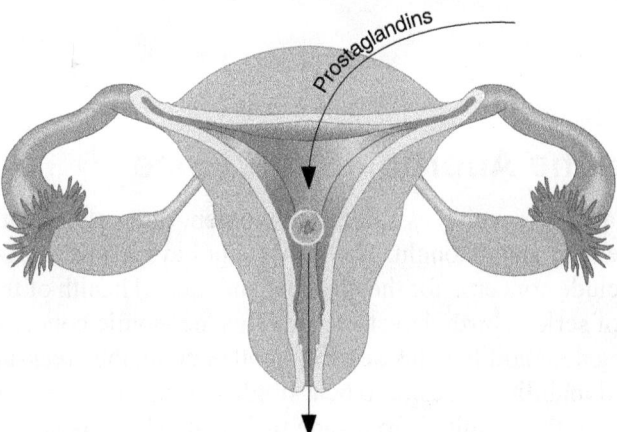

Prostaglandins, taken two days later, cause the uterus to contract and the cervix to soften and dilate. As a result, the fertilized egg is expelled in 97% of the cases.

Vacuum aspiration

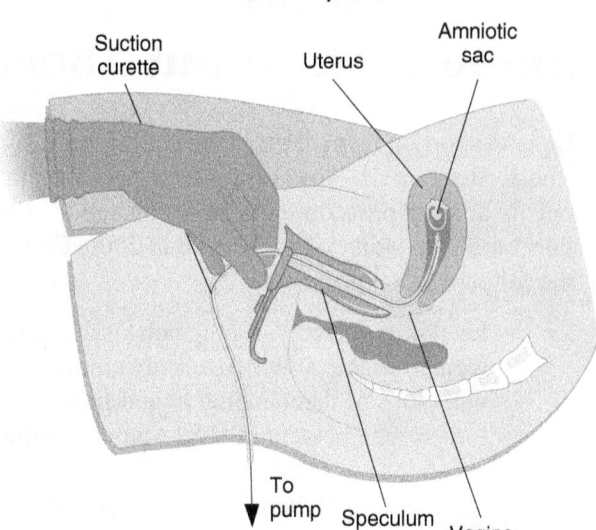

Figure 14.9 *Abortion Methods Used in Early Gestation*

sex in society 14.3
Some Facts About Abortion

Despite abortion being legal in the United States since Roe v. Wade in 1973, many women hesitate to talk openly about a procedure that an estimated 1.21 million American women experienced in 2006. Consider the following facts:

- Forty-nine percent of pregnancies among women in the United States are unintended, with 40% of them ending in abortion.
- Fifty-seven percent of U.S. women obtaining abortions are in their 20's, with teens representing 18 percent of those seeking abortions.
- Women who have never been married and are not living with a partner have 45% of all abortions
- Over 60 percent of abortions are among women who already have at least one child.
- Fifty-four percent of women having abortions used a contraceptive method during the month they became pregnant.
- Eight percent of women having abortions have never used a method of birth control, with nonuse greatest among those who are young, unmarried, poor, black, Hispanic, or poorly educated.
- Eighty-seven percent of all U.S. counties lack an abortion provider; 35% of all women live in these counties.
- The U.S. Congress has barred the use of federal Medicaid funds to pay for abortion except when the woman's life would be endangered by a full-term pregnancy or if the pregnancy resulted from rape or incest. Seventeen states do use public funds to pay for abortions for some women (Alaska, Arizona, California, Connecticut, Hawaii, Illinois, Massachusetts, Maryland, Maine, Montana, New Jersey, New Mexico, New York, Oregon, Vermont, Washington, and Wyoming).

Source: Alan Guttmacher Institute (2011a).

Reactions to the Abortion Experience

Deciding to terminate a pregnancy is a decision women, often along with their partners, make with great thought. The reasons for having an abortion are varied. They include concerns for the physical and mental health of the mother, discovery of serious birth defects in the fetus, economic concerns of a couple regarding their ability to take care of another child, the break-up of a relationship and inability or desire to be a single parent, and concerns related to a pregnancy that resulted from rape or incest. The reasons are many, yet the one similarity for all is that *this* pregnancy is unwanted. Most women report the immediate feeling of relief, with the abortion representing the end to a crisis pregnancy. Ideally women would not have to make this very difficult decision. Free access to birth control could be a way to help women avoid unplanned pregnancies. A 2012 study found that free access to birth control would prevent as many as half of all abortions in the U.S. (Pierpert, Madden, Allsworth & Secure, 2012).

Over the years those who oppose abortion have suggested that women suffer long term mental health issues after an abortion calling it "postabortion syndrome". Scientific evidence has never supported this and a new, large rigorous study in Denmark has found no higher rates of mental health problems among women in the 12 months after the abortion than in the 9 months prior to the abortion (Guttmacher, 2011 b). The American Psychiatric Association (2000) does not recognize "post abortion syndrome and it is not included in the most recent *Diagnostic and Statistical Manual,* which characterizes recognized psychological illnesses. Critics claim that much of the available data on the purported syndrome has come from "expert witnesses" in congressional hearings and anecdotal reports from physicians, clinicians, and women who have incurred ill effects after having abortions. In repeated studies since the early 1980's, leading experts have concluded that abortion does not pose a threat to a woman's mental health (Guttamacher, 2011).

Abortion follow-up includes referral for postabortion counseling and group therapy for women who need these services to cope with their distress. Postabortion counseling and support groups are viable options for women who have emotional distress related to their abortions.

The decision to have an abortion is not an easy one to make. It is a complex moral and ethical decision that most women (and men) take seriously. The decision has both immediate- and long-term consequences that need to be taken into account. Overall, the decision to terminate an unwanted pregnancy becomes one of the many decisions couples make over the course of their reproductive years.

Thought Questions

1. What are the differences among birth control, contraception, and family planning?
2. What are the five mechanisms of action for fertility control methods?
3. What is an acceptable level of risk of pregnancy for a fertility control method? Why?
4. What are the risks associated with pregnancy and childbirth for the various fertility control methods?
5. What category of fertility control methods offers the best protection against STDs? What are differences in STD protection among the methods in this category?
6. How do hormonal contraception measures work?
7. What risks are associated with the pill?
8. How do a person's (or couple's) fertility control needs change over the course of a lifetime?
9. What key questions should you ask yourself when evaluating any fertility control method?

Test Yourself!

1. Birth control methods are best described as techniques that enable couples to
   a. prevent births.
   b. prevent conception.
   c. prevent families.
   d. prevent implantation.
2. When couples choose a method of birth control, which issue is most critical to preventing a pregnancy?
   a. The theoretical effectiveness rate associated with the method
   b. Their willingness to use the method correctly and consistently
   c. Whether the method is prescriptive or over-thecounter
   d. Whether the method is hormonal or a barrier method.
3. To practice natural family planning effectively, a woman must
   a. be able to communicate with her physician.
   b. purchase an ovulation kit.
   c. understand her menstrual cycle and fertile periods.
   d. abstain from any sexual contact for 6 to 8 days per month.
4. All but which of the following are considered barrier methods of birth control.
   a. Condom
   b. Diaphragm
   c. Vaginal sponge
   d. IUD
5. A woman who has trouble remembering dates and time periods would be wisest to choose which of the following methods of birth control?
   a. IUD
   b. Evra
   c. Birth control pill
   d. NuvaRing
6. Students who are concerned with protection against pregnancy and STDs would be wisest to use which form of birth control?
   a. The Evra patch
   b. NuvaRing
   c. Vaginal sponge
   d. Condom
7. Emergency contraception is effective up to ____ days after unprotected sexual intercourse.
   a. 3
   b. 5
   c. 1
   d. 10
8. A tubal ligation as a method of birth control might be an attractive choice to
   a. a single woman under 30 without children.
   b. a lesbian in a long-term relationship.
   c. a woman over 35 with children.
   d. a woman conflicted about motherhood.
9. Men who have had a vasectomy
   a. no longer ejaculate.
   b. no longer get erections.
   c. no longer have sperm in the ejaculate.
   d. no longer produce sperm.

10. The majority of women who terminate their pregnancies
    a. go on to experience posttraumatic stress disorders.
    b. do so in the first trimester of their pregnancies.
    c. rely on nonsurgical techniques such as oral medications.
    d. make the decision to do so around the 14th week of pregnancy.

Journal article

Hollander, D. (2003, January–February). Availability of emergency contraception through student health centers is growing, but gaps remain. Perspectives on Sexual and Reproductive Health, 35 (1), 54–55.

Web Resources

Alan Guttmacher Institute
www.guttmacher.org

A nonprofit institute protecting and expanding reproductive choices of women and men, including preventing unintended pregnancies, guaranteeing freedom to terminate unwanted pregnancies, protecting reproductive capacity and promoting wanted pregnancies, fostering women's health throughout pregnancy and childbirth, and promoting the birth of healthy infants. The site provides the latest statistics and the latest policy papers concerning these topics.

Feminist Women's Health Center (FWHC)
www.fwhc.org

A nonprofit organization that promotes and protects a woman's right to choose and receive reproductive health care, including keeping abortion safe, legal, accessible, and acceptable. Articles are accessible on women's health, birth control, abortion, breast cancer, menopause, and resources.

Birthright International
www.birthright.org

A support organization to girls and women who experience distress from unplanned pregnancy. Provides alternatives to abortion; free pregnancy tests; legal, medical, financial, and legal assistance; referral to social agencies; and maternity and baby clothes.

NARAL Pro Choice America
www. naral.org

This organization, previously known as NARAL (National Abortion and Reproductive Rights Action League), is a key political action and educational organization designed to promote reproductive freedom. Its specific mission has been

Successful Contraception
www.arhp.org

A site of the Association of Reproductive Health Professionals, an interdisciplinary group composed of professionals to track laws at the federal and state levels, educate voters, and keep legislators and the courts prochoice.

Planned Parenthood Federation of America (PPFA)
www.plannedparenthood.org

Planned Parenthood is both an advocacy group for reproductive rights as well as a major provider of reproductive health care services. It is also committed to providing comprehensive sexuality education.

American College of Obstetricians and Gynecologists
www.acog.com

The certifying organization of physicians who specialize in reproductive health. Its Web site provides information on birth control as well as providers.

References

Advocates for Youth. (2003). Contraceptive choices: Intrauterine device [Online]. Available: www.advocatesforyouth .org/teens/health/contraceptives/iud.htm.

Alan Guttmacher Institute. (2003, January). Nowhere but up: Rising costs for Title X clinics. *Issues in Brief, 1.*

American Psychiatric Association. (2000). *Diagnostic and statistical manual* (4th ed., text revision). Washington, DC: Author. 2), 75–84.

Christin-Maitre, S., Bouchard, P., &Spitz, M. (2000). Medical termination of pregnancy. The New England Journal of Medicine. 342 (13), 946–954.

Consumers Union. (2009, December). Seven of 20 condoms tested earned a perfect score: extra protection. Consumer Reports.

Cutie, C. & Dorgara, T. (2013). Vasectomy (beyond the basics). Patient information. Available: www.uptodate.com/contents/vasectomy-beyond-the-basics

Davis, C. Blank, J. Lin, H. & Bonillas, C. (1996). Characteristics of vibrator use among women. Journal of Sex Research, 33(4). 313–321.

Food and Drug Administration. (2003, September 5). FDA approves Seasonale oral contraceptive [Online]. FDA Talk Paper, T03-65. Available: www.fda.gov.

Guttmacher Institute (2011a, August). Facts on induced abortion in the United States. Available: http://www.guttmacher.org/pubs/fb-induced-abortion.html

Guttmacher Institute (2011b, January, 31). Comprehensive new study finds no causal link between abortion and mental health problems. Available : http://www.guttmacher.org/media/inthenews/2011/01031/index.html

Guttmacher Institute (2011, February 16). Title X–supported family planning services nationally in each state. Available: http://www.guttmacher.org

Hatcher, R. A., Trussel, J., Stewart, F.Nelson, A, Cates, W., Kowal, D. & Policar, M. (2011). *Contraceptive technology* (20th ed.). New York: Arden Media.

McDonough, P., (1995, September/October). The safest sex. Psychology Today, pp.47–49.

Murphy, R., & Allina, A. (2003, January/February). Improving access to emergency contraception. *Network News.*

Norris, K, (1996, September). Celibate passion. Utne Reader, pp.51–53.

Organon Inc. (2003). NuvaRing FAQs [Online]. Available: www.nuvaring.com/consumer/faqs.

Ortho-McNeil Pharmaceutical. (2003). Ortho Evra [Online]. Available: http://birthcontrol.orthoevra/faqs/faqs.html.

Piepert, J, Madden, T., Allsworth, J. &Secura, G. (2012). Obsterics & Gynecology. 120(6):1291–7.

Planned Parenthood Federation of America (2007). Emergency Contraception. [Online]. Available: www .plannedparenthood.org

Planned Parenthood Federation of America (2013). OrthoEvra. Available: www.plannedparenthood.org

Planned Parenthood Federation of America (2013). Contraceptive implants. Available: www.plannedparenthood.org

Planned Parenthood Federation of America (2013). Abortion. Available: www.plannedparenthood.org

Planned Parenthood Federation of America (2013). Essure. Available: www.plannedparenthood.org

Planned Parenthood Federation of America (2013). Contraceptive sponge. Available: www.plannedparenthood.org

VCF Contraceptive (2012). VCF contraceptive film. Available: VCFContraceptive.org

chapter

fifteen

Sexually Transmitted Diseases (STDs)

Student Learning Objectives

After reading this chapter, students will be able to

- Describe the major STD trends of the past decade.
- Diagram and describe the Pyramid of Risk for STD/HIV infection.
- Explain how demographic variables are related to STD/HIV risk.
- Describe how sexual orientation affects STD/HIV risk.
- Describe the characteristics of core transmitters of STD, including HIV.
- Evaluate the relationship between sexual/medical history and STD/ HIV risk.
- Assess a variety of sexual lifestyles and the continuum of risk for STD that they represent.
- Evaluate the risks inherent in a variety of sexual behaviors.
- Develop a personal plan for reducing the risk for STD/HIV infection.
- Describe the major modes of STD/HIV transmission.
- Describe the major symptoms associated with STD/HIV infection.
- Describe the epidemiology of a variety of STDs.

---

activity teaser: Why should you wait to have sex? Find out with the Personal Exploration Activity on page 548.

Introduction

Sexually transmitted diseases (STDs), also known as sexually transmitted infections (STIs), are infections that are almost always contracted through sexual contact. More than 110 million people in the United States are currently infected with a sexually transmitted disease (see table 15.1). Among those infected approximately 51,000,000 are men and 59,000,000 are women. Each year an additional 20 million people develop new cases of one or more of the 25 diseases categorized as STDs (CDC, 2013). Roughly half of the STD cases are incurable, lifelong infections (Division of STD Prevention (DSTD, 2011). STDs represent 87 percent of all of the cases of disease reported to the Centers for Disease Control and Prevention. It costs the US Healthcare System approximately 15.6 billion dollars to treat and manage the STD **epidemic** (CDC, 2013).

The STD epidemic is really a series of epidemics since we are really talking about over two dozen different types of infections, many of which are asymptomatic (without symptoms). Because of the asymptomatic nature of many STDs, many of those who are infected go undiagnosed (Fortenberry, 2002). This situation has led public health officials to refer to the problem as the "hidden epidemic" (DSTD, 2000). Tracking the hidden epidemic is difficult to do because individuals with asymptomatic diseases do not even know they are infected. Their infections go undiagnosed as they continue to infect others. In addition, not all STDs are reportable by law. Consequently, surveillance of these diseases by public health officials requires periodic surveys of health care providers to assess the full magnitude of the problem (DSTD, 2000).

Although STDs theoretically can be transmitted via any form of sexual contact, vaginal and anal intercourse are much more *efficient* modes of transmission than is oral-genital sexual contact. Some STDs, such as HIV and hepatitis B, also are transmitted by contaminated blood through needle sharing associated with injection drug use (Eng & Butler, 1997). Wasserheit

Table 15.1 Estimated Prevalence of the Most Common STDs

Disease	Estimated Prevalence*
Genital Warts (HPV)	79,100,000
Genital Herpes (HSV)	24,100,000
Trichomonal Vaginitis	3,710,000
Chlamydia	1,570,000
HIV(all stages)	908,000
Hepatitis B	422,000
Gonorrhea	270,000
Syphilis (all stages)	117,000
Total estimated cases	110,197,000

*included new and existing, reported and surveyed cases

Source: (CDC, 2013). National Center for HIV/AIDS, Viral Hepatitis, STD, and TB Prevention.

case study 15.1

Yolanda: Assessing the Risk

Yolanda, 22, single, identifies as Latina.

Yolanda, a student in a human sexuality class, expressed the following concerns about finding out about her sex partners' medical histories:

It looks like I'm going to have to spend a lot more time getting to know my sex partners before I take a chance of having sex with them without condoms. Up until today I thought I was a responsible lady because I'm on the pill and take responsibility for my sexuality. I always thought the pill would protect me against STDs. Boy, was I wrong. I never realized that there was so much to find out about a guy before you could tell if he was a threat to you.

I used to try to sneak a look to see if he had any symptoms, but now you're saying there are lots of other things that are important about his sexual past that I need to know about. I'm not sure what I'm going to do, but I know I'll never let any guy in there bareback until I can answer all those questions about him.

Critical Thinking

As Yolanda points out, reducing risk for acquiring an STD involves both personal action and understanding the risks posed by your partner. Understanding your partner's sexual lifestyle and medical history in order to make an informed decision regarding their STD threat is not an easy task. What specific steps would you take to find out about your partner's sexual lifestyle and medical history? How long do you think this process would take? How would this process impact your sexual activities with that person?

(1992) coined the term **epidemiological synergy** to refer to the effects of infection with one STD on the transmission of another. An example of this synergistic effect would be between a genital ulcer disease such as syphilis where the ulcerative lesions caused by the disease provide an entry point for HIV. Someone who has a genital ulcer and has sex with a person who is infected with HIV is more likely to become infected as a result (Rosen, 2003, Kassutto & Sigall, 2004).

Another problem associated with understanding and tracking STD trends relates to how they are tabulated and reported. STD statistics are generally presented as **rates** instead of raw numbers. Raw numbers represent the actual number of cases reported. Rates standardize the raw numbers of cases by factoring in the size of the population affected. This allows public health officials to analyze disease trends and compare the magnitude of the problem between one area and another.

The raw numbers of cases used to calculate rates come from reported cases or estimated cases. The reporting of some STDs such as Syphilis is required by law and tabulated by state and federal health authorities. The reporting of other STDs such as Genital Herpes is not required by law and disease data is obtained through national surveys of hospitals, private physicians, and other sources (Timreck, 2002). There are two types of rates: (a) **incidence rates,** which measure new cases and assess the risk of the spread of new cases of disease, and (b) **prevalence rates,** which measure the prevailing number of old and new cases and are a good barometer on the full impact of the condition as a public health problem. Acute infections that

Epidemiological synergy The distribution of disease caused by the effects of infection with more than one condition

Rates Statistics calculated by dividing the number of cases of disease by the population at risk of infection

Incidence rates Rates of new infection used to measure the likelihood of becoming infected

Prevalence rates Rates of prevailing infection used to measure the extent of the overall threat faced by the public

can be cured with antibiotics, such as syphilis, gonorrhea, and chlamydia, are typically reported and analyzed using incidence rates. Chronic diseases that can be treated but not cured such as HIV/AIDS, genital herpes, and genital warts (HPV) are often reported and analyzed using prevalence rates. (Weinstock, Berman, & Cates, 2004).

STD Transmission, Signs, and Symptoms

STDs can be grouped in several ways to study their transmission, symptoms, treatment, and prevention. Table 15.2 provides a summary of the transmission, symptoms, diagnosis, and treatment of the most common STDs. One simple way to group STDs is by the nature of transmission. The main modes of STD transmission are as follows:

- Direct sexual contact (sexual contact with someone's STD symptoms, such as genital ulcers) or sexual contact with someone's infected semen, vaginal lubricant, blood, and other body fluids
- Maternal transfer (mother to fetus during pregnancy or childbirth)
- Sharing contaminated needles through injectable drug use

Minor STDs, such as crabs and scabies, can be passed through direct sexual contact with infected persons or, in rare cases, their contaminated bedding, items of clothing, and similar objects. Some STDs (such as HIV and hepatitis B) can be spread both by sexual contact and by injectable drug use.

During sexual exposure to genital ulcers or other symptoms (such as genital warts), the uninfected person is exposed to infectious organisms that are present in the **serous fluid** of the lesions. During sexual contact, these pathogens are transmitted through the thrusting and grinding of sexual activity. The organisms are introduced into tiny breaks in the skin that commonly occur during sexual activity.

During sexual exposure to semen, vaginal lubricants, blood, and other body fluids, the infected partner passes the infection through unprotected vaginal or anal intercourse or oral sex. During sexual exposure to contaminated blood, STD organisms that live in the blood are passed between individuals as they exchange this body fluid. Blood is exchanged from person to person most commonly through (a) sexual contact with someone who has open lesions or ulcers that bleed during sex or (b) sexual contact that involves un-lubricated anal intercourse and some vaginal intercourse.

STD micro-organisms can be passed by maternal transfer two ways:

- During pregnancy, STD micro-organisms in the mother's blood pass through the placenta and enter the bloodstream of the fetus.
- During labor and delivery, the newborn is exposed directly to disease-causing germs present in the birth canal.

Any type of shared injectable drug use is capable of transmitting blood-borne STDs. The transmission could be by an athlete shooting steroids and then passing the unsterilized needle to a friend to use, or it could

Serous fluid A fluid that has the characteristics of serum

Table 15.2 Common STDs, Their Source, Symptoms, Diagnosis, and Treatment

Name	Source	Signs and Symptoms	Diagnosis	Treatment
Chlamydia	Bacterium	Male: Watery discharge; pain when urinating Female: Usually asymptomatic; sometimes a similar discharge to men's; leading cause of pelvic inflammatory disease (PID)	Men: Culture of discharge from urethra Female: Cervical culture	Antibiotics other than penicillin
Gonorrhea (clap)	Bacterium	Male: Pus discharge from urethra; burning during urination Female: Usually asymptomatic; can lead to PID and sterility in both men and women	Male: Culture of discharge Female: Cervical culture	Antibiotics (ceftriaxone)
Genital herpes	Virus	Blisters in genital and rectal area	Presence of blisters and laboratory identification of virus in fluid of blister	Zovirax (acyclovir prescription)
Venereal warts	Virus (HPV)	Cauliflower-like growths in genital and rectal areas	Presence of lesions	Removal of lesions by laser surgery or chemicals
Syphilis	Bacterium (spirochete)	Primary: Chancre Secondary: Rash Latent: Asymptomatic Late: Irreversible damage to central nervous system, cardiovascular system	Blood test	Penicillin or other antibiotic
HIV/AIDS	Virus	Asymptomatic at first; opportunistic infections	Blood test, usually none in initial stages	AZT (now called ZDV; not a cure)
Chancroid	Bacterium (*Bacillus*)	Male: Painful irregular chancre on penis Female: Chancre on labia	Smear/stain and microscopic identification	Tetracycline
Pubic lice (crabs)	Metazoan	Intense itching of areas covered with pubic hair	Presence of lice and nits (eggs) on pubic hair	Prescription or over-the-counter shampoo

be by a heroin addict doing the same. The risk is in the sharing, not the drug of choice.

In most cases, infestation with scabies and crabs occurs during sexual contact. A person whose genitals are infected with the lice pass on the crabs or scabies during sexual contact with an uninfected sex partner. Lice also are able to live on clothing and bedding and, in rare cases, can be spread via these inanimate objects.

Diagnosis, Treatment, and Epidemiology of Common STDs

The following section takes a more detailed look at several STDs. Specifically, we'll consider how they are diagnosed and treated and look at **epidemiological** issues around each one.

Genital Warts (HPV)

Diagnosis

Genital warts, also known as venereal warts, are caused by infection with the **human papilloma virus (HPV).** There are at least 46 known varieties of HPV. Of these, at least 12 types of the virus are associated with genital infection. The virus is spread through direct contact with an infected person's genital warts during sexual contact.

The average incubation period for genital warts is 3 months from the time of exposure. The initial warts can be isolated or appear in clusters on the genitals and perianal area. The warts vary in size from 1/8 inch to considerably larger, and in some cases growths become so large that they cause deformity of genital structures. Growths can **autoinnoculate** adjoining tissue. These "kissing lesions" are often found on the labia or under the foreskin of uncircumcised men. Infection with warts is not painful, but continued growth can cause a painful obstruction of the vaginal, anal, or urethral opening.

Estimates of infection with no symptoms vary from 10 to 45 percent of infected individuals. Most HPV infections are temporary, and symptoms resolve by the body's immune response. Although studies have shown that most cases of HPV are undetectable after 2 years, reactivation of the virus can occur (DSTD, 2013a), (Ho, Bierman, Beardsley, Chang, & Burk, 1998).

The major concern associated with HPV is the increased risk for cancer. Cervical infection with HPV is associated with at least 80 percent of all cervical cancer cases (Schiffman, 1992; Woodman et al., 2001). Women with HPV infection of the cervix are 10 times more likely to develop cervical cancer than women without the infection (Schiffman, 1992). As many as 10 percent of women with cervical HPV infections will develop **cervical intraepithelial neoplasms (CINs)** within 1 year. HPV types 16, 18, and 31 have been found in all types of genital cancers. HPV 16 is responsible for more than half of all cases of cervical cancer. Four HPV types, 16, 18, 31, and 45, account for 80 percent of all cervical cancer associated with HPV (Ciaran et al., 2003; DSTD, 2000).

Treatment

No medication is available to cure a person of asymptomatic HPV infection because it is a viral infection (DSTD, 2011a). Various forms of treatment, however, are used to treat genital warts. Factors that influence selection of treatment include wart size, wart number, anatomic site of the wart, patient preference, cost of treatment, convenience, adverse effects, and provider experience. The primary reason for treating genital warts is reduction of symptoms and ultimately, removal of the warts. Treatment regimens are classified into patient-applied and provider-applied medications. Patient-applied

---

Epidemiological Dealing with incidence, distribution, and control, as in STDs

Genital warts An STD caused by the HPV or human papilloma virus

Human papilloma virus (HPV) A condition spread through direct contact with an infected person's genital warts during sexual contact

Autoinnoculate To self inflict the spread of disease from one body part to another

Cervical intraepithelial neoplasms (CIN) Tumors or growths within the cervical membrane tissues

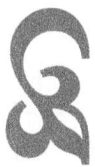

healthy sex hints 15.1

Making Sense of the HPV Vaccine

Deciding to get the HPV vaccine is a personal decision. The answers to the following questions will help you decide if it is the right decision for you.

What is the HPV vaccine?

On June 8, 2006, the FDA's Advisory Committee on Immunization Practice (ACIP) officially recommended the first vaccine designed to prevent Human Papiloma Virus (HPV) infection and reduce the risk for genital warts and cervical cancer. The vaccine, brand name, Gardasil®, protects against four types of HPV (types 6,11,16, & 18). Together, these four types of HPV cause about 70% of cervical cancers and 90% of genital warts in women. The vaccine does not offer protection against the remaining types of HPV. The vaccine is administered through a series of three shots over a 6-month period. The second and third doses ideally are administered 2 and 6 months after the first dose.

Who should get it?

HPV vaccines are routinely recommended for 11 and 12 year old girls and boys. Both vaccines are administered as a 3-dose series. The vaccine series can be started beginning at age 9 years. Vaccination is also recommended for 13 through 26 year-old females, and 13 through 21 year-old males who have not completed the vaccination series. Males aged 22 through 26 years may be vaccinated. HPV vaccine is also recommended for gay and bisexual men (or any man who has sex with men) and persons with compromised immune systems (including HIV) through age 26, if they did not get fully vaccinated when they were younger.

How long does it last?

Although the full duration of vaccine protection is not yet known, studies indicate that it is effective for at least five years. There is no evidence of any lessening of immunity during the five years following complete vaccination.

What does it cost?

The list price cost of the vaccine is $119.75 per dose or about $360 for the full series. Check with your health care provider for the actual cost as this may vary from the list price. Many states provide free or low-cost vaccines at public health department clinics to people without health insurance coverage for vaccines. Check with your state and local health department for availability of free clinics. While some insurance companies may cover the vaccine and cost of administration, others may not. Check with your insurance carrier for coverage.

Should I continue to get regular check-ups?

The HPV vaccine does not protect you against all forms of cervical cancer therefore you should continue to get your regular check up and cervical cancer screening test. National cervical cancer screening recommendations have not changed for females who receive the HPV vaccine.

Do I still need to practice safer sex?

If you are sexually active you should continue to practice the protective sexual behaviors (abstinence, monogamy, limiting the number of sex partners, using condoms etc.) discussed in this chapter and chapter 14. The HPV vaccine does not protect you against all HPV types and other sexually transmitted diseases.

Continues.

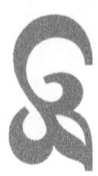 **healthy sex hints 15.1—Continued**

Making Sense of the HPV Vaccine

Does the HPV vaccine work for boys and men?

Experts do not yet know if the vaccine works for boys or men. Studies are now being conducted to test the vaccine in males. When more information is available, this vaccine may be licensed and recommended for boys and men as well.

Source: CDC (2012). HPV and HPV Vaccine - Information for Healthcare Providers. Available online at: http://www.cdc.gov/std/HPV/STDFact-HPV-vaccine-hcp.htm.

medications are preferred by some patients because they can be administered in the privacy of their own homes. To ensure that patient-applied modalities are effective, patients must comply with the treatment regimen and must be capable of identifying and reaching all genital warts.

Epidemiology

An estimated 79 million Americans are infected with HPV (CDC, 2013). Each year approximately 14 million new people are infected in the United States (DSTD, 2013a). Recent estimates, based on studies of diverse popu-

Table 15.3 Recommended Regimens for External Genital Warts

Patient-Applied:
Podofilox 0.5% solution or gel
OR
Imiquimod 5% cream
OR
Sinecatechins 15% ointment
Provider–Administered:
Cryotherapy with liquid nitrogen or cryoprobe. Repeat applications every 1–2 weeks.
OR
Podophyllin resin 10%–25% in a compound tincture of benzoin
OR
Trichloroacetic acid (TCA) or Bichloroacetic acid (BCA) 80%–90%
OR
Surgical removal either by tangential scissor excision, tangential shave excision, curettage, or electrosurgery.

Source: DSTD (2011b). Centers for Disease Control and Prevention, National Center for HIV/AIDS, Viral Hepatitis, STD, and TB Prevention, Division of STD Prevention

lations ranging from adolescent high school girls and female students attending college health centers to STD clinic patients, indicate that approximately 1 percent of all Americans are infected with HPV (Moscicki et al., 2000; DSTD 2000). Women and individuals in the 20- to 24-year-old age bracket constitute the bulk of the visits. Routine testing of women for HPV in four locations yielded the following infectivity percentages; between 9 percent and 45 percent of women attending health services in a university health center had positive test results; 23 percent of women attending family planning clinics were positive; 82 percent of street prostitutes in a select study had the virus (Quinn & Cates, 1993).

Moscicki et al. (2000) found that over 50 percent of adolescent girls who were HIV-positive and over 30 percent of those who were HIV-negative

The genital warts associated with HPV infection can get large enough to block the openings of the urethra, vagina or anus. *Source:* Centers for Disease Control and Prevention, National Center for HIV/AIDS, Viral Hepatitis, STD, and TB Prevention, Division of STD Prevention

tested positive for HPV. HPV may become an even more serious problem among HIV-infected persons than other groups. These individuals have a greater susceptibility to precancerous lesions on the cervix (among heterosexual women) and anus (among gay men) than their non-HIV-infected peers. In one HIV study of gay men, HPV infection was found in 60 percent of those who were HIV-negative and almost 100 percent of those who were HIV-positive (DSTD, 2000).

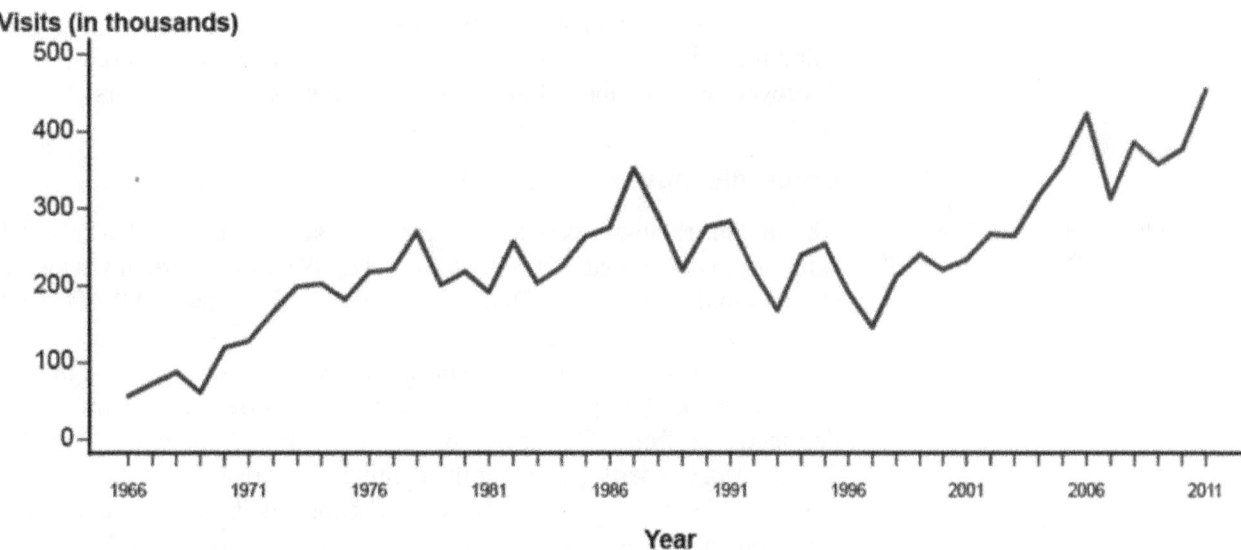

Genital Warts—Initial Visits to Physicians' Offices, United States, 1966–2011

Figure 15.1 *Genital Warts Consultations* The number of visits to physicians for genital warts has increased steadily in the past decade.

Source: DSTD (2012a). Centers for Disease Control and Prevention, National Center for HIV/AIDS, Viral Hepatitis, STD, and TB Prevention, Division of STD Prevention

Chlamydia

Diagnosis

Chlamydia is a sexually transmitted disease caused by the *Chlamydia trachomatis* organism. It is transmitted through contact with infected semen or cervical mucus. It also can be passed through oral contact (usually fellatio) with infected mucus patches in the throat.

During sexual contact, the organisms are passed by person-to-person contact with the infected ejaculate or mucus. Incubation is from 1 to 30 days. The initial symptoms of chlamydia in men are a scanty, clear to milky-white discharge from the penis, and burning upon urination. Some women notice a scanty, clear to milky-white discharge and irritation of the vulva. Seventy-five percent of women and 50 percent of men usually have no symptoms for chlamydia. This is why screening sexually active women and their sex partners for chlamydia in a variety of health care facilities that serve them is the basis for the government's prevention program for the disease.

In the 1960s and 1970s, chlamydia infection was believed to be a relatively minor problem. Men with the infection were often referred to as having "nonspecific urethritis" and were not counseled extensively regarding the necessity to have their sexual partners examined. Chlamydia, however, was discovered to be a major source of **PID** (pelvic inflammatory disease). Up to 20 percent of all women with *C. trachomatis* infection will develop PID. PID can result in chronic pain, ectopic pregnancy, and sterility, and in rare instances it is fatal. More than half of all PID is caused by *C. trachomatis*. Infection in men rarely leads to major complications. Less than 1 percent of men infected with *C. trachomatis* develop epididymitis (Morse et al., 1990).

Treatment

Chlamydia infection is relatively easy to treat. Azithromycin (1 gram, taken orally in a single dose) or doxycycline (100 milligrams, taken orally twice a day for 7 days) are the two recommended treatments. The organism is destroyed by a number of antibiotics and alternative treatments (DSTD 2011c).

Epidemiology

Chlamydia trachomatis is the most prevalent sexually transmitted bacterial pathogen in the United States. In 2011, 1,412,791 cases of chlamydia were reported to the Centers for Disease control from 50 states and the District of Columbia (DSTD, 2012c). The chlamydia rate for 2012 was 457.6 cases per 100,000 persons. This represents an increase of 8.0% from the rate of 423.6 in 2010. During 1991–2011, the rate of reported chlamydial infection increased from 179.7 to 457.6 cases per 100,000 population (DSTD, 2012c). Most experts agree that the continuing increase in reported cases of chlamydia is due to increased screening for this infection and also the development and use of more sensitive screening tests (DSTD, 2012c). Figure 15.2 shows the rapid climb in rates during the years 1991-2011.

Chlamydia rates continue to rise and represent a serious disease threat because of the asymptomatic nature of infection (DSTD, 2012c). Seventy-five percent of women and 50 percent of men usually have no symptoms

PID The acronym for *pelvic inflammatory disease,* a generic term that can apply to any STD that produces the characteristic symptoms of infection

Chlamydia trachomatis The most prevalent sexually transmitted bacterial pathogen, causing the STD chlamydia

Chlamydia—Rates by Sex, United States, 1991–2011

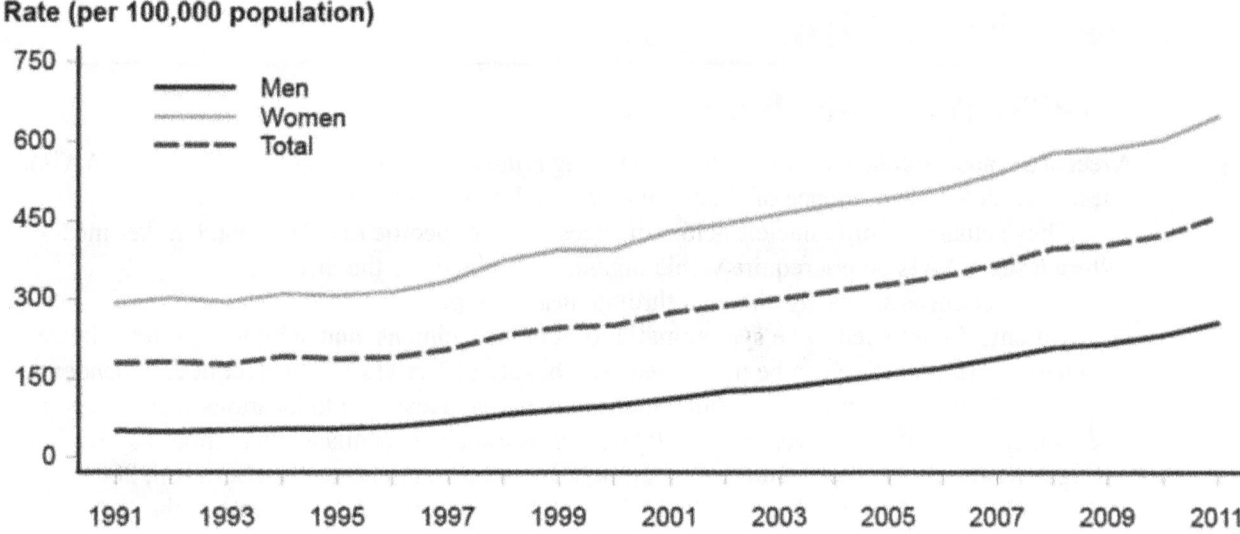

Figure 15.2 *Chlamydia Morbidity* The number of new cases of chlamydia infection in men and women continues to rise every year.

Source: DSTD (2012d). Centers for Disease Control and Prevention, National Center for HIV/AIDS, Viral Hepatitis, STD, and TB Prevention, Division of STD Prevention.

for chlamydia. This is why screening sexually active women (and their sex partners) for chlamydia in a variety of health care facilities that serve them is the basis for the government's prevention program for the disease. Most public STD and family planning clinics routinely screen all gonorrhea patients for infection with chlamydia trachomatis, since roughly 50 percent of all gonorrhea patients have coexistent infection with chlamydia. In 2011, the overall rate of reported chlamydial infection among women in all 50 states and the District of Columbia (648.9 cases per 100,000 females) was over two and a half times the rate among men (256.9 cases per 100,000 males), a reflection of the nation's commitment to screening women for this infection (DSTD, 2012c). Chlamydia rates by race/ethnicity show a slightly lower rate for whites than for all other racial/ethnic groups. As with many STDs, rates are highest in the South than in other regions (DSTD, 2012c; Karon et al., 2001; Guaschino & DeSeta, 2000).

Genital Herpes Infection

Diagnosis

Genital herpes infection is caused by exposure to the herpes simplex virus type 1 (HSV 1) or herpes simplex virus type 2 (HSV 2) through sexual contact. HSV 1 initially was associated with oral infection and HSV 2 with genital infection. Over the past 25 years, however, the increased popularity of oral sex has led to an almost equal probability of contracting either form from the genital area.

Genital herpes An infection caused by exposure to the herpes simplex virus type 1 or type 2 through sexual contact

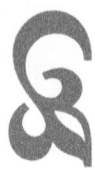

healthy sex hints 15.2

NAATs: Tests for Chlamydia

A recent advance in chlamydia and gonorrhea testing is the nucleic acid amplification tests (NAATs). These tests detect the presence of chlamydia through DNA testing.

They actually identify nucleic acid sequences that are specific to chlamydia. Unlike smear or culture tests, NAATs do not require viable organisms to diagnose the disease.

The specimens are easily obtained through urine samples.

Patients do not need to be symptomatic to obtain specimens, and samples can be collected anywhere urine collection can be performed. The beauty of NAATs is that it reduces dependence on invasive tests and allows public health programs to expand testing into locations such as schools where other means of testing were unacceptable. A classic study in a Philadelphia school-based clinic setting demonstrated a yield of more than 20 percent among students tested (Bertrami, 2002).

Another advantage of NAATs is their ability to test for gonorrhea infection at the same time using the same specimen. The same Philadelphia study found that almost half of students infected with chlamydia had coexistent gonorrhea infection. These gonorrhea infections would often go undetected with traditional tests that only checked for chlamydia. The ability to test for both infections simultaneously using an easy-to-obtain urine specimen represents a major breakthrough in STD testing and a major tool in the prevention of gonorrhea and chlamydia (MMWR, 2002).

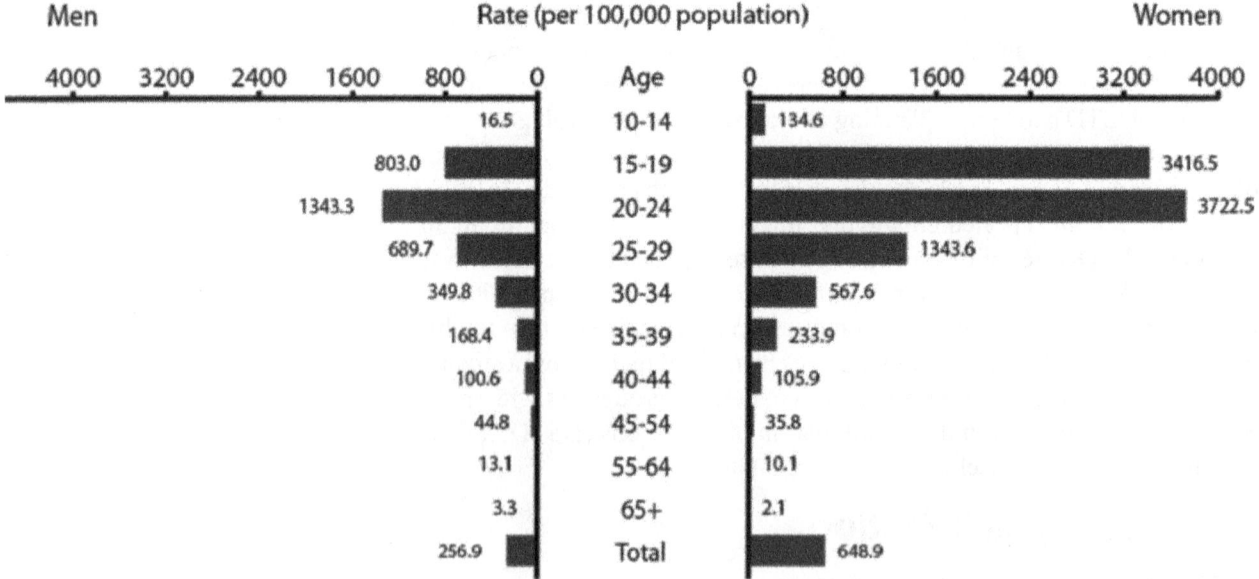

Figure 15.3 *Chlamydia—Rates by Age and Sex, United States, 2011*

Source: DSTD (2012e). Centers for Disease Control and Prevention, National Center for HIV/AIDS, Viral Hepatitis, STD, and TB Prevention, Division of STD Prevention.

A 2- to 12-day incubation period follows transmission of the virus. The initial symptoms (also known as the primary outbreak) start as discrete grouped **vesicles.** After a short time (a few hours to a few days), the vesicles break open, merge with each other, and form painful ulcers, which drain and crust over. The entire first episode takes 15 to 20 days. Often, a systemic, flulike syndrome accompanies the primary outbreak. The symptoms of this syndrome, known as the **prodrome,** include aches, fever, and malaise.

Vesicles Fluid-filled blisters

Prodrome A systemic, flulike syndrome that accompanies genital herpes infection

Recurring outbreaks occur in most sufferers on an average of five to eight times per year and last approximately 10 days per episode. Recurrences often are preceded by the same prodromal syndrome that accompanies the primary episode. The frequency and severity of recurring episodes diminish with time.

Genital herpes in adults tends to be a self-limiting, albeit painful, STD. It is a much more serious condition among newborns (infected as they pass through the birth canal) and those whose immune systems are compromised because of HIV infection (DSTD, 2013b).

Treatment

Genital HSV infection has no cure but can be managed successfully with the use of antiviral drugs. Advances in antiviral therapies, such as acyclovir, have made drugs available that shorten the duration of outbreaks and reduce the number and likelihood of recurrent episodes. Treatment regimens differentiate between initial outbreaks and recurrent episodes of the disease. Table 15.4 describes the recommended treatment for initial outbreaks.

Systemic antiviral drugs such as acyclovir can also be used as daily suppressive therapy (suppress the likelihood of an outbreak) for the prevention of recurrent outbreaks. Suppressive therapy reduces the frequency of genital herpes recurrences by 70%–80% in patients who have frequent recurrences. Treatment also is effective in patients with less frequent recurrences. Safety and efficacy have been documented among patients receiving daily therapy with acyclovir for as long as 6 years and with valacyclovir or famciclovir for 1 year (DSTD. 2011d). Table 15.5 describes the recommended suppressive therapy for recurrent outbreaks.

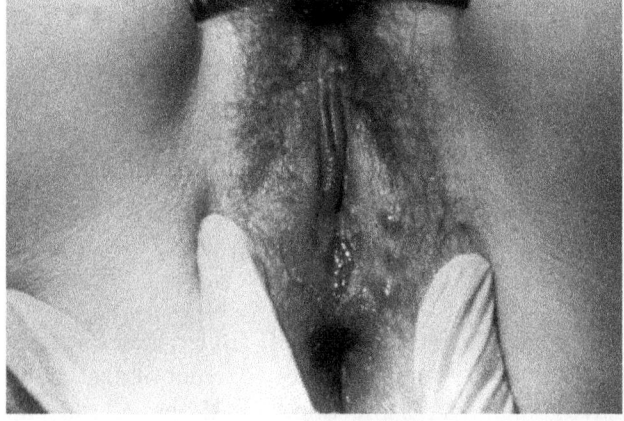 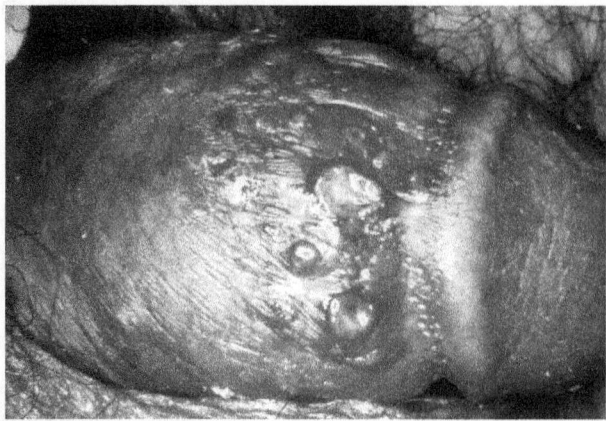

The primary symptoms of herpes are fluid-filled vesicles that break open to form painful, highly infectious ulcers. *Source:* Centers for Disease Control and Prevention; Division of STD Prevention

Table 15.4 Antiviral Treatment for Initial Genital HSV Infection

Recommended Regimens*
Acyclovir 400 mg orally three times a day for 7–10 days
OR
Acyclovir 200 mg orally five times a day for 7–10 days
OR
Famciclovir 250 mg orally three times a day for 7–10 days
OR
Valacyclovir 1 g orally twice a day for 7–10 days

*Treatment can be extended if healing is incomplete after 10 days of therapy.

Source: DSTD (2011d). Centers for Disease Control and Prevention, National Center for HIV/AIDS, Viral Hepatitis, STD, and TB Prevention, Division of STD Prevention

Table 15.5 Antiviral Treatment for Suppressive Therapy

Recommended Regimens*
Acyclovir 400 mg orally twice a day
OR
Famiciclovir 250 mg orally twice a day
OR
Valacyclovir 500 mg orally once a day*
OR
Valacyclovir 1 g orally once a day

* Valacyclovir 500 mg once a day might be less effective than other valacyclovir or acyclovir dosing regimens in patients who have very frequent recurrences (i.e., ≤10 episodes per year).

Source: DSTD (2011d). Centers for Disease Control and Prevention, National Center for HIV/AIDS, Viral Hepatitis, STD, and TB Prevention, Division of STD Prevention

As with the other viral STDs, most treatment regimens focus on slowing the replication of the virus and boosting the immune system. Treatment also includes techniques to speed drying and healing of the vesicles and blisters associated with the infection.

Epidemiology

It is estimated that, annually, 776,000 people in the United States get new herpes infections. About 16.2%, or approximately one out of six, people aged 14 to 49 years have genital HSV-2 infection. Over the past decade, the percentage of persons with genital herpes infection in the United States has remained stable (DSTD, 2013b). Initial consultations with private physi-

Genital Herpes—Initial Visits to Physicians' Offices, United States, 1966–2011

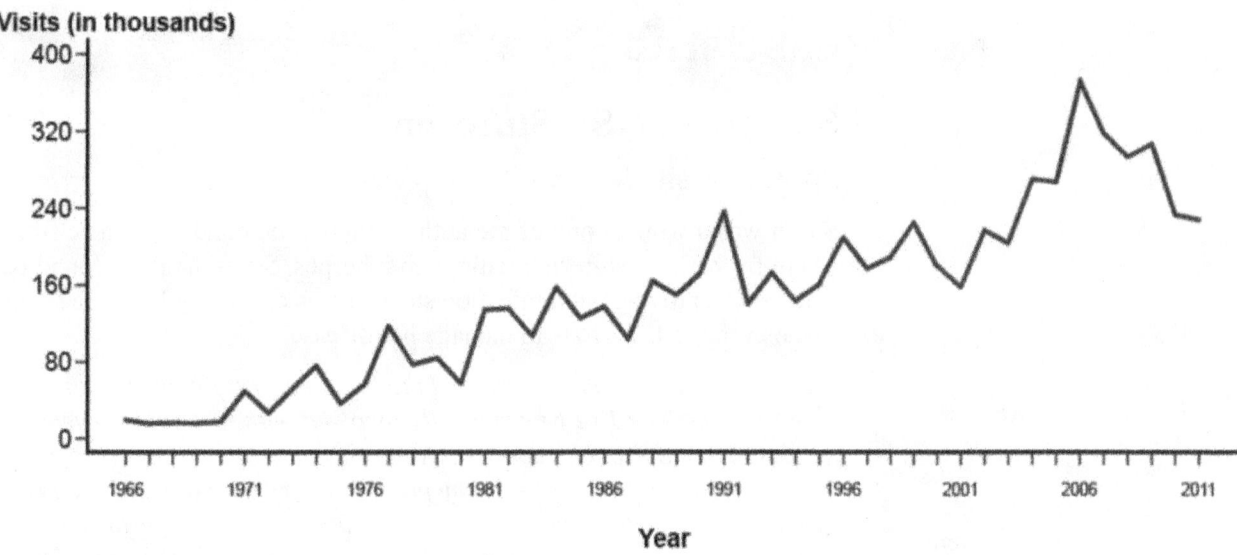

Figure 15.4 *The number of visits to physicians for genital herpes has increased significantly over the past 40 years.*

Source: (DSTD 2012d). Centers for Disease Control and Prevention, National Center for HIV/AIDS, Viral Hepatitis, STD, and TB Prevention, Division of STD Prevention

cians for genital herpes increased from fewer than 25,000 in 1996 to about 350,000 in 2006. Consultations then dropped and have stabilized since 2011 (see Figure 15.4) (DSTD,2012b) The majority of those infected do not have clinical disease. Women are at a greater risk than men for acquiring the infection. It is suggested that this is due to the greater efficiency of male to female transmission (DSTD, 2013b).

HIV/AIDS

Diagnosis

AIDS represents the end stage of **HIV.** Figure 15.5 traces the natural progression of HIV infection. As you can see, AIDS can develop within 2 years of exposure but typically takes longer. HIV infection is caused by person-to-person transmission of the human immunodeficiency virus.

The most common modes of transmission are (a) sexual contact (vaginal or anal intercourse are most efficient), (b) sharing contaminated needles (through injecting drug use), and (c) maternal-to-fetal transfer. Once the virus has been transmitted, it enters the bloodstream, where it incubates from 8 weeks to 6 months, when it will show positive on a blood test.

A person who elects to take a blood test for HIV is given a screening test, called the *ELISA* (enzyme-linked immunosorbent assay), which detects the presence of antibodies to the HIV. If this test is negative, the person is counseled to come back for a second ELISA in a few months, to make sure the maximum incubation period has elapsed. If a person tests positive on the initial ELISA, he or she is given a second test, called the *Western blot,* to confirm infection. If this test comes back positive, the person is diagnosed as having HIV infection. Besides taking a traditional blood test OraSure

AIDS The acronym for *acquired immunodeficiency syndrome,* the end result of HIV infection

HIV The acronym for *human immunodeficiency virus,* the infection that leads to AIDS

case study 15.2

Susan, an HSV Sufferer

Susan, 23, single, is white.

Susan was a woman one of the authors met while conducting a self-help group for persons suffering with genital herpes. Susan had just found out that the ulcerative genital infection she had was caused by HSV. She came to the group to learn how to manage her disease.

I was shocked when my doctor told me I had herpes. I couldn't figure out how I got it, since I've been sexually involved with just my boyfriend for the past 6 months and he doesn't have any symptoms.

The doctor explained that my present boyfriend might not even have given it to me. [The doctor] explained that since I had several other sex partners since beginning to have intercourse at 19 years old, any of those guys could have given it to me. He said I might not have had any initial symptoms or might have missed them because they were so mild.

Now, because I've been stressed out—a new job, graduate school, getting engaged, moving into a house—the herpes is coming back. He suggested that I come here and learn about how to cope with it if I keep getting recurrences. I'm so stressed, but I know this is also the worst thing for me if I want to help my body keep it under control. Please help me!

Critical Thinking

What makes the potential transmission of a past viral condition such as herpes different from a past bacterial infection such as gonorrhea?

Opportunistic infection An infection that is able to develop as a result of the body's weakened immune status

Technologies has developed a mouth swab that can be administered at home and provides results in 20 minutes. A positive result with this test does not mean that a person is definitely infected with HIV, but rather that this test should be followed up with a confirmatory Western blot test performed in a medical setting (OraSure, 2012).

HIV infection is essentially a disorder of the immune system. The virus weakens the body's immune system, making the person susceptible to other infections and chronic diseases. These are called **opportunistic infections** because they take advantage of the body's weakened state to attack and cause disease. When people with a fully functioning immune system come in contact with opportunistic organisms, they normally repel them.

People with HIV cannot fight off opportunistic infections and eventually die from them. Most people with HIV infection are completely free of symptoms for more than 10 years. Others deteriorate rapidly and develop symptoms and AIDS within 2 to 4 years.

Early symptoms of HIV infection stem from infections that begin to invade the body because of its weakened immune status. When the immune system begins to fail, the following symptoms begin to occur: fatigue, diarrhea, fever, night sweats, skin rashes, sudden weight loss, dry cough, swollen lymph nodes, and vaginal yeast infection. These symptoms can be present for weeks, months, or even years without opportunistic infections taking hold.

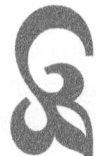

healthy sex hints 15.3

Self-Help for People with Genital Herpes

Most people with genital herpes are able to manage their infections and prevent spreading their infection to others.

The following tips will help you do just that.

1. If you are taking acyclovir or other herpes medication on a maintenance schedule and it helps reduce recurring episodes of infection, continue taking the medicine as prescribed.
2. At the first hint of prodromal symptoms, consider yourself infectious and capable of spreading your infection. During this time, abstain from intercourse, engage in non-genital sexual pleasuring, or use condoms.
3. Treat any outbreak as you would the flu (another viral infection), with bed rest and over-the-counter pain relievers.
4. Keep your genitals clean and dry. Take short baths, pat your genitals with a towel, and use a hair dryer to dry the area thoroughly.
5. Avoid pantyhose, tight underwear, and binding clothes until the blisters crust over and dry up. If you can, take a day or two off during the worst symptoms, stay in bed, and avoid wearing clothes.
6. Do not cover the blisters with petroleum jelly or other cream that blocks air from drying the area.
7. Minimize stress, as it delays healing.

With treatment, many people with HIV can prevent these symptoms from ever occurring. And aggressive treatment can return symptomatic individuals to a symptom-free state. Although the medication doesn't kill the virus, it slows or stops viral replication and thereby boosts **immunocompetence.** If an opportunistic infection does take hold, the person moves from being infected with HIV to being diagnosed as having AIDS. In 1993, the CDC broadened the definition of AIDS to include 26 opportunistic infections. Infection with any one of these combined with being HIV-positive leads to a diagnosis of AIDS.

Immunocompetence The level of efficiency of the immune system

Mortality The number of deaths during a specific time period

Treatment

In recent years, potent combination antiretroviral therapies (ART) have been developed that have altered the landscape of HIV/AIDS treatment. Antiretroviral therapies, typically consisting of three or more antiretroviral (ARV) drugs, have greatly improved the health and survival rates of people infected with HIV. More than 20 individual ARVs in six different classes are available in the United States. These can be combined to construct a number of effective treatment regimens tailored to individual patients. In past years, many of the available ARVs presented problems related to issues such as adverse effects, pill quantity, and dosing frequency. Given these issues, much attention was devoted to estimating the point at which the potential benefits of ART outweighed the potential risks of ART. Today, the newer ARV regimens are for most patients, simple, tolerable, and effective.

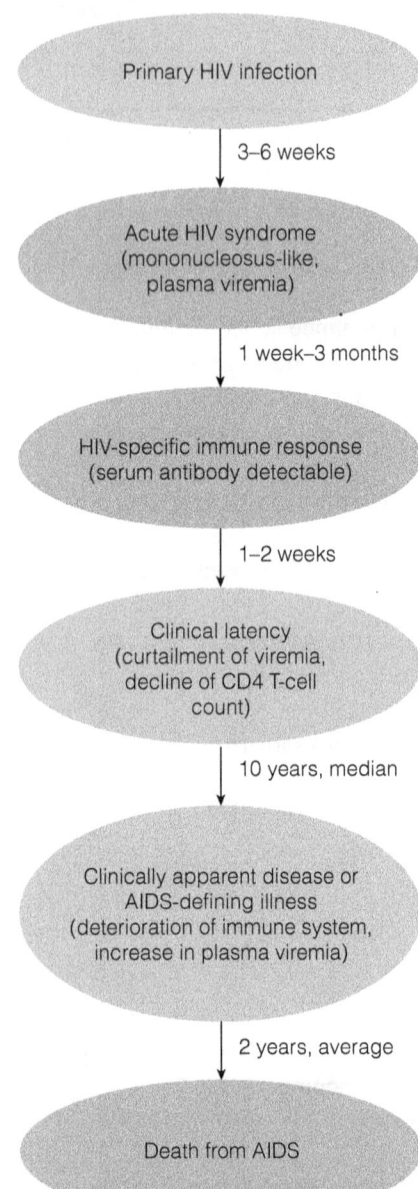

Primary HIV infection

↓ 3–6 weeks

Acute HIV syndrome
(mononucleosus-like,
plasma viremia)

↓ 1 week–3 months

HIV-specific immune response
(serum antibody detectable)

↓ 1–2 weeks

Clinical latency
(curtailment of viremia,
decline of CD4 T-cell
count)

↓ 10 years, median

Clinically apparent disease or
AIDS-defining illness
(deterioration of immune system,
increase in plasma viremia)

↓ 2 years, average

Death from AIDS

Figure 15.5 *The Natural History of HIV* It may take several years for a person infected with HIV to develop AIDS.

As a result of both the availability of ARV regimens that are less toxic and easier to administer, and the increasing appreciation of the adverse impacts of untreated HIV, most HIV experts recommend earlier initiation of treatment, and many recommend ART for all people infected with the virus unless there are compelling reasons not to treat (Coffey, 2011).

HIV/AIDS treatment is not a cure. The multitude of new combination antiretroviral therapies do not kill all of the HIV, as antibiotics kill bacteria. Antiviral therapy prevents or slows the unchecked replication and growth of HIV, helping the infected person's immune system keep the virus in check. This prevents the person from contracting opportunistic infections. Other treatments focus on killing the opportunistic infections that take hold (DHAP, 2013). It is beyond the scope of this textbook to describe the more than 20 forms of antiretroviral therapy in six classes that are currently available in the United States. The current treatment options allow persons infected with HIV to live longer and more productive lives. In a sense, HIV has become more of a chronic disease as evidenced in the declining death rate for AIDS.

Epidemiology

Since initial AIDS reporting began in 1981, the Division of HIV/AIDS Prevention (DHAP) at the Centers for Disease Control and Prevention (CDC) has developed a comprehensive program of HIV surveillance to collect, analyze, and disseminate data on HIV infection and AIDS. Through HIV surveillance, DHAP monitors many facets of the trends in HIV in the United States. By 1986, all 50 states, the District of Columbia, and several U.S. dependent areas had instituted AIDS case reporting. Beginning in 1985, many states implemented HIV case reporting as part of an integrated HIV and AIDS surveillance system. As of 2008, all states had implemented confidential, name-based HIV reporting (DHAP 2013).

CDC estimates that 1,148,200 persons aged 13 years and older are living with HIV infection. Over the past decade, the number of people living with HIV has increased, while the estimated annual number of new HIV infections has remained relatively stable at about 50,000 new HIV infections per year (see Figure 15.6). Two groups, men who have sex with men (MSM) and African Americans continue to represent the greatest number of new cases of HIV infection (DHAP, 2013).

Although MSM represented about 4% of the male population in the United States in 2010, this group accounted for 78% of new HIV infections among males and 63% of all new infections. MSM accounted for 52% of all people living with HIV infection in 2009, the most recent year these data are available. African Americans continue to experience the most severe burden of HIV, compared with other races and ethnicities. African Americans represent approximately 12% of the U.S. population, but accounted for an estimated 44% of new HIV infections in 2010. They also accounted for 44% of people living with HIV infection in 2009, the most recent year these data are available (DHAP, 2013).

Heterosexuals accounted for 25% of estimated new HIV infections in 2010 and 27% of people living with HIV infection in 2009 the most recent year these data are available (DHAP, 2013). New HIV infections among women are primarily attributed to heterosexual contact (84% in 2010) or injection drug use (16% in 2010). Women accounted for 20% of estimated new HIV infections in 2010 and 24% of those living with HIV infection in 2009. The 9,500 new infections among women in 2010 reflect a significant 21% decrease from the 12,000 new infections that occurred among this group in 2008 (DHAP, 2013).

The number of AIDS deaths has been steadily declining since 1996. The decline in AIDS deaths is consistent across all regions and all risk groups and can be attributed mostly to the success of the newest generation of AIDS medications. The lowered AIDS death rate has resulted in more people with AIDS surviving the disease than at any time in the past. Lowering the death rate resulted in a slight increase in the prevalence of the condition as more existing cases add into the new cases each year (ONAP, 2010).

Gonorrhea

Diagnosis

Gonorrhea infection is very similar to Chlamydia clinically. Following sexual exposure, the organism incubates from 1 to 30 days. Most people who develop symptoms notice them within 1 to 3 days. The initial symptoms are the same as those associated with Chlamydia. Discharge and burning upon

Gonorrhea A sexually transmitted disease caused by the bacteria *Neisseria gonorrheae*

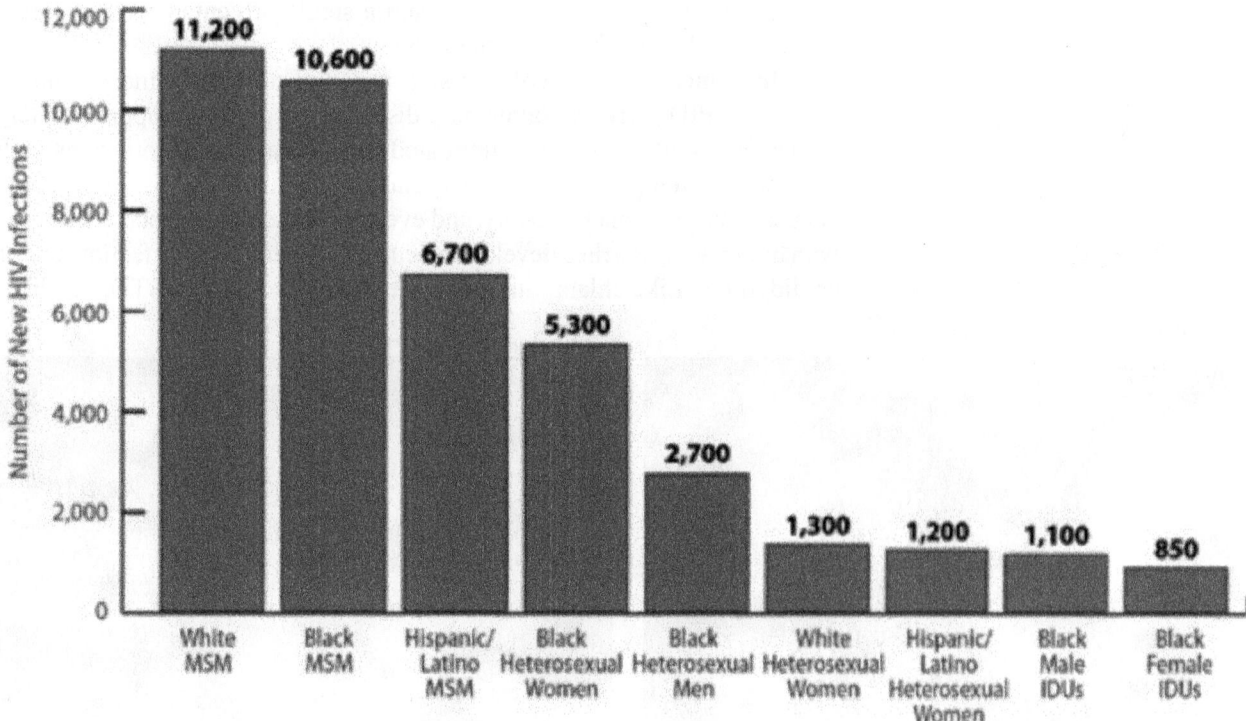

Figure15.6 *Estimated New HIV Infections in the United States, 2010, for the Most Affected Subpopulations*

Source: DHAP (2013). Centers for Disease Control and Prevention, National Center for HIV/AIDS, Viral Hepatitis, STD, and TB Prevention, Division of HIV/AIDS Prevention

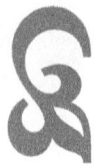

healthy sex hints 15.4

Should You Take the AIDS Test?

The question about whether to get tested for HIV has concerned many individuals. Where HIV infection and AIDS are concerned, clouds of fear, suspicion, and misunderstanding still loom large in many communities. Fears of being ostracized by family and friends, being kicked out of school, or losing a job have kept many people who suspect exposure to HIV from being tested. In some cases, people simply cannot face the possibility of a positive test and do not want to know.

If you are considering having a screening test for HIV, keep these tips in mind:

- Take your test anonymously in an alternative-site facility where you will be given a number and your name will not be used (some facilities do confidential, not anonymous, testing).
- Make sure the testing site does counseling before and after the test.
- Many college health centers offer HIV testing. Students can also get tested through Planned Parenthood, health departments, and other facilities specifically designed for HIV/STD testing.

urination are the most common symptoms in men. Gonorrhea symptoms—heavy discharge, yellowish-green in color, and severe burning are usually are more severe than those associated with Chlamydia. The symptoms usually are enough to cause men with the infection to seek treatment. Up to 20 percent of men have no symptoms. About 50 percent of women infected with gonorrhea are asymptomatic, and a small percentage will notice a discharge or have irritation of the vulva.

In women, gonorrhea often results in complications, the most common of which is PID (pelvic inflammatory disease)—occurring in approximately 15 percent of all women with untreated gonorrhea. These women, as with those who develop PID from chlamydia, have an increased risk for chronic pain, ectopic pregnancy, sterility, and even death. Less than 1 percent of men with untreated gonorrhea develop disseminated gonococcal infection and/or epididymitis. Like chlamydia, gonorrhea is easy to treat (DSTD, 2013c).

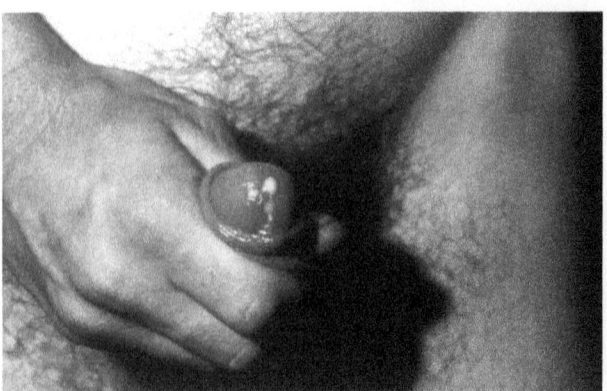
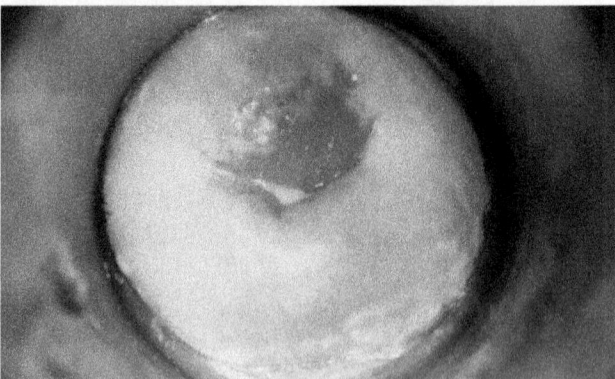

Gonorrhea infection typically produces a profuse, thick, yellow-green discharge, but it can also mimic the milder symptoms of chlamydia. Infection in the cervix, throat, or rectum is often asymptomatic.

Source: Centers for Disease Control and Prevention, Division of STD Prevention

Treatment

Increases in drug-resistant strains of gonorrhea, particularly those acquired in Asia or the Pacific, including Hawaii, require have treatment regimens be changed to inhibit the development of antibiotic resistant strains of *N. gonorrhoeae*. Patients infected with *N. gonorrhoeae* frequently are co-infected with *C. trachomatis;* this finding has led to the recommendation that patients treated for gonococcal infection also be treated routinely with a regimen that is effective against uncomplicated chlamydial infection. Because most gonococci in the United States are susceptible to doxycycline and azithromycin, routine co-treatment might also hinder the development of antimicrobial-resistant *N. gonorrhoeae* (DSTD, 2011e).

Epidemiology

Gonorrhea is one of the most common STDs. There were 321,849 cases of gonorrhea reported to the CDC in 2011 (DSTD, 2013c). Because it can be easily diagnosed clinically in a physician's office, public health officials estimate that gonorrhea might be underreported by as much as 50 percent. CDC estimates that approximately 820,000 people annually are infected with gonorrhea (DSTD, 2013c).

From 1975–1997, the national gonorrhea rate declined 74% after implementation of the national gonorrhea control program in the mid-1970s. In 2009 gonorrhea rates decreased further to 98.1 cases per 100,000, the

Table 15.6 Treatment of Uncomplicated Gonococcal Infections of the Cervix, Urethra, and Rectum

Recommended Regimen
Ceftriaxone 250 mg in a single intramuscular dose
PLUS
Azithromycin 1 g orally in a single dose
or doxycycline 100 mg orally twice daily for 7 days*
Alternative Regimens
If ceftriaxone is not available:
Cefixime 400 mg in a single oral dose
PLUS
Azithromycin 1 g orally in a single dose
or doxycycline 100 mg orally twice daily for 7 days*
PLUS
Test-of-cure in 1 week
If the patient has severe cephalosporin allergy:
Azithromycin 2 g in a single oral dose
PLUS
Test-of-cure in 1 week (DSTD, 2011 e).

Source: (DSTD, 2011e). Centers for Disease Control and Prevention, National Center for HIV/AIDS, Viral Hepatitis, STD, and TB Prevention, Division of STD Prevention

Gonorrhea—Rates, United States, 1941–2011

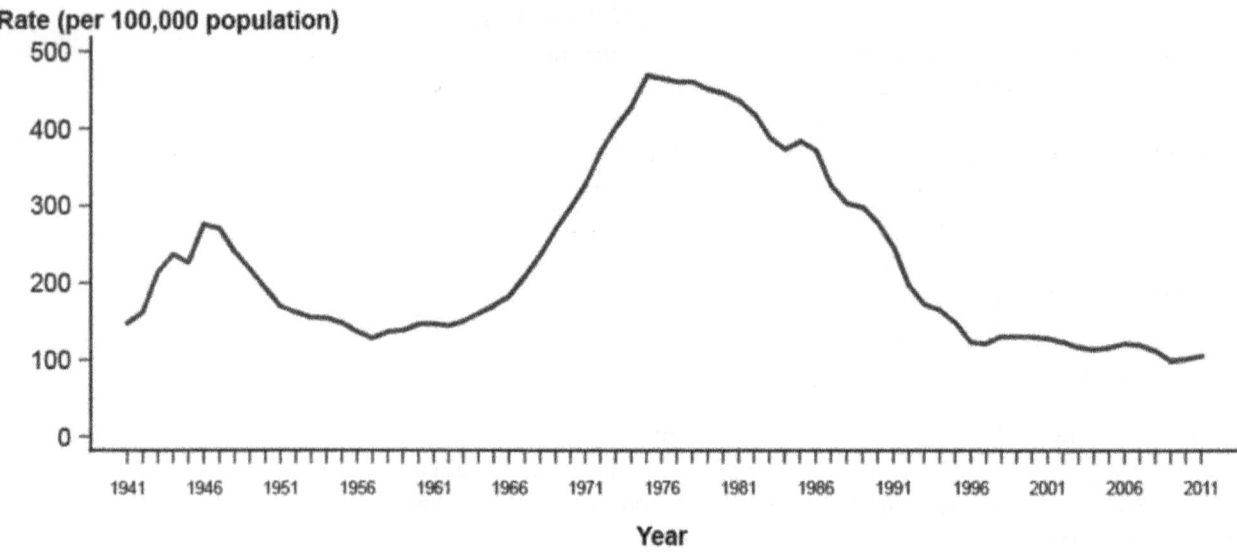

Figure 15.7 *Gonorrhea rates have leveled off since 1996.*

Source: DSTD (2012g). Centers for Disease Control and Prevention, National Center for HIV/AIDS, Viral Hepatitis, STD, and TB Prevention, Division of STD Prevention

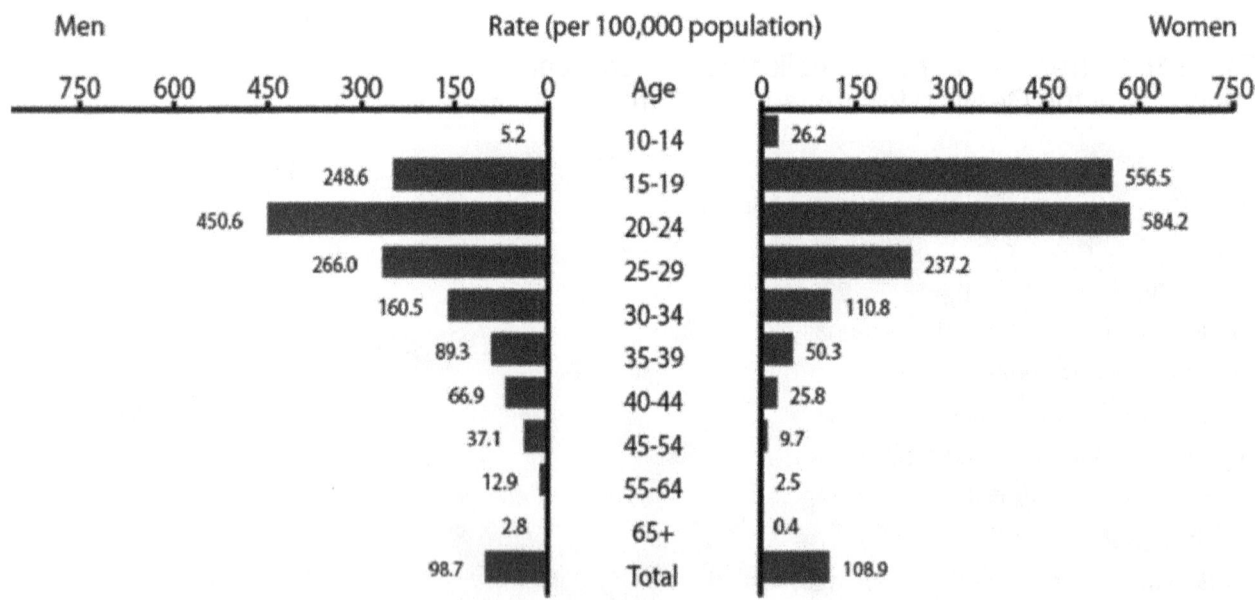

Figure 15.8 *Gonorrhea rates by Age and Gender*

Source: (DSTD 2012h). Centers for Disease Control and Prevention, National Center for HIV/AIDS, Viral Hepatitis, STD, and TB Prevention.

lowest rate since recording of gonorrhea rates began (see Figure 15.7). The rate increased slightly in 2010 to 100.2 and increased again in 2011 to 104.2 per 100,000 population, with a total of 321,849 cases reported in the United States in 2011 (DSTD, 2012f).

As depicted in Figure 15.8, gonorrhea rates are highest in the 15-19 and 20-24 year-old age groups for both men and women. The high-

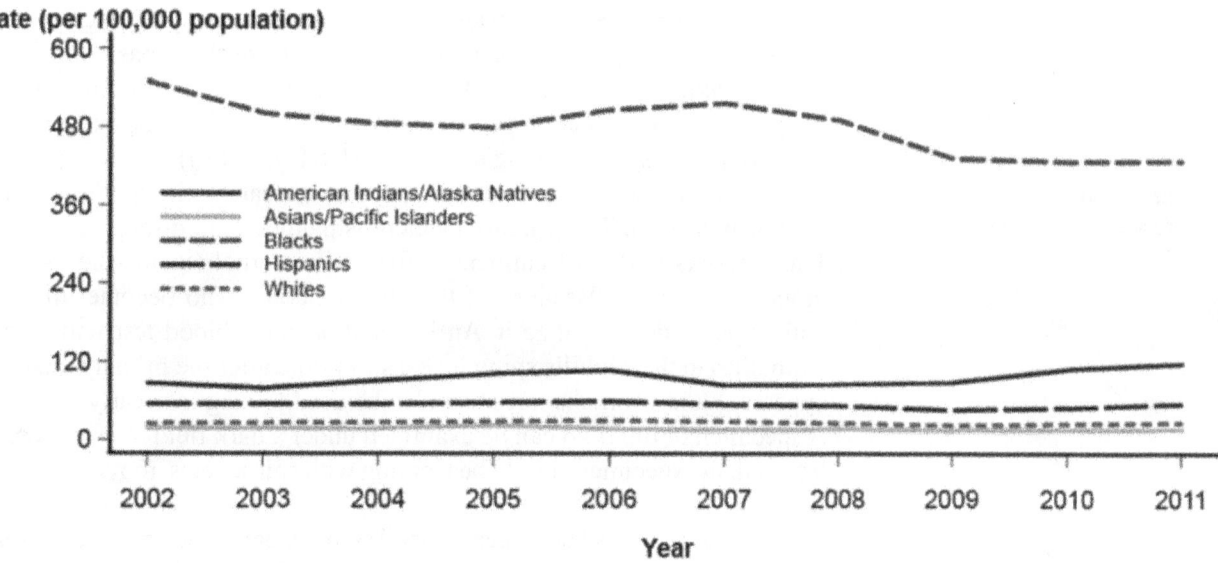

Figure 15.9 *Gonorrhea—Rates by Race/Ethnicity, United States, 2002–2011*

Source: DSTD (2012i). Centers for Disease Control and Prevention, National Center for HIV/AIDS, Viral Hepatitis, STD, and TB Prevention.

est overall rate is among young women between 20 and 24 years old (DSTD 2012h).

As shown in Figure 15.9, gonorrhea rates have remained relatively steady among all racial/ethnic groups since 1997.

> ❧ *Intellectual and Emotional Wellness* ❧
>
> High-level intellectual wellness is the cornerstone of effective prevention of STDs. Knowing the risks and how to reduce them is critical to preventing STDs. This knowledge includes information about personal behavior and also about lifestyles and demographic risks. Intellectual wellness also fosters enhanced decision making. Reducing the risks for STD is all about personal choice. Because STDs are sexually transmitted, their prevention and control are more than just a medical matter. STDs involve our most intimate emotions. Knowing about prevention and seeking treatment are one thing. Working through the anxiety, fear, and guilt, and a host of other emotions that interfere with clear thinking about STDs is another thing. Emotional health can help us deal with the emotions that can cloud rational thinking.

Syphilis

Diagnosis

Syphilis is a blood-borne STD caused by infection with *Treponema pallidum,* a corkscrew-shaped bacterium. A **spirochete** type of bacteria, the *T. pallidum* is easily killed by penicillin and other broad-spectrum antibiotics. It is unique among STD organisms because its corkscrew shape and motility facilitate its entry into the bloodstream.

Syphilis An STD caused by the spirochete bacterium *Treponema pallidum*

Spirochete A mobile, flexible, corkscrew-shaped bacterium of the genus *Spirocheta,* one type of which causes syphilis

Chancre A painless, indurated primary lesion of early syphilis

After exposure to the bacterium, it enters the body through breaks in the skin or by penetrating intact skin, and from there passes into the bloodstream. Once in the bloodstream, it can move freely throughout the body. The usual incubation period for syphilis is 3 to 4 weeks, but it can be as short as 10 days or as long as 90 days (DSTD, 2013d).

After the incubation period, a **chancre** appears at the spot where the organism entered. The primary chancre is painless and disappears within 1 to 5 weeks without treatment. Often it is internal (inside the vagina, mouth, or rectum). Because of this, many people who become infected with syphilis don't realize it. An infected person's blood test will detect antibodies to the syphilis spirochete a short time after the primary chancre appears. Fluid from chancres can also be used to diagnose early syphilis. A specimen of the fluid can be examined under a dark field microscope. If infected, the specimen should be teeming with spirochetes, moving in their typical corkscrew motion (DSTD 2011e).

About 6 weeks later a generalized rash appears. The rash varies from being highly noticeable, covering the entire trunk, to a mild eruption on the hands or feet. As with the chancre, the rash disappears without treatment after 2 to 6 weeks.

In about 25 percent of the cases, a second rash appears and also goes away without treatment. At this point, those who are infected enter the latency period, during which time they are infected but have no symptoms. Although asymptomatic, they are capable of transmitting the infection only by donating blood. However, since all blood drawn on patients in the United States is tested for syphilis, no cases of the disease have been detected this way in decades. Syphilis can also be passed across the placenta by a pregnant woman passing the infection to her developing fetus, resulting in **congenital syphilis.** A requirement of routine prenatal care is a blood

Congenital syphilis The disease acquired by the fetus in the womb and present at birth

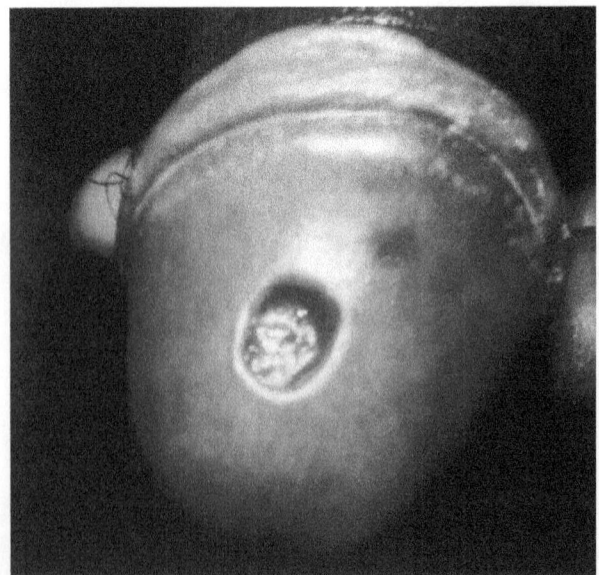 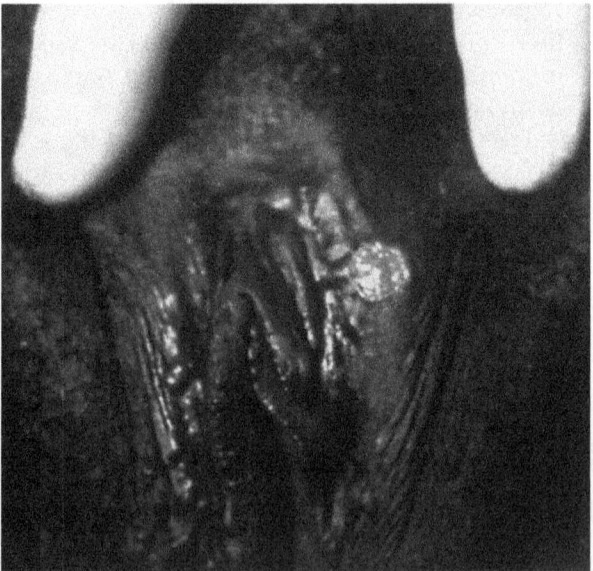

The typical chancre of primary syphilis is round with raised edges and painless; it is often internal and goes unobserved.

Source: Centers for Disease Control and Prevention, Division of STD Prevention

test for syphilis. Most adult women with health insurance get this test early in their pregnancies. If it is positive, they can be treated. Treatment of the mother almost always results in treating her developing fetus (DSTD, 2011e).

Treatment

Treatment of early syphilis is relatively straightforward. Injections of penicillin are sufficient to treat most early cases of syphilis. One shot is administered to those who have been infected for less than 1 year. Those having infections more than 1 year are given three injections, each spaced 1 week apart (DSTD, 2011f).

Epidemiology

The rate of P&S syphilis reported in the United States has steadily decreased over the past several decades. In 2000, the rate was the lowest since reporting began in 1941. The low rate of P&S syphilis and the concentration of the majority of syphilis cases in a small number of geographic

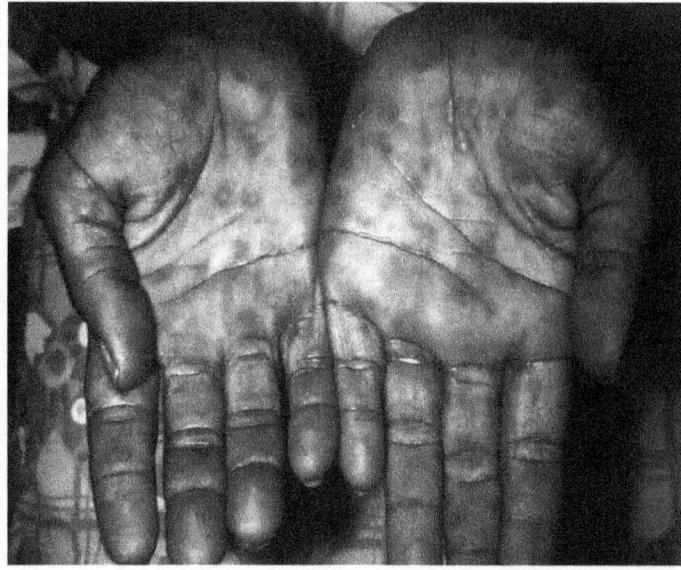

The typical rash associated with secondary syphilis is bilateral (on both hands or feet instead of just one), discolored, and raised.

Source: Centers for Disease Control and Prevention, Division of STD Prevention

areas in the United States led to the development of a national plan to eliminate Syphilis in the country. Although the rate of P&S syphilis in the United States declined 89.7% during 1990–2000, the rate increased annually during 2001–2009 before decreasing again in 2010. The 2011 rate remained unchanged. Overall increases in rates were observed primarily among men (increasing from 3.0 cases per 100,000 population in 2001 to 8.2 cases in 2011 (DSTD, 2012j).

Syphilis remains a major health problem among men who have sex with men (MSM). In recent years, young MSM have accounted for an increasing number of syphilis cases in the United States (see Figure 15.10). Cases among MSM have been characterized by high rates of HIV co-infection and high-risk sexual behaviors. The estimated proportion of P&S syphilis cases attributable to MSM increased from 7% in 2000 to 72% in 2011 (DSTD, 2012j). The occurrence of this syphilis epidemic among urban MSM is believed to be associated with a relaxation of safe sex behavior and coexisting HIV infection (DSTD, 2005d). Many of these men suffer from what experts call "AIDS burnout," the relapsing back to unsafe sexual activity due to years and years of exposure to prevention messages and

Table 15.7 Recommended Treatment for early Syphilis

Recommended Regimen for Adults
Benzathine penicillin G 2.4 million units IM in a single dose
For individuals who are allergic to penicillin, doxycycline or tetracycline, taken for a minimum of 14 days, is recommended for the treatment of early syphilis (DSTD, 2011f).

Source: (DSTD, 2011f).Centers for Disease Control and Prevention, National Center for HIV/AIDS, Viral Hepatitis, STD, and TB Prevention.

Primary and Secondary Syphilis—by Sex and Sexual Behavior, 2007–2011

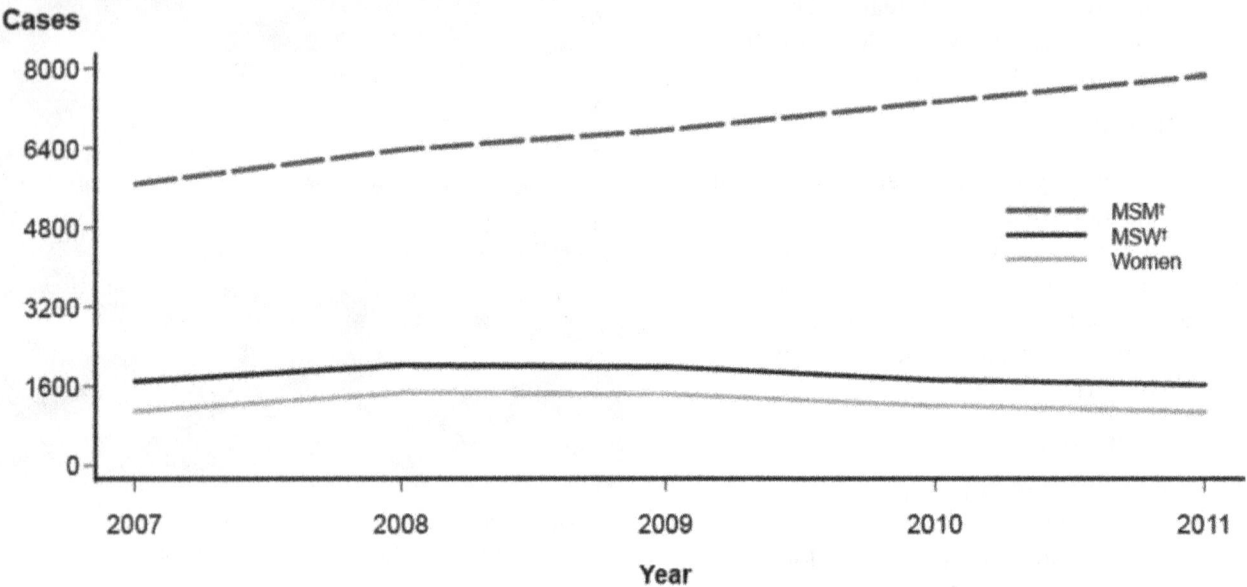

Figure 15.10 *Primary and Secondary Syphilis—by Sex and Sexual Behavior, 2007–2011*
While Primary and secondary syphilis rates for heterosexual men and women have steadily declined, the rate for men who have sex with men has steadily increased since 2007.

Source: DSTD (2012k). Centers for Disease Control and Prevention, National Center for HIV/AIDS, Viral Hepatitis, STD, and TB Prevention.

compliance with safe sex behaviors. Advances in AIDS treatment may be a factor in undermining adherence to safer sex practices, encouraging the perception that safer sex is no longer so important (Taylor et al., 2005).

After an 18% increase in the rate of congenital syphilis during 2006–2008, the rate of congenital syphilis decreased during 2008–2011 (from 10.5 to 8.5 cases per 100,000 live births). In 2011, a total of 360 cases were reported, a decrease from 387 cases in 2010 and 429 cases in 2009. This recent decrease in the rate of congenital syphilis is associated with the decrease in the rate of P&S syphilis among women that has occurred since 2008 (DSTD, 2012j, Golden et al., 2003).

Since 1990, the decline in early syphilis also led to a corresponding decrease in congenital syphilis rates. The current rate of 8.8 cases per 100,000 women is lower than it has been in over a decade (DSTD, 2012j).

Other Minor STDs

Chancroid

Diagnosis

Chancroid An STD named for the irregular and painful genital lesions it produces, caused by the bacterium *Haemophilus ducreyi*

Chancroid is often confused with syphilis because both present with an initial genital ulcer as the primary symptom. The ulcers associated with

Sex in Society 15.1

The Tuskegee Study: It Couldn't Happen Here—or Could It?

In 1932, the U.S. Public Health Service (USPHS) embarked on one of the most tragic experiments ever conducted by a government on its own people. From 1932 to 1970, in Macon County, Alabama, the USPHS conducted a study under the guidance of the Tuskegee Institute (which, ironically, is one of the nation's most prestigious black academic institutions) on the history of syphilis in blacks.

Syphilis, it was hypothesized, progressed differently in blacks than whites. The study originally was intended to be a short-term investigation (6 to 9 months' duration) but evolved into a 40-year project that followed the subjects well beyond the initial stages of their disease through latency into complications and ultimately to their deaths.

Much of what we know about the disease, how it spreads, its complications, and how it attacks the body and kills comes from the Tuskegee Study.

The study followed 600 black subjects (399 infected men and 201 uninfected controls) for 40 years. Treatment was withheld intentionally from these men, even after they were diagnosed with serious, life-threatening complications of the disease. None of them benefited from penicillin as the effective treatment of choice in 1951. The USPHS devised elaborate plans to keep track of these men (and to continue to withhold treatment) even after they moved from Alabama to other states.

In 1966, Peter Buxtun, an investigator for the USPHS, brought the matter before the then-director of the Division of Venereal Diseases, Peter Brown. Given the moral climate and racial turmoil of the 1960s and the immorality of such an experiment, Buxtun pleaded that something be done. A special committee was impaneled within the USPHS to discuss the study. The committee ruled in favor of continuing the study to its natural end point.

Buxtun's pleas went unheeded, and the experiment continued. Not until Buxtun leaked his story to an Associated Press writer and it broke on the front pages of the *Washington Post* in 1972 was something done. In 1973, a special subcommittee of the U.S. Congress, chaired by Edward Kennedy (D-MA) began to investigate the matter.

The committee found the USPHS culpable, the study was terminated, and special regulations concerning conducting government experiments were drawn up. These regulations now serve as guidelines for handling human subjects in any government-financed study. Surviving participants of the Tuskegee Study and their heirs filed a $1.8 billion class action lawsuit. The government settled the suit out of court for $10 million (Jones, 1993).

---

chancroid, however, are irregular in shape and painful (versus symmetrical and painless for syphilis).

The typical incubation period is 4 to 10 days, after which the ulcer appears. After their initial appearance, the ulcers progress to become beefy, granular, painful erosions. The ulcers are accompanied by painful, swollen, lymph glands in the groin.

Like syphilis, chancroid is diagnosed through the presence (or history) of symptoms and the results of a blood test. It is often diagnosed in part, ruling out infection with syphilis. A negative test for syphilis focuses the diagnosis on looking for antibodies to the causative organism, *Haemophilus ducreyi,* or isolating it in a biological culture (DSTD, 2011f).

Treatment

Chancroid is easily treated with antibiotics taken either orally or through an intramuscular injection.

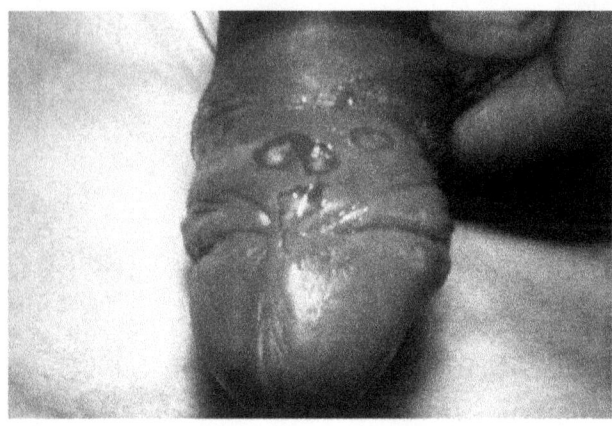

Unlike syphilis, the ulcers of chancroid are irregular in shape and painful.

Source: Centers for Disease Control and Prevention

Hepatitis B virus (HBV) A disease caused by contact with infected blood; often associated with unprotected sex with multiple partners

Carriers Individuals who have a given disease and are capable of passing it on but have no apparent symptoms

Epidemiology

Reported cases of chancroid had declined steadily from 1987 - 2001 when there was a slight increase. In 2011, a total of 8 cases of chancroid were reported in the United States. Only six states reported one or more cases of chancroid in 2011 (DSTD, 2012k).

Hepatitis B Virus (HBV)

Diagnosis

Hepatitis B virus (HBV) infection is another blood-borne disease transmitted through activities that involve percutaneous (i.e., puncture through the skin) or mucosal contact with infectious blood or body fluids (e.g., semen, saliva), including

- Sex with an infected partner
- Injection drug use that involves sharing needles, syringes, or drug-preparation equipment
- Birth to an infected mother
- Contact with blood or open sores of an infected person
- Needle sticks or sharp instrument exposures
- Sharing items such as razors or toothbrushes with an infected person

HBV is not spread through food or water, sharing eating utensils, breastfeeding, hugging, kissing, hand holding, coughing, or sneezing (DSTD, 2012L).

HBV is a serious viral disease that attacks the liver and can cause extreme illness and even death. HBV can cause acute infection or not be apparent. To most people, infection with hepatitis B is not clinically apparent. Between 10 and 68 percent of all cases are chronic **carriers;** the infected individuals have the disease and are capable of spreading it but have no

Table 15.8 Treatment for Chancroid

Recommended Regimens
Azithromycin 1 g orally in a single dose
OR
Ceftriaxone 250 mg intramuscularly (IM) in a single dose
OR
Ciprofloxacin* 500 mg orally twice a day for 3 days*
OR
Erythromycin base 500 mg orally three times a day for 7 days (DSTD, 2011f).

*Ciprofloxacin is contraindicated for pregnant and lactating women.

Source: (DSTD, 2011f). Centers for Disease Control and Prevention, National Center for HIV/AIDS, Viral Hepatitis, STD, and TB Prevention.

noticeable symptoms. When they do notice their symptoms, they usually have jaundice, dark urine, fever, malaise, and moderate liver enlargement with tenderness.

Diagnosis is made through a combination of a clinical examination and a blood test indicating the presence of hepatitis B surface antigen (HBsAG). Chronic infection can lead to cirrhosis of the liver and liver cancer (DSTD 2012L).

The following populations are at increased risk of becoming infected with HBV:

- Infants born to infected mothers
- Sex partners of infected persons
- Sexually active persons who are not in a long-term, mutually monogamous relationship (e.g., >1 sex partner during the previous 6 months)
- Men who have sex with men
- Injection drug users
- Household contacts of persons with chronic HBV infection (DSTD, 2012L).

Treatment

HBV infection has no cure because, like HIV, it is caused by a virus. For acute infection, no medication is available; treatment is designed to reduce the pain and suffering associated with the symptoms.

For chronic infection, several antiviral drugs (adefovir dipivoxil, interferon alfa-2b, pegylated interferon alfa-2a, lamivudine, entecavir, and telbivudine) are available. Persons with chronic HBV infection require medical evaluation and regular monitoring to determine whether disease is progressing and to identify liver damage or hepatocellular carcinoma.

A vaccine for HBV has been available since 1981. At first, the vaccine was recommended for use by those whose work caused them to come in contact with potentially contaminated blood (such as health care workers and those living with persons infected with HBV). It is now recognized that many other persons are potentially at risk through drug-related behavior and sexual activity with infected persons and should consider becoming vaccinated. The vaccine is now recommended that the following populations:

- All infants, beginning at birth
- All children aged <19 years who have not been vaccinated previously
- Susceptible sex partners of Hepatitis B surface antigen (HBsAg)-positive persons
- Sexually active persons who are not in a long-term, mutually monogamous relationship (e.g., >1 sex partner during the previous 6 months)
- Persons seeking evaluation or treatment for a sexually transmitted disease
- Men who have sex with men
- Injection drug users
- Susceptible household contacts of HBsAg-positive persons
- Health care and public safety workers at risk for exposure to blood or blood-contaminated body fluids

- Persons with end-stage kidney disease
- Residents and staff of facilities for developmentally disabled persons
- Persons with chronic liver disease
- Persons with HIV infection
- Travelers to foreign countries where HBV is common
- Unvaccinated adults with diabetes mellitus who are aged 19 through 59 years (discretion of clinicians for unvaccinated adults with diabetes mellitus who are aged ≥60 years)
- All other persons seeking protection from HBV infection—acknowledgment of a specific risk factor is not a requirement for vaccination (DSTD 2012 L).

Epidemiology

In 2009, 3,374 cases of acute Hepatitis B in the United States were reported to CDC. The overall incidence of reported acute Hepatitis B was 1.5 per 100,000 population, the lowest ever recorded (see figure 15.11). Because many HBV infections are either asymptomatic or never reported, the actual number of new infections is estimated to be approximately tenfold higher. In 2009, an estimated 38,000 persons in the United States were newly infected with HBV. Rates are highest among adults, particularly males aged 25–44 years (DSTD, 2012L).

The rate of new HBV infections has declined by approximately 82% since 1991, when a national strategy to eliminate HBV infection was implemented in the United States. The decline has been greatest among children born since 1991, when routine vaccination of children was first recommended (DSTD, 2012 L).

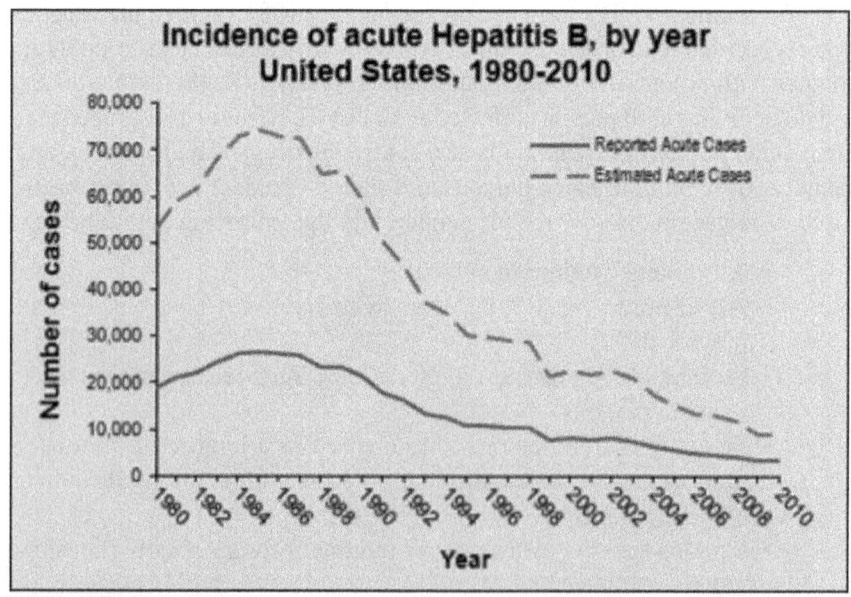

Figure 15.11 *Incidence of Acute Hepatitis B by Year United states, 1980-2010*

Source: (DSTD 2012 L). Centers for Disease Control and Prevention, Division of Viral Hepatitis

The risks associated with HBV infection are gender, age, sexual orientation, IDU status, and race/ethnicity. Men have a slightly higher incidence of HBV than women. Part of this is attributed to a higher risk among gay men. Eighteen percent of all HBV cases are among gay men. Hetero- sexuals (especially those with a history of STDs and multiple sex partners) accounted for 40 percent of all infections. Persons involved with IDU activities accounted for 15 percent of all cases. Health care workers accounted for 2 percent of all cases, and household contact with a person infected with HBV accounted for 3 percent of the cases (NCID, 2003).

Non-gonococcal Urethritis (NGU)

Diagnosis

Non-gonococcal urethritis (NGU) is diagnosed when *Neisseria gonorrhea* is ruled out as the causative agent of discharge and burning in a male. In most cases, a negative lab test for gonorrhea and the presence of symptoms is enough to diagnose NGU. NGU is also a surrogate measure of chlamydia in men, as more than half of all cases of NGU are attributable to *C. trachomatis*. In some cases, a test for *C. trachomatis* is done.

Non-gonococcal urethritis (NGU) An infection in the urethra of males, usually caused by chlamydia bacteria

Treatment

NGU presents the same symptoms as chlamydia infection in men and is treated using the same treatment schedule recommended for chlamydia.

Epidemiology

Visits to physicians for NGU peaked in 1990 and, except for a slight increase in 1999, declined steadily throughout the decade. Annual incidence of NGU is estimated at approximately 3 million cases annually in the United States (DSTD, 2011G).

Pubic Lice

Diagnosis

Infection with **pubic lice,** commonly called *crabs,* is caused by infestation of *Phthirius pubis*. The lice are transmitted during sexual contact from the infested pubic hair of one person to the other. In rarer instances, the lice are transmitted from contaminated bedding, clothing, and towels that people share.

Pubic lice *Phthirius pubis;* small insects (metazoan) that infest the host's pubic hair

Female lice lay eggs, called *nits,* which attach to the shaft of the pubic hair of the exposed individual. The incubation period for lice is between 24 and 48 hours, at which time the eggs hatch and another batch of lice spread throughout the pubic hair.

Symptoms of pubic lice are (a) visual confirmation of the lice, (b) intense itching of the pubic and perianal area, (c) skin irritation, and (d) secondary sores and erosions from scratching. Although infestation rarely leads to complications, persons with pubic lice sometimes develop secondary infections from their intense scratching (DSTD, 2011h).

Treatment

Treatment of lice consists of special shampoos that kill the lice on the skin and hair. The shampoos are applied to the affected areas, allowed to sit for up to 10 minutes, and rinsed off thoroughly. Bedding, clothing, and other contaminated articles must be washed and dried thoroughly under hot settings or dry-cleaned. Fumigation of the person's house is not necessary (DSTD 2011h).

Scabies

Diagnosis

Like crabs, **scabies** is caused by infestation with a mite. This mite, *Sarcoptes scabies,* is transmitted in the same way as pubic lice. Symptoms are similar with one notable exception: S. scabies actually burrows under the skin of an infected person and feeds on cellular matter (DSTD, 2011h).

Diagnosis usually consists of identifying the mite's burrows under the skin.

Treatment

Because of the burrowing of the mites involved in scabies, treatment involves applying a lotion (similar to the shampoos used in pubic lice) that is left on the skin for 8 to 14 hours before being washed off. More than one application of the lotion may be required (DSTD, 2011H).

STD Prevention and Risk Reduction

Personal health STD/HIV prevention programs focus largely on individual behavior as the basis for risk reduction. Many of these programs emphasize "safer sex" (using condoms consistently and correctly and verifying HIV status through testing) as the primary prevention approach (Crosby et al, 2003). Others stress abstinence from sexual intercourse as the preferred preventive approach (Howard & McCabe, 1990).

Community health prevention programs emphasize public health interventions designed to stop the diseases from spreading. Examples of activities are political lobbying to establish needle exchange programs, increased funding of STD/HIV services (for example, to allow expanded hours), free and confidential treatment, and socio-marketing to promote condom distribution and family planning services.

The problem with compartmentalizing STD/HIV risks is that it fails to acknowledge that personal and community risks have a synergistic effect. We propose a new way to conceptualize the relationship between community and personal risks as pyramidal in nature, consisting of various public and personal factors that build upon each other. Figure 15.12 illustrates this Pyramid of Risk.

Demographic Variables and the Distribution of STDs/HIV

The foundation of the pyramid is made up of **demographic** variables that influence STD/HIV risk. These are generally beyond our individual control. The next level of risk revolves around the sexual and medical history of ourselves or our partners. Because these risks are part of a person's past, they also cannot be changed. They are the history that each of us brings to any sexual encounter. The third level of risk represents a person's current **sexual lifestyle,** the interaction between the types and numbers of current sex partners. The last level of risk is the one most educators focus on: personal sexual behavior. Most risk reduction pamphlets provide a laundry list of sexual behaviors that range from low risk to high risk. Although the

Sexual lifestyle The interaction between types and numbers of current sex partners

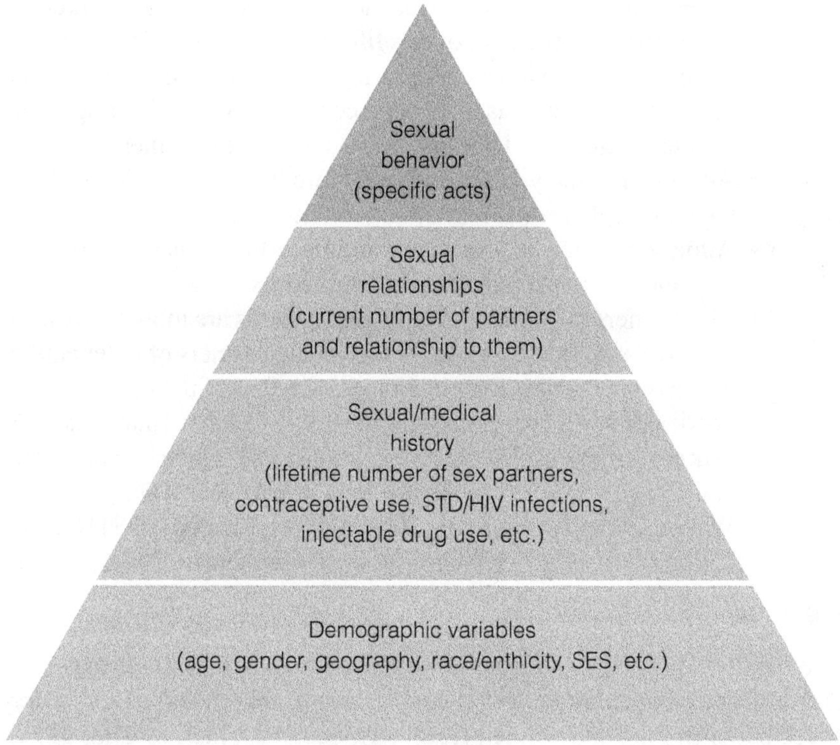

Figure 15.12 *A Pyramid of Risk for STDs* To assess one's true risk of acquiring STDs, demographic and sexual/medical history risks must be combined with behavioral and lifestyle factors.

four levels of factors influence STD/HIV risk independently, the interaction of levels can have a synergistic effect that can increase or reduce personal risk dramatically.

Seven major demographic variables that contribute to STD/HIV risk are age, gender, sexual orientation, injecting drug user (IDU; the clustering of injectable drug users in communities), geography, socioeconomic status (SES), and race/ethnicity.

Age

Estimates suggest that young people aged 15–24 years acquire nearly half of all new STDs.[1] Compared with older adults, sexually active adolescents aged 15–19 years and young adults aged 20–24 years are at higher risk of acquiring STDs for a combination of behavioral, biological, and cultural reasons (DSTD, 2012m).

Some age-related STD considerations are:

- People tend to have sex with partners in their general age groups. Since the 14-24 year old group has the highest rates of infection having sex with members of this group increases risk.
- The earlier the onset of intercourse (first time a person has sexual intercourse), the greater their potential exposure to different sex partners over their lifetime. There is an association between lifetime number of sex partners and increased risk of acquiring STDs.

- Individuals who initiate sexual activity earlier are more likely to have more sex partners over a lifetime (more than 25 percent of women initiating intercourse by age 15 had more than 10 lifetime sex partners, whereas only 6 percent of women initiating intercourse at age 20 or later had more than 10 sex partners).
- Adolescents and young adults are more likely than older adults to have multiple (sequential or concurrent) sexual partners.
- Adolescents and young adults are more likely than older adults to engage in unprotected sexual intercourse.
- The partners of adolescents and young adults are more likely to be at higher risk for having an STD than the partners of older adults.
- The transformation zone in women (the end of the cervix, where cervical tissue meets vaginal tissue) is most exposed during adolescence, and this tissue is most susceptible to STD infection in general and viral infection (cancer-causing) in particular (DSTD 2005c, Wallis, 2005, Bearman et al., 2004, Sipkin et al., 2003, DSTD, 2000; Quinn & Cates, 1993; Alan Guttmacher Institute, 1991).

Gender

The risk for STDs/HIV is different for men and women. Biological gender is a risk factor related to the genetic, anatomical, and physiological differences between men and women (Kennedy, Scarlett, Duer, & Chu, 1995). Women face a greater risk than men for both acquiring a sexually transmitted disease and developing complications for several reasons:

- Heterosexual women are receptive sexually—vaginally, orally, and anally. This greatly increases their risks for initial infection by exposing a greater surface area of mucosal tissue (Quinn & Cates, 1993). Once infected with most STDs, heterosexual women tend to be asymptomatic more often than heterosexual men. Most heterosexual men notice initial symptoms of infection, whereas about half of women are asymptomatic (Morse, Moreland, & Thompson, 1990).
- Because of the asymptomatic nature of STDs in women, more women than men do not seek treatment during the initial stages of infection. This delayed access to treatment results in progression of the disease and a greater likelihood of developing complications (Bonaviglia, 2000). For example, about 15 percent of women develop complications associated with gonorrhea or chlamydia versus less than 1 percent of men (Morse et al., 1990).
- Menstruation plays a role in facilitating the movement of pathogens from the lower reproductive tract (below the cervix) to the upper parts, facilitating the development of complications. Women face the added risk of passing on their infection to their developing fetus during pregnancy or newborn through childbirth (Smeltzer & Whipple, 1991). The likelihood of transmitting infections such as syphilis or HIV is greatly reduced if mothers attend routine prenatal screening and receive treatment.

Sexual Orientation

Risks for STDs are affected by a person's sexual orientation. The risks that heterosexual women face accrue as a result of their anatomy and physiology, which facilitate exposure to disease agents. Sexual exposure results in infection without symptoms, and menstruation facilitates infection.

Gay and bisexual men have some of the risks that heterosexual women do. They are receptive sexually and tend to have asymptomatic infections. This facilitates the development and spread of disease. In addition, certain diseases, such as HIV and hepatitis B, exist in **endemic** levels in the gay community (Bucharcz et al., 2005). These diseases are incurable and capable of causing death.

Endemic A 20 percent level of ongoing infection within a specific population

Heterosexual men are at less risk than heterosexual women and gay men for a variety of reasons. First, their symptoms tend to be more obvious because these men usually are the insertive sexual partners and develop external symptoms.

As an example, fewer than 1 percent of all heterosexual men infected with gonorrhea develop complications such as **epididymitis.** Also, female-to-male transmission of STDs is more difficult because heterosexual men are not receptive sexually, and vaginal fluids are less likely to transmit infection than is contaminated semen (Morse et al., 1990).

Epididymitis Inflammation of the small oblong body that rests upon and beside the surface of the testes

Of the four groups, lesbian women have the lowest rates of infection. Gay women tend to have fewer sexual partners over the course of their lifetime, and they do not engage in vaginal or anal intercourse (Kennedy et al., 1995).

IDU

The risk for STD/HIV is becoming increasingly related to the prevalence of **IDUs** (injectable drug users) in a community (Powelson et al., 2000, Bachmann et al., 2000). Drug use is associated with increased STD/HIV risk in two ways.

IDU The acronym for *injectable drug user*

- Psychoactive drugs impair users' ability to make good decisions regarding sexual behavior. Therefore, engaging in safer sex becomes less likely when a person is using psychoactive drugs. And good choice of partner(s) is impaired by psychoactive drug use.
- Injectable drug use often involves needle sharing between users. This facilitates the transmission of blood-borne infections such as HIV and hepatitis B if one of the users is infected.

The drugs most often involved are crack cocaine and injectable heroin. A vicious cycle of drug abuse, exchanging sex for money or other resources, unsafe sex, and infection with a variety of genital ulcer diseases has occurred since the mid-1980s. This cycle is intimately related to the resurgence of syphilis and other diseases in urban America. The effects are most notable among young, urban, black and Hispanic/Latino men and women (Finelli et al, 1993).

Urban/Rural and Geographic Differences

STDs including HIV are disproportionately higher in urban areas than in rural or suburban locations **(DSTD, 2005).** "Core urban populations" may be a major contributing factor for higher STD rates in urban communities and disproportionately high personal risk, despite individual behavior (Bearman et al, 2004, Wallis, 2005, Garnett & Anderson, 1996). The rate of acquisition of gonorrhea, for instance, in core urban populations is as

case study 15.3

Jim

Jim, 24, single, is white.

Jim was a student in Dr. Blonna's human sexuality class. Jim came to see him after class about some concerns regarding STDs.

You've got to help me. I made a mistake, and I'm super paranoid about what's going to happen to me. I was coming back to school last Friday night late, and I was cruising through Paterson [a large city adjacent to the town where the college campus is located]. I don't know what got into me, but I picked up a hitchhiker on Broadway and gave her a ride to the end of Paterson. She was really hot and offered to give me a blow job to thank me.

I said yes, and she went down on me in the parking lot where she lived. I don't know how to describe how I felt afterward—part ashamed, part stupid, part afraid. I'm so worried that I got AIDS from her.

On Monday in class, you talked about demographic risks, and the whole thing got me freaked.

My girlfriend wanted to have sex last night, and I used a condom with her. She freaked out. She's on the pill, and we never use condoms. I broke down and had to tell her what I did. Am I going to die of AIDS?

Critical Thinking

Although the female –to- male transmission of the HIV virus through oral sex is much less efficient than through vaginal or anal intercourse, what demographic and other factors influenced the risk of this act for Jim?

---

much as 300 times higher than in the rest of the population (Rice, Roberts, & Handsfield, 1991).

With a high level of infection and prevalence of deadly diseases, any sexual activity (even so-called safer sex) between or with members of this population carries a higher degree of risk than the same behavior with non–core group people.

❧ *Intellectual and Emotional Wellness* ❧

STDs used to be called "social diseases" because of the nature of sexual transmission.

Social wellness is a major preventive strategy against STDs. Being in a mutually exclusive, monogamous, disease-free relationship is the best prevention against STDs. In the United States, the quality of one's social environment seems to be directly proportional to socio-economic status (SES). As SES rises, most Americans seek out safer, healthier communities, and safe communities carry much lower risk for STDs. High-risk/low-wellness communities should be targeted for STD prevention and treatment services and programs.

Socioeconomic Status

(SES) To a large extent, STDs mimic other chronic diseases. SES can either facilitate or hinder access to preventive and interventive STD health care. People of lower SES tend to lack enabling factors related to prevention and treatment of STDs such as health care insurance and access to treatment services (Gallet, 2002, Santelli et al., 2000). Even though free public clinics are available, they may not be utilized promptly because poor people often lack access to transportation, don't have sick days if they are employed, or are unaware of the availability of free care (Donelan et al., 1996).

Also, people of lower SES often do not perceive themselves to be at great risk for STDs/HIV and tend not to respond to symptoms promptly or consistently practice preventive behavior (Ramos, Shain, & Johnson, 1995). Poverty and lower SES, too, contribute to higher levels of drug use—a major risk factor for STDs/HIV (Potterat, Rothenberg, Woodhouse, Muth, Pratts, & Fogle, 1985).

Race/Ethnicity

African Americans and Hispanics continue to have the highest rates of STD infection in the United States. Rates for almost all STDs are substantially higher for these groups than for whites. Risk for certain STDs like gonorrhea and syphilis are as much as 30 times higher for African Americans than for whites (DSTD, 2005). Part of that disparity is attributed to the higher use of public health clinics by African Americans than whites. Public clinics tend to have more complete reporting of STDs than private health care providers (DSTD, 2000).

Although disease rates in general are higher for blacks and Hispanics than whites, racial/ethnic differences are often markers for social class and poverty (Navarro, 1990). Poverty, especially that which affects the urban poor, is the true risk factor. The increased problem of STDs in minority populations in inner cities may stem in part from the unequal distribution of poverty, not race or ethnicity (Navarro, 1990). A greater proportion of blacks and Hispanics/Latinos live at or below poverty than whites. Socioeconomic differentials (often referred to as *class differentials*) are larger than race differentials in **morbidity.** When studies control for SES differentials, racial differences in disease distribution drop markedly. The problem of STDs in minority populations in inner cities is a result, in part, of the unequal distribution of SES (Fortenberry, 2002, Navarro, 1990).

Morbidity The relative incidence of a disease

Sexual/Medical History

The next level of risk on the pyramid is sexual medical history. This is something we cannot control because it has occurred in the past. Yet, a person's sexual and medical history can greatly influence the present level of risk for STDs/HIV (Manhart et al., 2004, Holloway, 2005). The following are sexual/medical factors most associated with the current risk for STDs/HIV:

> *Lifetime number of sexual partners.* In general, the greater the number, the higher the risk. Threshold levels of "safe" sexual activity have been identified (Greenhalgh, 2000). Once the threshold number of sexual partners is reached, the risk for disease increases exponentially.

Incidence The number of new cases of a disease during a specific time period

Contraceptive use. Barrier contraceptive users have the lowest rates of infection. They are followed by other contraceptive users and nonusers, who have the highest risk (Manhart et al., 2004).

History of IDU. Persons with a history of IDU have an increased **incidence** of infection with blood-borne diseases, particularly HIV and hepatitis B (Alter & Margolis, 1990; Finelli et al., 1993).

Prior STD history. Persons who have been infected with STDs in the past are more likely to become infected again than those who have never been infected **(Manhart et al, 2004).**

Sexual Relationships

Sexual relationship refers to the connections between people rather than the specific behaviors in which they engage. In general, the risk for STDs/HIV decreases as sexual relationships move away from multiple, anonymous, sexual encounters toward monogamous (with uninfected partner), trusting partnerships (Wallis, 2005, Bearman et al., 2004, Metzler et al., 2000, Lauman et al., 1994,).

STD/HIV sexual relationship risks are specifically related to overall numbers of partners and the quality of the relationship (trust, understanding, and knowledge of one's partner). Figure 15.13 shows the continuum of risks for sexual relationships. There are two dimensions of lifestyle of partner risk: familiarity risk and exclusivity risk.

Familiarity risk. Familiarity risk is synonymous with *anonymity.* Laumann et al. (1994) operationally defined the extent of familiarity along a continuum that measured how long the study subjects knew their partners before having sex with them. Studies show that the less familiar one is with the sex partner (the greater the anonymity), the greater is the risk. Anonymity is a risk factor because it influences the ability to make an informed choice about the risk for STD/HIV (Manhart et al, 2005, Bearman et al, 2004, Laumann et al, 1994).

Exclusivity risk. Laumann et al. (1994) call the second variable *exclusivity*—the quality of the sexual relationship. Exclusivity, they believe, has to be examined for *both* partners. If one partner

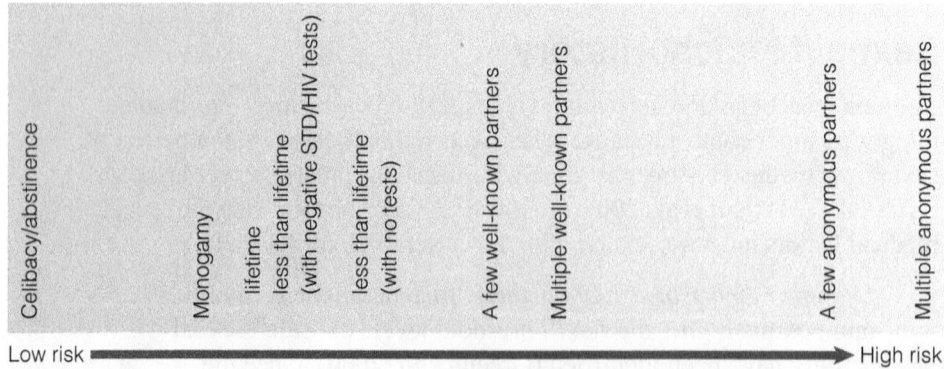

Figure 15.13 *Continuum of Risk for Sexual Relationships STD risks increase as relationships become less familiar and exclusive.*

sex in society 15.2

Core Transmitters of STDs

STDs seem to be much more common in certain pockets of the population. These pockets occur mostly in urban areas among specific subpopulations of sexually active people called *core groups*. People in core groups (mostly urban African American and Latino lower-SES young men and women) have a disproportionate risk for acquiring STDs. The risk of transmission of STDs among a core group is 300 to 600 times greater than among the U.S. population in general. The following factors are related to transmission of STDs in the core population:

Endemic levels of infection (20 percent or more of the population infected) (Eng & Butler, 1997)

High concentrations of infected persons in small geographic areas (DSTD, 2000). Only 5.9 percent of census tracts accounted for 51 percent of cases of STDs, and an additional 9 adjacent census tracts accounted for 72 percent of cases and 74 percent of sexual contacts) (Garnett & Anderson, 1996).

High levels of intergroup sexual activity and socializing (Bearman et al., 2004, Wallis,

2005, Piot & Islam, 1994). Of those infected with STDs, 51 percent had picked up their sexual partners in the same location (only 2 percent of all the bars and clubs in town) (Webster et al., 1993).

High levels of repeat infections. Small percentages of infected individuals accounted for large percentages of multiple infections (Garnett & Anderson, 1996).

High levels of multiple STD infections (coexisting infection with gonorrhea and chlamydia; syphilis and HIV; HIV and chancroid) (Nakashima et al., 1996).

Longer than average duration of infectivity (because of a delay in seeking treatment) and *rate of asymptomatic infection among core group members* (Garnett & Anderson, 1996).

High levels of substance abuse and higher levels of sex for drugs than non–core group patients (Finelli et al., 1993).

is monogamous but the other is not, the benefits of exclusivity are lost. Furthermore, if an uninfected person is monogamous with someone who has an STD, exclusivity can actually increase the risk by increasing the extent of exposure. For exclusivity to work, both partners have to be uninfected and monogamous. Subjects (and partners) who were not sexually exclusive were at increased risk for acquiring an STD (Manhart et al, 2005, Bearman et al, 2004, Lauman et al., 1994).

The highest risks were associated with the "interaction of risky partners" (lack of exclusivity and familiarity) and many partners. This sexual lifestyle, which combines multiple partners with anonymous sexual encounters, creates a deadly synergy that increases the risk exponentially (Manhart et al, 2005, Bearman et al, 2004, Lauman et al., 1994).

Sexual Behavior

At the top of the Pyramid of Risk is sexual behavior. In general, as illustrated in Figure 15.14, the risks increase as behaviors incorporate unprotected

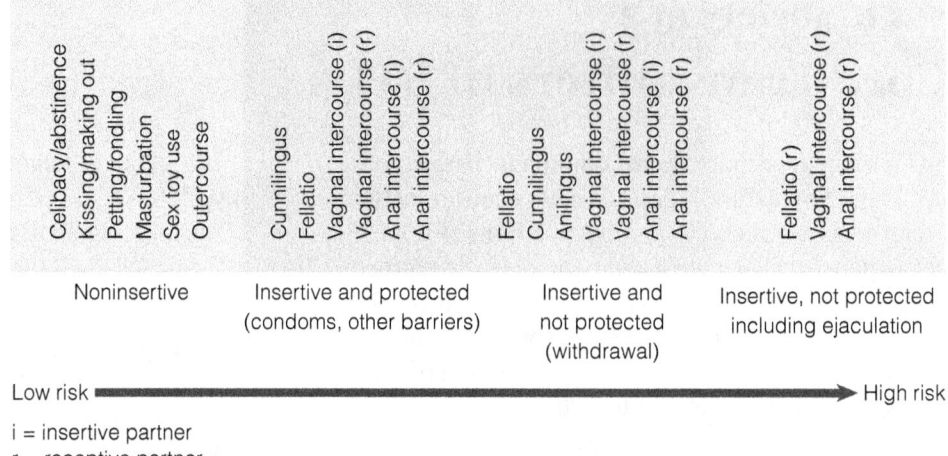

Figure 15.14 *A Continuum of Risk for Sexual Behaviors* STD risks increase as sexual activities become unprotected and receptive.

insertion and ejaculation. The lower-risk behaviors are non-penetrative and do not involve an exchange of bodily fluids. As we move along the continuum of risk, the behaviors reflect attempts to utilize barrier protection against infectious agents. The highest risk behavior is receptive anal penetration including ejaculation, which consists of unprotected ejaculation of semen into the delicate, non-lubricated tissue of the rectum. This allows direct access of infectious STD/HIV agents to the bloodstream.

Theoretically, as Figure 15.14 illustrates, the risk for STD/HIV is greater for the receptive partner of any sexual activity (MMWR, 2001, Manhart et al, 2005)

A Closer Look at Sexual Behaviors and STD Risk

Much remains to be known about the relative safety of various sexual behaviors. For instance, a wealth of literature documents the degree of protection condoms provide in preventing STDs. Little, however, has been written concerning the effects of non-penetrative sexual activity and withdrawal. Some of these activities now are included in "safer sex" methods, instead of "safe sex" behaviors because of the lack of adequate documentation on their effectiveness.

The effects of some of the more bizarre techniques haven't been documented at all. Consider the recommendation of some safe sex educators of the use of dental dams and clear plastic food wraps to prevent the transmission of STDs through cunnilingus, fellatio, and vaginal intercourse. We do not advocate these measures because they are untested and not intended for those purposes. No evidence is available to suggest that they work. In fact, the American Dental Association issued a disclaimer concerning using dental dams (square pieces of latex designed to be used over the mouths of dental patients) for any circumstances other than dental hygiene. Clear plastic food wraps are an even more vivid example of safe sex gone mad. The notion of covering one's genitalia with plastic wrap and then having intercourse or oral sex would be comical if the potential results weren't so dangerous.

case study 15.4

Lillie's Risk

Lillie, 43, divorced, is white.

Lillie is a continuing student who made these comments in class:

Thank you! Finally, someone has said what I believed all along: It's not just sexual behavior that's the risk. It's the behavior in the context of a relationship that determines risk. I was always so annoyed and insulted when sex educators told me that I should always insist that my partner wear a condom and that any woman who is sexually active is at equal risk of becoming infected.

I always felt that as long as I had one uninfected partner, and the two of us were monogamous, I was at low risk.

It's funny because even though I'm not married, my boyfriend (of 3 years) is less of a threat to me than my husband used to be. My ex-husband was always cheating on me, and I was worried that even though I was monogamous, he'd bring something home to me.

I fully trust my current boyfriend. We've been monogamous (though unmarried) for 3 years, and I've never felt safer. We spent a lot of time building the trust and commitment in our relationship. I have great sex with him because I can fully relax and trust him, even though I've never gone down the list of things I need to know about his sexual past. We did talk about whether either of us ever had a viral STD, because viruses are forever.

Critical Thinking

Do you agree with Lillie's assessment of her STD risk? Why or why not?

For those who choose to have sexual intercourse, barrier methods provide the best protection. For those who do not want to have intercourse, a variety of non-penetrative sexual activities offer close to 100 percent effectiveness against STDs.

Condoms

If worn properly and used consistently, condoms (both male and female) help protect the wearer against some STD infection by preventing direct contact between the penis and cervical, vaginal, rectal, or pharyngeal secretions or lesions. They also protect against exposure to penile lesions, discharges, and infected semen. Proper use for preventing STDs requires putting them on prior to any sexual contact, and they must remain intact throughout sexual activity.

Condoms are more effective against sexually transmitted infections such as gonorrhea, chlamydia, trichomoniasis, and HIV, which are transmitted by fluids from mucosal surfaces and from semen (and therefore captured or blocked by the condom) than STDs transmitted by skin-to-skin contact such as HPV, herpes simplex virus (HSV), syphilis, and chancroid (MMWR 2001). The organisms of the latter diseases and others live in outcrops of blisters, warts, and lesions that could exist in areas that condoms do not protect (MMWR, 2001). In laboratory studies, male latex condoms have been shown to block the larger bacterial pathogens (gonorrhea and chlamydia) and, to a lesser extent, smaller viral organisms (such as HIV, HSV, and HPV) (Grimes & Cates, 1990; Conant, Hardy, Sernatinger, Spicer, & Levy, 1986; Minuk, Bohme, & Bowen, 1986). Similar findings have not been found for natural membrane condoms. Although they block the passage of sperm and are similar in their ability to prevent pregnancy, their pores are large enough to allow the passage of some STD organisms. Natural membrane condoms should not be the first choice for the prevention of STDs unless one is allergic to latex (MMWR, 2001).

In human studies, condoms also have been shown to be effective in reducing the risks for contracting STDs. Studies from all over the world, with diverse populations of users, have consistently documented that condoms reduce the risks for spreading STDs. Research as far back as the 1940s studied the use of condoms by troops in World War II and the Korean and Vietnam conflicts. In all three conflicts, soldiers and seamen using condoms had significantly lower rates of infection than their peers who did not use condoms (Hart, 1974).

More recent studies of college men, men and women attending STD clinics, sex workers in Kenya and Zaire, and many others document that condoms provide **consistent protection** against a host of STDs (Manhart et al., 2004, Anderson, 2003, Crosby et al., 2003, Darrow, 1989; Cameron et al., 1991; Mann et al., 1987). Although use of condoms does not provide 100 percent protection against STDs, the studies we have mentioned have reduced risk by 50 to 80 percent in actual users (Cates & Stone, 1992).

Condoms lubricated with Nonxynol 9 (N-9) spermicides have not been found to be any more effective than other lubricated condoms in protecting against the transmission of HIV and other STDs (Richardson, 2002). Additional findings regarding condoms lubricated with N-9 are; spermicide-coated condoms cost more, have a shorter shelf-life than other lubricated condoms, and have been associated with urinary tract infection in young women (MMWR 2001).

Women-Centered Barriers

Although the male condom is the most reliable form of barrier protection against STDs/HIV, studies show that the women who stand to benefit the most do not use them consistently and correctly. The least consistent users of the male condom are adolescent women, women with a history of STD infection, and lower-SES women (who generally have less power and equality in their sexual relationships with men and have less negotiating skill) (Rosenberg & Gollub, 1992). This problem could be dramatically lessened, if not eliminated, if more women were to use female barriers consistently and correctly.

Clinical studies of the effectiveness of female condoms in preventing STDs are very limited **but** their theoretical effectiveness against STDs is high (Green & Gollub, 2003). Laboratory studies have demonstrated the effectiveness of the female condom in blocking viruses. Female condoms are recommended for use when male condoms cannot be used properly (Green & Gollub, 2003).

Personal Exploration Activity
My Most Persuasive Reasons to Wait to Have Sex

Although there are many great reasons to have sexual intercourse, there are also some really good reasons to wait. One of the best ways to avoid an STD is to limit your sexual partners. This activity will help you practice being assertive about why you want to wait to have sex.

This will be more fun if you can find a friend to role-play this with you. It will be even more fun if you find a friend of the opposite sex. Tell your friend that you would like for him or her to act out the following scenario with you. You are playing the parts of a couple who disagree when to become sexually active. One partner is ready to become sexually intimate, but the other partner wants to stay monogamous and to wait at least 4 months to be tested for HIV/AIDS and STDs before becoming intimate. Your friend will play the role of trying to persuade you to have sex, and your role is to give your friend all of the good reasons that you two should wait. Once you have finished, decide who was the most persuasive and discuss other good arguments you could have used. The more we practice assertively telling a partner what we need, the more likely we are to do it in our "real" relationships.

In both laboratory and STD clinic studies, the following rates of effectiveness were reported for the sponge, diaphragm, and spermicides:

- An overall reduced STD infection rate among barrier users compared to non-barrier users
- Lower STD infection rates (87 percent lower) for women using barriers and attending health maintenance organizations (HMOs) than nonusers
- Lower STD infection rates (61 percent lower than nonusers) for women attending STD clinics who used barriers
- Up to 70 percent effectiveness against gonorrhea when using barriers
- Up to 40 percent effectiveness against chlamydia when using barriers

Even though condoms have a higher rate of theoretical effectiveness against STDs, the women who need them the most use them less consistently and correctly. Woman-centered barriers, though theoretically less effective against STDs, provided greater actual effectiveness for women who used them instead of the male condom (Rosenberg & Golub, 1992).

Non-penetrative Sexual Behaviors

The effectiveness of non-penetrative sexual activity in preventing STDs is relatively undocumented. Effectiveness in preventing STDs is generalized from the hypothesized ability of these methods to prevent unintended pregnancy by preventing the deposit of live sperm into the vagina. Because these methods exclude penetration and ejaculation, their ability to prevent pregnancy is very high (theoretically close to 100 percent).

Methods such as masturbation, use of sex toys, and even oral-genital sexual contact in preventing the transmission of STDs have not been scientifically studied and documented. Do they work? No one knows for sure. When theorizing about their ability to prevent STDs, one can say that, because they do not involve penetration and ejaculation, they must offer a high level of protection against STDs as well. We are not as totally convinced of this hypothesis as some other safer sex educators are.

The major difference in the ability of these activities to prevent STDs would be the presence or absence of genital symptoms that potentially could spread pathogens even in the absence of penile penetration and ejaculation. Also, STD organisms, in rare instances, could be passed from genital ulcers to the eyes via contaminated fingers. For instance, if a person who had genital lesions associated with herpes were to engage in mutual masturbation with his or her partner, and then rubbed the eyes, the herpes virus could be spread to this site.

These facts are why we present sexual behaviors on a continuum of risk from low to high. No behavior except celibacy is completely risk-free. Viewing sexual activity in this way will allow you to examine the risk of specific behaviors in the context of other sexual activities. You also must evaluate any behavior within the context of the relationship you have with your partner. The less you know about your partner, the more risky any behavior becomes.

Using the Pyramid to Reduce Risks

The pyramid model presented earlier in the chapter shows that the risk for STDs/HIV combines personal lifestyle and behavior, past sexual history, and demographic factors. Focusing on just one set of factors and ignoring the others isn't enough. Though a person can never dismiss personal behavior as crucial to the success of prevention activities, other factors affect personal risk despite the most exemplary personal behavior. For example, in certain core areas, individuals have 300 times more risk for acquiring infection simply by virtue of community risk factors **(Potterat et al., 1985)**. Even if you are rather conservative in your behavior, if you live and interact sexually in such an area, engaging in any sexual activity carries a higher risk of becoming infected and engaging in risky sexual behavior may be life-threatening. This demographic influence might make risk reduction measures much different from someone who lives in a lower-risk area.

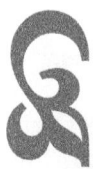 **healthy sex hints 15.5**

Reducing the Risk for STDs: Some Basic Guidelines

Although no universal solutions will work equally well for everyone, here are a few guidelines for reducing your risk for acquiring an STD.

1. *Become comfortable with your own sexuality.* Learn as much as you can about your sexuality. This will make you more accepting of who you are and what you need. You will be less likely to give in to doing something risky if you know and respect yourself.
   This includes choosing to abstain if that's what you desire.

2. *Check yourself for signs and symptoms of STDs.* This goes hand in hand with item 1. If you are comfortable with your body and your sexuality, you will be more aware of changes that signify possible STD infection. If you or your partner has the sores, rashes, discharges, itching, or pain associated with STDs, avoid sex.

3. *Develop a repertoire of low-risk sexual outlets.* Learn how to enjoy a low-risk sexual outlet. It's perfectly OK to say no to unprotected intercourse and yes to masturbation or massage.

4. *Work on your communication skills.* Practice how to initiate a dialogue about STD risk reduction. You'll need to find out a lot about your partner to assess and reduce your personal risk. The only way to do this is to be able to talk openly about your sexual lifestyle.

5. *Understand your demographic risks.* Find out about the area in which you live. You can get information about the level of STDs in your community from your local and state health departments.

6. *Know your partner's sexual/medical history.* Take time and care to find out the things you need to know about your partner, or develop the level of trust in the relationship that will allow you to make some judgments about your risk. In the meantime, if you choose to have sex with your partner, use condoms and non-intercourse options to reduce your risk.

7. *If you are at risk, seek regular checkups.* If you have a very high-risk profile, go in for an STD checkup every 3 months. If you are in a lower risk category, go in at least twice a year. Most states have a list of free public clinics in your area.

8. *If you are not in a mutually monogamous, disease-free relationship, protect yourself.* Do not rely on your partner to look out for your health. All forms of sexual activity carry some degree of risk for spreading STDs. Gauge the level of risk you are willing to assume.

9. *Strive to be in a mutually satisfying, disease-free relationship with one person.* If both you and your sex partner are monogamous and disease-free, you will not be at risk for STDs. Two mutually exclusive, uninfected partners can enjoy sex without fear of infection.

sex in society 15.3

Interactions Among Geographic Differences, Sexual Behavior, and Disease Infectivity

Pinkerton, Chesson, and Layde (2002) found that the risk of acquiring STDs varies significantly according to the interaction of four major risk factors: (a) disease infectivity (the ease with which a disease is transmitted through penile-vaginal intercourse), (b) the level of infection within a community, (c) the number of different sex partners, and (d) the number of unprotected sex acts (consistent condom use).

Pinkerton et al. (2002) found that in geographic areas with high morbidity of very infectious diseases such as gonorrhea and chlamydia, the best way to reduce risk was to decrease the overall number of sexual partners. This was found to be more protective than the overall number of protected sex acts. In other words, by decreasing the overall number of different sex partners, one decreased their risk more than by using condoms consistently with multiple sex partners. Because highly infectious diseases are relatively easy to acquire with even one sexual exposure, lowering the number of potential exposures (by decreasing the overall number of partners) was found to be the best way to reduce risk.

In contrast, in geographic areas with high morbidity of less infectious diseases such as HIV, the best way to reduce risk was to increase the number of protected sex acts. Having fewer partners was less protective than using condoms with each sex act.

Because HIV is more difficult to spread through penile- vaginal intercourse than gonorrhea and chlamydia, being exposed to a single episode of intercourse with different partners (most of whom might be uninfected) might pose less of a risk of infection with HIV than being consistently exposed to a single, infected partner. Consistent exposure to a single infectious partner therefore required more consistent condom use (decreasing the overall number of unprotected sex acts).

The same dynamic can hold true for sexual/medical history. If the sex partner has a high-risk past (used injectable drugs and might be HIV-positive, for instance), the other partner's personal behavior might be much different from that of someone whose partner has no history of infection. If the personal history includes a risk such as prior infection with gonococcal pelvic inflammatory disease (PID), for instance, a woman might take extra precautions against becoming infected with gonorrhea again as it could increase the risk for developing PID again. Each individual has to develop a personal plan for STD risk reduction based on his or her (and the partner's) pyramid.

Plans will vary according to the individuals involved. Although reducing risks this way takes a little more thought, it also respects individuality.

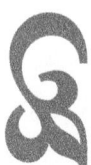 **healthy sex hints 15.6**

Are You Really Sleeping with Your Partner's Partners?

Probably the most overused myth associated with sexual lifestyle is the notion that when you "sleep with someone, you sleep with everyone they have ever had sex with." We're sure you all have heard this at one point or another during your lives. Here are seven reasons why we disagree with this message:

1. For the most part, it is an anti-sex, fear-based message. It targets guilt and a sense of helplessness. None of these are part of healthy sexuality.
2. It uses incorrect terminology. You will rarely get any STDs (except maybe crabs or scabies) by merely *sleeping* with someone. You must engage in some kind of sexual activity with the person to acquire an STD.
3. You do not "have sex" with anyone but the *person* you actually come in physical contact with. Any explanation other than this is nonsense (actually, it's a metaphor to induce fear).
4. Most non-viral STDs are cured when a person receives treatment. If your partner had a non-viral STD and was properly treated, the infection stopped there.
5. If your partner's partner was infected with an STD but did not pass it on to your partner, it *cannot infect you* under any circumstances.
6. Even viral STDs such as genital herpes can be controlled with treatment. *You* are not at risk for your partner's partner who had a viral STD unless this person infected your lover, who then passes the infection on to you.
7. Being exposed to your partner's antibodies to past sex partners is *not the same* as being exposed to disease producing germs (although research shows that people can develop antibodies in response to *being exposed* to human semen, this is not the same thing as being infected with a disease).

Based on the data we just presented, do you still think you are sleeping with everyone your partner has slept with when you have sex with him or her?

Personal Assessment

A Pyramid of Risks for STDs

As we discussed in this chapter, your risk for becoming infected with a Sexually Transmitted Disease is influenced by a combination of factors described in the Pyramid of Risk Model. The pyramid describes four levels of risk factors. Some of these factors such as sexual/medical history and the demographic variables age, race, and gender, are beyond your ability to control. Others such as your sexual behavior and relationships are within your control.

Instructions

1. Read the section of Chapter 15 that describes Blonna's Pyramid of Risk Model.

2. Evaluate how each of the four levels of risk proposed in the model impacts your personal vulnerability to infection.

3. Factor in the two levels of risk (sexual/medical history & demographic variables) that cannot be changed but still affect your personal vulnerability to infection.

4. Assess your current relationship status and the behaviors you engage in with your sex partner(s).

5. Describe your own risk using this model.

Thought Questions

1. What are the various modes of transmission associated with STDs/HIV?

2. What are four major trends associated with STDs over the past two decades?

3. What is the underlying premise of the Pyramid of Risk for STDs?

4. How are demographic variables related to the risk for STD/HIV?

5. What are five important things to know about a potential sex partner's sexual history as related to STD/HIV risk?

6. How do sexual lifestyles and sexual behavior work together to increase or decrease risk?

7. What are the major signs and symptoms of STDs in men and women?

8. Why do gay men and heterosexual women have a similar risk profile?

Test Yourself!

1. Which group is not experiencing an increase in STD morbidity and mortality?
   a. Urban, heterosexual, African Americans
   b. Rural homosexual men
   c. Hispanic adolescents
   d. Female partners of HIV-infected intravenous drug users

2. *Epidemiological synergy* refers to
   a. the proliferation of STDs that cause damage to the epidermis.
   b. a synergistic effect caused by two different germs.
   c. the increased risk for acquiring an STD if already infected with one.
   d. a pattern of rampant disease spread through populations.

3. The Pyramid of Risk for STDs assumes that
   a. there are four levels of STD risk; some can be changed, some cannot.
   b. disease risk is like a pyramid or iceberg.
   c. those at the top of the risk pyramid have the greatest chance of becoming infected.
   d. there are five levels of risk that correspond to demographics.
4. Which best characterizes the risk associated with sexual lifestyle and sexual behaviors?
   a. They are two separate risk categories that do not relate to each other.
   b. The lower your STD lifestyle risk, the less attention you need to pay to specific sexual behaviors.
   c. The higher your STD lifestyle risk, the less attention you need to pay to specific sexual behaviors.
   d. Sexual medical history does not impact sexual lifestyle risk.
5. Which of the following is *not* an STD risk associated with one's sexual medical history?
   a. Number of lifetime sexual partners
   b. History of contraceptive use
   c. Immunization status
   d. Age of onset of sexual intercourse
6. The belief that "when you sleep with someone, you sleep with everyone they have slept with" is inaccurate because
   a. it is a simplistic metaphor.
   b. your partner's sex partners had sex with him or her, not you.
   c. being exposed to antibodies that your partner produced in relation to their sex partners is not the same thing as having sex with those people.
   d. all of the above

7. Which of the following is not a viral STD?
   a. Syphilis
   b. HIV
   c. HPV
   d. Genital herpes
8. Why do gay men and heterosexual women share a similar STD risk profile?
   a. They both are sexually attracted to heterosexual men who carry most STDs.
   b. They are insertive sexually.
   c. They are receptive sexually.
   d. Their primary sex partners are men.
9. Which of the following is most responsible for the pattern of decreasing AIDS mortality?
   a. The sexual behavior of HIV high-risk groups has changed.
   b. Cocktail AIDS drugs are used.
   c. Less virulent strains of HIV now predominate.
   d. Most people with AIDS have already died.
10. Which STD is making a comeback in selected major U.S. cities after being on the verge of extinction in the past 5 years?
    a. Smallpox
    b. Syphilis
    c. Scabies
    d. Chancroid

Web Resources

The Division of STD Prevention
www.cdc.gov/std/

The Division of STD Prevention, at the Centers for Disease Control and Prevention, provides national leadership through research, policy development, and support of effective services to prevent STDs (including HIV infection) and their complications such as enhanced HIV transmission, infertility, adverse outcomes of pregnancy, and reproductive tract cancer.

The Division of HIV/AIDS Prevention
http://www.cdc.gov/hiv/dhap.htm

CDC's HIV mission is to prevent HIV infection and reduce the incidence of HIV-related illness and death, in collaboration with community, state, national, and international partners.

American Social Health Association (ASHA)
http://healthfinder.gov/FindServices/Organizations/Organization.aspx?code=HR0966

A nonprofit organization dedicated to stopping sexually transmitted diseases and their consequences. The site offers excellent links and information to other ASHA programs. It provides STD information, facts and questions, sexual health glossary, and support groups sections.

Gay Men's Health Crisis
http://www.gmhc.org/

A nonprofit organization providing support services to men, women, children, and their families with AIDS in the New York City area, as well as education and advocacy nationwide.

References

Alan Guttmacher Institute. (1991). *Sex and America's teenagers.* New York: Author.

Alter, M., & Margolis, H. (1990). The emergence of hepatitis B as a sexually transmitted disease. *Medical Clinics of North America, 6,* 1529–1541.

Anderson, J.E. (2003). Condom Use and HIV Risk Among US Adults *American Journal of Public Health* v. 93 no. 6 (June 2003) p. 912–14.

Bachmann, L.H., Lewis, I., Allen R. (2000). Risk and prevalence of treatable sexually transmitted diseases at a Birmingham substance abuse treatment facility. *American Journal of Public Health* v. 90 no. 10 (October 2000) p. 1615–18.

Bearman, PS, Moody, J., Stoval, K. (2004). Chains of infection: the study of adolescent romantic and sexual networks. American Journal of Sociology. Vol. 110, (1), July 2004 pgs 44–91.

Bertrami, R. (2002, November). *Chlamydia screening in the Philadelphia public schools.* Paper presented at the annual Meeting of the American Public Health Association, Philadelphia.

Bonavoglia, A (2000).Making love in the dark. *Ms.* v. 10 no. 5 (August/September 2000) p. 54–9

Cameron, D. W., et al. (1991). Condom use prevents genital ulcers in women working as prostitutes: Influences of human immunodeficiency virus infection. *Sexually Transmitted Diseases, 18,* 188–194.

Cates, W., & Stone, K. M. (1992). Family planning, sexually transmitted diseases and contraceptive choice: A literature update—Part I. *Family Planning Perspectives, 24*(2), 75–84.

CDC (2013). CDC Fact Sheet: Incidence, Prevalence and Cost of Sexually Transmitted Infections in the United States. Atlanta: US Department of Health and Human Services, Centers for Disease Control and Prevention, National Center for HIV/AIDS, Viral Hepatitis, STD, and TB Prevention. Available online at: http://www.cdc.gov/std/stats/STI-Estimates-Fact-Sheet-Feb-2013.pdf

CDC (2006). HPV and HPV Vaccine-Information for Healthcare Providers. Available online at: http://www.cdc.gov/std/HPV/STDFact-HPV-vaccine-hcp.htm.

Ciaran, B. J., Woodman, S. C., Rollason, T. P., Winter, H., Bailey, A., Yates, M., & Young, L. S. (2003, January 4). Human papillomavirus type 18 and rapidly progressing cervical intraepithelial neoplasia: Mechanisms of disease. *The Lancet, 361*(9351), 40.

Coffey, S. (2011). *Antiretroviral Therapy.* Health resources and Services Administration. Rockville MD. available online at: http://hab.hrsa.gov/deliverhivaidscare/clinicalguide11/

Conant, M., Hardy, D., Sernatinger, J., Spicer, D., & Levy, J. (1986). Condoms prevent transmission of AIDS-associated retrovirus. *Journal of the American Medical Association, 255,* 1706.

Crosby, R.A., DiClemente, R.J., Wingood G.M. (2003). Value of Consistent Condom Use: A Study of Sexually Transmitted Disease Prevention Among African American Adolescent Females. *American Journal of Public Health* v. 93 no. 6 (June 2003) p. 901–2.

Dan, B. D. (1996). Sex and the singles whirl: The quantum dynamics of hepatitis B. *Journal of the American Medical Association, 256*(10), 1344.

Darrow, W. W. (1989). Condom use and use-effectiveness in high-risk populations. *Sexually Transmitted Diseases, 16,* 157–162.

DHAP (2013). Surveillance brief: Surveillance Systems Supported by the Division of HIV/AIDS Prevention. Atlanta GA: Centers for Disease Control and Prevention, National Center for HIV/AIDS, Viral Hepatitis, STD, and TB Prevention, Division of HIV/AIDS Prevention. available online at: http://www.cdc.gov/hiv/statistics/recommendations/publications.html

DSTD (2000). *Tracking the hidden epidemics: Trends in STDs in the United States 2000.* Atlanta: Public Health Service. Atlanta GA: Centers for Disease Control and Prevention, National Center for HIV/AIDS, Viral Hepatitis, STD, and TB Prevention, Division of STD Prevention.

DSTD (2013a). *Genital HPV Infection-CDC Fact Sheet.* Atlanta GA: Centers for Disease Control and Prevention, National Center for HIV/AIDS, Viral Hepatitis, STD, and TB Prevention, Division of STD Prevention. available online at: http://www.cdc.gov/std/HPV/STDFact-HPV.htm

DSTD (2013b). *Genital Herpes- CDC Fact Sheet.* Atlanta GA: Centers for Disease Control and Prevention, National Center for HIV/AIDS, Viral Hepatitis, STD, and TB Prevention, Division of STD Prevention. available online at: http://www.cdc.gov/std/Herpes/STDFact-Herpes.htm

DSTD (2013c). *Gonorrhea- CDC Fact Sheet.* Atlanta GA: Centers for Disease Control and Prevention, National Center for HIV/AIDS, Viral Hepatitis, STD, and TB Prevention, Division of STD Prevention. available online at: http://www.cdc.gov/std/Gonorrhea/STDFact-gonorrhea.htm

DSTD (2013d). *Syphilis- CDC Fact Sheet.* Atlanta GA: Centers for Disease Control and Prevention, National Center for HIV/AIDS, Viral Hepatitis, STD, and TB Prevention, Division of STD Prevention. available online at: http://www.cdc.gov/std/syphilis/STDFact-Syphilis.htm

DSTD (2012a). *2011 Sexually Transmitted Disease Surveillance Report: Genital Warts.* Atlanta GA: Centers for Disease Control and Prevention, National Center for HIV/AIDS, Viral Hepatitis, STD, and TB Prevention, Division of STD Prevention. Available online at: http://www.cdc.gov/std/stats11/figures/53.htm

DSTD (2012b). *2011 Sexually Transmitted Disease Surveillance Report: Genital Herpes.* Atlanta GA: Centers for Disease Control and Prevention, National Center for HIV/AIDS, Viral Hepatitis, STD, and TB Prevention, Division of STD Prevention. Available online at: http://www.cdc.gov/std/stats11/figures/55.htm

DSTD (2012c). *2011 Sexually Transmitted Disease Surveillance Report: Chlamydia.* Atlanta GA: Centers for Disease Control and Prevention, National Center for HIV/AIDS, Viral Hepatitis, STD, and TB Prevention, Division of STD Prevention. Available online at: http://www.cdc.gov/std/stats11/chlamydia.htm

DSTD (2012d). *2011 Sexually Transmitted Disease Surveillance Report: Chlamydia Rates by Sex.* Atlanta GA: Centers for Disease Control and Prevention, National Center for HIV/AIDS, Viral Hepatitis, STD, and TB Prevention, Division of STD Prevention. Available online at: http://www.cdc.gov/std/stats11/figures/1.htm

DSTD (2012e). *2011 Sexually Transmitted Disease Surveillance Report: Chlamydia Rates by Age and Sex.* Atlanta GA: Centers for Disease Control and Prevention, National Center for HIV/AIDS, Viral Hepatitis, STD, and TB Prevention, Division of STD Prevention. Available online at: http://www.cdc.gov/std/stats11/figures/5.htm

DSTD (2012f). *2011 Sexually Transmitted Disease Surveillance Report: Gonorrhea.* Atlanta GA: Centers for Disease Control and Prevention, National Center for HIV/AIDS, Viral Hepatitis, STD, and TB Prevention, Division of STD Prevention. Available online at: http://www.cdc.gov/std/stats11/gonorrhea.htm

DSTD (2012g). *2011 Sexually Transmitted Disease Surveillance Report: Gonorrhea Rates-United States.* Atlanta GA: Centers for Disease Control and Prevention, National Center for HIV/AIDS, Viral Hepatitis, STD, and TB Prevention, Division of STD Prevention. Available online at: http://www.cdc.gov/std/stats11/figures/16.htm

DSTD (2012h). *2011 Sexually Transmitted Disease Surveillance Report: Gonorrhea rates by Age and Sex.* Atlanta GA: Centers for Disease Control and Prevention, National Center for HIV/AIDS, Viral Hepatitis, STD, and TB Prevention, Division of STD Prevention. Available online at: http://www.cdc.gov/std/stats11/figures/21.htm

DSTD (2012i). *2011 Sexually Transmitted Disease Surveillance Report: Gonorrhea Rates by race and Ethnicity.* Atlanta GA: Centers for Disease Control and Prevention, National Center for HIV/AIDS, Viral Hepatitis, STD, and TB Prevention, Division of STD Prevention. Available online at: http://www.cdc.gov/std/stats11/figures/24.htm

DSTD (2012j). *2011 Sexually Transmitted Disease Surveillance Report: Syphilis.* Atlanta GA: Centers for Disease Control and Prevention, National Center for HIV/AIDS, Viral Hepatitis, STD, and TB Prevention, Division of STD Prevention. Available online at: http://www.cdc.gov/std/stats11/syphilis.htm

DSTD (2012k). *2011 Sexually Transmitted Disease Surveillance Report: Other Sexually Transmitted Diseases; Chancroid.* Atlanta GA: Centers for Disease Control and Prevention, National Center for HIV/AIDS, Viral Hepatitis, STD, and TB Prevention, Division of STD Prevention. Available online at: http://www.cdc.gov/std/stats11/other.htm

DSTD (2012L). *Hepatitis B Facts for Health Professionals.* Atlanta GA: Centers for Disease Control and Prevention, National Center for HIV/AIDS, Viral Hepatitis, STD, and TB Prevention, Division of STD Prevention. Available online at: http://www.cdc.gov/hepatitis/HBV/HBVfaq.htm#overview

DSTD (2012m). *STDs in Adolescents and Young Adults.* Atlanta GA: Centers for Disease Control and Prevention, National Center for HIV/AIDS, Viral Hepatitis, STD, and TB Prevention, Division of STD Prevention. Available online at http://www.cdc.gov/std/stats11/adol.htm

DSTD (2011a). *Sexually Transmitted Disease Treatment Guidelines: Human Papillomavirus (HPV) Infection.* Atlanta GA: Centers for Disease Control and Prevention, National Center for HIV/AIDS, Viral Hepatitis, STD, and TB Prevention, Division of STD Prevention. Available online at: http://www.cdc.gov/std/treatment/2010/hpv.htm

DSTD (2011b). *Sexually Transmitted Disease Treatment Guidelines: Genital Warts.* Atlanta GA: Centers for Disease Control and Prevention, National Center for HIV/AIDS, Viral Hepatitis, STD, and TB Prevention, Division of STD Prevention. Available online at: http://www.cdc.gov/std/treatment/2010/genital-warts.htm

DSTD (2011c). *Sexually Transmitted Disease Treatment Guidelines: Chlamydial Infections.* Atlanta GA: Centers for Disease Control and Prevention, National Center for HIV/AIDS, Viral Hepatitis, STD, and TB Prevention, Division of STD Prevention. Available online at: http://www.cdc.gov/std/treatment/2010/chlamydial-infections.htm

DSTD (2011d). *Sexually Transmitted Disease Treatment Guidelines: Genital HSV Infections.* Atlanta GA: Centers for Disease Control and Prevention, National Center for HIV/AIDS, Viral Hepatitis, STD, and TB Prevention, Division of STD Prevention. Available online at: http://www.cdc.gov/std/treatment/2010/genital-ulcers.htm

DSTD (2011e). *Sexually Transmitted Disease Treatment Guidelines: Gonococcal Infections.* Atlanta GA: Centers for Disease Control and Prevention, National Center for HIV/AIDS, Viral Hepatitis, STD, and TB Prevention, Division of STD Prevention. Available online at: http://www.cdc.gov/std/treatment/2010/gonococcal-infections.htm

DSTD (2011f). *Sexually Transmitted Disease Treatment Guidelines: Diseases Characterized by Genital, Anal, or Perianal Ulcers.* Atlanta GA: Centers for Disease Control and Prevention, National Center for HIV/AIDS, Viral Hepatitis, STD, and TB Prevention, Division of STD Prevention. Available online at: http://www.cdc.gov/std/treatment/2010/genital-ulcers.htm#syphilis

DSTD (2011g). *Sexually Transmitted Disease Treatment Guidelines: Ectoparasitic Infections.* Atlanta GA: Centers for Disease Control and Prevention, National Center for HIV/AIDS, Viral Hepatitis, STD, and TB Prevention, Division of STD Prevention. Available online at: http://www.cdc.gov/std/treatment/2010/urethritis-and-cervicitis.htm#nongonococcal

DSTD (2011h). *Sexually Transmitted Disease Treatment Guidelines: Diseases Characterized by Urethritis and Cervicitis.* Atlanta GA: Centers for Disease Control and Prevention, National Center for HIV/AIDS, Viral Hepatitis, STD, and TB Prevention, Division of STD Prevention. Available online at: http://www.cdc.gov/std/treatment/2010/ectoparasitic.htm

DSTD (2005). Trends in Reportable Sexually Transmitted Diseases in the United States, 2004. National Surveillance Data for Chlamydia, Gonorrhea, and Syphilis. Available online at: http://www.cdc.gov/std/stats/trends2004.htm

Donelan, K., Blendon, R. J., Hill, C. A., et al. (1996). Whatever happened to the health insurance crisis in the United States? Voices from a national survey. *Journal of the American Medical Association, 276,* 1346–1350.

Dunn, R. A., & Rolfs, R. T. (1991). The resurgence of syphilis in the United States. *Current Opinions in Infectious Diseases, 4,* 3–11.

Eng, T. R., & Butler, W. T. (Eds.). (1997). *The hidden epidemic: Confronting STDs.* Washington, DC: Academy Press, Institute of Medicine.

Finelli, L., Budd, J., & Spitalny, K. (1993). Early syphilis: Relationships to sex, drugs, and changes in high-risk behavior from 1987–1990. *Sexually Transmitted Diseases, 2,* 89–95.

Fortenberry J.D. (2002). Clinic-based Service Programs for Increasing Responsible Sexual Behavior. *The Journal of Sex Research* v. 39 no. 1 (February 2002) p. 63–6.

Gallet, C.A. (2002). A note on the determinants of sexually transmitted disease rates. *The Social Science Journal* v. 39 no. 4 (2002) p. 613–16.

Garnett, G. P., & Anderson, R. M. (1996). Core-group transmission of STDs. *Sexually Transmitted Diseases, 20*(4), 181–191.

Golden et al. (2003). HIV/STD Risks in Young Men Who Have Sex With Men Who Do Not Disclose Their Sexual Orientation—Six U.S. Cities, 1994–2000. JAMA v. 289 no. 8 (February 26 2003) p. 975–7.

Green, Y., Gollub, E (2001). CDC promotes the female condom for HIV/STD prevention. *American Journal of Public Health* v. 91 no. 11 (November 2001) p. 1732–3.

Greenhalgh, T. (2000). The STD codes. *Accountancy International* v. 125 no. 1277 (January 2000) p. 60

Grimes, D. A., & Cates, W. (1990). Family planning and sexually transmitted diseases. In K. K. Holmes, P. A. Mardh, P. F. Sparling, P. Wiesner, W. Cates, S. M. Lemon, & W. E. Stamm (Eds.), *Sexually transmitted diseases* (2nd ed., pp.1087–1094). New York: McGraw-Hill.

Guaschino, S., & DeSeta, F. (2000). Update on *Chlamydia trachomatis* [review]. *Annals of the New York Academy of Science,* 900, 293–300.

Hart, G. (1974). Factors influencing venereal infection in a war environment. *British Journal of Venereal Disease, 50,* 68–72.

Ho, G. Y. F., Bierman, R., Beardsley, L., Chang, C. J., & Burk, R. D. (1998). Natural history of cervicovaginal papilloma virus infection in young women. *New England Journal of Medicine, 338,* 423–428.

Holloway, L.R. (2005). What You Should Know Before Having Sex. *Ebony* v. 60 no. 10 (August 2005) p. 118, 120, 122–3.

Howard, M., & McCabe, J. B. (1990). Helping teenagers postpone sexual involvement. *Family Planning Perspectives, 22,* 21–26.

Jones, J. (1993). *Bad Blood: The Tuskegee Study—A Tragedy of Race and Medicine.* New York City, NY; Free Press.

Karon, J. M., Fleming, P. L., Steketee, R. W., & DeCock, K. M. (2001). HIV in the United States at the turn of the century: An epidemic in transition. *American Journal of Public Health, 91*(7), 1060–1068.

Kassutto, S, Doweiko, JP. (2004). Syphilis in the HIV Era. *Emerging Infectious Diseases* v. 10 no. 8 (August 2004) p. 1471–3

Kennedy, M. B., Scarlett, M. I., Duer, A. C., & Chu, S. Y. (1995). Assessing HIV risk among women who have sex with women: Scientific and communication issues. *Journal of the American Medical Women's Association, 50,* 103–107.

Kodner, CM., Nasraty, S. (2004). Management of Genital Warts. *American Family Physician* v. 70 no. 12 (December 15 2004) p. 2335–42.

Kuyoh, M.A., Toroitich-Ruto, C., Grimes D.A., Schulz, K.F., Gallo, M.F. (2003). Sponge vs. diaphragm for contraception. *Contraception,* Jan2003, Vol. 67 Issue 1, p15–19.

Laumann, E. O., Gagnon, J. H., Michael, R. Y., & Michaels, S. (1994). *The social organization of sexuality: Sexual practices in the United States.* Chicago: University of Chicago Press.

Manhart, L.E., Aral S.O., Homles , K.K. (2004). Influence of Study Population on the Identification of Risk Factors for Sexually Transmitted Diseases using a Case-Control Design: The Example of Gonorrhea. *American Journal of Epidemiology* v. 160 no. 4 (August 15 2004) p. 393–402.

Mann, J., Quinn, T., et al. (1987). Condom use and HIV infection among prostitutes in Zaire [letter]. *New England Journal of Medicine, 316,* 345.

Metzler, C.W., Biglan, A., Noell, J. (2000). A randomized controlled trial of a behavioral intervention to reduce high-risk sexual behavior among adolescents in STD clinics. *Behavior Therapy* v. 31 no. 1 (Winter 2000).

Minuk, G., Bohme, G., & Bowen, T. (1986). Condoms and hepatitis B virus infection. *Annals of Internal Medicine, 104,* 584.

MMWR (2001). Revised guidelines for HIV Counseling, testing and referral.

Morbidity and Mortality Weekly Report. U.S. Government Printing Office (GPO), Washington, DC 20402-9371. November 9, 2001 / 50(RR19); pgs.1–58. Available online at: http://www.cdc.gov/mmwr//preview/mmwrhtml/rr5019a1.htm

MMWR. (2002, October 18). Screening tests to detect chlamydia and gonorrhea infections. Morbidity and Mortality Weekly Report, 51 (RR-15). Atlanta: U.S. Department of Health and Human Services, Centers for Disease Control and Prevention, Division of STD.

MMWR. (2002, May). 2002: Sexually transmitted disease: Treatment guidelines. *Mortality and Morbidity Weekly Report, 51* (RR-6).

Morse, S., Moreland, A., & Thompson, S. (1990). *Sexually transmitted diseases.* New York: Gower Medical.

Moscicki, A. B., Ellenberg, J. H., Vermund, S. H., Hooland, C. A., Darragh, T., Crowley-Nowick, P. A., et al. (2000, February). Prevalence of and risks for cervical human papillomavirus infection and squamous intraepithelial lesions in adolescent girls. *Archives of Pediatrics & Adolescent Medicine, 154*(2), 127.

Nakashima, A. K., Rolfs, R. T., Flock, M. L., et al. (1996). Epidemiology of syphilis in the United States, 1941–1993. *Sexually Transmitted Diseases, 23*(1), 16–23.

National Center for Infectious Disease. (2003). Hepatitis surveillance 1980–2001 [Online]. Available: www.cdc.gov/ ncidod/diseases/hepatitis/resource/dz_burden02.htm.

Navarro, N. (1990). Race or class: Mortality differentials in the United States. *Lancet, 336,* 1238–1240.

ONAP (2010). *National HIV/AIDS Strategy for the United States.* Washington DC: The White House Office of National AIDS Policy. available online at: http://www.cdc.gov/hiv/pdf/policies_nhas.pdf

OraSure (2012). OraQuick In-Home HIV Test. Bethlehem: PA. available online at: http://www.oraquick.com/Home

Pinkerton, S. T., Chesson, H. W., & Layde, P. M. (2002, September). NIMH prevention trial group: Utility of behavioral changes as markers of STD risk reduction in sexually transmitted disease/HIV prevention trials. *Journal of AIDS, 31*(1), 71–79.

Piot, P., & Islam, M. Q. (1994). Sexually transmitted diseases in the 1990s: Global epidemiology and the challenges for control. *Sexually Transmitted Diseases, 21* (Supplement 2), 7–13.

Potterat, R., Rothenberg, R., Woodhouse, D. E., Muth, J. B., Pratts, C. I., & Fogle, J. S. (1985). Gonorrhea as a social disease. *Sexually Transmitted Diseases, 1,* 25–32.

Powelson, M., Fletcher, JF. (2000). Sexually transmitted diseases, drug use, & risky behavior among Miami-Dade County jail detainees. *Corrections Today* v. 62 no. 6 (October 2000) p. 108–13, 122

Quinn, T., & Cates, W. (1993). Epidemiology of STDs in the 1990s. In T. Quinn (Ed.), *Sexually transmitted diseases.* New York: Raven.

Ramos, R., Shain, R. N., & Johnson, L. (1995). Men I mess with don't have anything to do with AIDS: Using ethnotheory to understand sexual risk perception. *Sociology Quarterly, 36,* 483–505.

Rice, R. J., Roberts, P. L., & Handsfield, H. H. (1991). Sociodemographic distribution of gonorrhea incidence: Implications for prevention and behavioral research. *American Journal of Public Health, 10,* 1253–1257.

Richardson B.A. (2002). Nonoxynol-9 as a vaginal mircrobicide for prevention of sexually transmitted infections. *JAMA* 2002;287:1171–2.

Rosen, T (2003). Update on Genital Lesions. JAMA v. 290 no. 8 (August 27 2003) p. 1001–5.

Rosenberg, M. J., & Gollub, E. L. (1992). Commentary: Methods women can use that may prevent sexually transmitted disease, including HIV. *American Journal of Public Health, 82*(11), 1473–1478.

Santelli, J.S., Lowry, R, Brener, ND (2000). The association of sexual behaviors with socioeconomic status, family structure, and race/ethnicity among US adolescents *American Journal of Public Health* v. 90 no. 10 (October 2000) p. 1582–8.

Schiffman, N. H. (1992). Recent progress in defining the epidemiology of human papillomavirus infection and cervical neoplasia. *Journal of National Cancer Institute, 84,* 394–398.

Smeltzer, S., & Whipple, B. (1991). Women & HIV. *Journal of Nursing, 4,* 249–256.

St. Louis, M. E., & Wasserheit, J. N. (1998). Elimination of syphilis in the United States. *Science, 281,* 353–354.

Taylor, M., Prescott, L. Brown, J., Wong, W., Allen, M., Broussard, D., Lori, P. (2005). Activities to increase provider awareness of early syphilis in men who have sex with men in 8 cities, 2000-2004. *Sexually Transmitted Diseases,* Oct, 2005 Supplement, Vol. 32, p S24–S29.

Timmreck T.T. (2002). *Introduction to Epidemiology.* Sudbury Mass: Jones & Bartlett Publishers.

Ungvarski, P. J. (1997). Update on HIV infection. *American Journal of Nursing, 97*(1), 44–51.

Wallis, C (2005). A Snapshot of Teen Sex. *Time* v. 165 no. 6 (February 7 2005) p. 58.

Wasserheit, J. (1992). Epidemiological synergy. *Sexually Transmitted Diseases, 2,* 61–77.

Webster, L. A., Berman, S. M., & Greenspan, M. (1993), Surveillance for gonorrhea and primary and secondary syphilis among adolescents United States, 1981–1991. *Mortality and Morbidity Weekly Report,* 42(SS-3), 1–10.

Weinstock H., Berman S, Cates W. Sexually transmitted diseases among American youth: incidence and prevalence estimates, 2000. *Perspectives on Sexual and Reproductive Health* 2004; 36(1):6–10.

Woodman, C. B., Collins, S., Winter, H., Barley, A., Ellis, J., Prior, P., et al. (2001). Natural history of cervical human papillomavirus infection in young women: A longitudinal cohort study. *Lancet, 357*(9271), 1831–1836.

chapter
sixteen

Sexual Coercion

Student Learning Objectives

After reading this chapter, students will be able to

- ♥ Define *sexual coercion* and *sexual victimization* and the three forms highlighted in this chapter: harassment, rape, and child sexual abuse.
- ♥ Explain and give examples of the three conditions that constitute sexual harassment.
- ♥ Describe the dynamic of power over subordinates in determining sexual harassment.
- ♥ Define *rape,* and differentiate it from other forms of sexual aggression.
- ♥ Describe the typical pattern of rape by a stranger, and develop a personal plan to reduce the risk for this form of rape.
- ♥ Define *acquaintance rape* and identify the risks.
- ♥ Develop a personal plan for reducing the risk for date rape.
- ♥ Describe the risks associated with the major "date rape" drugs.
- ♥ Assess the impact of alcohol abuse in coercive sex.
- ♥ Describe the characteristics of rapists.
- ♥ Evaluate common myths associated with rape and rapists.
- ♥ Describe the preconditions of child sexual abuse.
- ♥ Evaluate ways to reduce the risks for child sexual abuse.

activity teaser: What is the message in the music? Learn more in the Personal Exploration Activity on page 618

case study 16.1

Marc: Learning That No Means No

Marc, 23, identifies as Italian American.

Marc, a senior, was a student in one of Dr. Blonna's human sexuality classes. He submitted a written assignment about how he learned the difference between yes and no.

I'm embarrassed to write this, but I think the story needs to be told. I grew up learning that when a woman said no, she really meant yes. My brother and his friends explained it to me by saying that women do this so they can remain ladies but still get laid. It made sense to me then, even though I now realize this kind of thinking is crazy.

I didn't encounter this with the first two women I had sex with. They both willingly went along. I went out with my second girlfriend for almost 2 years. When we broke up, I had to start dating again and didn't get anywhere with the first two girls I went out with. They didn't even let me get to first base.

The third woman was very sexy. I met her at a frat party, and she was hot. We danced a little and had a couple of beers, and then she wanted to leave. I walked her back to her room, and she invited me up. Her roommates had gone home for the weekend, and we started making out on the couch. She was so sexy, and I thought she really wanted to have sex. She let me feel her breasts and put my hand in her pants, but every time I tried to unzip her jeans, she pulled away and said no. I figured she was just teasing and really wanted me to continue, so I kept pushing the limit.

After about 20 minutes of this, she suddenly pushed me off of her and literally dumped me on the floor. She screamed at me, "Look, I told you no five times! I don't want to fuck you. Now get out before I call the campus cops!" I was shocked and very upset. I really didn't want to rape her, just push her until she gave in. I felt embarrassed and wanted to explain how I felt, but she told me if I didn't leave immediately, she'd call the police. I ran out of there zipping up as I left. I've seen her on campus, but she won't even look at me. I learned that no really means no!

Sexual coercion Any nonconsensual sexual behavior that occurs as the result of arguing, pleading, and cajoling, and includes, but is not limited to, force

Sexual victimization Depriving a person of free choice and forcing him or her to endure, observe, or comply with sexual acts

As we have seen in the case of Marc, there is a fine line between pursuing sex assertively and sexual coercion. Marc learned firsthand that "No means no," or that line is crossed. **Sexual coercion** is any nonconsensual sexual behavior that occurs as a result of arguing, pleading, and cajoling, in addition to force. **Sexual victimization** occurs when a person is deprived of free choice and is forced to endure, observe, or comply with sexual acts. Coercive sex can take many forms. The commonality is the element of power and victimhood. In this chapter, we focus on three forms: rape (also called sexual assault), sexual harassment, and child sexual abuse. We will start our examination with a look at rape.

Rape

The dictionary definition of **rape** is "sexual intercourse without the consent of the man/woman and effected by force, duress, intimidation, or deception as to the nature of the act" (Benton, 1996). The word *rape* comes from the Latin term *rapere,* which means to steal, seize, or carry away. Rape has been a common theme in literature, art, and popular culture throughout history.

Chilling examples of rape occur regularly in cartoons, comic strips, and other "children's entertainment." The caveman, replete with club and knuckles dragging the earth, is out and about to find a mate. When he spies the female he desires, he hits her with the club, knocks her out, and drags her away by her long hair (presumably to make her his wife).

More than 95 percent of rapes are committed by men against women or other men (Rand, 2008). Although 9 of 10 rapists are men, this does not mean that all men rape, nor are all men potential rapists. If you were to take a sample of 100 rapists, more than 90 would be men. If you were to take a random sample of 100 men, fewer than 10 would be rapists or potential rapists. The statistic does mean, however, that most of the rapes are committed by a small percentage of men who achieve power over women and other men by forced sexual aggression.

Rape is a form **sexual aggression,** a broader term that encompasses all forms of nonconsensual physical sexual activity against men, women, children, and gay people as victims (Cate & Lloyd, 1992). It includes fondling, oral sex, and anal sex, as well as vaginal intercourse. **Sexual coercion,** the broadest term, covers all nonconsensual sexual behavior that results from arguing, pleading, and cajoling, in addition to force.

The term *victim* is gradually being replaced by words such as *target* and *survivor,* in some contexts. This language avoids further degradation of the person who was raped. The new terminology connotes the encouragement for survivors to reclaim control over their lives.

In most states, to be considered rape, the target's body (usually the vagina) has to be penetrated. Forced oral sex and the insertion of fingers and other objects into the vagina, anus, or mouth don't automatically qualify as rape. Although these sexually aggressive acts are still illegal and can result in prosecution, they are tried as less serious offenses than is rape. Rape includes acquaintance rape (also known as date rape), stranger rape, marital rape, gang rape, and statutory rape. A last category of rape, male rape, usually is committed by men against other men but does occur, rarely, with women as the perpetrators.

Rape Illicit sexual intercourse without consent

Sexual aggression Any form of forced sexual contact, including but not limited to intercourse, without the person's consent

❧ *Physical Wellness* ❧

Men who engage in coercive sex often use their physical strength to intimidate, threaten, and/or overpower their victims. High-level physical wellness may empower women and help prevent becoming victims of coercive sex. Activities such as lifting weights to develop strength and practicing self-defense skills can help women repel would-be attackers. Feeling physically stronger and more prepared to fight might also send nonverbal messages to would-be attackers. Perpetrators are less likely to target women who appear strong, self-assured, and able to defend themselves.

Here are some common myths associated with rape:

Myth: Rape is a sexual act, not a violent one.

Fact: Although the rapist achieves sexual gratification through his actions, the rape is first and foremost an act of violence. If sexual release were all that a rapist desires, he could achieve that by finding a willing partner, masturbating, or paying a prostitute for sex. The rapist seeks to dominate his victim, to exert power, and to humiliate by using threat and violence. In contrast, sex is a consensual act of pleasure, not a violent act of power.

Myth: Women secretly want to be raped.

Fact: Even though many men and women have rape fantasies, there is a world of difference between using fantasy to become sexually aroused and actually desiring to be assaulted, forced to submit to another's sexual onslaught, and humiliated or beaten in the process. In a fantasy, you control the situation, orchestrate the script, and create the happy ending. In a rape, someone assaults you and controls you. Women do *not* want to be raped.

Myth: A woman can't be raped if she really doesn't want to be.

Fact: The logic of this myth revolves around the difficulty surrounding inserting a penis into a vagina that is thrashing to and fro. Men who rape use force to hurt women, to injure them to the point of submission. They have been known to break a woman's hip to stop it from moving. Rape is not about two lovers playfully teasing each other into submission. Rape is about force, domination, and pain.

Myth: Women "ask for it" by the way they act and dress.

Fact: Women don't dress provocatively to invite rapists. The idea of a woman wanting to attract a man and initiate a sexual liaison by acting in a sexy way is much different from the notion of a woman dressing in revealing clothing because she wants to be raped. If a woman intentionally acts and dresses provocatively to attract a man, that style doesn't give any man the right to rape her.

Myth: *No* really means *yes.*

Fact: Where does the notion that *no* means *yes* come from? Is it a rationalization, made up by men, to justify their domination and overpower women into submission? Or is it a leftover piece of baggage from the Victorian era, reminding women that ladies are not supposed to enjoy sex? In that line of thinking, because a lady can't ask for sex, she has to say no even though she means yes. That way she can have it both ways: maintain her status as a lady and still have sex ("He did it to me"). Wherever this belief came from, it's time to stop it and realize that *no* means *no.* When in doubt, don't continue.

Myth: Rape is justifiable under certain circumstances.

Fact: Rape is never justifiable. No one—husband, lover, boyfriend, father, or any man—ever has the right to force sex on anyone.

Myth: Most rapists are crazy.

Fact: Most rapists are not crazy. They are similar to the average man except for three distinguishing characteristics: (a) They are hostile toward women and have a harder time handling it; (b) they have more traditional beliefs about gender roles; and (c) they are more willing to use force to achieve their ends.

Myth: Women are responsible for preventing rape.

Fact: *Everyone* is responsible for preventing rape.

Posttraumatic Rape Syndrome

An estimated 70 percent of adults in the United States have experienced a traumatic event at least once in their lives, and up to 20 percent of these people go on to develop **posttraumatic stress disorder (PTSD).** PTSD can occur in either victims or witnesses of traumatic events ranging from natural disasters to rape [American Psychiatric Association (APA), 2000]. The three main diagnostic criteria for PTSD are (a) re-experiencing the event through dreams, flashbacks, and other means; (b) persistent avoidance of stimuli associated with the event; and (c) persistent symptoms ranging from difficulty falling asleep to irritability and outbursts of anger (APA, 2000).

Posttraumatic stress disorder (PTSD) A syndrome developing after exposure to an extremely traumatic event. Symptoms include anxiety, sleeplessness, eating disorders, depression, and hyperactive nervous system activity

An estimated 1 out of 10 women will get PTSD at some time in their lives. Women are about twice as likely as men to develop PTSD. This incidence may be due to the fact that women tend to experience interpersonal violence (such as domestic violence, rape, or abuse) more often than men.

Burgess and Holmstrom (1974) coined the term *rape trauma syndrome (RTS)* to identify a cluster of emotional responses to the extreme stress experienced by victims of rape. RTS has two phases. The first is the acute (initial) phase, which usually lasts anywhere from a few days to a few weeks after the attack. The next phase is the reorganization phase, which usually lasts anywhere from a few weeks to several years after the attack.

Acquaintance rape, also known as *date rape*, is a form of rape defined as forced sexual intercourse by a dating partner. Many experts consider acquaintance rape to be the most common and least reported of all forms of rape (Cate & Lloyd, 1992). Previous research has shown that college campuses, contrary to public opinion, are not safe havens from sexual coercion. College women are at a greater risk for rape and other forms of sexual assault than women in the general population or in a comparable age group (Fisher, Koss, Gidycz, & Wisnewski, 1987). This is due in part to the nature of the college environment where large concentrations of young women come into contact with young men in a variety of public and private settings at various times on and off their college campuses. Fisher, Cullen, and Turner (2000), in a national study of 4,446 college women, found that almost 3 percent (2.8%) of study participants experienced a completed or attempted rape during the academic year. They estimate that women at a college that has 10,000 female students could experience more than 350 rapes a year.

Acquaintance rape Forced intercourse by a person, other than a spouse, whom the victim knows

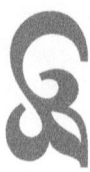

healthy sex hints 16.1

What to Do If You Are Raped or Sexually Assaulted

What to Do If You Have Been Raped

1. Go to a safe place away from your attacker.
   - Your first concern is your personal safety.
2. Call a friend, family member, or someone else you trust, and ask her or him to stay with you.
3. Go to a hospital emergency department immediately.
   - Preserve all physical evidence of the assault. Do not shower, bathe, douche, brush your teeth, or change your clothes before you go to the hospital.
   - Hospital staff will provide medical care for sexual assault victims.
   - Even if you think that you do not have any physical injuries, you should still have a medical examination and discuss with a health care provider the risk of exposure to sexually transmitted diseases and the possibility of pregnancy resulting from the sexual assault.
4. If you want to report the assault, call your local police department from the hospital.
   - The police department will have trained rape crisis personnel to help you.
   - Reporting the crime can help you regain a sense of personal power and control, and can also help ensure the safety of other potential victims.
5. If you suspect that you may have been given a rape drug, ask the hospital or clinic where you receive medical care to take a urine sample.
   - The urine sample should be preserved as evidence.
   - Rape drugs, such as Rohypnol and GHB, are more likely to be detected in urine than in blood.
6. Write down as much as you can remember about the circumstances of the assault, including a description of the assailant.
7. Talk with a counselor who is trained to assist rape victims about the emotional and physical impacts of the assault.
   - It will be difficult, but it is important to talk with someone who understands the trauma of rape and knows how to help.

Source: American Academy of Family Physicians (2003).

The Sexual Victimization of College Women

Fischer et al's (2000) study, "The National College Women Sexual Victimization Study (NCWSV)," was chartered by the National Institute of Justice, the research arm of the United States Bureau of Justice Statistics. The study is noteworthy for several reasons relating to design, sampling, and questioning methodology.

The NCWSV was designed to overcome the shortcomings of previous studies that attempted to estimate the incidence of sexual victimization of college women. Previous studies were flawed by small sample sizes, nonrandom sampling techniques, delimitating types of sexual victimization studied, and confusing labeling of both the types of sexual victimization under study and the details of the specific incidents reported by subjects.

The study was designed as a telephone survey of 4,446 female college students. Each subject was interviewed over the phone by a trained female interviewer. The study greatly expanded the types of sexual victimization (incidents) under study, including (a) completed rape, (b) attempted rape, (c) completed sexual coercion, (d) attempted sexual coercion, (e) completed sexual contact with force or threat of force, (f) attempted sexual contact with force or threat of force, (g) completed sexual contact without force, (h) attempted sexual contact without force, (i) threat of rape, (j) threat of contact with force or threat of force, (k) threat of penetration with force, and (l) threat of contact with force. These terms are defined in Table 16.1.

The sample for the NCWSV was composed of undergraduate and graduate women attending 2- or 4-year institutions across the United States during the fall 1996 semester. The sample was stratified to include students from all sized institutions (1,000–2,499; 2,500–4,999; 5,000–19,999; and 20,000 or more) and locations (urban, suburban, and rural). Schools were randomly chosen from a probability proportional to total female enrollment. Subjects were then randomly chosen from the institutions picked for the study (Fisher et al., 2000).

A key methodological issue that is credited for the study's success was its use of a two-tiered questioning approach. Subjects were initially queried with a set of "screening" questions that identified whether the subject had experienced a sexual victimization event.

Screening questions were very graphic in their depiction of the potential sexual victimization events. For instance, the first screening question was "Since school began in fall 1996, has anyone made you have sexual intercourse by using force or threatening to harm you or someone close to you? Just so there is no mistake, by *intercourse* I mean putting a penis in your vagina." No previous sexual victimization surveys used such specific screening questions that, in a sense, operationally defined the event under study. Such specific wording left little doubt for subjects regarding the nature of the question being asked and contributed to higher response rates. If a woman answered yes to the screening question, the interviewer asked a series of "incident report" questions that described in detail the nature of the event.

Incident report questions covered all aspects of the event, ranging from the relationship of the perpetrator to the subject, the environment in which the event occurred, whether the victim used force to repel the perpetrator, and additional details.

Key Findings of the NCWSV

As previously mentioned, the most startling finding of the study was the overall high incidence of sexual victimization and attempted sexual victimization among college women. Overall, 2.8 percent of the sample had experienced either a completed rape (1.7%) or an attempted rape (1.1%). This accounts for a rape victimization rate of 27.7 rapes per 1,000 female students (Fisher et al., 2000). The actual rate of the overall incidence of rape was actually 35.3 rapes per 1,000 women. This is due to the fact that some women in the study were actually raped or had experienced attempted rape more than one time during the 7-month study period. The 35.3/1,000 rate is what projects out to an estimated 350 rapes per year among 10,000 college women in any given university (Fisher et al., 2000).

Table 16.1 Descriptions of Types of Victimizations

Type of Victimization	Definition
Completed rape	Unwanted completed penetration by force or the threat of force. Penetration includes penile-vaginal, mouth on your genitals, mouth on someone else's genitals, penile-anal, digital-vaginal, digital-anal, object-vaginal, and object-anal.
Attempted rape	Unwanted attempted penetration by force or the threat of force. Penetration includes penile-vaginal, mouth on your genitals, mouth on someone else's genitals, penile-anal, digital-vaginal, digital-anal, object-vaginal, and object-anal.
Completed sexual coercion	Unwanted completed penetration with the threat of noncoercion physical punishment, promise of reward, or pestering/verbal pressure. Penetration includes penile-vaginal, mouth on your genitals, mouth on someone else's genitals, penile-anal, digital-vaginal, digital-anal, object-vaginal, and object-anal.
Attempted sexual coercion	Unwanted attempted penetration with the threat coercion, physical punishment, promise of reward, or pestering/verbal pressure. Penetration includes penile-vaginal, mouth on your genitals, mouth on someone else's genitals, penile-anal, digital-vaginal, digital-anal, object-vaginal, and object-anal.
Completed sexual contact with force or threat of force	Unwanted completed sexual contact (not penetration) with contact with force or force or the threat of force. Sexual contact includes touch, threat of forcing, grabbing or fondling of breasts, buttocks, or genitals, either under or over your clothes; kissing, licking, or sucking; or some other form of unwanted sexual contact.
Completed sexual contact without force	Any type of unwanted completed sexual contact (not contact without force penetration) with the threat of nonphysical punishment, promise of reward, or pestering/verbal pressure. Sexual contact includes touching, grabbing, or fondling of breasts, buttocks, or genitals, either under or over your clothes; kissing, licking, or sucking; or some other form of unwanted sexual contact.
Attempted sexual contact with force or threat of force	Any type of unwanted attempted sexual contact (not penetration) with contact with force or the threat of force. Sexual contact includes touching, grabbing, or fondling of breasts, buttocks, or genitals, either under or over your clothes; kissing, licking, or sucking; or some other form of unwanted sexual contact.
Attempted sexual contact without force	Unwanted attempted sexual contact (not penetration) without force the threat of nonphysical punishment, promise or reward, or pestering/verbal pressure. Sexual contact includes touching, grabbing or fondling of breasts, buttocks, or genitals, either under or over your clothes; kissing, licking, or sucking; or some other form of unwanted sexual contact.
Threat of rape	Threat of unwanted penetration with force and threat of force. Penetration includes penile-vaginal, mouth on your genitals, mouth on someone else's genitals, penile-anal, digital-vaginal, digital-anal, object-vaginal, and object-anal.
Threat of contact with force or threat of force	Threat of unwanted sexual contact with force and threat of force. Sexual contact includes touching, grabbing force or fondling of breasts, buttocks, or genitals, either under or over your clothes; kissing, licking, or sucking; or some other form of unwanted sexual contact.
Threat of penetration without force	Threat of unwanted penetration with the threat of non-physical punishment, promise of reward, or pestering/verbal pressure. Penetration includes penile-vaginal, mouth on your genitals, mouth on someone else's genitals, penile-anal, digital-vaginal, digital-anal, object-vaginal, and object-anal.
Threat of contact without force	Threat of unwanted sexual contact without the threat of force, physical punishment, promise or reward, or pestering/verbal pressure. Sexual contact includes touching, grabbing or fondling of breasts, buttocks, or genitals, either under or over your clothes; kissing, licking, or sucking; or some other form of unwanted sexual contact.

Source: Fisher, Cullen, and Turner (2000, p. 8).

Table 16.2 Rates of Sexual Victimization

Type of Victimization	Victims			Incidents	
	# of Victims in Sample	% of Sample	Rate per 1,000 Female Students	# of Incidents	Rate per 1,000 Female Students
Completed or attempted					
Completed sexual coercion	74	1.7	16.6	107	24.1
Attempted sexual coercion	60	1.3	13.5	114	25.6
Completed sexual contact with force or threat of force	85	1.9	19.1	130	29.2
Completed sexual contact without force	80	1.8	18.0	132	29.7
Attempted sexual contact with force or threat of force	89	2.0	20.0	166	37.6
Attempted sexual contact without force	133	3.0	29.9	295	66.4
Threats					
Threat of rape	14	0.31	3.2	42	9.5
Threat of contact with force or threat of force	8	0.18	1.8	50	11.3
Threat of penetration without force	10	0.22	2.3	50	11.3
Threat of contact without force	15	0.34	3.4	75	16.9
Total	568			1,161	

Source: Fisher et al. (2000, p. 16).

Another disturbing finding of the study was the small percentage of women who actually defined their victimization as rape (even though they said yes when asked whether someone had "by force or threat put their penis into your vagina"). Fisher et al (2000) explain that this reluctance may be due to reasons such as feeling embarrassed, not clearly understanding the legal definition of rape, or being reluctant to label someone they are intimate with and who victimized them as a rapist (Fisher et al., 2000).

A third finding of the study was the overall incidence of other forms of sexual victimization. As Table 16.2 shows, when other forms of sexual victimization were studied, the rates varied from 9.5 to 66.4 cases per 1,000 women. The types of sexual victimization ranged from threats of rape and sexual contact to completed sexual coercion. Figure 16.1 shows that the overall percentage of women who were sexually victimized in the study exceeded 15 percent (Fisher et al., 2000).

A fourth finding of the study was the relationship of the perpetrator to the victim. For both completed and attempted rape, 9 out of 10 women knew the perpetrator. The relationships most often cited were a boyfriend, ex-boyfriend, classmate, friend, acquaintance, or coworker. College professors were not cited in any of the completed or attempted rapes (Fisher et al., 2000).

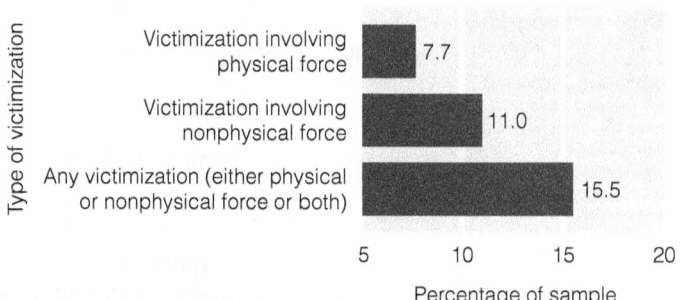

Figure 16.1 *Percentage of Women Sexually Victimized*

Source: Fisher et al. (2000, p. 17).

The vast majority of the rapes occurred after midnight and on campus in the victim's residence, in other living quarters on campus, or at a fraternity house. Risk factors positively associated with rape were (a) frequently drinking to get drunk, (b) being unmarried, (c) having a history of a previous sexual assault, and (d) living on campus. The vast majority of women reported that they did not suffer physical or emotional injuries as a result of the completed or attempted rape.

About one in five reported being injured (20%). The percentages for other forms of sexual victimization were lower, ranking from 0 percent (completed sexual contact without force) to 17 percent (threatened rape) (Fisher et al., 2000).

> ∾   *Environmental Wellness*   ∾
>
> High-level environmental wellness implies safety, security, and respect. A safe home environment includes appropriate parenting, setting boundaries for behavior, and getting help with emotional problems. A neighborhood that offers high-level environmental wellness is well lit and policed, and it has neighbors looking out for one another. The schools are safe and do not tolerate sexual harassment and discrimination. The community has safe playgrounds and parks that are well patrolled and not inviting for sex offenders. A college that offers high-level environmental wellness is a microcosm of any community. It has policies and procedures in place for dealing with harassment and discrimination and offers safety and protection. Its students don't fear walking to their cars after class or attending social functions. In addition, enforcement is swift, fair, and equal for all on campus.

Drinking and Date Rape

Many college students use alcohol and other drugs to "fit in," cope with college stressors, and reduce inhibitions related to dating and sex. Unfortunately, alcohol consumption is often linked to sexual coercion and other forms of violence. The National Advisory Council on Alcohol Abuse and Alcoholism's Report on College Drinking estimates that more than 70,000 students are the victims of alcohol-related sexual victimization (sexual assault and rape) (Task Force, 2002).

Often, this alcohol is consumed in large quantities for the express purpose of getting drunk. Weschler, Davenport, Dowdell, Moeykens, and Castillo (1994) coined the term **binge drinking** to describe such a pattern of alcohol consumption. Binge drinking is operationally defined as "having five or more drinks in a row, at least once during the previous 2 week period" (Weschler et al., 1994, p. 1673). The greatest predictors of binge drinking were living in a fraternity or sorority house, engaging in drinking games, and living a "party-centered" lifestyle (Weschler et al., 1994).

Bingeing on alcohol often becomes part of the social fabric of the college experience. Weschler et al (1994) studied the binge drinking behavior of more than 17,000 students on 140 four-year college campuses across the United States. About one in six (16%) of all the respondents were nondrinkers (15% of the men, 16% of the women). About two in five (41%) were

Binge drinking Having five or more drinks in a row, at least once during the previous 2 week period

drinkers but did not binge. Almost half (44%) of all the students were binge drinkers. About one in five (19%) were frequent binge drinkers (17 % of the women and 23% of the men). These students had three or more binge drinking episodes within the past 2 weeks.

Weschler and colleagues found binge drinking to be associated with unplanned and unsafe sexual activity, physical and sexual assault, other criminal violations, physical injury, interpersonal problems, and poor academic performance. Binge drinkers were more likely than non-binge drinkers and abstainers to engage in unplanned sexual activity, not use protection when having sex, get hurt or injured, damage property, argue with friends, miss classes, get behind in schoolwork, and do something they later regretted. Frequent binge drinkers were 10 times more likely than bingers to have unplanned and unprotected sex, get into trouble with campus police, and get injured or damage property. When asked to evaluate the seriousness of their bingeing and its repercussions, less than 1 percent of the binge drinkers designated themselves as problem drinkers (Weschler et al., 1994).

In a follow-up study, Weschler, Eun, Kuo, Sebring, Nelson, and Lee (2002) found that 1 percent of students living in residence halls or fraternity and sorority houses were victims of alcohol-related sexual assault and/or rape. About 20 percent of students experienced alcohol-related threats and and/or attempted sexual contacts.

Despite the overall decline in drinking among all adults in the United States over the past two decades, drinking on college campuses fails to show a corresponding drop-off. Drinking by college students often revolves around its social nature. College women perceive drinking as a way of being around others and seeking the acceptance of peers (Gleason, 1994). Alcohol is consumed more for social than for personal reasons (Montgomery, Benedicto, & Hammerke, 1993).

Students reported using alcohol more for the purpose of meeting members of the other sex than for personal reasons, although alcohol did make them feel better about themselves. Drinking behavior that elsewhere would be characterized as alcohol abuse is often socially acceptable and even desirable behavior on certain college campuses (Weschler et al., 1994). "Party schools" foster reputations and environments in which binge drinking is part of the fabric of college life. Conversely, institutions that do not have alcohol outlets within 1 mile of campus and colleges that prohibit alcohol use for everyone (even those older than 21 years of age) have lower rates of alcohol bingeing.

Other Date Rape Drugs

Many other drugs, used alone or in consort with alcohol have been implicated in sexual victimization. Marijuana, cocaine, gamma hydroxybutyrate (GHB), benzodiazepines, ketamine, barbiturates, chloral hydrate, methaqualone, heroin, morphine, LSD, and other hallucinogens have all been used to facilitate rape (Higher Education Center, 2003). When combined with alcohol (which they often are), many of these drugs cause reduction of inhibitions, weakness, memory loss, and blackout. These incapacitating effects are used by sexual victimization perpetrators to take advantage of their targets (Higher Education Center, 2003).

Rohypnol A depressant drug also known as the "date rape drug," because it causes loss of memory and makes women vulnerable to uninvited sexual intercourse

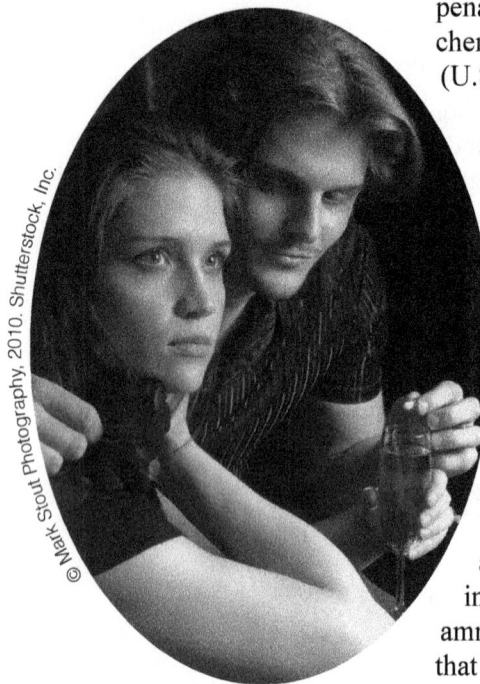

Rohypnol and GHB, available in liquid or pill form, are often mixed into the drinks of unsuspecting victims.

Two drugs in particular, **Rohypnol** and GHB, have been dubbed "date rape drugs" because of their increased use and association with sexual assault and rape. Rohypnol was the key target in the Drug-Induced Rape Prevention and Punishment Act of 1996. This legislation was developed in response to the threat posed by Rohypnol. The act established harsher penalties for the use of even the smallest quantities of flunitrazepam (the chemical name of Rohypnol) for the purpose of facilitating a violent crime (U.S. Congress, 1996).

Rohypnol—also known as roofies, rophies, Mexican valium, ropies, and the "forget me" drug (to name a few)—is the trade name for flunitrazepam, a benzodiazepine. Benzodiazepines are depressant drugs. Rohypnol is similar to Valium in its effects on the body, only 10 times more powerful. The United Nations Commission on Narcotic Drugs has transferred Rohypnol from a Schedule IV to a Schedule III drug. Several states in the United States have already moved Rohypnol to Schedule I [Office of National Drug Control Policy (ONDCP), 2002b].

Rohypnol is a tasteless, odorless, clear drug available in powder form. It mixes easily in liquids and is virtually undetectable when mixed in alcoholic beverages (its preferred delivery by date rape perpetrators). When swallowed, it takes effect in 15 to 20 minutes, and its effects last for more than 12 hours. Users experience a slowing of psychomotor performance, muscle relaxation, sleepiness, and/or amnesia. Rohypnol leaves the body after 72 hours and is undetectable after that time (ONDCP, 2002b).

GHB—also known as cherry meth, liquid X, organic Quaalude, and fantasy, to name a few—is similar in its nature and effects to Rohypnol. It is also a tasteless, odorless, clear, depressant drug. It is available in either powder or liquid form, and easily mixes in alcoholic beverages, where it is undetectable. GHB is not produced legally in the United States. It is produced in clandestine laboratories. Users claim it can produce euphoric, hallucinogenic states, and act as a growth hormone that stimulates muscle growth. Because of this latter claim, GHB is often marketed through the same channels (gyms, health clubs, rave clubs, and so forth) where anabolic steroids are sold (ONDCP, 2002a).

Both drugs have been implicated in date rape in the United States. Both drugs, besides having classic depressant drug characteristics (slowing central nervous system functioning), can cause memory loss and loss of consciousness. Because of this, women who have been assaulted and raped while under the influence of these drugs are unable to resist the perpetrator or recall any of the details concerning the incident. The assailant mixes the drug into the drink of the unsuspecting woman, allows it to take effect, takes advantage of her, and denies any knowledge of the event if the woman realizes or suspects what has happened. Because both drugs pass through the victim's system within 72 hours, she typically does not have the opportunity to get tested for the drugs (ONDCP 2002a, 2002b).

Stranger Rape

Stranger rape Forced intercourse by a person who is unknown to the target person

Stranger rape is rape by a person whom the target does not know. The overwhelming majority of rapes reported to the police and resulting in prosecution are stranger rapes. Although stranger rape can involve a pre-

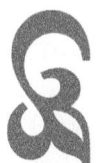

healthy sex hints 16.2

Reducing Risks for Date Rape

The following are specific strategies for women to reduce their risks for date rape:

- Arrange for your first date to be in a public place or as part of a larger group.
- Arrange your own transportation, or go with your friends.
- In the earliest stages of the relationship, suggest paying for yourself. This will derail any notion that your date thinks you owe him something. It also will give you an opportunity to assess his views about women.
- Pay attention to your date's attitudes and behavior. Is he controlling? Does he want to make all of the decisions?
- Avoid using alcohol and other drugs if you don't want to become involved in intimate sexual activities.
- Do not accept *any* drinks from another person. Pour your own drink or only drink from sealed bottles.
- Don't send mixed messages or anything that can be perceived as "teasing." If kissing is acceptable but you don't want to go any farther, state this clearly: "I'd like to hug and kiss, but I don't want to let things go any farther than this."
- If things begin to get out of control, resist. Use more and more emphatic verbal resistance: "I said *no!*" If this doesn't work, use physical force: punch, slap, kick.
- Men are much more likely to believe you if you use physical force when you're saying no. Push him away, stand up, open the door, ask him to stop, or leave. If this doesn't work, say, "This is rape. I'm calling the police."
- Run away. If he persists, escape. Get away. Go to a public place, and call the police.

meditated assault with an anonymous assailant descending upon the victim totally without warning, statistics prove otherwise. Most cases of stranger rape seem to spring out of chance meetings that create the potential for assault. The assailant targets the victim in a park, a shopping mall parking lot, while driving in a car, and so on. The perpetrator initiates contact, appears friendly and "safe," and lulls the victim into relaxing her (usually the victim is female) guard, allowing the perpetrator to strike. The assailant maneuvers the target to one or the other of their cars or lures the victim into an alley, stairwell, or other remote location, then commits the rape.

Stranger rapes are more likely to involve guns, knives, and other weapons than other forms of rape (Rand 2008). Older persons are more likely to be raped in their homes than in public places, and the assailant often gains access by overpowering. A relatively recent type of stranger rape involves targeting women who are driving by themselves. The perpetrators intentionally rear-end the cars of their potential victims, forcing them to pull off the road, where they are assaulted when they leave their car to investigate the accident. Often the rape is combined with stealing the woman's car.

Marital Rape

For many years, police were reluctant to investigate and prosecute marital rape. In a landmark case from 1978, Greta Rideout of Oregon filed charges against her husband for nonconsensual sex, bringing marital rape to national

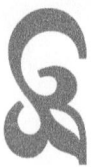 **healthy sex hints 16.3**

Reducing Risks for Stranger Rape

Personal Preparation

1. *Plan in advance.* Be aware of where you are, areas of possible trouble, and escape routes.
2. *Avoid dark and isolated areas.* Park in well-lit areas, as close to stores as possible. Avoid dark side streets, back roads, and the like, whenever possible. Jog and bicycle only in busy or public places.
3. *Arrange for an escort.* Have someone leave work, school, or an event with you and walk you to your car. Avoid empty stairwells and elevators unless you are accompanied by your escort.
4. *Use technology.* Carry an airhorn or whistle. If you can afford it, install automatic door locks and alarms in your car. Buy a cellular phone and carry it with you. Install your local police department number as a quick-dial memory number.
5. *Take a self-defense course.* Know how to defend yourself. A few simple techniques can make a difference.
6. *Remain vigilant.* Don't let your guard down. You are a potential victim any time you go anywhere by yourself.

What to Do If You Are Attacked

1. *Run away if you can.*
2. *Resist if you can.* Be as active and loud as possible: Scream, curse, yell, and cause a scene. If you have a whistle or horn, blow it.
3. *Fight back.* Kick, punch, bite, scratch, vomit, and spit. Use your keys, umbrellas, rolled-up newspapers, and books to jab for the eyes, throat, and face. There are no rules, and fighting back may reduce the abuse you might sustain without increasing your risk of injury. Carry keys in your hand as a weapon.
4. *Stall for time.* If you can't fight back, talk to your attacker—by name, if you know it. Express "empathy." Get him talking. Try to escape at the first distraction.

In the Car

1. *Always drive with your doors locked.*
2. *Lock your doors immediately after you park.*
3. *Approach your car with your keys in your hand* (have them sticking out like brass knuckles), and check the backseat to make sure no one is hiding there before you let yourself in.
4. *If you break down, do not leave the car.* Leave only to quickly tie a white rag to the antenna, then lock yourself in, and wait for the police. If someone other than the police arrives, ask this person to call the police or a local garage. Don't open the door.
5. *If your car is hit from behind, don't leave the car.* Put your flashers on and wait for the police to arrive.
6. *Buy a cellular phone, if you can afford it.* It will enable you to call the police immediately.

At Home

1. *Don't list your full name in the phone book, over the doorbell, or on the mailbox.*
2. *Install secure locks on all windows and doors.* Change locks if you lose your keys, move, or change your living situation (a roommate, husband, or boyfriend leaves).
3. *Install a peephole and safety chain and bar* on your door.
4. *Don't let people in your home unless you can verify who they are.* All service representatives (gas company, police, and so on) have identification. Request that they hold it in front of the peephole so you can see it. When in doubt, call the agency and verify who they are.
5. *Leave a light on near the entrance* when you know you will be returning home after dark.
6. *Organize or join a neighborhood watch program* for your block, building, or complex.
7. *Get a dog.* Perpetrators are less likely to attack you if you have a dog with you.

attention. Approximately 13 percent of married women have been raped by their husbands (Russel, 1990). In most cases, the husband used force (84%) or the threat of force (9%). The rape was an isolated incident for 31 percent of the victims. Another 31 percent reported being raped more than 20 times, and the rest fell somewhere in the middle (Russel, 1990).

Perpetrators of marital rape share some of the same personality traits as other rapists—namely, anger, power, and sadism. Husbands who rape are also more likely to abuse their wives verbally, psychologically, and physically. More than 30 percent of wives who were raped also reported having been targets of physical abuse during their marriage (Frieze, 1983).

Verbal and psychological abuse often prove more damaging than physical abuse. The verbal and psychological abusers create an environment of endless criticism, suspicion, and torment. Abusers often undermine their mates' confidence and self-esteem through constant criticism of everything from the way they look to their level of competence in performing simple household tasks. Abusers are extremely jealous and turn even the most casual remark or involvement with another person into suspicions of flirting or having an affair. This constant flow of criticism, insults, and accusations is tormenting and can result in a host of psychological problems (Marano, 1996).

Survivors of marital rape suffer after-effects that are similar to those of women who have been sexually assaulted by someone they know (date rape). Because they know their assailants intimately and have an established history of trust, they feel especially betrayed, humiliated, and angry.

Statutory Rape

Statutory rape refers to sexual intercourse between a person older than the legal age of consent with a partner who is younger than the legal age of consent. The legal age of consent in the states varies from 12 to 21 years of age. Traditionally, most states' original legal wording of definitions of statutory rape defined perpetrators as males and victims as females. Revised definitions of statutory rape are more gender-neutral and describe adult perpetrators and victims under the legal age of consent.

Statutory rape A person older than the legal age of consent having intercourse with a partner who is younger than the legal age of consent

The recent high-profile case of 34-year-old teacher Mary Kay Letourneau, convicted of the statutory rape of her 12-year-old student/lover, illustrates the importance of these revisions. Letourneau received national attention when the former elementary school teacher was convicted of having sex with (and becoming pregnant by) her former student. Even though the two claimed to be in love and the sex was consensual, the courts convicted her of statutory rape. In statutory rape cases, consent of the underage partner has little bearing in the case. In the eyes of the law, people under the age of consent are not considered legally capable of making an informed decision concerning their sexual behavior.

Incidence of Rape

The true incidence of rape in the United States is unknown. There are two primary national sources of data regarding rape in the United States: the Federal Bureau of Investigation (FBI) Uniform Crime Reports and the Bureau of Justice's National Crime Victimization Survey.

Case Study 16.2

Donna: A Saga of Spousal Abuse

Donna, 33, divorced, identifies as African American.

Donna is a continuing education student and the mother of two daughters, 10 and 11 years of age. She related her story to one of the authors in a diary detailing her sexual development.

My father was an alcoholic. I didn't realize it as a young child, but by the time I was a teenager, I understood why my dad had lost his driver's license a couple of times, had a hard time holding down a steady job, and was so angry all of the time. Of course, by then it was too late. I loved him so much and felt so guilty about admitting to myself that he was an alcoholic. I blamed myself a lot for his behavior. "Maybe it's my fault Daddy drinks so much," I thought. "Maybe if I was a better daughter, he'd be OK." Often Dad's anger was directed at Mom. He'd come home drunk after stopping off for "a few beers" after work and just be itching for a fight. The least little thing Mom would do would set him off, and he'd smack her with the back of his hand. My sister and I would run for our lives and dive under our bed or lock ourselves in the closet until he'd pass out. We'd hear Mom getting hit but would be too afraid to do anything.

Afterward Mom would try to comfort us by saying that Daddy was really a "good man" and "cared" about her, but he just couldn't hold his liquor. She said that sometimes a woman has to stand by her man even when things weren't going well. I think about those words now, and I shudder. Sometimes he'd turn on us if we tried to help Mom. He broke my arm once during one of these outbursts, and I had to go to the hospital to have a cast put on. To this day I can't believe that the hospital staff didn't know what was happening and intervene. Not only was my arm broken, but I had black-and-blue marks all over from where Dad hit me with his belt and his hand. I ran away when I was 18. I guess it wasn't really running away since I was legally an adult, but to me it was because I wasn't leaving—I was escaping (at least I thought I was). I bounced around the country for a couple of years, in and out of jobs as well as relationships with men.

My first real love was a guy who reminded me a lot of my father. I guess I felt like a victim and was attracted to a guy who allowed me to be a victim. I needed to be punished to feel good, and he was up to the task. He'd treat me like dirt, constantly tell me I wasn't pretty and was terrible in bed, couldn't do anything right, and on and on. He drank, just like my dad, and beat me just like my dad beat my mom.

Fate saved me from him, however. He was a real bad guy and was arrested for stealing a car and crashing it into a storefront. He was sent to jail for 5 years, and I wasn't into waiting around, so I took off and wound up in a neighboring state.

I met my husband shortly after arriving. I was working as a barmaid, and he came into the bar late one night. I was very attracted to him and wound up going home with him that night. I moved in after about a month

Critical Thinking

How could Donna's early experiences with her mother and father have resulted in different choices she made in her life after she left home at 18?

and got pregnant with my first child about 6 months later. He liked to drink, but it didn't seem to affect him at first. He was a pretty good guy until times got tough.

After the baby was born, we got married and he lost his job the next week. He couldn't find another job and had to go on unemployment for 6 months. He couldn't handle this and began to take it out on me. I was pregnant with our second child at the time. He started really abusing me for my size (I gained a lot of weight) and began hitting me. I almost miscarried one night after he hit me and knocked me down. When he sobered up, he felt really bad and apologized. He told me he'd never do it again. He said he loved me.

I felt trapped and didn't know what to do. I was pregnant, had a 1-year-old baby, had no education, no real job skills, no money in the bank, and few real friends to turn to. I continued to live with him but began to fear for my safety and that of the kids. I started to try to think of a way out. Something deep within me didn't want to wind up like my mother. He must have sensed it because he got very controlling. He tried to limit my involvement with any friends, checked my mail, scrutinized the phone bills. The beatings were coming more often, and he began to hit the kids more and more.

Things finally came to a head one night. After a particularly savage fight, a neighbor called the police. When the police arrived, they saw what he had done to me and locked him up. My children and I were examined, and I pressed charges for domestic and child abuse. To make a long story short, the kids and I found refuge in a battered women's shelter, and he got 3 years in prison.

As soon as I was able, I filed divorce papers, went back to work, saved a few dollars, and left the state. I located my sister, also divorced with two kids, and we moved in together. We've both been working our way back slowly ever since—caring for each other and our kids, trying to put our lives back together. I'm in a support group for survivors of spousal abuse and have been dating a very nice man for about a year.

The FBI collects actual crime reports sent in from the individual states. These crime reports confirm to operational definitions established as part of the FBI's Uniform Crime Reporting (UCR) system. The UCR is a nationwide program that includes over 17,000 city, county, and state law enforcement agencies. It reports crime data that represent about 92 percent of the population of the United States (USDOJ, FBI, 2008).

Traditionally, the UCR has labeled rape as forcible rape and defined it in the following way: "the carnal knowledge of a female forcibly and against her will. Rapes by force and attempts or assaults to rape regardless of the age of the victim are included. Statutory offenses (no force used—victim under the age of consent, are excluded)" (USDOJ FBI, 2008). Sex crimes other than prostitution were reported under the category "sex offenses."

The UCR underwent major revisions starting in 1982, when the FBI decided to assess and upgrade its crime-reporting system. A new system, the National Incident- Based Reporting System (NIBRS), started phasing in on a voluntary basis at the end of 1987. NIBRS expanded the number of reportable offenses, revised and refined how these offenses were defined, and collected detailed information surrounding the incidents. Under NIBRS, the FBI not only continued to gather data on forcible rape and sex offenses but added new "group A" offenses: sex offenses—forcible, and sex offenses—nonforcible. This expanded data base provided additional information on sex-related offenses.

Unfortunately, the conversion to the NIBRS system has been slow and incomplete. The collection of states and law enforcement agencies that have implemented the program do not constitute a representative sample of law enforcement agencies or states, and therefore NIBRS data cannot be generalized to the entire nation. NIBRS agencies covered only 17 percent of the U.S. population and 22 states in 2002. Not all agencies within these states submit data in NIBRS formats. Only 7 of the 22 states fully report all NIBRS statistics. Most of the reporting law enforcement agencies that participate in NIBRS represent smaller population areas with no agency representing a population center of more than one million people. The largest participator is The Fairfax County Virginia Police Department covering a population of 948,050 (Addington, 2008).

The Bureau of Justice, National Crime Victimization Survey (NCVS), is a biannual telephone survey of over 89,000 people over the age of 12 conducted by the Census Bureau. It provides an estimate of the volume of violent and nonviolent crime in the United States. It differs from the UCR system because it is a survey and not a tabulation of actual crime reports filed by the police.

> *The Uniform Crime Reporting (UCR) Program and National Crime Victimization Survey (NCVS) were designed to complement each other. The UCR Program's primary objective is to provide a reliable set of criminal justice statistics for law enforcement administration, operation, and management, as well as to indicate fluctuations in the level of crime in America. The NCVS was established to obtain and provide previously unavailable information about victims, offenders, and crime (including crime not reported to the police). While the two programs employ different methodologies, they measure a similar subset of serious crimes. (FBI, 2001).*

Because studies that use reported incidents as their measure may greatly underestimate the true incidence of rape, independent researchers conduct survey research studies on smaller samples of women and extrapolate the findings to the population as a whole (similar to the NCWSV survey discussed previously). Often these independent studies define rape differently, use differing methodologies, and mix incidence and prevalence measures, making meaningful comparisons of their data almost impossible (Koss, 1996).

In 2007, the estimated *number* of forcible rapes (90,427) decreased 2.5 percent from the 2006 estimate. This represents a 3.7 percent decrease from 2003 levels and a 2.9 percent decline from 1998 levels. The estimated *rate* of forcible rapes in 2007 was 59.1 offenses per 100,000 women, a 3 percent decrease from the 2006 estimated rate of 60.9. (USDOJFBI, 2008).

The National Crime Victimization Survey reported an estimated 248,300 rapes in 2007. The rate of rape for 2007 was 100 per 100,000 persons age 12 or older. While the estimated number of rapes increased significantly in the past decade, the rate actually decreased due to the increase in population. The rate of rape in 1998 was 150 cases per 100 persons age 12 or older. This represents an estimated 33 percent decrease from 1998–2007 (Rand, 2008).

Although the actual numbers of cases in these two sets of data are greatly disparate, most experts (police and civilian) agree that the actual number of rapes is probably much higher than the reported or estimated numbers that usually show up in reports or in the press. Rape is one of the least reported of all crimes in the United States. Between 10 and 50 percent of all rapes may go unreported to the police (Williams, 1984).

If we use the 2007 FBI reported cases as a baseline, that means that almost 50,000 additional cases went unreported that year. Rape survivors are reluctant to report the crime for several reasons: fear of retaliation by the rapist; embarrassment or shame; fear of rejection by husband, boyfriend, or family; a desire to protect the rapist; and a lack of confidence in the judicial system (Koss, 1992).

In a study of 246 rape victims, the following six variables were found to be related to whether a victim reports a rape (Williams, 1984):

- The relationship between the victim and the rapist
- How the two came together
- Threat of force
- Use of force
- Extent of injury
- Use of medical treatment

Victims were more likely to report when the rapist was a stranger or acquaintance rather than a friend or relative, had broken into her house or had assaulted her in a public place (versus a party or other social situation), had threatened to use force (versus not threatening her), did use force (less likely to report if no actual force), had caused substantial injury (versus little physical harm), and had sought medical care for her injuries (versus not seeking medical care).

A close look at the variables related to a greater likelihood of reporting indicates that women are much more likely to report a rape when evidence of the attack was available. This could consist of observable or clinical evidence of injury and the need for medical attention, when the woman clearly was not at fault (forced entry or a public place, didn't know the perpetrator or didn't know him well), and she felt emotionally distant from the rapist.

The variables found to be unrelated to the reporting of a rape were the victim's age, race, employment, living situation, the rapist's age, race, number of rapists, and place of assault (Williams, 1984). Perhaps more rape victims would come forth if they didn't feel that they were responsible for providing the burden of proof that the crime occurred. This attitude in part stems from the myths associated with rape that persist despite years of efforts to clear up misconceptions about the crime by individuals and organizations concerned about rape.

Characteristics of Rapists

Most of what we know about men who rape comes from research conducted on convicted rapists. It is estimated that less than 10 percent of all rapists are convicted of this crime. FBI statistics in 1992 on convicted rapists,

sex in society 16.1
A Historical Look at Rape

In *Against Our Will,* one of the most definitive works on the subject, author Susan Brownmiller (1975) described the evolution of our current attitudes toward rape and the laws against it. According to Brownmiller, rape has a long, sordid history. In antiquity, women were considered one of the spoils of war, objects to be taken and used in whatever way one wished. After a battle, the conquering army routinely rounded up all female survivors and had free rein to do what they wanted with them. Women who resisted were routinely slaughtered. Women who were spared were often sold off as slaves once their captors became bored with them.

Although rape seems to have been a part of all cultures, it has not always been considered a crime against a person. The earliest statutes against rape were laws related to property. Women were not considered persons. Instead, they were valued as property. They could provide labor and bear children—two important commodities in an agrarian economy dependent on the availability of workers.

Under Hammurabi's Code (a Babylonian law approximately 4,000 years old), a woman was not considered to be a free, independent human being. She was considered to be some man's (father's, husband's) property. Therefore, if someone violated the woman, he committed a crime against that man's property and was prosecuted accordingly.

Women also were categorized according to their marital status and virginity. Virgins were considered purer than nonvirgins in relation to sex-related crimes. The purest of all virgins were those engaged to be married. A man convicted of raping a betrothed virgin was put to death and his victim set free. A man convicted of raping a married woman also was put to death. His victim, however, also was put to death because she was considered a willing victim or accomplice in the crime. Presumably, the feeling was that she somehow led the rapist on, or consented to the act. The two early beliefs briefly described here about women and rape—that a woman is a man's property and that rape cannot occur unless a woman somehow consents—still exist and form the foundation of much of the legislation and belief systems that people share about rape.

---

similar to those for perpetrators of other serious crimes, indicate that most are under 25 years of age, are from single-parent or foster parent homes, are marginally employed, have a low income, and have little formal education.

Because less than 10 percent of all rapists are ever convicted of their crimes, several researchers have studied populations of men who rape who have not been convicted or incarcerated. In one of the most comprehensive reviews of the literature, Cate and Lloyd (1992) identify seven characteristics of men who rape:

1. They are much more likely than their nonrapist peers to hold traditional beliefs about women and women's roles and female stereotypes. These beliefs range from nonsexual views concerning a woman's place (in the home) to sexual beliefs that men are the initiators during sex and that women want men to initiate.
2. They believe in rape-supportive myths—women secretly want to be overpowered during sex; they like it rough; *no* really means *yes*— and other stereotypical beliefs about women.
3. They use exploitative techniques such as coercing women into sex using alcohol and other drugs.
4. They accept the use of violence as a way to solve problems and dominate others.

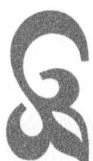

healthy sex hints 16.4

Helping a Friend Who Has Been Raped

Even though trained rape crisis professionals are available in most communities, the first contact a survivor has is often a friend, roommate, or family member. If someone you care about has been raped, here are some tips to help you support her:

- *Accept her.* Be nonjudgmental about what happened. Tell her she is not to blame for the incident.
- *Listen.* Encourage her to tell you what happened. Listen actively and give her positive feedback.
- *Offer shelter and support.* Tell her you'll be there for her (and be sure you are). Offer her a safe haven until her ordeal is over. Care for her needs (food, clothing, a shoulder to cry on).
- *Have empathy.* Tell her you're sorry for what happened but glad she's alive and her injuries aren't worse.
- *Encourage action.* Tell her it's important that she report what happened to the police and go to the hospital.
- *Accompany her to the police station and hospital.*
- *Keep your own feelings in check.* She will remain calmer if you do.

5. They are more likely to vent their anger and express their need to dominate sexually rather than find other outlets for these feelings.
6. They devalue all that is feminine. They are hostile toward "feminine" personality attributes such as nurturance and collaboration, and devalue traditional female pursuits such as child care and homemaking.
7. They are generally more sexually active than their peers who do not rape.

Malamuth, Sockloski, Koss, and Tanaka (1991) studied the sexual behavior of college men. Using a large, representative sample (their sexual histories were unknown) instead of convicted rapists, they found four characteristics of men who rape:

1. *Hostility toward women.* Men who rape have a deep-seated hostility toward women and feminine traits. They devalue traits such as nurturance and equality and value dominance, power, and aggression.
2. *Hostile home environment.* Men who rape grew up in households where violence, battering, sexual abuse, and hostility between family members were the norm.
3. *History of delinquency.* Men who rape associate with peers who are delinquent and reinforce the same hostile, aggressive behaviors that were modeled in their homes and that contributed to their own delinquency.
4. *Sexual promiscuity.* Contrary to the perception that men who rape are sexually deprived, rapists generally are more sexually active than nonrapists but report much higher levels of dissatisfaction with their sex lives than their nonraping peers.

Malamuth et al's and Cate and Lloyd's work seem to confirm Sanday's (1987) findings concerning hostility toward women, stereotypical perceptions about women, and the devaluation of women and all things feminine as key attributes of rapists and societies that are "rape-prone."

Characteristics of Targets

Any female can be the target of rape. The woman can be young or old, attractive or unattractive, dressed provocatively or conservatively. Most targets tend to be under 30 years of age and single. Age and marital status may have more to do with the likelihood that these women travel, shop, walk, and live alone rather than some other factor.

Women who are the targets of rape are no different from non-targets in terms of personality attributes, lifestyle, or behavior. Attempts to characterize targets as being different from other women only serves to blame the victim rather than understand that it is the men who rape through their own actions.

Sexual Harassment

Title VII of the Civil Rights Act of 1964 stipulates that it is an unlawful employment practice for a labor organization to exclude or to expel from its membership or otherwise to discriminate against any individual because of his or her race, color, religion, sex, or national origin. Sexual harassment has been deemed to be a form of discrimination based on sex.

The issue of sexual harassment leaped onto the television screens and front pages of the United States in 1992 with the much-publicized Clarence Thomas-Anita Hill sexual harassment hearings by the U.S. Congress, after President George H. Bush had nominated Thomas to the Supreme Court (see Sex in Society 16.2). Thomas had been Hill's boss at the Equal Employment Opportunity Commission (EEOC). Hill came forward at the time of Thomas's nomination with claims of sexual harassment.

These hearings brought sexual harassment out of the closet and forced people to examine this dark side of human sexual behavior. Since then, the number of sexual harassment complaints filed with the EEOC has increased from 6,000 in 1990 to 15,475 in 2001 (EEOC, 2003). Of the 15,475 charges filed, 7,309 were dropped due to no reasonable cause, 4,628 were closed administratively due to a variety of causes (inability to locate charging party, failure to respond to EEOC communications, and so forth), and 1,389 were withdrawn by the charging party because the claimant received desired benefits. Approximately 4,768 claims merited resolution, with 1,568 settled by the EEOC with the charging party receiving the desired benefits, and the rest being resolved in the charging party's favor through a variety of ways (EEOC, 2003).

U.S. Supreme Court rulings have made it easier to sue (and win) sexual harassment cases because victims no longer have to prove psychological harm, just that sexually inappropriate behavior took place (Kaufman, 1997).

According to the EEOC, sexual harassment consists of unwelcome sexual advances, requests for sexual favors, and other verbal or physical conduct of a sexual nature. These constitute **sexual harassment** when

(1) submission of such conduct is made explicitly, or implicitly a term or condition of an individual's employment or academic advancement, (2) submission or rejection of such conduct by an individual is used as the basis for academic or employment decisions affecting the individual, or (3) such conduct has the

Sexual harassment Unwelcome sexual advances, requests for sexual favors, and other verbal or physical conduct of a sexual nature in the workplace or educational setting

sex in society 16.2

The Clarence Thomas–Anita Hill Hearings

The Thomas–Hill Congressional hearings in 1992 had effects far beyond the matter of deciding whether Clarence Thomas should sit on the U.S. Supreme Court. As a result of these hearings, the issue of sexual harassment came to the fore and led to a whole new zeitgeist of how people are to conduct themselves in the workplace. The hearings were also noteworthy in that this event involved two prominent blacks—Thomas, a judge, and Hill, a law professor at the time of the hearings—with opposing political ideologies.

In her testimony, Hill described her position as an employee of Thomas at the Equal Employment Opportunity Commission (EEOC). She claimed that, beginning in 1982, Thomas had pressured her to go out on dates, and that he had made lewd comments to her, including references to a pubic hair on a Coke can and the size of his penis. She stated that, because Thomas was well connected and could help advance her career, she was reluctant to speak out at the time. She produced three witnesses who testified to Hill's having told them that she was being harassed, though they did not recall Hill's having accused Thomas by name.

Hill's critics charged that she waited too long (10 years) to speak of the harassment, and that she had agreed to testify to members of committee only under condition of anonymity. Her detractors took this as an indication that she made the charges only to try to derail Thomas's chances to gain a Supreme Court berth. They produced a number of witnesses who had worked for Thomas at the same time as Hill did, and these witnesses testified that they had observed no evidence of harassment and were not harassed themselves. Finally, Hill's critics questioned why she had followed Thomas to another job subsequent to the alleged harassment.

Thomas denounced the charges as completely untrue and a "high-tech lynching." In a close vote, he was confirmed to the Supreme Court. Irrespective of the outcome, the legacy of the hearings was far-reaching and has an enduring symbolic value. Major changes include the recognition of sexual harassment in the workplace, its definition, and enactment of legislation making sexual harassment easier to prove. Monetary awards and settlements also increased dramatically. In 1990, sexual harassment awards handled through the EEOC totaled $7.7 million; by 1996, settlements had reached $27 million.

Awakened by the prospects of costly lawsuits, the public and private sectors alike have gone on the defensive. Sexual harassment training is becoming common. Formal policies now are the rule rather than the exception in the workplace. More women (and men) are filing suit and supporting the victims of harassment. As a result of the Thomas–Hill hearings, public attitudes and actions regarding sexual harassment were irrevocably changed.

purpose or effect of unreasonably interfering with an individual's work or academic performance or creating an intimidating, hostile, or offensive working or educational environment. (EEOC, 2003)

Sexual harassment has two facets:

- Unwanted sexual attention or advances
- A hostile environment (work or school) in which the person faces daily stress and oppression because of the unwanted sexual attention

Although the two often go together, they can exist independently. Sexual harassment relates in part to how males are socialized. Men tend to interpret women's friendliness as a sign of sexual interest, as an invitation to pursue sexual involvement (Johnson, Stockdale, & Saal, 1991; Stockdale, 1993). Men and women perceive sexual harassment differently. Men are much less likely to perceive certain behaviors as harassing than women are (Jones & Remland, 1992). Thus, men have difficulty judging their behavior and its potential for harassment. The courts, too, have trouble determining whether certain actions cross the line between aggressive courting and sexual harassment.

> ❧   *Environmental/Occupational Wellness*   ❧
>
> A work environment with high-level environmental wellness is a place where workers coexist without fear of abuse, discrimination, or harassment. Policies to guard against harassment and discrimination are in place and are enforced swiftly, fairly, and equally for all levels of workers. Healthy workplaces are environments where people pursue their occupations in a safe and supportive atmosphere. Sexual harassment exists in exactly the opposite environment—one that is hostile, where those in power use their positions to take advantage of others. Each person has the responsibility to report coworkers and bosses who abuse the work site and thus turn it into a hostile environment for everyone.

Conditions of Sexual Harassment

Sexual harassment has three attributes that transcend individual perception and set the context for any interaction between individuals:

- A power differential in the relationship
- Inappropriate approach
- Pressure after expression of disinterest

A hallmark of sexual harassment is the use and abuse of power to secure sexual favors. Power differentials exist in the workplace and the classroom based on roles and responsibilities. The boss, supervisor, and professor have power over workers and students by the nature of their roles and authority. A boss or supervisor is responsible for evaluating work performance, giving assignments, and the like. A professor evaluates papers, tests, and exams, and ultimately assigns a grade to students in the class.

When someone holds power over another by virtue of a "superior" role, the subordinate person has a harder time refusing the advances. The subordinates fear reprisal—in a poor performance review, no raise, undesirable work assignments, even termination. In a school environment, the students fear a less objective review of their work and lower grades. Also, being approached in a respectful, inquiring way is vastly different from being approached in a harassing way.

Finally, if the pursuing person stops the pursuit once the subordinate has expressed noninterest or displeasure, it's not harassment. Persistence and an attempt to pressure the other person into responding, however, are more likely to be considered harassment, especially if the first two criteria are also present.

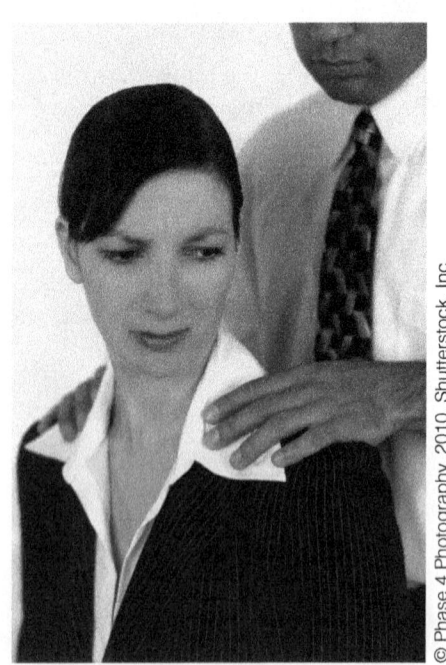

Physical intimidation often plays a big part in creating a hostile environment.

© Phase 4 Photography, 2010. Shutterstock, Inc.

Sexual Harassment Among LGBT People

The original language of the Civil Rights Act of 1964 that governs the EEOC's handling of sexual harassment cases was directed at discrimination

case study 16.3

Linda and Beth: Sexual Harassment Victims

Linda, 27, married, identifies as Filipino; Beth, 33, single, is white.

Linda, a secretary for a medium-sized trucking company, is being harassed by her boss, John. He takes every opportunity to position himself around Linda to maximize the opportunity for physical contact. John leans over her desk, puts his arm around her chair, places himself in a doorway through which she must pass, and uses these opportunities to brush against Linda. He has made comments about the size of her breasts, her shapely legs, and how he could really show her a good time in bed. Both John and Linda are married, and she has told him she is not interested in having an affair with him.

Beth is a driver for a local bus company, one of two women who drive for this company. The other 48 drivers are men. All drivers report to the local garage, where the buses are parked. The garage has two locker rooms, restrooms, a cafeteria, and administrative offices. Beth has complained to her supervisor (a man) that the work environment is not conducive to her well-being and may even be hostile. The male drivers are fond of soft- and hard-core pornography and have pinned-up pictures of naked women on the walls of the garage. They also leave these magazines out on the tables in the cafeteria.

Besides the print materials, the male drivers congregate in the cafeteria and tell sexually degrading jokes about women. They generally refer to women in derogatory terms when Beth is alone with them and when the other female driver is there. Although no one has made any direct advances toward her (she is living with her boyfriend and uninterested), she feels the work environment is hostile to women.

Both of these women are victims of sexual harassment—Linda, who is the victim of unwanted sexual advances from her boss, and Beth, who hasn't been personally confronted but is forced to work in a hostile environment created by her coworkers.

> *Critical Thinking*
>
> When does one worker's sexually open workplace become another's hostile environment?

based on sex. It was never intended to provide similar protections based on sexual orientation. Quittner (2002) identifies several recent court cases where the plaintiffs filed sexual harassment charges with the EEOC against their employers for discrimination based on sexual orientation.

In all of the cases, convincing cases were made for portraying work sites that were indeed hostile environments and denial of promotions based on sexual orientation. In one case, a butler at a prestigious Las Vegas hotel was subjected to taunts, catcalls, physical assaults (grabbing his crotch, poking his genitals, and so forth), and threats. He became afraid to go to work and was eventually fired from the job.

He filed a sexual harassment suit against the hotel. He lost his case, the courts citing that while the law clearly prohibits a gay man or woman from sexually harassing a heterosexual (that is, an opposite-sex) coworker, there were no protections for same-sex sexual harassment in the workplace.

Quittner (2002) cites another case of a male correctional officer in New York State being forced to leave his job after repeated incidents of verbal abuse from fellow heterosexual officers escalated into physical violence. The officer was denied by the District of New York federal court from suing his employer for same-sex sexual harassment. Such cases highlight the need for additional legislation to protect against harassment. In some states and cities, harassment based on sexual orientation is protected under broader antidiscrimination statutes.

Sexual Harassment Involving Children and Teens

One of the outcomes of the Thomas-Hill hearings and subsequent legislation is an attempt to define and prevent harassment at all levels. This has extended into all segments of society, including the elementary school.

Sexual Harassment in Elementary Schools

Sexual harassment in the schools goes way beyond mere teasing. Although poking fun and teasing can be emotionally painful and stressful, they do not constitute sexual harassment. In childhood, teasing peers of the other sex is a developmentally appropriate form of gender validation and, if not carried to an extreme, actually can strengthen the bonds little boys and girls have with their friends. Most of it is innocent and not discriminatory.

When the teasing is sexual in nature, it is a different matter. Uninvited sexual advances, lewd comments, ogling, and catcalls are different from simple putdowns ("Boys are better than girls," and vice versa) and nonsexual teasing. Even if they are not outright sexual acts directed at a child, they are capable of creating a climate of hostility that characterizes sexual harassment.

Often the focus of childhood teasing is sexual orientation. Children sometimes tease same- or opposite-sex peers with taunts of "queer," "homo," "fag," "lesbo," "dyke," and the like. Whether the perception is accurate or not, it creates a hostile environment for these children, making daily interactions with peers painful.

Several noteworthy court rulings have been made regarding sexual harassment by elementary school students (LeLand, 1996). In Lexington, North Carolina, in 1966, 6-year-old Jonathan Prevette was suspended for kissing a classmate in an incident that the court ruled was sexual harassment. In response, the boy's parents threatened to sue if their son was not reinstated and the policy changed. The school board reviewed the case and agreed that the incident wasn't sexual harassment and that the policy required retooling.

In another case, in New York, 7-year-old De'Andre Dearinge was charged with sexual harassment for kissing a student against her will and pulling a button off her skirt. Again, the school board intervened and reinstated the child.

What both of these examples illustrate is the difficulty in determining whether specific incidents involving students constitute sexual harassment or represent something else. Obviously, singular, isolated incidents have to be evaluated differently from repeated acts that are more in keeping with creating a hostile climate and failing to stop when the other person expresses a desire to halt the sexual overtures or remarks.

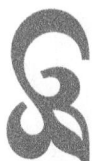

healthy sex hints 16.5

Sexual Harassment: How to Fight Back

The following guidelines may be helpful in fighting back if you think you have been the victim of sexual harassment on campus or at work.

1. If the harassment includes rape or attempted rape, file criminal charges against the perpetrator.
2. If the act does not include rape or attempted rape, confront the person who is harassing you. Write a letter to the offender, and follow up with a meeting. Be as clear and specific about the offender's actions as possible.
   - Be specific about the incidents, times, and dates. A history and pattern of events are important. Most harassers are repeat offenders.
   - Describe exactly what happened, your feelings about the incidents, and how you reacted. Include a short statement indicating your desire for the harasser to stop.
   - Sign and date the letter, and make duplicate copies.
   - Send a copy to the perpetrator, and indicate that if the behavior doesn't stop immediately, you will press charges using the letter as evidence.
3. Seek support. Don't hide what happened.
   - Talk to coworkers, fellow students, and people identified with the issue. This may help put pressure on the offender to stop.
   - Contact a local support group, and talk to others who have experienced the same problem.
   - Relate your incidents to your significant other.
4. If the behavior doesn't stop, meet with the offender's supervisor. Discuss the incidents and give a copy of your letter to the supervisor
   - In a work setting, this is the offender's immediate supervisor.
   - In a college setting, this person may be the department chairperson, the student center director, a member of the sexual harassment panel, or the dean of students.
5. Know your rights. Sexual harassment is against the law. You do not have to put up with it.
   - Obtain the company's/school's sexual harassment policy. Read it thoroughly, and make sure you follow its guidelines for handling your case.
   - Identify the administrative office and person responsible for handling sexual harassment violations in your workplace or school.

Although it may seem frightening, it's better to act quickly than to wait and see what happens. Harassers rarely stop their activities if they are not challenged.

Some child development authorities think that most 6- and 7-year-olds like the ones publicized in North Carolina and New York are too young to understand the concept of sexual harassment. Their behavior might be better labeled as a form of bullying in which they use power over another inappropriately. Some child development experts view this as a sort of testing the waters, and children (both perpetrator and victim) need to be educated about how to handle the situation rather than take it out of their hands. By having the proper authorities (such as school officials) step in, the victim relinquishes the ability to develop a repertoire of assertive behavior that could be used to fend off future would-be harassers (LeLand, 1996).

personal exploration activity
Coercive Sex in the Media

We all know that it is immoral to push, coax, or force someone to have a sexual interaction when they do not want to be sexual. However, this type of behavior is fairly common in today's music. The music we listen to may influence the way we think and act, so it is important to recognize the messages we are receiving. This activity will help you start to critically analyze the impact of the music in your life.

For the next week, list all the songs you hear on a sheet of paper in two columns: sexually coercive lyrics and nonsexual or healthy sexual lyrics. To really analyze the songs, you will have to listen closely to the lyrics. If you cannot understand the words, try looking on the group's Web site for the lyrics. You may be quite surprised at the song's message when you see the actual words. At the end of the week, evaluate your choices of music. Is your favorite music reflecting a healthy, positive view of sexuality or a negative, destructive one? Are you willing to reduce or eliminate the songs that reinforce the idea that sex is to be gotten at all cost and replace these with songs that reflect a healthy, positive approach to sexuality?

Prosecutors would counter this defense by claiming that abuse of power is the first step in harassment. If a 6- or 7-year-old thinks he or she can kiss or pull a button off a skirt of a classmate, the next act might be more overtly sexual in nature. Also, by stepping in quickly, school officials are bringing the issue to the students' (and parents') awareness.

In response to these and a host of other lawsuits being filed around the country, the U.S. Department of Education's Office for Civil Rights issued a new policy entitled "Sexual Harassment Guidance: Harassment of Students by School Employees, Other Students, and Third Parties." The document attempts to bring standards for determining sexual harassment in line with the guidelines used for evaluating adult cases. The policy defines the same two types of sexual harassment used in adult rulings: quid pro quo (say, sexual favors for advancement) and hostile environment (Chmielewski, 1997).

Sexual Harassment in College

Over the past decade, many colleges have instituted sexual harassment policies, in response to concerns of students, faculty members, and administrators. Most sexual harassment in college is between male professors and female students. Although the reverse (female professor harassing a male student) or same-sex harassment can happen, both are much less common.

Between 15 and 50 percent of undergraduate and graduate-level college women report having been the victim of sexual harassment by a professor. Furthermore, between 10 and 20 percent of male undergraduates have been the victims of sexual harassment (Benson & Thomson, 1990). This behavior encompasses either unwanted sexual advances or the creation of a hostile environment.

case study 16.4

Bethany: A Proposition from Her Professor

Bethany, 23, lesbian, is white.

Bethany, a college senior, was having trouble with one of her classes and went to see her professor, a 35-year-old married man.

When I went to see him, I was a little surprised that he shut the door. It was after our late-afternoon class, and there wasn't anybody around in his department. He had this weird little smile on his face when he asked me to sit down. I sensed something was wrong and should have left then, but I didn't. When I sat down, his first remark was about how good I smelled. I smiled and thanked him but thought to myself that the comment was totally inappropriate.

I explained to him that I was there because I was worried about my grade for the semester. I had gotten a D on the last test and didn't want to lower my grade below a B–. He told me not to worry; he didn't like to see me so sad. Again I smiled but thought that this remark was also inappropriate. He said he'd take care of me, that I was one of his favorite students. With that, he slid his hand over the table and began rubbing my hand with his.

I was getting very uncomfortable by now and moved my hand away. He said, "Don't be so tense; let me rub your shoulders." He started to get up, but I stood up and said, "I don't think that's necessary. I must be going." He said, "Sit down. I thought you wanted to talk about your grade." I sat back down, and he proceeded to explain to me that he'd had his eye on me all semester and was hoping I'd come to visit him. He explained that other female students in the past had worked out "special arrangements" to boost their grades. I asked him, "What kind of special arrangements?" He said, "Come on now, Beth, don't be so naive. You're a very sexy girl. We could have lots of fun together." At this point, I was so flustered that I got up quickly and excused myself. I had to beat him to the door because he got up as if to block my exit, but I already had opened the door. He smiled and told me not to do anything foolish. I didn't tell anyone because I was afraid he'd flunk me. He kind of ignored me the rest of the semester but did wind up giving me a higher grade than I thought I earned.

> ### Critical Thinking
>
> Have you ever been in a situation where a grade was so important you said, "I'd do anything to get a better grade in this class?" What makes class grades this important?

In a study at the University of California-Berkeley, approximately one-third of female students reported at least one incident of sexual harassment on campus (Benson & Thomson, 1990). The NCWSV, although not designed to measure sexual harassment per se, found that approximately 11 percent of the 4,446 women studied had been sexually victimized (other than rape). These incidents included sexual coercion, sexual contact with or without force, threats of rape, sexual contact, and penetration. About 10 percent of the women had also been victimized in the past. Even more startling is the percentage of women who reported being stalked in the previous academic year. The NCWSV defined stalked as "repeatedly followed, watched, phoned, e-mailed, or communicated with in some way that seemed obsessive to you and made you afraid or concerned for your safety." Fully 13.1 percent of the women, using these criteria, reported being stalked in the previous academic year. Although none of these NCWSV data meet the classic criteria for sexual harassment, many would argue that this scenario could represent a hostile environment for some campus women (Fisher et al., 2000).

Child Sexual Abuse

Child sexual abuse Any sexual contact between an adult and a child who is under 18 years of age

Child sexual abuse is any sexual contact between an adult and a child under 18 years of age. Child sexual abuse runs the gamut from inappropriate fondling and touching, to masturbation, to oral sex, to penetration of the anus or vagina with fingers or a penis. These and other forms of sexual behavior are considered evidence of child sexual abuse despite the child's consent or sexual precociousness.

Often sexual abuse starts off as normal hugging, kissing, and playful behavior. It then progresses to more intimate touching, manual and oral stimulation, and finally intercourse. The perpetrator often tells the child that he or she is not doing anything wrong but "Don't tell anyone because they might not understand." The perpetrator often uses bribes and rewards to get the child to conceal the illicit behavior. Or, physical threats or threats of desertion scare the child into silence. Children also may not report abuse because of fear and guilt. They sense that something is wrong but can't bear the shame of others finding out. Often, fear of reprisals from the perpetrator or other family member stands in the way of the victim's reporting abuse. In many cases, even when children report the behavior to a parent, they are not believed.

Child molestation Abuse of a child by nonfamily members

Incest Child sexual abuse involving genetically related family members

Pedophile An adult who is sexually aroused by children and initiates contact with them out of sexual desire

Child molester One who makes indecent sexual advances to children

Child sexual abuse involving nonfamily members is generally referred to as **child molestation.** Child sexual abuse involving genetically related family members is called **incest.** Often, the perpetrators are adults who fall between the two forms, such as steprelatives, the mother's boyfriend, or a caregiver brought into the house to watch the children. As we discussed in Chapter 9, a **pedophile** is an adult who is sexually aroused by children and initiates contact with them out of sexual desire. A non-pedophilic **child molester** is not motivated by sexual desire but, rather, by power, the desire to control, or out of affection.

---

k   *Intellectual and Emotional Wellness*   k

As adults, we have the intellectual and emotional maturity to make informed choices regarding when and with whom we want to be sexual. Although "age of consent" is a gray area chronologically, theoretically it is the age where intellect and emotion work together in the mature person to make informed choices regarding their behavior. Society has long believed that children must be "protected" sexually from sexual predators until they are mature enough to make informed decisions regarding their behavior. Sexual predators are often very smart and develop elaborate plans for deceiving, luring, and trapping their victims. They observe and note their victim's behavior, patterns, and weaknesses. Their cognitive abilities, although they may be high-level, are without the self-regulating moral/ethical controls that most of us have.

Preconditions Related to Child Sexual Abuse

Child sexual abusers tend to be shy and lonely, and they have poor inter-personal skills with other adults (Bauman, Kasper, & Alford, 1984). They are conservative in their political and sexual beliefs, tend to be religious, and lack knowledge about sex (Segal & Marshall, 1985). **Child molesters** are more likely to be victims of child sexual molestation themselves, alcoholics, and likely to have severe marital difficulties (Johnston, 1987). Preconditions related to child sexual abuse have been identified (Finkelhor, 1984); these are explored in the following sections.

Motivation to Abuse

Three key variables influence the perpetrator's motivation to abuse: (a) emotional congruence, (b) sexual arousal, and (c) blockage of alterna-tive forms of sexual arousal. Whereas adults typically are attracted to, and seek emotional connections with, other adults in emotional congruence, pedophiles are drawn to children for this fulfillment. This may be a result of the perpetrator's arrested emotional development, a need to feel powerful and in control, or a reenactment of his own childhood abuse.

Typically, adults are sexually aroused by other adults and find chil-dren's bodies immature and nonarousing. Pedophiles feel the opposite. They are sexually aroused by children and not by adults. In addition to the perpetrators' own modeling of sexual relations experienced in their youth or their own childhood trauma, it may be influenced by erotic portrayals of children in advertising and media or exposure to child pornography.

A subgroup of child sexual abusers is **sociopaths** who have **psycho-ses** or other forms of mental illness. These abusers obtain gratification not only from sexual activity but also from inflicting pain and suffering on their victims. **Blockage** refers to child sexual abusers' inability to use other forms of sexual release and gratification. The abusers may be unable to form adult sexual relationships and be sexually naive. Their strict upbringing and sexual values may block their ability to use masturbation and fantasy as outlets for their sexual desire.

Sociopath A manifestly antisocial psychopath

Psychosis A severe form of mental disorder or disease affecting the total personality

Blockage A child sexual abuser's inability to use other forms of sexual release and gratification

Internal Inhibitions Against Abuse

Child sexual abusers find ways to overcome internal inhibitions against adult-child sexual relations. Whereas other adults may be curious or fanta-size about this activity, they stop short of actually doing it because of the strong cultural and social restrictions against such behavior. They have well-developed impulse control. Child sexual abusers, however, lack these inhibitions. Furthermore, they are more likely to use alcohol and drugs to overcome any inhibitions they do have.

Internal inhibitions Natural impulse control against adult–child sexual relations

External Inhibitions Against Abuse

External inhibitions against abuse include influences of family members, neighbors, friends, social connections, and household privacy. The greatest inhibitor of sexual abuse is the mother. Child sexual abuse is much more likely to occur in households where the mother is absent or neglectful, has emotional or physical problems, or is a victim of marital abuse.

In cases where the mother herself was a victim of child sexual abuse or is disengaged from her husband, she will turn her back on, or even use, her daughter as a buffer between herself and her husband (Browning & Boatman, 1977). This behavior clears the way for the father, stepfather, mother's boyfriend, or other dominant man to gain access to the child.

Children who are socially isolated (having few close friends or neighbors) also are more likely to be victimized. Household sleeping arrangements and crowding, too, may create opportunities for abusers to gain ready access to victims.

> ### ❧ Social Wellness ❧
>
> As we have just described, sexual predators do not have strong social relationships. Starting with their dysfunctional relationships with their own parents, sexual predators have not developed mature, egalitarian relationships based on caring, respect, and tolerance. From those who harass, to those who rape, to those who abuse children, a common thread is immature, dysfunctional, unsatisfying social relationships. Those who engage in coercive sex often have limited experience with relationships based on love and caring, trust, respect, mutuality, sharing, and commitment. Their relationships are exploitive, self-centered, and destructive. They use power differentials in relationships to take advantage and inflict pain and suffering. Their relationships are really not relationships at all. They are artificial arrangements set up to trap and abuse.

Children's Resistance

Child sexual abusers prey on any perceived child weaknesses. They are canny in using coercion, threat, punishment, or force to overcome any resistance a child may use. Children who are emotionally insecure, deprived, needy, and unsupported are prime victims for the abuser's offers, pleas, bribes, and threats. Children who lack education about sexual abuse and do not have good communication skills and caring adult support systems are easier for the abuser to manipulate.

Risks for Child Sexual Abuse

In a study of approximately 800 college students conducted in 1984, eight risk factors were related to an increased likelihood of childhood sexual abuse (Finkelhor, 1984):

1. Have a stepfather
2. Ever lived with mother alone
3. Not close to mother
4. Mother never finished high school
5. Sex-punitive mother
6. No physical affection from father
7. Income under $10,000 a year (although low income by itself is not a risk)
8. Two friends or fewer in childhood

The incidence of childhood sexual abuse was virtually nonexistent in subjects who did not have any of these risk factors. In contrast, two-thirds of the subjects reporting five or more of the risk factors were victims of childhood sexual abuse. The risk factor that was the greatest predictor of child sexual abuse was having a stepfather. This doubled a woman's risk of ever being abused. These findings confirmed those of Russel (1990), who found that 1 in 40 victims of child sexual victims were abused by their biological fathers versus 1 in 6 by stepfathers.

The second greatest predictor was having a sex-punitive mother. This type of mother was likely to scold or punish her daughter for asking questions about sex or engaging in behavior such as masturbation.

Hyde (1994) has speculated about child abuse being related to male psychosexual development. She asserts that men are socialized to be sexually attracted to partners who are smaller and younger than they are, whereas women receive the opposite messages. Women usually are sexually involved with, and attracted to, partners who are larger and older than them.

Incidence of Child Sexual Abuse

The actual number of cases of child sexual abuse is unknown. Like rape, child sexual abuse is often unreported for many reasons. However, following a sustained 15-year increase from 1977 to 1992, reported cases of child sexual abuse have been decreasing since then (Jones & Finkelhor, 2001). Numbers of cases of reported child sexual abuse reached an estimated peak of 149,800 in 1992. Since that time, cases declined 2 to 11 percent each year through 1998 (Jones & Finkelhor, 2001). In 1998, estimated cases of child sexual abuse reached a low of approximately 103,600, which represents a total decline of 31 percent over that 6-year period (Jones & Finkelhor, 2001). This sustained decline in the number of cases contrasts significantly with the 1980s, when the United States experienced 10 percent annual increases in the number of cases of child sexual abuse (Jones & Finkelhor, 2001).

Explanations for the Decline

Wilson (2001), reporting in the Office of Juvenile Justice bulletin, identifies several reasons for the decline in child sexual abuse cases. The past two decades have seen a dramatic increase in public information and information about child sexual abuse. There has been an increase in child abuse prevention programs. The increase in awareness and prevention has led to the arrest and incarceration of more sex offenders. With the onset of Megan's Law (which we will discuss in detail later), new laws have been passed in many states to increase and improve the monitoring of sex offenders (Jones & Finkelhor, 2001).

The decline in child sexual abuse parallels declines in other criminal offenses that may be related to victimizing children. As we mentioned previously, the number of cases of all violent crime, rape, sexual assault, and other types of female victimization are down nationally. Factors that may be related to the declines in these crimes could also be related to the declines in child sexual abuse (Jones & Finkelhor, 2001).

Effects of Child Sexual Abuse

Several factors have an impact on the future well-being of the victim. Four factors are related to the need for long-term treatment and the prognosis for the child (Krugman, Bays, Chadwick, Levitt, McMugh, & Whitworth, 1991). The closer the victim's relationship to the perpetrator, the longer the

case study 16.5

Lucy: A Victim of Child Abuse

Lucy, 16, single, identifies as Latina.

A 16-year-old girl was referred to the STD clinic by her high school nurse. The report showed a classic macular/papular rash on her hands and feet and a blood test confirming secondary syphilis. This girl, Lucy, probably used drugs, had a few boyfriends, and was a dropout candidate. Dr. Blonna saw these kids all the time. Here he relates Lucy's case.

When I first interviewed Lucy, I knew from the start that this was not a cut-and-dried case. She was young, fresh-faced, and preppy-looking in her Catholic schoolgirl's pleated skirt and white socks.

Lucy was quiet, almost sunken in her posture. She averted eye contact, obviously embarrassed. After my usual introduction, explaining why I needed to talk to her, I began to explain the nitty-gritty of sexually transmitted diseases and how they are spread. By the time I got around to asking her about her sexual contacts, she was on the verge of tears.

Lucy's initial response to my asking for the names of her sexual contacts was "There's only one—my boyfriend, Hector." When pressed for Hector's address and telephone number, Lucy hemmed and hawed, said she didn't know where he lived or went to school, and tried to move the interview along.

Finally, I had enough and said, "Look, I know you're lying to me. What's going on here?" It took but a second for Lucy to break down and the floodgates to open up, her tears pouring forth in a torrent followed by shakes, sobs, and near hyperventilation. She couldn't contain herself any longer. Between gasps of air and body-wracking sobs, she told her story. There was no boyfriend Hector. Rather, there was a 45-year-old man, Luis. Luis was the boyfriend of her mother, Maria. He mostly lived with them and had free rein to come and go. It seemed that he liked to come around when Maria was still at work and Lucy and her younger sister were home from school. Luis had started sexually abusing Lucy about 5 years ago. It started out with her sitting on his lap and his fondling her. It progressed to his exposing himself to her, demanding fellatio, and, for the past couple of years, vaginal intercourse. When it began, Lucy was confused, but Luis told her not to say anything to her mother. Lucy thought her mother knew what was going on because there were times when Lucy didn't want to be left home with Luis, but her mom made excuses for him and didn't let Lucy leave.

When Luis began to force fellatio and intercourse on Lucy, he warned her not to tell her mother or he'd leave them or, worse, hurt her mother and little sister. Lucy was beginning to worry about her little sister. She'd seen the way Luis was eyeing her sister lately, and Lucy didn't want her to have to go through the same thing that she did.

Critical Thinking

Social workers and other mental health professionals are trained to pick up on cues like the ones Lucy presented. Should these people be held liable for missing the same cues? Why?

I'm not sure how the story ended. I brought Lucy downtown to the child welfare agency that afternoon. I had to fill out forms and was still there when they returned with her little sister, afraid but unmolested. The social worker told me that they were removing Lucy and her sister from the home, arresting Luis and probably Maria, and would find a safe home for the girls. The last image I have of Lucy is her sitting on the wooden bench in the child welfare office, her arm around her little sister, smoothing the pleats on her school uniform, looking much older and more tired than her 16 years.

abuse, the more violent the contact, and the more intrusive the relationship, the greater is the need for treatment and the poorer the hope for an effective outcome.

As adults, child sexual abuse victims report extremely sad, pain-filled childhoods. They recollect feelings of betrayal, fear, and loss of innocence, painting a picture of a lost childhood (Felitti, 1991). Victims of child sexual abuse often have difficulty forming intimate relationships as adults. They have feelings of shame and guilt, depression, a lack of trust, and revulsion at being touched, and they often are alcohol and other drug abusers (Frazier & Cohen, 1992). When victims are able to form relationships, they are often characterized by a lack of emotion and sexual interest and gratification (Jackson, Calhoun, Amick, Maddeve, & Habif, 1990).

Megan's Law

On October 31, 1994, the New Jersey State Legislature enacted the Registration and Community Notification Laws (RCNL), also known as **Megan's Law.** The law is named after Megan Kanka, who was lured into the house of a neighbor, whose son, a convicted sex offender, raped and murdered her. Only one family, neighbors of the perpetrator, had any knowledge of him living on the block.

Megan's Law requires that certain convicted sexual offenders must register with law enforcement authorities and provide for community notification depending on the degree of risk that they represent to the community. The law applies to those who have been convicted of specified sexual offenses and has a grandfather's clause that includes offenders who were convicted of similar offenses prior to the passage of the law. The degree of risk that offenders pose to the community is measured by a "tiered system" (Brooks, 1996, p. 54).

> *Tier 1* applies where the risk of re-offense is low. Under Tier 1, all law enforcement agencies likely to encounter the offender must be notified as well as the victim(s) and his or her family.

> *Tier 2* applies where the risk of re-offense is moderate. Under Tier 2, all law enforcement agencies and schools (public and private) likely to encounter the offender must be notified as well as the victim(s) and his or her family. The statute also requires notification to organizations in the community, including religious and youth organizations, likely to encounter the offender. Under the

Megan's Law Legislation requiring notification that a sex offender has been released and is residing in a community

court's decision, individual determinations must be made concerning which institutions or organizations own or operate an establishment where children or women are cared for and are "likely to encounter" the offender. The notice to all such organizations must specifically direct them not to notify anyone else.

Tier 3 applies where the risk of re-offense is high. The statute requires that, in addition to the individuals, organizations, and institutions required to be notified by Tier 2, notification as to Tier 3 offenders must be sufficient to reach members of the public likely to encounter the person registered (individuals residing within a half-mile radius of the offender's home).

Over 40 states rushed to enact Megan's Laws of their own, and in May 1996, President Bill Clinton signed into law a federal version of the legislation. The federal version of Megan's Law was a revision of the Federal Violent Crimes and Law Enforcement Act of 1994. The revised law, entitled Megan's Law, required all states wishing to continue to receive federal funding for law enforcement to comply with its identification and notification of sex offenders criteria (*Economist,* 1997). The law came under intense scrutiny from civil libertarian groups, who claimed it denies convicted sex offenders their constitutional rights to privacy and protection (Brooks, 1996).

The various versions of Megan's Law all contain provisions for identifying convicted sex offenders and ranking them on the aforementioned three-tiered scale according to their likelihood to offend again. The level of community notification varies according to the offender's level. Tier 1 offenders must register with local authorities, but their status is not released to the community (Webby, 2003). High-risk residents (all day care center operators; supervisors of Boy Scouts, Big Brothers, Big Sisters; and the like) are notified of Tier 2 offenders. All immediate neighbors and others likely to come in contact with Tier 3 offenders are sent registered letters notifying them of the presence of the offender in their neighborhood (*Economist,* 2002). In addition to registered letters, other means of community notification include posting of pictures and descriptions of sex offenders; mailings to families, community groups, and organizations deemed at risk by local authorities; and postings on Internet bulletin boards.

Critics of Megan's Law legislation claim that, in addition to being unconstitutional, it does not work. Just knowing that a sex offender lives on your street is not sufficient to protect your children (Webby, 2003; Bai, 1997). Neighbors of Megan Kanka, for instance, knew that at least one sex offender (the roommate of Megan's killer) already lived on their street (Knight Ridder/Tribune Services, 2003). Other critics cite that the placement of convicted sex offenders on the tiers often arbitrarily places many people convicted of sex offenses other than child sexual abuse in the highest-risk tiers (Tiers 2 and 3) unnecessarily.

Part of the problem, according to Levenson and D'Amoura (2007) is the shaky theoretical foundation upon which most of the legislation rests. Instead of being based on empirical evidence related to perpetrators and corrective actions, the social policies designed to prevent sexual violence are often based on myths perpetuated by the media frenzy surrounding sensational individual cases. For example, none of the common policies passed in recent years (sex offender registration, community notification, ie. Megan's Law, residence restrictions, civil commitment, and electronic monitoring) have been based on empirical studies that have been proven to significantly reduce initial or repeat sexual offenses (Levenson & D'Amora, 2007).

Another problem, according to Levenson & D'Amora (2007), is lumping all sex offenders together and treating them the same way. For example, a repeat child molester poses a much more serious threat to society than does the young adult who had sex with his teenage girlfriend, yet they are both viewed and treated the same way by the courts and correctional system. Lifetime registration and community notification for all sex offenders works against reintegrating such low-risk offenders back into society because it limits their employment and educational opportunities, restricts where they can live and makes it harder for them to access the social support systems they need. Research shows that as the length of time living in the community offense-free increases, recidivism decreases. Some of these offense-free sex offenders could be allowed to re-integrate into society after five years, and pose very little risk for recidivism (Levenson & D'Amora, 2007).

In New Jersey, sex offenders are allowed to challenge their tiering. They have 14 days from being notified of their tier designation to challenge it in court. There have been 1,620 cases involving 3,515 specific objections of tier designations since passage of Megan's Law in New Jersey. These 1,620 cases have resulted in 672 tier changes. In 528 cases, a Tier 2 or Tier 3 placement was downgraded to a Tier 1, eliminating the need for community notification (New Jersey Law Network, 2003).

There is no way to identify potential child abusers and isolate them from children. Preventing child sexual abuse must revolve around empowering children by teaching them the warning signs of inappropriate adult sexual behavior, and the escape and communication skills necessary to protect themselves. Parents and other adult caregivers must convey to their children a sense of approachability. Children must feel free to discuss their concerns without fear of reprisal.

Strategies to Prevent Child Sexual Abuse

Parents, teachers, and other helpful adults might use the following strategies to help prevent child sexual abuse:

1. *Provide sex education.* One of the cornerstones of any good school-based sexuality education program is a child sexual abuse prevention component. The unit should be comprehensive and cover issues including self-esteem, communication skills, inappropriate adult physical contact, refusal skills, and escape skills. This unit should be presented early in the child's curriculum, as most sexual abuse begins before 8 years of age.

2. *Become an approachable parent.* Open lines of communication early with your children. Continually underscore the fact that your children can come to you with any question involving sex. Do not punish your children for asking questions.

3. *Discuss inappropriate sexual behavior with your children.* Let your children know that you do not approve of any adult-child sexual contact (explain kissing, hugging, and so forth). Tell them that you

would never punish them for telling on another adult (no matter how close their relationship-stepfather, baby-sitter, coach). Differentiate "good touch" and "bad touch" while letting your children know that they have the right to want "no touch."

4. *Let your children know they can decide how, when, and by whom they want to be touched.* Do not force them to hug, kiss, or be affectionate with adults with whom they do not want to behave this way. This reinforces their trust in their intuition about other people's sexual behavior.

5. *Discuss refusal skills.* Have your children practice how to say no in an assertive way. Teach them how to refuse an offer to engage in any behavior in which they do not want to be involved.

6. *Discuss escape skills.* Teach your children how to escape from potentially dangerous or abusive situations. Tell them it is OK to yell, scream, hit, and run away from any adult who does not stop touching them when asked to. Help children identify trusted friends, neighbors, and family members with whom they can seek shelter.

7. *Discuss telling.* Your children have to understand that they absolutely must tell you if they have been approached or touched inappropriately by any adult, no matter how close that person's relationship is with you. Children need to understand that this isn't tattle-telling and is the best way to deal with the situation.

Personal Assessment

Temper Test

Directions: A number of statements that people have used to describe themselves are given here. Read each statement and then circle the appropriate number to indicate how you generally feel.

	Almost Never	Sometimes	Often	Almost Always
1. I am quick-tempered.	1	2	3	4
2. I get annoyed when I don't receive recognition for doing good work.	1	2	3	4
3. I have a fiery temper.	1	2	3	4
4. I feel infuriated when I do a good job or study hard and get a poor evaluation or test score	1	2	3	4
5. I am a hot-headed person.	1	2	3	4
6. I get furious when I'm criticized in front of others.	1	2	3	4
7. I get angry when others' mistakes slow me down.	1	2	3	4
8. I fly off the handle easily.	1	2	3	4
9. When I get angry, I say nasty things to anyone around me.	1	2	3	4
10. When I get frustrated, I feel like hitting someone.	1	2	3	4

Total Points: _____

Scoring:

Add the points (1–4) from each item together to get your total score, somewhere between 10 and 40. A man who scores 17 or a woman who scores 18 is just about average. If you score below 13, you're well down in the safe zone. A score above 20 means you may be a hothead—scoring higher than three-quarters of those tested. If these tendencies cause you to take out your anger on anyone else, professional help is advised.

Personal Alcohol Use

Go to www.intox.com. Click on the "Drink Wheel" on the right side of the screen. Complete the test using the amount and the type of alcohol you usually drink when partying. If you do not drink, use a friend's drinking behavior to complete the assignment.

What were your BAC (blood/breath alcohol concentration) results?

Scroll down and click on "Pharmacology and Disposition of Alcohol in Humans" and "Stages of Alcohol Intoxication." Read the information contained in these links.

What did you learn from this activity?

Thought Questions

1. What sexual acts are covered by the umbrella term *coercive sex*?

2. What conditions are necessary to meet sexual harassment criteria?

3. What is a "hostile environment" in a sexual harassment case? Give an example of a hostile environment.

4. How does power over a subordinate factor into sexual harassment?

5. What are three variations of rape? Is it considered a sexual act? Why or why not?

6. What are three risk factors for acquaintance rape?

7. What are three ways to reduce the risk for acquaintance rape?

8. What are some personality characteristics of a typical child molester?

9. What is the difference between a child molester and a pedophile?

10. What is Megan's Law?

Test Yourself

1. *Coercive sex* is best defined as
   a. another name for rape.
   b. begging and pleading for sex.
   c. any nonconsensual sexual behavior.
   d. using coercion to set up sexual liaisons.

2. The Sexual Victimization of College Women study found that
   a. date rape is very rare among college women.
   b. about 35 out of every 1,000 college women were rape victims during the time of the study.
   c. about 3.5 out of every 1,000 college women were rape victims last year.
   d. about 3.5 out of every 10,000 college women were rape victims last year.

3. College women are most often raped
   a. in off-campus residences by strangers.
   b. in on-campus residences by strangers.
   c. in off-campus residences by intimate partners.
   d. in on-campus residences by intimate partners.

4. Under Rohypnol, a central nervous system depressant, victims
   a. relax, pass out, are sexually victimized, and suffer from amnesia.
   b. relax, lose their inhibitions, and want sex.
   c. relax, become sexually aroused, and solicit sex.
   d. relax, pass out, and are usually left alone.

5. 5. Under the 1996 Drug-Induced Rape Prevention and Punishment Act,
   a. penalties for Rohypnol and GHB use were made much harsher.
   b. penalties for Rohypnol and GHB use were brought into line with other drugs such as marijuana.
   c. penalties for Rohypnol and GHB use were lessened since they are most often taken for personal use, not major distribution like other drugs such as marijuana or cocaine.
   d. penalties for Rohypnol and GHB use were left unchanged.

6. Which behavior should you avoid if you find yourself the victim of an attempted stranger rape?
   a. Run away if you can.
   b. Try to reason with the perpetrator.
   c. Fight back
   d. Scream, yell, curse.

7. The two criteria needed to prove work site–based sexual harassment are
   a. a hostile environment and unwanted sexual attention.
   b. sex is made a condition for employment.
   c. sex is made a condition of promotion.
   d. hostile sex is part of the work environment.

8. Recent EEOC rulings governing sexual harassment have omitted which of the following groups?
   a. Hispanic women
   b. Homosexuals
   c. White males
   d. African American women
9. Most adults are attracted to, and seek emotional and sexual connections to, other adults. Pedophiles
   a. are attracted to, and seek emotional and sexual connections to, other adults and children.
   b. are attracted to adults but seek emotional and sexual connections to children.
   c. are attracted to, and seek emotional and sexual connections to, children.
   d. neither are attracted to nor seek emotional connections to the children they desire sexually.
10. Megan's Law was recently
   a. struck down in Alaska and Connecticut.
   b. watered down due to cases in Alaska and Connecticut.
   c. upheld due to ruling related to cases in Alaska and Connecticut.
   d. overturned due to cases in Alaska and Connecticut.

Web Resources

National Center for Victims of Crime
www.ncvc.org

A nonprofit organization providing resources and advocacy to victims of crime. The site offers safety strategies for victims of domestic violence and stalking, highlights of laws and public policy impacting crime victims at state and federal levels, information on crime victims, and finding a lawyer. Access to a virtual library with full-text publications, a directory of publications, recommended reading, bibliographies and a book review, plus links to victim-related sites.

National Organization on Male Sexual Victimization
www.malesurvivor.org

A group started in 1988 by mental health providers who wanted to better understand and treat adult male survivors of childhood sexual abuse. A section on prevention and education talks about how to prevent abused boys from becoming abusive men.

Rape Abuse and Incest National Network (RAINN)
www.rainn.org

A nonprofit organization's hotline providing 24-hour counseling service to survivors of sexual assault. This site also offers information, statistics, and a list of local crisis centers.

Sexual Assault Prevention
www.4women.gov/FAQ/sexualassault.htm

A site sponsored by the US Government. It provides information on prevalence, aftereffects, and treatment of rape and sexual assault and links with a specific focus on higher education.

References

Addington, L. A. (2008). Assessing the Extent of Non-response Bias on NIBRS Estimates of Violent Crime. *Journal of Contemporary Criminal Justice,* 2008; 24; 32

American Academy of Family Physicians. (2003). What to do if you are raped [Online]. Available: http://familydoctor.org/x1976.xml.

American Psychiatric Association. (2000). *Diagnostic and statistical manual of mental disorders* (4th ed., text revision). Washington, DC: Author.

Bai, M. (1997). A report from the front in the war on predators: Years after Megan's murder, her law is still on trial. *Newsweek, 129*(20), 67.

Bauman, R., Kasper, C., & Alford, J. (1984). The child sex abusers. *Corrective and Social Psychiatry, 30,* 76–81.

Benson, D., & Thomson, G. (1990). Sexual harassment on a university campus: The confluence of authority relations, sexual interest, and gender stratification. *Society for the Study of Social Problems, 29*(3), 236–251.

Benton, W. (Ed.). (1996). *Webster's new international dictionary.* Toronto: Encyclopedia Britannica.

Brooks, A. (1996). Megan's Law: Constitutionality and policy. *Criminal Justice Ethics, 15*(56), 51.

Browning, D., & Boatman, B. (1977). Incest: Children at risk. *American Journal of Psychiatry, 134* (1977), 69–72.

Brownmiller, S. (1975). *Against our will.* New York: Simon & Schuster.

Burgess, A. W., & Holmstrom, L. L. (1974). Rape trauma syndrome. *American Journal of Psychiatry, 131,* 981–985.

Cate, R. M., & Lloyd, S. A. (1992). *Courtship.* Newbury Park, Calif.: Sage.

Chmielewski, C. M. (1997). Sexual harassment meets Title IX: New federal rules to combat sexual harassment and place schools at the battlefront. *NEA Today, 16*(2), 25.

The Economist. (1997). Pointing the finger at Megan's Law. *342*(8004), 27–29.

The Economist. (2002, November 16). A scarlet letter: Megan's Law, changing the law for sex offenders. *365*(8299).

Equal Employment Opportunity Commission. (2003). Sexual harassment charges: EEOC and fair employment practices agencies (FEPA) combined, FY 1002-FY 2001 [Online]. Available: www.eeoc.gov/stats/harass.html.

Felitti, V. (1991). Long-term medical consequences of incest, rape, and molestation. *Southern Medical Journal, 84,* 328–331.

Finkelhor, D. (1984). *Child sexual abuse: New theory and research.* New York: Free Press.

Fisher, B., Koss, M. P., Gidycz, C. A., & Wisnewski, N. (1987). The scope of rape: Incidence and prevalence of sexual aggression and victimization in a national sample of higher education students. *Journal of Counseling and Clinical Psychology, 55,* 162–170.

Fisher, B. S., Cullen, F. T., & Turner, M. G. (2000). *The sexual victimization of college women.* Washington, DC: U.S. Department of Justice.

Frazier, P., & Cohen, B. (1992). Research on the sexual victimization of women. *Counseling Psychologist, 20,* 141–158.

Frieze, I. H. (1983). Causes and consequences of marital rape. *Signs, 8,* 532–553.

Gleason, N. A. (1994, May). College women and alcohol: A relational perspective. *Journal of American College Health, 42*(6), 279–289.

Higher Education Center. (2003). Sexual assault: Alcohol and other drugs [Online]. Available: www.edc.org/hec/pubs/factsheets/fact_sheet1.html.

Hyde, J. S. (1994). *Understanding human sexuality* (5th ed.). New York: McGraw-Hill.

Jackson, I., Calhoun, K., Amick, A., Maddever, H., & Habif, V. (1990). Young adult women who report childhood intrafamilial sexual abuse: Subsequent adjustment. *Archives of Sexual Behavior, 19,* 211–221.

Johnson, C. B., Stockdale, M. S., & Saal, F. E. (1991). Persistence of men's misperceptions of friendly cues across a variety of interpersonal encounters. *Psychology of Women Quarterly, 15*(3), 463–475.

Johnston, S. (1987, February). The mind of the molester. *Psychology Today,* 60–63.

Jones, L. M., & Finkelhor, D. (2001, January). The decline in child sexual abuse cases. *Juvenile Justice Bulletin.* Washington, DC: Bureau of Justice Statistics, Office of Juvenile Justice and Delinquency Prevention.

Jones, T. S., & Remland, M. S. (1992). Sources of variability in perceptions of and responses to sexual harassment. *Sex Roles, 27*(3–4), 121–142.

Kaufman, L. (1997). A report from the front: Why it's gotten easier to sue for sexual harassment. *Newsweek, 129*(2), 32.

Knight-Ridder/Tribune Services. (2003, January 13). Public must be involved to make Megan's law work. *San Jose Mercury News,* p. 7485.

Koss, M. P. (1992). The underdetection of rape: Methodological choices influence incidental estimates. *Journal of Social Issues, 48,* 61–75.

Koss, M. P. (1996). The measurement of rape victimization in crime surveys. *Criminal Justice and Behavior, 23*(1), 55–69.

Krugman, R., Bays, J., Chadwick, D., Levitt, C., McMugh, M., & Whitworth, J. (1991). Guidelines for evaluation of sexual abuse of children. *Pediatrics, 87,* 254–260.

LeLand, J. (1996). A kiss is just a kiss: Where should schools draw the line between normal childhood behavior and sexual harassment? *Newsweek, 128*(17), 71–72.

Levenson, J. S., D'Amora, M. S., Hern, A. L. (2007). Megan's Law and Its Impact on Community Re-Entry for Sex Offenders. *Behavioral Sciences and the Law,* (2007). 25: 587–602.

Malamuth, N. M., Sockloski, R. J., Koss, M. P., & Tanaka, J. S. (1991). Characteristics of aggressors against women: Testing a model using a national sample of college students. *Journal of Consulting and Clinical Psychology, 59,* 670–781.

Marano, H. E. (1996). Why they stay: A saga of spouse abuse. *Psychology Today, 29*(3), 56–66.

Montgomery, R. L., Benedicto, J. A., & Hammerke, F. M. (1993, December). Personal U.S. social motivation of undergraduates in using alcohol. *Psychological Reports, 960–962.*

Muram, D., Miller, K., & Cutler, A. (1992). Sexual assault of the elderly victim. *Journal of Interpersonal Violence, 791,* 70–76.

New Jersey Law Network. (2003, February 18). New Jersey law [Online]. Available: www.njlawnet.com/megan.html.

Office of National Drug Control Policy. (2002a). Gamma hydrobutyrate (GHB) [Online]. Available: www.whitehousedrugpolicy.gov/publications/factsh/tgamma/index.html

Office of National Drug Control Policy. (2002b). Rohypnol [Online]. Available: www.whitehousedrugpolicy.gov/publications/factsht/rohypnol/index.html

Quittner, J. (2002, December 10). Left out of the law: In the eyes of the court, just about everyone can be a victim of sexual harassment—except, perhaps, out gay men and lesbians. *The Advocate,* pp. 26–29.

Rantala, R. R., & Edwards, T. J. (2000, July). *Effects of the NIBRS on crime statistics.* Bureau of Justice Statistics Special Report (NJC 178890). Washington, DC: U.S. Department of Justice, Office of Justice Programs.

Rand, M. R. (2008). *National Crime Victimization Survey, 2008.* Bureau of Justice Statistics, National Crime Victimization Survey. Washington, DC: U.S. Department of Justice. http://www.ojp.usdoj.gov/bjs/pub/pdf/cv07.pdf

Ruskin, L. (2002, November 12). Sex registry goes to court; John Doe: Alaskans say law amounts to retroactive punishment. *Anchorage Daily News* p. 1.

Russel, D. E. H. (1990). *Rape in marriage.* Bloomington: Indiana University Press.

Sanday, P. (1987). The socio-cultural context of rape: A crosscultural study. *Journal of Social Issues, 37*(4), 5–27.

Segal, Z., & Marshall, W. (1985). Heterosexual social skills in a population of rapists and child molesters. *Journal of Consulting and Clinical Psychology, 53,* 55–63.

Stockdale, M. S. (1993). The role of sexual misperceptions of women's friendliness in an emerging theory of sexual harassment. *Journal of Vocational Behavior, 42*(1), 84–101.

Task Force of the National Advisory Council on Alcohol Abuse and Alcoholism. (2002). *A call to action: Changing the culture of drinking at US colleges.* NIH Publication 02-5010. Washington, DC: National Institute on Alcohol Abuse and Alcoholism.

United States Congress. (1996).The Drug-Induced Rape Prevention and Punishment Act of 1996. 21 USC 841(b)(7).

United States Department of Justice, Federal Bureau of Investigation (USDOHFBI) (2008). *Crime in the United States, 2007.* (September 2008). Available online at: http://www.fbi.gov/ucr/07cius.htm.

Webby, S. (2003, January 13). Lack of funding, personnel hinder enforcement of Megan's Law. *San Jose Mercury News,* p. 1058.

Wechsler, H., Davenport, A., Dowdell, G., Moeykens, B., & Castillo, S. (1994). Health and behavioral consequences of binge drinking in college. *Journal of American Medical Association, 272*(21), 1672–1677.

Weschler, H., Eun, L. J., Kuo, M., Sebring, M., Nelson, T. F., & Lee, H. (2002). Trends in college binge drinking during a period of increased prevention efforts: Findings from four Harvard School of Public Health college alcohol study surveys, 1993–2001. *Journal of American College Health, 50*(5), 203–217.

Williams, L. (1984). The classic rape: When do victims report? *Social Problems, 31,* 459–467.

Wilson, J. J. (2001, January). Explanation for the decline in child sexual abuse cases. *Juvenile Justice Bulletin.* Washington, DC: Bureau of Justice Statistics, Office of Juvenile Justice and Delinquency Prevention.

seventeen

The Business of Sex

Student Learning Objectives

After reading this chapter, students will be able to

- Explain the major historical events that have shaped current attitudes and practices related to sex for sale over the past three decades.
- Describe the significance of Madonna, Calvin Klein, Gary Hart, and Matt Drudge in shaping the sexual climate of today.
- Differentiate pornography, erotica, and obscenity.
- Discuss how technological advances have combined with other historical trends to create a new commercialization of sex.
- Describe some of the problems inherent in policing the Internet for sexual victimization and exploitation.
- Evaluate the effectiveness of blocking tools that parents can use to limit children's access to Internet- or television-based sexual material.
- Evaluate the effects of sexually explicit materials on sexual behavior.

activity teaser: Is sex being sold to you? Find out with the Personal Exploration Activity on page 659.

case study 17.1

Lisa: Addicted to Cybersex

Lisa, 42, married, is white.

Lisa is a continuing education student. She has been married for 22 years and is the mother of a 14-year-old daughter and 13-year-old son. She works part-time and is taking one of the author's human sexuality classes for personal enrichment.

Critical Thinking

What are your thoughts about cybersex being *real* sex or just fantasy sex?

I had a real problem with computer sex. I had to see a therapist because I was really addicted. My telephone and Internet bills were getting huge, and I was spending about 3 hours a night online. I've been in counseling for a couple of months and actually took this class to try to understand my sexuality a little better. I think my marriage was in jeopardy, and that scared me.

My addiction began innocently enough. I had a lot of time on my hands. My husband, whom I love very much, travels about half of the time. As the national sales manager for a small company, he is off on business at least 2 weeks a month. He earns a fabulous salary, and I don't have to work. The kids are both grown up and don't need me much except to drive them around. Other than my exercise class, I had no real time commitments.

We bought my son a new, powerful computer with Internet access, and he showed me how to go online and get into these chat rooms. I started to log on and chat with people. Before long, I found my way into a couple of chat rooms that were sexually oriented. I mean, the primary purpose was to discuss sexual fantasies. It was quite a turn-on. I was getting into these intimate discussions with all kinds of men. It started out as kind of generic. We talked about our sex lives and what we liked to do in bed. Then it got personal—what we'd like to do to each other.

At first I didn't think it was a problem, and I didn't feel guilty, but after a while I found that I was getting really worked up about these calls. I'd masturbate after hanging up. Sometimes I'd even make myself come while online. That's when I started to worry. I never wanted to meet these guys face-to-face, but I started to feel like I was still having sex with them. I was also worried about my kids walking in and seeing me playing with myself.

It all came to a head when my husband saw one of the Internet bills. It seems as though I used a toll number instead of one of the toll-free access ones, and the bill was over $550 for the month. I had to explain the whole thing to him, and he freaked out. He felt like I cheated on him, and he considered separation. It took several weeks to restore his trust and convince him that I still loved him. We moved the computer into my son's room, and I promised not to go online again. We started seeing a family therapist, and I got a part-time job to get me out of the house a little. I'm taking this class to try to learn a little about my sexuality.

As the case study points out, sex is definitely for sale on the Internet. The last 50 years have seen technology play an increasingly more significant role in selling sex. Prior to the 1960s, sexual themes in mainstream advertising were mostly covert and reflected the mores of the times. Advertisers were subjected to much more stringent controls concerning issues such as the verbal content of advertisements, overt pictorial displays of nudity, and implied sexual themes. Modesty prevailed, as cleavage, bare midriffs, and other examples of exposing the human body were not allowed. Using sex in advertising was limited to full-bosomed "sweater girls" to promote cigarettes, appliances, and cars.

Besides the lack of overt sexuality in advertising, it was noticeably absent from other forms of entertainment and media. Few mainstream books, television shows, magazines, movies, and other media included sexual content. Although Kinsey's studies had been conducted and disseminated to the professional community, sexual information was not readily available to the general public.

Changes in the 1960s

These cultural conditions all began to change in the 1960s. The peace, prosperity, and contentment of the post–World War II 1950s began to give way to the rebelliousness of the baby boom generation of the 1960s.

Many social, economic, technological, and political forces came together to create a synergy that changed the course of history. As Petersen (1999) notes, a number of firsts came together during 1960s. The sixties saw the birth control pill, the IUD, Freedom Riders, be-ins, sit-ins, love-ins, the Peace Corps, topless bathing suits, topless bars, water beds, lava lamps, *Hair* (the play), hippies and yippies, Playboy Clubs, Stonewall, and Woodstock all converge in a turbulent decade of social change. Nowhere was change more evident than in issues related to sexuality.

Technological advances in contraception brought widespread availability of the birth control pill. This gave women newfound freedom and control of their fertility, and enabled them to reenter the workforce in ever-increasing numbers. The number of women taking birth control pills rose from 408,000 in 1961 to 6 million in 1966 (Petersen, 1999).

Masters and Johnson (1966) released their breakthrough research regarding sexual response and sexual pleasure. Men and women learned about the clitoris and multiple orgasms. Other research followed when the interest in information about sexuality became an outcry. Popular magazines of the 1950s, such as *Playboy,* were joined by *Penthouse, Screw, Cosmopolitan,* and others to meet this need (Petersen, 1999).

All of these developments helped spawn a **women's movement,** which began to question many long-standing cultural assumptions regarding the roles of men and women in society. The women's movement brought to the forefront issues such as equal rights, abortion, child care in the workplace, sexual assault, and a host of others. The ensuing debate forever changed the way men and women perceived themselves and their roles as citizens.

Women's movement A force to gain full educational, social, and economic opportunities and rights for women equal to those that men are traditionally understood to have

Styles, too, began to change. The Broadway play *Hair* focused attention on changing sex roles for men and women. It rejoiced in a newfound androgyny that liberated men from their clean-cut image and women from their bras. Men began to grow long hair and wear beads, and some women discarded their bras and exposed their midriffs. Attitudes and values about sexuality were changing faster than the society could adapt to the change.

One of the most telling legacies of the 1960s was the growing mainstream acceptance of sex as a topic of discussion. Books, films, magazines, newspapers, posters, and the evening news began to increase the level and realism of sexual content. Self-help books about sexuality proliferated. Academicians, feminists, and politicians began to seriously discuss the implications of sexuality and gender research for social policy and laws. While this was going on, average Americans were beginning to discuss their own sexuality. One of the most interesting byproducts of the women's and sexual revolutions of the 1960s and early 1970s was how comfortable people became in discussing sex (Hunt, 1974; Hite, 1976).

Changes in the 1970s and 1980s: Three Illustrative Examples

The 1970s and 1980s saw a continued increase of sexual themes in the media. Not only did the amount of sexual information increase, but the content, too, became more diverse. Subjects such as homosexuality, bisexuality, and interracial sex were becoming much more noticeable in mainstream media. This new wave of sexual permissiveness was marked by changing rules about what previously had been considered private information. Three well-known media figures serve as examples here: actress/singer Madonna, designer Calvin Klein, and 1988 presidential candidate Gary Hart.

The Material Girl

Although now a mother in her 40s, Madonna ushered in a new era of mainstream hedonism and me-generation narcissism in the 1970s. Madonna's "material girl" embodied all of the elements of post-1960s sexuality: open acceptance of sexual desire, the pursuit of sex and passion, a focus on self-fulfillment, glorification of the human body as a sensual and sexual object, permission to explore bisexuality, interracial sex, and personal adornment and clothing that transcended gender conventional style. Madonna combined all of these things into one package and put that package on display in American living rooms. She represented the disparate elements of the tumultuous 1960s, the self-centered 1970s, and the androgynous 1980s in a synergistic, in-your-face assault on American sexual mores.

Although not a self-professed "women's libber" or political figure, Madonna has been one of our most visible and enduring symbols of the post-1960s-1970s American sexual revolution. While the Britney Spears and Christina Aguileras come and go, Madonna has managed to reinvent herself in each of the past three decades and remains an icon of American sexual liberation. She embodies all of the issues that many people have been struggling with most of their lives. She is part caricature, part best friend, part you or me. Almost anyone who identifies with any of the vast changes in American sexual values of the past three decades can see something of himself or herself in Madonna.

Calvin Klein's Clothing Ads

Calvin Klein has been one of the most influential businesspersons in the United States, responsible for increased acceptance of homosexuality, bisexuality, and **androgyny.** Through his clothing and, more important, his advertising, Klein ushered in an acceptance of alternative sexual lifestyles without ever conducting a study, publishing research, or delivering a speech. Klein has pushed the limits of acceptability and taste to the maximum for 25 years.

Androgyny Exhibiting both male and female traits

Klein's clothing style almost single-handedly transformed the boundaries of acceptable standards of dress for men. Klein ushered in denim chic. His casual look helped men (and women) introduce the casual look into the social scene and the workplace. Today, we often see men in denim shirts or dress shirts and ties with jeans or a casual sport coat in the fanciest of locations—the ballet, opera, theater, and most restaurants and clubs. Klein-influenced attire is accepted in all but the most formal of workplaces. This represents a milestone in gender role expectations for men. More and more, men are realizing that being a man doesn't have to include strict adherence to a dress code of the past.

Klein's advertising, however, had even more of an impact on the fabric of sexuality than his clothing did. From the start, Klein's ads pushed the advertising industry to the limits. He exposed flesh—exposed naked backs, buttocks, and breasts. He posed his models suggestively, and flaunted the merchandising of products through sex. Even when he wasn't exposing flesh, he was emphasizing the allure of young, nubile bodies; the curve of a hip in skin-tight jeans, the slope of a neck from a denim shirt wide open at the collar, the span of a set of shoulders, or the bulge of a bicep. All of these images are Klein trademarks.

Another of Klein's impacts was with his models. He imprinted first homosexuality, then bisexuality, and most recently androgyny onto the American advertising and marketing scene. Klein's male models of the 1970s were hunks—well-built, with bulging arms and chiseled abdomens. His men of the 1970s turned on male and female viewers alike. His eroticism was always double-edged: It mimicked the sex role behavior of gay men and was a turn-on to heterosexual women. Gay men admired Klein's hunks with their tight buns, broad shoulders, and clean-shaven, healthy look. Straight women admired them for the same look.

Klein's more recent group shots left lingering questions about who was cavorting with whom in the ads. Were the men cavorting with the women, the other men, or both? Were the women wistfully admiring the men or the other women, or both? It was clear who the men were and who the women were. The object of their affection, however, was in doubt.

One of Klein's more recent advertising themes is of a sort of emaciated androgyny. The men and the women are cast in muted tones—blacks, blues, grays. Most of the models look thin and in need of some personal grooming. This has been referred to as a "heroin chic" look.

A 1995 Klein campaign raised the ire of media watchdog groups that claimed he crossed the line from bad taste into harmful promotion

sex in society 17.1

Reactions to the Lady Gaga

Students' reactions to Lady Gaga tend to be polarized. Love her or hate her, she is a current icon of a changing society.

"Lady Gaga—wow, is she hot." (male, age 22)

"Lady Gaga—I love her. She does what she wants, says what she wants. She's a real bitch, but cool." (female, age 21)

"She's hot, but I wouldn't screw her. She probably has AIDS." (male, age 22)

"I love her. She's definitely a '90s woman." (female, age 19)

"What a slut." (female, age 19)

"I wish I could be more like her. She's so confident and assertive. She knows what she wants and goes after it." (female, age 18)

"I think she's gross. She'd sleep with anybody." (female, age 29)

"I like her attitudes about sex. She's exploring all of the possibilities and apologizing for nothing. She's got guts." (female, age 35)

"She's my ultimate fantasy lady, but I don't think I'd want to marry her." (male, age 23)

of a life-threatening lifestyle and look. This advertising campaign used adolescent boys in various seductive poses amid backdrops reminiscent of someone's den. An anonymous voice in the background asked the boys, "Do you like to pose?" The campaign, critics claim, bordered on "kiddie porn" and smacked of pedophilia (Martin, 1995). Whatever one feels about Klein and his various campaigns over the past two decades, his images and ideas undoubtedly helped shape American perceptions about what is sexy and sensual.

❧ *Physical Wellness* ❧

Critics of media portrayals of what is sensual, beautiful, and sexual claim these set unrealistic standards of perfection and a physical ideal that is unattainable for most people. Proponents of sexy media themes and personalities view these positively.

The widespread interest in lifting weights, exercising, and eating healthfully comes in part from images of physical beauty personified by models and popular media personalities (such as Madonna), who promote these behaviors as contributing to their sexiness. You can scarcely pass a women's or men's magazine that doesn't portray the virtues of working out to sculpt a "sexy" body. In a sense, then, the fitness craze, which generally enhances physical wellness, is fueled by the same sexual climate that has also produced many negative sexual images.

Monkey Business

A presidential aspirant finishes our trilogy of symbols of an evolving American sexuality of the past 30 years. Gary Hart was a Democratic Party candidate for president of the United States in 1988. One of the front-runners in the campaign, he had a good chance to earn the Democrats' endorsement for president. All of that changed on the fateful morning of May 3, 1987, when the headline of the *Miami Herald* read, "Miami Woman Linked to Hart" (Bradlee, 1997).

Gary Hart—candidate for president, respectable congressman, businessman, husband, father, with all-American good looks and a charismatic personality—was caught by photographers with Donna Rice, his associate, sitting on his lap on the deck of the yacht *Monkey Business.* Reporters revealed that Rice had stayed overnight in Hart's Capitol Hill house.

This may not seem like a big deal today. As a culture, we seem to have been desensitized to such carryings-on. In 1988, however, it represented a tremendous change in the evolution of American sexual values and the way in which the media covered events and the lives of public figures. Prior to Hart's affair, the personal sex lives of political and other (such as sports) figures were off-limits. The media stayed away from reporting on sexual behavior, especially if this activity was out of public view. It was not allowed on air, in print, or as a subject of an interview.

Stories that we've read about in recent years, such as the Governor of New York's involvement with a prostitute, former President Clinton's affair with his intern, and numerous others involving powerful people never would have been aired in the past. We would not know about them. The unwritten rules of the game were that certain aspects of celebrities' lives were off-limits to the media and not available to the public.

That all changed with the Gary Hart case. Leaking of the story and the subsequent in-depth coverage, complete with front-page photos, broke new ground. The rules had changed. One newspaper's decision about allowing the story to be printed changed the way the U.S. media would report the news from then on. It also set the stage for how information of that nature would be handled in the future.

It also opened the floodgates for a new way of sexual information to be disseminated to the American public. Sexual behavior, drug use behavior, and the like, began to be carried over the airwaves into every small town, big city, and suburban living room. This was the beginning of the in-your-face talk shows, newsmagazine programs, and shock jocks that now are prominent on the American media landscape.

Madonna, Klein, and Hart broke new cultural ground by pushing sexual standards to the limit. They set the stage for allowable behavior and media coverage. What makes their emergence as sexual standard-bearers different from those that came before them is timing. The sweeping changes they created in entertainment, advertising, and media reporting came at a time when the United States was ushering in the first wave of massive technological changes.

Changes in the 1990s and 2000s: Two Illustrative Examples

Two events more than any that occurred during this period of American sexual history have defined sex for sale at the end of the 20th century and the beginning of the 21st century. Both involve money—specifically, the huge amounts of money to be made from subscription Internet services. The first was the use of one such service, *The Drudge Report,* to release speculation of the Bill Clinton–Monica Lewinsky affair. The second is the proliferation of Internet subscriber pornography sites. To understand both, we first need to understand the impact of technological innovations over the past 20 years.

The Impact of Technological Innovations

Stern and Handel (2002) propose that the one constant in the relationship between sexuality and the changing technological landscape is sexuality. Americans have been interested in exploring their sexuality since they landed on the shores of the new world.

Sexuality has historically been expressed through all forms of communication technology, from print (magazines, newspapers, books, and the like), to telegraph, telephone, radio, television, movies, non-Internet computer, and most recently the Internet (Stern & Handel, 2002). Americans' interest in sexuality hasn't changed; it has merely evolved and become more visible as new technologies have emerged and evolved. As Petersen (1999, p. 486) points out, "From Edison's kinetoscope, which had given us the nickel image of *The Kiss,* to today's seemingly unlimited Internet potential, Americans have increasingly made sex visible. The electric lights that had taken sex out of the shadows now provided not a sewer but a pulsing, sensuous, sane environment, a carnal consensus for the millennium."

The 1990s and early 2000s brought a new wave of information technology that included affordable cable television, videocassette and digital videodisc (DVD) players, personal computers (PCs), home videocassette recorders, and high-speed Internet access. These new technologies were different from all those that had preceded them.

The three qualities that set them apart from all the others were power, personal use, and low cost. Cable television brought the world into our living rooms. With hundreds of channels at our disposal we are literally flooded with visual information and data from around the world. For the first time in history, with the Gulf War in 1990, we were spectators in one of our wars as we watched it unfold on television on real time as it actually happened. There were no time delays, no papers to read, nothing to mull over. We simply sat back and watched our country wage war, without editing or tape delay as in Vietnam and previous conflicts.

In 1999, a national survey found that over a third of all 2- to 7-year-olds and over two-thirds of all 8- to 18-year-olds had a television in their own bedrooms. Many of those televisions were hooked up to cable TV services and videocassette recorders (Roberts, 2000). The number of people in the United States who subscribe to cable television has risen steadily over the past few years. In 2000, 70 percent of all homes in the United States had direct to home pay cable television service (U.S. Department of Labor, 2003). Sales of cable television services in the United States rose by 16 percent in 2001. Worldwide, close to 50 million homes had direct to home cable television service. Sales are projected to reach 80 million (U.S. Department of Labor, 2003). Home VCR costs have decreased markedly in the past decade. In 1996, more than 84 percent of all homes in the United States owned at least one VCR, and 39 percent owned two or more.

In addition to the power of the media, these technologies ushered in a new era of personal accessibility and efficiency in delivering sexual content. Cable television and personal computers have become as common as the telephone. Cable television made available pay-per-view movies, X-rated programming, and a host of other innovations that have the potential to bring sexual content along with other topics into our homes 24 hours a day.

The Flattening of the World

In *The World is Flat* (Friedman, 2007), Pulitzer Prize-winning author and *NY Times* foreign affairs columnist Thomas L. Friedman describes the ten key world events and technologies of the late 1990's that leveled the technological playing field of the world. A flat world, according to Friedman, is one where information, products, and services are available equally on a competitive basis to all countries and individuals. Once the world became flat it was inevitable that the creation, sales, and marketing of sexual goods and services would follow.

One of the key flatteners that set the stage for everything is what Friedman refers to the "new Age of Connectivity." Prior to the 1990, the emerging Internet and World-Wide-Web were a mish-mash of disparate technologies. The Internet was divided into various segments of "turf", each controlled by a type of computer (PC vs. Mac) or browser (Netscape vs. Windows 95, etc.). Sharing information, goods, and services was difficult because these different Internet **protocols** and **platforms** did not communicate with each other. To share files with someone in a different location you had to be sure that your computer and the other person's could "talk" to each other.

On top of this, connecting to the Internet meant using a dial-up telephone connection which was very slow and had limited **bandwidth.** Assuming you could connect with the person or organization you wanted to share information with, it was virtually impossible to share large files (especially pictures, photographs, movies, or charts) because of the incredible amount of time needed to upload and download the files.

All of this changed when the New Age of Connectivity was ushered in. Government regulating agencies, corporations, and individuals, realizing the incredible potential of the Internet and World Wide Web, converged to bring down the walls and regulations that separated the technologies. One of the key factors responsible for ushering in this new age was the

Protocols standardized computer language and systems for developing computer platforms

Platforms computer operating systems that determine how computers operate and interpret and communicate information

Bandwidth a measure of the amount of information a fiber-optic cable can transmit

Telecommunications Act of 1996. This bill launched the fiber-optic boom of the 1990s. Prior to this act, most connections to the Internet involved copper telephone wires and dial-up modems. This ensuing connection was inefficient, slow, and subject to security breaches because it was easy to tap into. Fiber-optic cable, on the other hand, was lightening–fast, reliable, and secure. The Telecommunications Act of 1996 allowed long-distance and local telecommunications companies to get into any business they chose. Realizing that laying fiber-optic cable would allow them to move information, goods and services cheaply, and to compete on a world-level, telecommunications companies around the world dumped billions of dollars into laying fiber-optic cable across the globe. These two occurrences, standardizing protocols and platforms and wiring the world for the coming digital revolution set the stage for the next flattener, switching to digital signals.

Digitization is the process of converting words, music, pictures and raw data into combinations of 1s and 0s

Digitization is the process of converting words, music, pictures and raw data into combinations of 1s and 0s. Digitizing words, music, pictures, and raw data allows large files to be uploaded and downloaded by individuals, companies, and governments using a variety of computers and servers. In other words, using a Windows XP-enabled PC from home, individuals could upload and download massive amounts of information previously unavailable to them. Individuals from around the globe could compete with each other, small businesses could compete with large businesses, and emerging countries could compete with first-world industrialized giants. In order to start up a small, Internet–based business, all one needed was a computer, fiber-optic connection, and a small amount of start-up capital. The "dot com" bubble (and subsequent bursting) of the late 1990s and early 2000s refers to this proliferation of small, Internet-based businesses that sprang up under these conditions.

Companies like E-Bay changed the way Americans and the world did business. No longer did you need a store, a showroom, or a warehouse to move goods and services. Everything could be handled online. Once again, sex-based information, goods, and services were quick to take advantage of the new technology.

Armed with a lightning-fast, high-speed Internet connection the power of the home computer grew and continues to grow. The personal computer took the nation by storm in the early 1990s, and introduction of the Internet offered Americans the opportunity to connect instantly with millions of users worldwide. The personal computer industry has grown more than 400 percent since 1990. In 1996, 40 percent of U.S. homes had at least one personal computer (Lagnado, 1996). In 1999, more than half of all U.S. households had at least one personal computer, and more than 56 percent of all households were online (Brown, 2002). By 2003, 79 percent, or roughly 83 million American households, owned at least one personal computer (Seitz, 2003).

The sweeping acceptance of these technologies and their sheer power and ability to move volumes of information and images into U.S. homes opened the floodgate to another wave of sexual communication. Stern and Handel (2002) consider this new state of technological evolution provided by high-speed Internet connectivity as very efficacious in delivering sexuality-related information, entertainment, and services.

One positive aspect of this second wave is its ability to provide accurate, nonbiased information on sexuality (Edwards, 1996). As Fisher and Barak (2002) point out, Internet-based sexuality education programs can offer significant resources and expert instruction, and they can reach massive audiences in a very cost-effective manner. The Internet also opens up many exciting venues for conducting sex research. Mustanski (2002) explains that the anonymity and accessibility of the Internet, along with access to very large sample sizes, make sexual survey research very attractive.

On the down side, the Internet is so large and powerful that it is almost impossible to police. It brings graphic, sadomasochistic, live video clips into the living room. It connects 45-year-old pedophiles with potential victims through **chat rooms.** Couple this technology with a much more permissive culture, and you have an entirely different sexual landscape today than at any time in U.S. history. It is a no-holds-barred culture in which almost anything goes—and much of it goes into our living rooms, bedrooms, and offices via these new technologies. Although all of these things existed before 1990, now the low cost has allowed Americans to be exposed to almost any sexual idea, theme, or image in the privacy of the home. Nearly anything goes—especially if it sells. Our two examples give contrasting views of this new climate.

Chat rooms Live e-mail discussion lines in which a person can communicate with others by typing messages

The Drudge Report

One key element of a flatter world was the new-found ability of individuals to upload information quickly and easily and make it available to others across the globe in a split-second. No longer did would-be journalists, political commentators, or the average person next-door have to be without a voice. Prior to the flattening of the world, if someone wanted to express a political opinion they had to write a "Letter to the Editor" of their local or other newspaper and hope that it would get published a week later. If that was to slow they could take to the streets with signs and hope for a 15-second sound bite on television.

The flattering of the world changed all of this forever. Now, all you needed to have your message heard was a personal computer and a broadband Internet connection. This created a entirely new phenomenon, blogging. With a blog, anyone could create a forum for sharing their ideas. None of the material needed to be pre-screened, approved, or unfortunately, checked for accuracy. With blogging a person could upload a column, picture, or video clip, and have it available to anyone *across the world* instantly. This changes the rules for political (and sexual) discourse completely and permanently. With no censorship and an instant world-stage, bloggers seized a large chunk of the political and sexual landscape previously unavailable to the average person.

One such blogger, 30-year-old computer geek Matt Drudge, burst onto the American scene on January 18, 1998, when he published a story in his online gossip column, *The Drudge Report,* about the then-alleged affair between President Bill Clinton and Monica Lewinsky. What makes this case unique isn't the details of the affair. As we know, for decades, presidents have been having affairs and using their power, influence, and office to attract women. What is unique about this particular affair is that it was released to the world through an entirely new medium: a subscriber-based online news outlet, *The Drudge Report.*

In 1995, Drudge, a man with a dream of becoming the first nationally recognized online gossip columnist, started his business from scratch. Working from his apartment, his newsletter (www.drudgereport.com) grew to include an estimated 85,000 paid subscribers. Drudge was signed by America On-Line (AOL), at the time one of the nation's largest Internet service providers, to publish the newsletter for it. Drudge gained notoriety for many cases, particularly one where he made allegations that a well-known White House aide, Sidney Blumenthal, was a wife beater.

Critics of Drudge cite his admitted "80 percent" accuracy rate as sub-standard for mainstream news reporting. Most mainstream media outlets will not publish a story with a 20 percent margin for error. Furthermore, they claim that anyone with a penchant for gossip, a computer, and a Web site can post such "news" on the Internet. The Internet, with the potential to reach billions of subscribers worldwide in an instant, is a relatively unsupervised medium. Anyone can create a Web site and post news, without peer review or supervision. Proponents of online news outlets claim that mainstream media outlets are too conservative, sit on stories too long, and protect political and other figures.

⁍ *Emotional Wellness* ⁌

Not only is sexual information available in unprecedented amounts, but sexual counseling, therapy, and self-help also are within the average person's reach. As sex comes into the open, so does sexual healing. Online chat rooms, self-help groups, and other computerized services offer increasing opportunities for dealing with sexual concerns and problems.

Web sites are available catering to all people and interests. Gay people who need help to come out of the closet can find help and link up with others around the country or around the corner. Transgendered people no longer have to feel alone. They have their own Web sites and referral networks a mere mouse-click away. Although electronic resources will never take the place of a live helping relationship, the technological innovations and resources available to average individuals can greatly improve their emotional wellness by providing easy access to information and services that were not available a decade ago.

In the Clinton-Lewinsky case, Drudge's claim that the media was sitting on the story (he found out about the affair through unnamed reports of supposed tapes Linda Tripp had made of telephone conversations with Monica Lewinsky) proved true. It was only after the public furor created by Drudge's report that the mainstream news media released the story. Drudge's popularity worldwide soared following the release of the story. Subscriptions to his newsletter soared, and his new-found notoriety included his reporting being picked by Agence France Presse (the world's oldest news wire service) as one of the century's top 10 media events.

Subscriber Internet Services

One of the most fascinating outgrowths of the new technologies regarding sexuality is the burgeoning development of subscriber Internet services. Subscriber Internet services are similar to cable television premium channels and pay-per-view services.

With cable television, subscribers can pay for a menu of related channels (a group of movie channels, for instance) or an individual channel (Home Box Office (HBO) is a good example). In addition, subscribers can pay for a single event (pay-per-view) available to all subscribers to the service, or just to subscribers of a specific channel (who can buy a boxing match, auto race, specific movie, and so forth).

Adult-oriented Internet sites are following the same model. Most of these sites allow "visitors" to enter their sites and sample their wares. In most cases, the sites provide enough tantalizing X-rated samples of pages included in the overall site to give the visitor a sense of what lies within the entire site. If the person likes the site, he or she can "subscribe" for a monthly fee. Fees range from a few dollars a month to over $50 for some of the more exotic sites.

For the price of a subscription, most sites provide members with the following features: X-rated still photos, short video clips, full-length video films, chat rooms (to chat with the site sponsor and/or other members), dating services, merchandise (sex aids, books, magazines, videos, and more), and links, to name the most common. In most cases, the site sponsor usually is featured in the photos, videos, and chat. Sites are sponsored by porn stars, swinging couples, exotic dancers and strippers, and a host of "amateurs" (self-proclaimed "boy and girl next door" types). All sites are blocked to nonmembers and those under the age of consent (varies from 18 to 21 years old).

Membership sales to subscriber adult Internet sites have become the next frontier in sex for sale in the United States and the world. Danni Ashe, a former stripper and a pioneer in this medium, hosts one of the most widely subscribed sites on the Web. Ashe started Danni's Hard Drive in 1995 from her bedroom as a hobby. It has grown into a medium-sized corporation with 42 employees, a 15,000-squarefoot office/studio, and over 4.5 million users per month. In 2001, Danni's Hard Drive was expected to make between $7 and $8 million in profit (Lewis, 2001). In 2009, Danni's Hard Drive receives 7–10 *million* hits per/day (Danni.cash, 2009).

Danni's Hard Drive is by no means a fluke. Rather, it is a harbinger for how sex will be sold in the future. Subscriber Internet sex sites are among the most profitable forms of business being conducted either on or off the Web. What makes them unique is that they do not rely on advertising. Instead of being driven by selling advertisements and the needs and wants of advertisers, subscriber sites turn enough profits to be self-sustaining.

Indeed, most premier subscriber sex sites have profit margins of more than 20 percent (which is unheard of in most sales-related businesses). Start-up costs are generally low, and most subscriber sex sites turn profitable after just 6 months. In comparison, Amazon.com, probably the most well-known retail site on the Web, was still nowhere near profitable 4 *years* after it started (Lewis, 2001).

More than 200,000 sexually explicit Internet sites were available in 2001, and experts estimated that 40 percent of adult Internet users spent at least 90 minutes per week online viewing porn. According to Greg Clayman, the president of Video-secrets.com, a company that provides streaming video to Danni's Hard Drive and other large-scale Internet subscriber sites, it seems that people use the Internet to do three primary things: check e-mail, check investments, and check pornography (Lewis, 2001). Of the $2 billion paid for online content in the United States last year, $1.4 billion was for pornography.

Internet subscriber sex sites have survived the crash of the dot.com economy, a severely depressed stock market, a weak economy, and war in the Middle East, to thrive when other e-businesses are shutting down. Many business analysts find such success a mystery, but when you view it as part of the evolving sex-for-sale phenomenon that has been with us since the dawn of recorded history, it makes perfect sense. Consumers of these products can shop at home. They can preview what they might be interested in buying, and purchase it online without leaving their house. They can view, interact with, and download sexually explicit material in the privacy of their own homes where the average buyer feels most comfortable. A flat world makes the uploading and downloading of sexually explicit materials inexpensive and easy to do.

Although both Internet subscriber sex sites and *The Drudge Report* illustrate the most recent evolution of sex for sale adapting to technological innovation, we fully expect that by the time we go to press, yet another technological breakthrough will have emerged, with those who sell sex following closely on its heels.

❧ *Social Wellness* ❧

Many argue that the current sexual climate in the United States impacts negatively on our social wellness as individuals and as a culture. Everything from child-rearing to productivity in the workplace, they say, becomes harder as parents, employers, and government have to compete against the lure and distraction of sexual availability. It is more difficult, they argue, to uphold standards of decency and social relationships in the face of a no-holds-barred societal attitude toward sex. Others disagree. They argue that greater sexual freedom and availability of sexual information and services empowers people and fosters understanding of their sexuality. Social wellness, they say, is thereby enhanced because sexuality, a natural part of life, is allowed its full expression. This allows people to understand their sexuality better and develop higher levels of social wellness.

Pornography, Erotica, and Obscenity

One of the major concerns about the increasing availability of sexual information and images in the media and over the Internet is the easy access to pornography, erotica, and obscene materials. In past decades, restricting access to this material was much easier than it is today. Back then, keeping material away from minors and adults who did not desire that type of exposure was simple. Today it is much more difficult. The debate concerning what is pornographic, erotic, or obscene has reopened and intensified. Although *pornography, erotica,* and *obscenity* have been used interchangeably, these terms mean entirely different things.

Pornography

Derived from the Latin roots *porne* (prostitute) and *graphos* (depicting), the literal translation of **pornography** is a depiction in writing or pictures of prostitutes or prostitution.

Pornography A depiction of lewd material or erotic behavior designed to cause sexual arousal

It refers more commonly to any depiction of lewd material or erotic behavior designed to cause sexual arousal. In U.S. culture, the connotation of pornography and pornographic materials is usually negative, even though most people admit they get sexually excited while viewing it.

Erotica

Derived from the Greek word *erotikos* (love poem), **erotic** means devoted to or tending to arouse sexual love or desire. Erotic materials depict beauty, love, sensuousness, voluptuousness, and the like. In U.S. culture (and most others around the world), the depiction of erotica and erotic materials tends to be positive. This judgment is subjective, however. Some people do not distinguish pornography from erotica, and lump them together.

Erotic Devoted to arousing sexual love or desire

In real life, separating some pornographic materials from erotica is difficult. Often, the context of the material helps to define it. For instance, one could view two films, an X-rated porn film and a sex ed video. Each film portrays a heterosexual couple having sex. Both films have graphic displays of nudity, masturbation, oral sex, and intercourse in various positions. What is the difference? Are the films pornographic or erotic?

The porno film makes little mention of love or expressions of caring. The relationship between the partners may be unknown or casual. The sexual acts may be forced or seemingly initiated by one partner for his or her own gratification. The genitalia are overemphasized, with close-ups of the coupled genitalia. Most porn films end with a mandatory, degrading ejaculation in the face of the female.

The sex education video emphasizes communication. The couple talks to each other. They ask what each one desires, whether something feels good, and the like. They take their time. Their intent is mutual pleasuring. They equally participate and initiate. The narration describes what is happening. The partners proceed through the various acts and show their appreciation, caring, and kindness. These videos do not include genital close-ups and orgasm. They do not show "in-your-face" ejaculation.

One could almost use a continuum to evaluate sexually explicit materials. Pornographic materials would represent one extreme and instructional sex education materials would be at the other end, with erotica in the middle. To complicate matters, one must also consider whether the material is obscene.

Obscenity

Obscenity Material that is abhorrent to moral virtue and accepted norms of social behavior

Obscenity is derived from the Latin word *obscenus,* which means dirty, filthy, and disgusting. Obscene materials repel the senses and are abhorrent to morality, virtue, and accepted norms of societal behavior. In 1966, the U.S. Supreme Court defined obscene materials as meeting three criteria:

- The dominant theme had to appeal to a purely erotic interest in sex.
- The material had to be offensive to contemporary community standards.
- The material had to be without serious literary, artistic, political, or scientific value.

This definition posed serious difficulties in interpretation, and numerous challenges have been brought to bear. In 1973, the Supreme Court reversed its ruling using the three original criteria. In *Miller v. California,* the Court decided that only one criterion was necessary to define obscenity: local community standards. Each community had to decide for itself whether specific materials were offensive by its standards. The producers, actors, distributors, and sellers of materials that a community defines as obscene are all subject to prosecution even if the materials were produced in another community. This criterion is still in effect today. It is troubling because it gives a vocal minority in a community the ability to declare anything from skimpy bathing suits to Michelangelo's *Venus de Milo* obscene.

In general, materials described as erotic are not perceived as obscene and usually are not the target of prosecution. Obscene materials, in contrast, are considered to be subcategories of pornography. The overwhelming majority of Americans believe that adults should have access to sexually explicit material, both erotic and pornographic, depicting sexual activity between consenting adults (Diamond & Dannemiller, 1989).

Support for obscene materials is much less. These materials usually depict themes other than sexual activity between consenting adults. Materials that involve children, rape, sadomasochism, and similar themes are more often those that fail to meet community standards.

Prostitution

Prostitution The exchange of sexual services for money

Prostitution has been around since the dawn of civilization. The earliest written accounts are in the Bible. Jesus himself took time to protect a prostitute from a stone-throwing crowd who would persecute her. Prostitution is illegal in the United States except in Nevada, where it is regulated and limited to certain counties.

In Nevada and other places where prostitution is legal, prostitutes are called *sex workers,* and they are employed in the sex worker industry. Prostitution is legal in many European, Asian, African, and South American countries, where it is considered a victimless crime.

Small numbers of prostitutes in the United States have organized in an attempt to try to legalize it in all 50 states. Legalization, they believe, will help protect prostitutes, ensure better working conditions, extend benefits such as disability and Social Security, and help them reduce their risk for contract-

sex in society 17.2

Ain't Nobody's Business If We Do

Peter McWilliams's book *Ain't Nobody's Business If We Do* is based on a single idea: You should be allowed to do whatever you want with your own person and property, as long as you don't physically harm the person or property of a non-consenting other.

Simple. Seemingly guaranteed to us by that remarkable document known as the United States Constitution and its even more remarkable Bill of Rights. And yet, it's not the way things are.

Roughly half of the arrests and court cases in the United States each year involve consensual crimes— actions that are against the law but directly harm no one's person or property except, possibly, the "criminal's."

More than 750,000 people are in jail right now because of something they did, something that did not physically harm the person or property of another. In addition, more than 3 million people are on parole or probation for consensual crimes. Furthermore, more than 4 million people are arrested each year for doing something that hurts no one but, potentially, themselves.

The injustice doesn't end there, of course. Throwing people in jail is the extreme. If you can throw people in jail for something, you can fire them for the same reason. You can evict them from their apartments. You can deny them credit. You can expel them from schools. You can strip away their civil rights, confiscate their property, and destroy their lives—just because they're different.

At what point does behavior become so unacceptable that we should tell our government to lock people up? The answer, as explored in this book: We lock people up only when they physically harm the person or property of a non-consenting other.

Go to McWilliams's Web site for the book: www.mcwilliams.com to read more about his ideas regarding our sexual (and other) personal freedoms and how they are threatened.

How do you feel about laws that target consensual behavior that harms no one? What are you willing to do to protect these freedoms?

ing a variety of sexually transmitted diseases, including HIV (Shrage, 1996; Prostitutes' Education Network, 2003). It also will free police to spend more time on other forms of crime, relieve the courts of a tremendous burden, and allow women to use their bodies the way they want to.

Although people tend to assume that all prostitutes are women, men and women alike engage in exchanging sex for money, food, shelter, drugs, or other resources. They can be subcategorized. Prostitutes who literally solicit clients off the streets are called *hookers* (females) and *hustlers* (males), although the labels could apply to either gender. These prostitutes also are known as *streetwalkers*. They generally are at the lower end of the social order of prostitutes.

Street hustlers and hookers are frequently addicted to drugs, are runaways, or have other economic or personal problems that force them into the often violent world of streetwalking.

Street prostitutes solicit customers who walk or drive by them. Streetwalkers usually negotiate with their clients and then have sex with them either in their car or at a local hotel or motel where short-stay rooms are available at reasonable rates. Some hustlers and hookers solicit clients in truck stop parking areas and have sex with their clients in their rigs.

In urban areas, many street hookers and hustlers are runaways— adolescents who have run away from home or have been forced out by their

case study 17.2

Edgar: Paying for Sex

Edgar, 43, married, identifies as Hispanic.

Married for 20 years, Edgar has two children, ages 13 and 16. He is a middle manager in an insurance company. He describes his relationship with his wife as intimate and committed but feels the passion in their relationship died several years ago. Although they have sex about once a week or every other week, it isn't very exciting and he wants more. He frequents massage parlors about twice a month, paying for a massage that includes masturbation and usually fellatio.

I guess you could say that sex for me has never been all that exciting. Except for the prostitutes I used to pay for when I was in Vietnam, I was sexually inexperienced. I didn't have sex until I enlisted in the army at 18 and went to Vietnam. When I returned, I got a job in an insurance company and went to college at night.

I met my wife at the insurance company during the first month I worked there, and we got married about a year after that. The first year or so, things were OK. My wife wasn't very interested in sex, and we probably had intercourse about once a week that first year. She's pretty conservative and isn't into oral sex or anything kinky. I really didn't know what to expect of married life. My dad never really talked about sex with me, and I was too embarrassed to talk to my friends about it in much detail. My first son was born after a year, and things slowed down a little more with my wife.

I was in New York for a training program for my current job. I guess it was about 10 years ago. I remember walking around Times Square and going into the bookstores and bars. I passed a massage parlor, and the guy out front was passing out coupons for a special deal. I said, "What the heck," and went in. I had been curious about these massage parlors and was feeling horny. No one there knew me, so I took a chance. I picked out my masseuse and went into our little room.

After undressing, she started to rub my back, and before long her touches became a lot more intimate. She asked if I wanted her to jerk me off, and I said yes. I had to pay her a little more but it was worth it. The next night I went into a different place and found out I could get a blow job for about $20. The masseuse there was unattractive, but, boy, could she give head. It reminded me of my experiences in Vietnam.

When I returned home to Virginia from my training program, I began to seek out massage parlors in Richmond and other places within a reasonable drive from my home. I've been doing this at least once a month more than 10 years. My wife doesn't know, and the cost isn't too much. I'm basically happily married and love my kids. I wish I had more sex with my wife and she was into oral sex, but I don't think she'll change. She won't even talk about seeing a sex therapist, so I keep doing what I'm doing. I don't have a problem with it, and it probably keeps my marriage going.

sex in society 17.3

The HIV Highway

They call it the HIV highway. In reality, it is a transcontinental highway linking the several sub-Saharan African countries. It is more like a dirt road than a highway. It is a symbol of the old Africa, where time has stood still and traditions live on. The HIV highway got its name because of health officials' belief that it has been a main conduit of infection with the deadly virus. The highway has countless roadside stops where prostitutes ply their trade.

This is the same trade they have pursued throughout the history of the road. The main difference is that now most of them are infected with HIV. These factors make sex along the trans-Africa highway a deadly behavior:

- Condom use by the truck drivers and the prostitutes is practically nonexistent.
- Anal intercourse is common.

- The coexistence of genital ulcer disease (STDs that cause genital ulcers such as chancroid and syphilis) is common in the women and their customers.
- A final tragic note is the reluctance of these men to use condoms with their wives once they have been notified of their HIV seropositivity. Many of them perceive condom use as both unmanly and a sure sign of promiscuity.

The governments of sub-Saharan nations have instituted a massive STD/HIV prevention program to try to combat the problem. They have literally set up prevention service on the road. They have worked with the prostitutes to try to have them organize and institute greater compliance with use of condoms. They have used educational strategies ranging from one-to-one counseling to massive governmental media campaigns.

parents or caregivers. Many have run away from abusive home environments and are willing to risk the dangers of the streets over the sure harm of the environments from which they escaped. Many of the gay youth hooking and hustling on the streets ran away from persecution for their sexual orientation.

Streetwalking has many unwritten rules, which concern respecting other prostitutes' work areas (also known as "turf"), outwitting undercover police officers, avoiding sadists and murderers, and trying to avoid STDs/HIV. Because of these "rules," streetwalkers often work for pimps (a type of business agent) who help control some of these problems in exchange for a share of the profits.

Street pimps vary in their approach to working with hookers and hustlers. Some provide valuable protection and care for their workers to some extent. Others are thinly disguised sadists and criminals who dominate their hookers and hustlers through drugs, violence, and fear. In the netherworld of streetwalking, violence and death are never far away.

Brothels

Prior to 1920, large **brothels** could be found in every major American city. Many were elegant facilities where customers (overwhelmingly male) could have a drink, eat dinner, play cards, socialize with peers and the prostitutes, and have sex.

Typically, brothels were set up like hotels, with socializing downstairs and sex negotiated in upstairs rooms. Repeat business was the norm, and clients were generally recruited by word of mouth (Petersen, 1999). As a

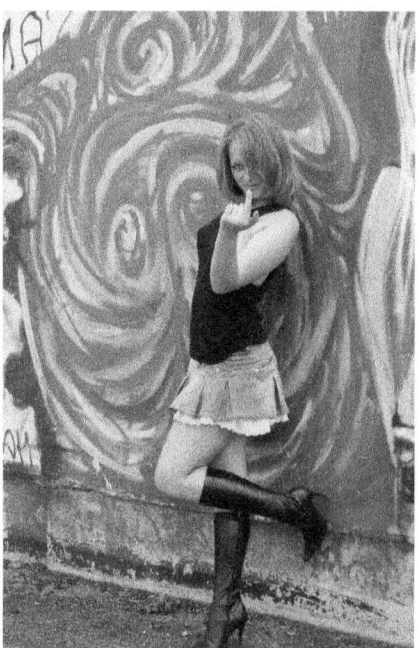

Prostitution is one of the world's oldest professions.

Brothel A house of prostitution

result of legislation and the sweeping moral reform of the early 1920s, most brothels were closed, driving prostitution into the streets or the massage parlors. Brothels still exist in Nevada and, on a much smaller scale, most major metropolitan areas.

Massage Parlors

Prostitutes who work in massage parlors are referred to as *hookers* and *hustlers* but also may be known as *masseuses*. Most massage parlors are fronts for houses of prostitution, where, in addition to a massage, clients are able to receive masturbation, oral sex, and sometimes sexual intercourse.

Most clients of massage parlors walk in off the street and pay cash for a massage and either masturbation or oral sex. Their visit usually lasts 30 minutes and costs anywhere from $20 to $50. Massage parlors usually have procedures that help screen for potential undercover police activities. For example, they require that customers sign a form indicating that they are not police officers. Clients pay for the massage in advance, with no mention of sexual "extras" until the later stages of the massage. The overwhelming majority of prostitutes working in massage parlors are female.

Escort Services

In theory, escort services involve the legal practice of "escorting" a client to dinner, a show, a political affair, and the like, for a fee. In reality, most escort services derive their primary business through "out-call" male and female prostitution.

Escort services advertise in telephone books, newspapers, and magazines. Many clients are referred by other satisfied customers. Customers call and are matched with the type of "escort" they desire. Escorts come to the client's residence or hotel and negotiate sexual activity (O'Kane, 1994).

Prostitutes who work for escort services are referred to as *call girls* or *call boys,* as well as escorts. Escort services may be run by a pimp or madam who works the phones and arranges the meetings. Some escort services are run by groups of prostitutes who schedule appointments based on availability and referral. Many call girls and call boys work independently after they establish their own client base.

In general, call girls and call boys are at the top of the status hierarchy of prostitutes. They typically charge from $50 to $200 an hour or between $500 and $1,000 a night. Call girls and call boys work through telephone calls, personal meetings, and referrals. Because they are not on the street, they are not subject to the control and fees associated with pimps. If call persons are not in business for themselves, they have a madam or pimp scheduling for them.

Periodically, high-priced call girls are arrested, and their high-profile clients make the headlines. Ashley Dupre is an example. In 2008, her well-publicized affair with then NY Governor Elliot Spitzer was on the front page of every newspaper in America. She told the story of an enterprising entrepreneur who earned a living catering to the sexual needs of the rich and famous. Her clientele included famous actors (and actresses), politicians, judges, businesspersons, and assorted celebrities as well as the governor.

Exotic Dancers, Strippers, and Live Sex Performers

Bars and clubs dedicated to providing adult entertainment from dancers have proliferated in the 1990s. These may be bars (which have licenses to sell and offer alcoholic beverages and are open to the general public) or "gentlemen's clubs" (which do not have licenses to sell liquor and are open to members only). The activities of establishments licensed to sell liquor are regulated by agencies such as the Bureau of Alcohol, Tobacco and Firearms (AFT). These establishments usually are under a stricter code than clubs, which usually are regulated by local ordinances. Because of this, clubs usually tend to offer more risqué forms of entertainment ranging from totally nude dancing to lap and couch dancing.

About 2,500 gentlemen's clubs have been established around the United States. The industry has gotten so large that it has its own trade publication, *Stripper* magazine. The revenues generated from these clubs are staggering: from $500,000 a year for the average club to more than $5 million for a well-run club. Once called *go-go dancers,* the entertainment provided by strippers and exotic dancers has changed in the 1990s. Go-go dancers and strippers of the past usually performed on a stage, or literally in a cage, separated from their customers. Appreciative customers sometimes threw money onto the stage or offered to buy the dancer a drink and offer a tip.

In the 1990s, dancers have come off the stage and cages and onto the bars, tabletops, couches, and laps of customers in these clubs. Nowadays, exotic dancers typically dance along the bar, discarding items of clothing as they stop to tease customers, who are allowed to slip their tips (usually folded dollar bills) into the dancer's top or G-string (a skimpy thong covering her pubic area). Dancers (at least those desiring larger tips) usually allow customers to feel their breasts, buttocks, and vulva fleetingly while passing along their tips.

Most dancers earn between $10 and $20 an hour and rely heavily on tips to make up the bulk of their earnings. Many of the larger gentlemen's clubs employ big-name, hard-core film actresses as feature performers. The nation's top five or six porn actresses can earn $15,000 to $20,000 per week (four shows a night) to dance at the larger clubs. The next half-dozen famous actresses earn about $8,000 to $15,000 to dance in these clubs. Club owners use film credits and magazine spreads to market their performers (Schlosser, 1997).

Many states have laws regulating a dancer's attire and may require her to wear pantyhose and keep her top on or at least hold it up against her breasts. Customers are not allowed to fondle the dancers, with the exception of inserting dollar bills into their G-strings or tops. Any sexual exchange between dancer and customer is not allowed, as this behavior constitutes prostitution, and bars usually hire bouncers to ensure that neither customers nor dancers violate this rule. Exotic dancers in clubs often leave the bar to dance one-on-one with customers.

Lap dancers usually straddle a customer and dance suggestively against his crotch. Couch dancers usually take a customer to a private couch, where they kneel on top of him or over him and dance suggestively

case study 17.3

Kim: Working Her Way Through College as an Exotic Dancer

Kim, 23, single, lesbian, identifies as Korean American.

Last year my lover Danielle convinced me to apply for a job as an exotic dancer at a local men's club.

She had been doing it for a few months, and the money was great. She said that with my exotic Asian looks I'd make a fortune in tips if I was willing to act a little. I didn't want to do it, but Danielle said she'd be there a lot to make sure nobody hassled me when I danced. Besides, she said, if I got the job, they occasionally had two girls dance at the same time, and we could try this if I wanted to.

I got the job, and the money really was good, and the bouncers kind of adopted me because they knew I was Danielle's lover. I was a nervous wreck the first night I had to dance. The first set was a near-disaster. I didn't want to make eye contact with the customers because I thought they'd know I wasn't straight, and I was worried that they'd really be obnoxious. I didn't dance too well, either. I think I earned about $7 in tips, mostly out of sympathy.

The next night was better. I had a couple of drinks before going on, and Danielle was there, so I danced for her. She told me to relax and fantasize that she was the only person in the bar. It started to be a real a turn-on, and I relaxed and really got into the music. The guys in the bar went crazy and were all holding dollar bills to stick into my G-string. That was a real turn-off, but the manager and the bouncers made sure that things didn't get out of hand. They told me to smile, and if I let the guys touch my breasts and butt, I'd get more tips. I took their advice and brought home close to $300 that first night. I average about $150 in tips on a typical night.

I don't really like it when the customers proposition me, but it comes with the territory. I'd say about 30 percent of the guys hit on me, but I've learned how to cope with it by smiling, telling them I like guys but love women, and move on. Most of them can deal with that, and it probably feeds their fantasies when they go home and jerk off or have sex with their wives.

Danielle and I have talked about opening a bar of our own when we graduate this year. We want to do something upscale that caters to women's fantasies and dance in the club together as well as manage the place. There is a ton of money to be made in this line of work.

Critical Thinking

Dancers and club operators would describe what they do as providing erotic entertainment and not engaging in sexual activities with customers. How would you characterize Kim's behavior at work?

---

in a more private ambiance. The objective of lap dancing and couch dancing in many instances is to offer the customer the opportunity literally to be masturbated to the point of orgasm by the dancer's motions without her ever using her hand. Such dancing usually requires an extra fee ($20 and up) and is timed (if the customer hasn't "come" or wants more stimulation, he has to buy more time).

Live sex shows usually take place in a theater environment but often occur in a bar or club. One or more couples literally have sex on stage, on the floor, or on the bar while the customers watch, often masturbating as they become aroused.

Although dancing and live sex shows are not the same as prostitution, the performers often are prostitutes and are willing to arrange sex for pay sessions with customers at a later time. Live sex shows now are available on the Internet. A customer can sign on in Iowa and be a member of the audience in a live sex show in Amsterdam.

❧ Environmental/Occupational Wellness ❧

Some communities have organized to restrict sex industry outlets to nonresidential sectors rather than eliminate X-rated bookstores, bars, and other establishments. Other communities have banned them outright. The issue of community boundaries regarding the sex industry directly affects sex workers themselves.

Sex workers are employed in a variety of work sites. Some, such as X-rated movie houses, bookstores, massage parlors, and escort services, are legal and protected under law. Others, such as prostitution and nude dancing, are illegal in most states. Sex workers, particularly those working illegally, are at increased risk for a variety of problems ranging from disease to unfair labor practices. Many sex workers are calling for unionization as a way to increase work-site-based protections. In the majority of non-sex-based business, participating in sexually oriented activities (Internet use, telephone sex, and the like), even on lunch or break time, is grounds for dismissal. Many corporations and other workplaces routinely screen workers' computer and telephone records to monitor such activities.

Tech Sex

Whereas prostitution entails sexual contact with a live person, tech sex—sexual activity that connects with some form of technology—is masturbatory sex. It is designed to excite and arouse, leading to release of tension through masturbation.

The same technological innovations that make sexual information available have opened new World-Wide outlets for purveyors of impersonal sex for sale. These include sex talk lines, interactive cable TV sex, interactive computer sex, and computer sex chat rooms. These differ from ordinary pornography and erotica because the customer connects to a live human being via the phone, television, or computer. It is the ultimate sex of the 1990s–2000s technological revolution. Just ponder these statistics:

Every second—$3,075.64 is being spent on pornography

Every second—28,258 Internet users are viewing pornography

Every second—372 Internet users are typing adult search terms into search engines (Family Safe Media, 2009).

Tech sex is a very lucrative international business. The pornography industry is larger than the revenues of the following companies combined: Microsoft, Google, Amazon, eBay, Yahoo!, Apple, Netflix and EarthLink. In 2008 world-wide pornography revenues topped 97 *billion* dollars. The top earners were; China (over $ 27 billion), South Korea (over $25 billion), Japan (over $19 billion) and the United States (over $13 billion) (Family Safe Media, 2009).

Telephone Sex

Every night, between the hours of 9:00 P.M. and 1:00 A.M., approximately 250,000 people in the United States dial a commercial phone sex number. The average call lasts 6 to 8 minutes and costs anywhere from $0.89 to $4 a minute. In 1996, Americans spent between $750 million and $1 billion on telephone sex (Schlosser, 1997).

A customer buys telephone sex by dialing a 900 number. A new scam uses a free 800 number to mask a 900 pay-per-call service. When the 800 number is called, the caller is identified through caller ID, and the 900 pay-per-call provider bills the incoming number for the call ("Call for a Crackdown," 1994).

In 1991, the Federal Communications Commission (FCC) restricted the type of calls that could be made using 900 numbers. It banned all domestic calls it considered "obscene communications for commercial purposes." Because the ban does not extend to overseas calls, however, this loophole has created a burgeoning foreign market for telephone sex. Phone sex calls are routed to out-of-the-way places such as Aruba, the Mariana Islands, Guyana, and the Dominican Republic, where operators are standing by to take your call and cater to your every whim (Schlosser, 1997).

In 1993, telephone companies earned nearly $900 million from international services. An estimated 90 percent of those revenues came from phone-sex lines. These foreign revenues are shared among the domestic American company, its foreign phone company, and telephone sex providers. Some small countries have started their own telephone companies to get a bigger chunk of the market (*Economist,* 1994; "Adult Video," 1995).

Once customers' connections are established, they are billed per minute to their telephone bill. A person can engage in heterosexual talk, homosexual talk, bisexual talk, or group talk. It is anonymous, graphic, expensive—and an illusion. Phone sex practitioners are trained to keep customers talking, to cater to their every fantasy. Because it is impersonal and anonymous, they are tempted to say things that normally are taboo.

The typical telephone sex customer is a "lonely heart" seeking conversation. Often, the sexual content of the call is of secondary importance. Anyone, however, is capable of becoming hooked on phone sex. Most telephone "actresses"— as they are referred to—are housewives, accountants, secretaries, bank tellers, senior citizens, and various other women seeking to earn a little extra income (Schlosser, 1997).

Although it is a seemingly innocent form of sexual contact, telephone sex has become a major problem. It is a difficult form of sexual exchange to control. Minors have easy access to these services, and the costs can add up. The media are full of stories of parents opening up their phone bills and being surprised by Junior's 900-number bill for hundreds of dollars. Also, pedophiles and other sex offenders often use Internet access to identify and lure their victims. They can gain access to potential victims by establishing relationships with phone sex providers to illegally trace their victim's telephone numbers through caller ID.

personal exploration activity
Is Sex Selling to You?

Most states have laws that forbid selling sex. But there are definitely no laws forbidding using sex to sell. You are constantly bombarded by ads using sex to grab your attention. This activity will help you increase your awareness of just how often sex is used to sell a product to you and help you decide whether you want to support the products using this tactic.

For the next month, every time you thumb through a magazine, look at the newspaper, or view any other print material that has advertisements, look for the ads that use sex to sell. The sex part may be in the form of a couple embracing, a sexy guy wearing no shirt, and so forth. Evaluate what they are trying to sell and whether the product is really related to the picture. Put a Post-it or some type of marker on the page with your evaluation and stack all evaluated material in one place. At the end of the month, look at all of the pages you have marked. Were the majority of ads just using sex to sell the product? Do you agree with this technique? If not, are these products you will avoid buying because of their blatant use of sex in a commercial way? Are these ads influencing the way you view sexuality?

Commercial Television

Two trends within commercial television programming are of note concerning the dissemination of sexually explicit material and messages: the relaxation of restrictions on presenting sexual themes (particularly regarding the spoken word) and the creation of music video. Commercial television closely regulates overt visual sexual programming.

Total frontal nudity and sexual behavior without clothes are prohibited. Partial nudity is regulated but has a much wider berth than it did 20 years ago.

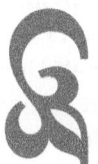

healthy sex hints 17.1

Television Rating Guide

In response to the 1996 Telecommunications Law, a voluntary committee made up of executives from the television and movie industries was established. In December 1997, the task force, led by Jack Valenti, the chief of the Motion Picture Association of America (MPAA), presented a set of guidelines to rate television programs.

Valenti's group presented ratings that are remarkably similar to those used in evaluating motion pictures. These, and the proposed TV ratings, evaluate programming by age-appropriateness. Those contesting such a rating system prefer a more content-based rating system similar to that used in Canada. The Canadian system evaluates programming based on the strength of content using a 1 to 3 scale on V (violent content), S (sexual content and nudity), and L (adult language). A program could get mixed ratings —L-1, V-3, or S-1—for instance.

These guidelines have sparked controversy among children's and parents' rights groups. The groups' major complaint centers on the ambiguity of the ratings, which are age, not content, based.

Sources: Bash (1997); Kent (1997); "U.S. TV Ratings System" (1996).

Shows such as *Baywatch* and the morning workout shows feature scantily clad lifeguards and athletes with bulging swimsuits and plunging tank tops. In soap operas, lovemaking is depicted but involves the participants in bed under the covers, or the camera cuts away as clothes begin to be shed. Although partial nudity is common, it is restricted to non-genital displays.

In 1997, under pressure from the federal government, the entertainment industry proposed a set of voluntary standards to rate television programming. The spoken word and sexual posturing while clothed are subject to much less regulation. Talk shows and soap operas are permitted to use all but the most graphic language (*fuck* is still banned, but *balls* and *screw,* among others, are permissible). Participants on panel talk shows and audience participation programs bare their soul while discussing everything from adultery to zoophilia.

The most unique addition to prime-time commercial television sex is the music video. This medium combines the power of music with implied and overt sexual themes. Undulating bodies (many partially clad) combine with seductive melodies and lyrics to offer a powerfully erotic presentation. In other cases, music combines with a kaleidoscope of disjointed violent images ranging from smashing guitars to drive-by shootings. Illicit drug use is often thrown into the mix, creating a unique mélange of sex, drugs, and music.

Cable Television, DVDs, and Videocassettes

A leading product that cable television subscribers request is pay-per-view and subscription sex services. The adult video market, personified by sex-on-cable providers such as Playboy, Spice, and the Adam and Eve Channel, grew from $521 million in 1994 to $664 million in 1995, with projections for continued growth ("Adult Video," 1995). In 2002, revenues from the Playboy Channel (the pay-TV Playboy service) surged by 30 percent, with sales exceeding $23 million. This surge in pay-TV services offset losses from Playboy's print and other operations (Devaney, 2002).

Recognizing the fortunes to be made in adult entertainment online, major corporations are going after these markets. For instance, General Motors earns over $150 million in revenue from adult channels on its Direct TV cable television venue. AT&T, which has withdrawn from the scandalous 900 pay telephone sex lines, is heavily invested in cable television. It handles several pay-per-view adult television channels, including the very profitable Playboy's Hot Network (Devaney, 2002).

The advent of cable television and home DVD/VCRs has almost single-handedly caused the near-extinction of the "porno movie theater." Cable television has literally brought the world of soft-core and hard-core pornography into Middle America's living room. Twenty years ago, viewing pornography entailed either a trip to the local X-rated movie house or threading a super-8 film into the old family projector, setting up the screen, and hoping kids (or parents) wouldn't discover you watching the movie.

Today, virtually every cable television service provider has at least one soft-core channel that serves up late-evening viewing of "non-penetrative" (penetration and ejaculation scenes have been edited out) versions of X-rated films. Many of the larger metropolitan-area cable television companies also offer X-rated (penetration and ejaculation are shown) channels for home viewing. These channels typically are offered for an extra charge (premium) that rarely exceeds $15 per month, thereby ensuring access to nearly all markets. In 1996, the Federal Telecommunications Law was passed, limiting the hours for airing these channels to between 10 P.M. and 6 A.M. All companies also are required to provide devices that deny transmission without a code that can be entered to activate the service.

The cost of the average DVD/VCR player has dropped to well below $200, putting it in the range of affordability for most households. The boom in DVD/VCR player sales of the 1980s and 1990s created a massive audience for marketing home movies. The fastest-growing segment of the home video market is the adult video consumer. The number of hard-core sex video rentals in the United States rose from 75 million in 1985 to 490 million in 1992. It reached an all-time high in 1996, with rentals of more than 665 million X-rated sex videos (Schlosser, 1997).

Purchases of adult videos in the United States approached that of rentals over the past decade. The X-rated video segment of the film industry is one of the most profitable and reliable forms of film production. In California alone, more than 8,000 new hard-core video titles are produced annually (Gardetta, 1988).

"Adult entertainment" has grown into a multibillion-dollar a year industry. In 2001, Americans rented more than 750 *million* adult films and watched millions more on cable and satellite TV and in hotel rooms (Devaney, 2002). The industry has prospered during the past 5 years, despite recessions, terrorism, and economic uncertainty. In the past few years, dozens of new studios have been popping up throughout California's San Fernando Valley, the seat of the adult film industry in the United States (Gardetta, 1998).

This dramatic rise in home video rentals and purchases has shifted the focus of consumption of these products from the seedy adult movie houses of 20 years ago to the home. It also has provided easier access for adolescent viewers.

Computer Sex

As we mentioned, more than half of U.S. households own at least one personal computer, and over 56 percent (over 30 million users) of Americans are Internet users. Most of these users are experienced PC owners who access the Internet with their home computers (Richards, 1997). Web TV (a type of Internet TV) and other non-PC Internet access devices introduced in the U.S. marketplace in 1998 are expected to add an additional 250,000 to 300,000 users. If this technology catches on, the average non-computer-literate person will have access to the World Wide Web and Internet (Richards, 1997).

The world of personal computers has opened up two primary access points to sexually oriented materials and adult-oriented Web site connections via the Internet and X-rated software. Until recently, the word *sex* was the most popular search term (it was supplanted by *MP3*) on the Internet (Lewis, 2001). Fisher and Barak (2002) report that the top eight Internet searches involve pornography.

Rimm's (1995) controversial study, "Marketing Pornography on the Information Superhighway," surveyed 917,410 sexually explicit pictures,

case study 17.4

Jon: Watching X-rated Videos

Jon, 18, single, gay, is white.

Jon is a college freshman in one of the author's online human sexuality classes. His written comments were composed in response to the author's queries concerning Jon's exposure to X-rated videos as an adolescent.

The first time I ever saw an X-rated video was over at my friend Tom's house. Tom had a collection of straight and gay porno and kept them hidden in the back of his closet. Tom invited me and a couple of other friends over one night and when his parents were out, we watched one. We watched a few videos on everything including fucking, oral, anal, group, straight, gay, and interracial sex.

It was kind of weird watching it with these guys. Nobody knew I was gay, and I got real turned on by the gay scenes but was able to disguise it because of all the other stuff on the tape. I made a copy of the tape and watched it until I wore it out. I must have jerked off a couple of hundred times to that tape.

Since then I have found an X-rated video store that has gay tapes and DVDs that I rent every once in a while. I have to be very careful because nobody knows I'm gay, and I've got to hide the stuff from my roommate. I like to watch the tapes and masturbate. I don't think there is anything wrong with this. The only thing I worry about is getting caught by my roommates who are straight.

Critical Thinking

Is Jon's use of X-rated videos a healthy way for him to explore his homosexuality or does it keep him from coming out as a gay man?

---

descriptions, short studies, and film clips available on the Internet. Critics of this study point out that Rimm didn't actually view or count actual images on the Internet. He studied dozens of private (available to subscribers only) adult bulletin boards sites and described how sexual images were described, *not* the images themselves.

From the organization of content on these private, adult bulletin boards, Rimm generalized to the Internet as a whole. This approach would be like, as Petersen (2002) puts it, studying a dozen adult bookstores in New York's Times Square and generalizing their inventory to *all* bookstores such as Barnes & Noble and Borders. In fact, for consenting (and often paying) adults, the Internet makes downloading hard-core pictures, movie clips, and stories easy.

Unfortunately, the Internet also provides access to hard-to-find materials that aren't readily available and are often illegal. This cornucopia of sexually explicit materials includes pedophilia, bondage, sadomasochism, and sex with animals (Elmer-Dewitti, 1995).

Internet-based sexually oriented materials are difficult to supervise. With more than 40 million sites (the number grows by thousands daily) and nearly universal access, the Internet provides global access to sexually oriented material. A consumer who has a connection to the Web can access sexually oriented chat rooms, still pictures (X-rated stills of anything

case study 17.5

Ed

Ed, 41, married, is white.

Ed, a continuing education student, recalls his response to finding an X-rated video in the VCR in the family room after a sleepover his 14-year-old son had the night before.

I was cleaning the basement family room. The VCR light was on, so I ejected the film and, much to my surprise, found an X-rated video in it. I figured my son and his friends had watched it the night before, so I talked with him about it when he came home from school. I asked him if it was his, and he said it was one of his friend's father's tapes. His buddy had brought it over for the guys to watch.

I told him that I was more upset over him leaving it in the basement where his 10-year-old brother could have viewed it than the fact that he had seen it. I asked him what he thought of the movie, and he told me that it was a real turn-on.

I reemphasized to him that his mother and I still didn't want him to begin having intercourse until he was older and found a girlfriend he cared about and it would be exclusive. I also reassured him that I understood his natural curiosity about sex and sexual behavior and that masturbation was an acceptable outlet. I also wanted to be sure that he understood that X-rated films are fantasy sex and that he shouldn't confuse what he saw on some of these tapes with reality. I explained that these tapes are designed to cater to our fantasies but that real sex between two people involves talking, negotiating, and caring.

He said he understood and didn't really expect that sex would be like the film. He said that some of the stuff on the film was too kinky for him anyway. I sometimes worry that my approach is too casual, but Ed is a very responsible boy and seems to treat girls with respect. I feel that if I make too big a deal out of this, it will become a forbidden-fruit deal and he'll want to watch them even more.

> ### Critical Thinking
> Is Ed helping or hurting his son's healthy sexual development in his approach to viewing X-rated materials?

desired, including kiddie porn), video clips (short sections of sex films), and live sex shows (the viewer becomes part of the audience from his or her living room) that can originate from anywhere around the globe.

A person can connect with a live sex show from Denmark, a sadist or masochist from Asia, or a housewife selling still pictures of herself engaging in fellatio with her husband in Australia. Although this may sound too good to be true to an adult who enjoys pornography, it can cause much concern for the average parent of a teenage son or daughter. Technology is available to block minors' access to adult Internet sites. These barriers, however, work only if parents and other adults using home PCs install them and check up on them regularly. Problems remain, however, even with these technological aids in place.

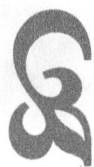

healthy sex hints 17.2

Computer Blocking Software

Several blocking software packages are available for use with personal computers to selectively block Internet sites that transmit sexual material intended for adults. These products average about $35 retail and must be installed on the computer's hard drive. Each works in a slightly different way.

PC Magazine rated seven products and found that no single screening tool will meet the needs of every user (Kunro, 1997). The tools ranged from simple to complex to install and use. The more complex software seems to provide more comprehensive blocking capability, allowing parents to control Web sites, chat rooms, e-mail, and other applications. Some allow parents to control the amount of time children spend online and to monitor the sites visited.

All of the tested products performed well in their intended functions. *PC Magazine* found, however, that a foolproof blocking software product is impossible to develop because of the subjective nature of what parents consider objectionable and the ever-changing nature of the Internet.

Nonetheless, these products do offer a tool to help parents monitor their children's computer activity. As with all software applications, parents must continually upgrade and monitor the products to ensure that they are performing at optimal efficiency.

Sources: Munro (1997); "Is Your Kid Caught Up in the Web?" (1997); "Guarding Young Web-Surfers" (1997).

Computer chat rooms share many of the characteristics of telephone sex lines. They allow intimate but non-personal interaction over telephone lines. Users of computer chat rooms sit at a keyboard and "chat" by typing in messages and sharing them with other users in the "room." The relative safety of sitting at a keyboard creates an environment in which "chatter" is often personal and graphic in its sexual content (Topp, 1997).

Software

The production of computer software has undergone a renaissance over the past few years. The primitive, sexually oriented software of the 1980s, which featured cartoonlike animation, has given way to the crystal-clear CD-ROM-based X-rated interactive software of the 1990s. The newest software features sound, color, lifelike graphics, and the ability to move the characters into a limitless variety of sexually explicit interactions. Software technology is increasing in sophistication and quality with such speed that, by the time this page is printed, the X-rated software on the shelves of your local computer or "adult" store will be outdated.

X-rated and soft-core software is available in stores, through the mail, or can be downloaded directly onto a personal computer. It is a huge industry that is difficult to supervise. Innovative software peddlers market their wares through chat rooms on the Internet, computer and sex magazines, and shareware (public domain software that is exchanged without cost) (Silberg, 1996).

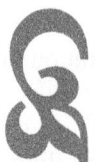

healthy sex hints 17.3

Safe Internet Use

The Internet offers the world at your fingertips. It personifies the best and the worst of technological innovation. With a little common sense and some specific safeguards, it can be a great source of sexual information and materials. The following tips can help you surf safely.

1. Install site-blocking software. Some things on the Internet are best kept away from children.
2. Monitor your family's use of the Internet. Computers were never intended to take the place of live human interaction.
3. Establish online guidelines, and limit the amount of time children stay online.
4. Think of the computer as you would a television set. You don't want to (or want your family to) spend hours mesmerized in front of the screen. Take a walk; shoot baskets; do something interactive, such as playing Scrabble or cooking together.
5. Never give out your real name and address over the Internet, for any reason (especially on chat lines).
6. Never agree to unsupervised personal meetings with people you "meet" over the Internet. Let the person know you will meet in a neutral public place and that you will be bringing a friend.
7. If you use online sex services (view erotic materials, chat, and so forth), realize that this is fantasy sex. The reason it is a turn-on relates in part to the anonymity of the sex.
8. Like all fantasy sex, recognize that you may not want to actually experience what you discuss or view on the Internet.
9. If someone you met on the Internet has found out who you are and where you live and is trying to establish contact with you against your will, call the police immediately. Internet use is not illegal, but stalking is.
10. If you find yourself becoming addicted, disconnect, drop your online service, and get professional help.

Effects of Pornography and Sexually Explicit Material

As long as pornography has been available, there have been attempts to regulate it, citing that it leads to a variety of social maladies including rape, sexual harassment, degradation and exploitation of women, and weakening of the moral fiber of America. Two presidential commissions on pornography and obscenity have been impaneled over the past 25 years to examine the effects of viewing such material.

The first commission was designated in 1970 by President Richard Nixon. The commission was charged with examining whether exposure to pornography could cause personal harm or lead to sexual violence. It found that exposure to pornography and obscene materials did not cause personal harm or contribute to sexual violence.

The second commission, impaneled by President Ronald Reagan in the early 1980s, had a similar charge. The Meese Commission found that exposure to nonviolent pornography was not harmful and did not lead to sexual aggression and violence (Attorney General's Commission on Pornography, 1986; Petersen, 1999).

A secondary finding of the commission, however, touched off a great deal of controversy among human sexuality professionals. This finding was the claim that the most prevalent forms of pornography were violent in nature and that exposure to this material had a causal relationship to sexual violence.

℘ Spiritual Wellness ℘

Our nation's *moral fabric* is a term used by all presidents (including George W. Bush as well as Nixon and Reagan) to describe our standards as a society. It refers to our values, attitudes, and beliefs about moral issues that reflect our spiritual health as a nation. Religious leaders and others concerned with the moral fabric of America claim that the widespread availability of pornography, both online and through other sources, reflects our moral bankruptcy as a society. Our spirituality, they say, suffers when sex becomes a commodity instead of an intimate bond that connects people through love and commitment. Those who represent the opposing view cite the absence of evidence connecting greater sexual availability and permissiveness with moral decay.

These claims were instantly refuted by sex researchers and professional organizations (Board of Directors, 1987). Researchers argued that studies of the sexual content of samples of pornographic material revealed that between 4 and 16 percent contained violent themes or scenes depicting violence (Slade, 1986). Professional organizations decried the supposed causal link between viewing violent pornography and sexual violence, citing the lack of substantiating evidence within the commission's report or in the professional literature.

℘ Intellectual Wellness ℘

One positive outcome of greater accessibility to sexual resources coupled with the technological innovations of the past decade is the incredible explosion in information technology. Our ability to conduct research, gather information, process what we've found, and share resources has never been better. Average people working from home on a personal computer can tap into the greatest minds of our time without leaving home. This has the potential to greatly enhance our intellectual well-being. We have unprecedented access to information about any facet of sexuality, in the privacy of our own home.

Personal Assessment

Private Lives of Public People

1. Do the media (or anyone) have the right to divulge a private citizen's personal sexual information under any circumstances?   yes _____ no _____

2. Do the media (or any person) have the right to divulge a public figure's (person running for office, sports figure, entertainer, and so forth) personal sexual information under any circumstance? yes _____ no _____

   If you answered yes to question 1 or 2, please describe those circumstances.

   _____

3. Does a person's personal sexuality influence his or her professional behavior?
   yes _____ no _____

4. If you answered yes to question 3, please describe how.

   _____

5. Should some sexual things be kept private regardless of the circumstances?
   yes _____ no _____

6. If you answered yes to question 5, please describe these things and why you feel this way.

   _____

Cyber-Sex Addiction Screening Test (c-SAAT)

This is an assessment developed by Shannon O'Hara, a marriage and family therapist from Los Angeles. It is designed to assess sexually compulsive Internet behavior. More than three positive answers indicate a possible need to seek help from a professional counselor specializing in this area.

1. Spending increasing amounts of time online focused on sexual or romantic intrigue or involvement

2. Involvement in multiple romantic or sexual affairs in chat rooms

3. Not considering online sexual or romantic "affairs" to be a possible violation of spousal/partnership commitments

4. Failed attempts to cut back on the frequency of online or Internet sexual and romantic involvement or interaction

5. Online use interferes with work (tired or late due to previous nights use, online while at work)

6. Online use interferes with primary relationships (minimizing or lying to partners about online activities, spending less time with family, partners)

7. Intense engagement in collecting Internet pornography

8. Engaging in fantasy online acts or experiences that would be illegal if carried out (for instance, rape, child molestation)

9. Decreased social or family interactive time due to online fantasy involvements

10. Being secretive or lying about the amount of time spent online or type of sexual/ romantic fantasy activities carried out online

11. Engaging with sexual or romantic partners met online, while also involved in marital or other primary relationship

12. Increasing complaints and concern from family or friends about the amount of time spent online

13. Frequently becoming angry or extremely irritable when asked to give up online involvement to engage with partners, family, or friends

14. Primary focus of sexual or romantic life becomes increasingly related to computer activity (including pornographic CD-ROM use)

Thought Questions

1. How are pornography, obscenity, and erotica different?

2. What is the significance of the Gary Hart scandal in establishing a new *zeitgeist* concerning the media and sexuality?

3. What impact has technology had on the availability of sexuality explicit material and services?

4. What are the arguments for and against legalization of prostitution?

5. What is Peter McWilliams's position on sex laws?

6. What are some of the sexual problems associated with the Internet, and how can they be addressed?

Test Yourself

1. Madonna's sexual significance as a media icon is that
   a. she brought the me-generation's pursuit of sex, passion, and self-fulfillment into mainstream culture.
   b. she had 10 platinum albums in the 1970s.
   c. she was the first pop singer to appear nude in *Playboy.*
   d. she was the first female pop singer to publish a book on S&M.

2. Gary Hart's contribution to using sex to sell newspapers, magazines, and television advertising is that
   a. he was the first politician to be caught in bed with his secretary.
   b. he was the first national-level politician to have his private sexual activities aired by mainstream media.
   c. he was the first presidential candidate to have sex with a campaign worker.
   d. he was the first national-level politician to father a child out of wedlock.

3. Calvin Klein was one of the first designers to use ____, the intentional blurring of gender roles in national advertising campaigns.
   a. bisexuality
   b. homosexuality
   c. androgyny
   d. omnisexuality

4. Matt Drudge ushered in a new era of media coverage of the sexual exploits of public figures with his ____ coverage of the Bill Clinton–Monica Lewinsky affair.
   a. sordid
   b. satellite
   c. documentary
   d. Internet

5. According to Petersen, Americans' pursuit of sexuality-related goods and services has always
   a. driven technological innovation.
   b. lagged behind technological innovation.
   c. been a function of good economic times.
   d. been driven by fear of law.

6. Obscene materials are generally illegal. The Supreme Court has long believed that the best judge of obscenity is
   a. the Supreme Court.
   b. local religious leaders.
   c. local community standards.
   d. the U.S. Postal Service.
7. Prostitution is legal ____ in the United States.
   a. in all states
   b. in Nevada
   c. in New York, California, and Nevada
   d. nowhere
8. Which of the following statements best characterizes the selling of sexually explicit materials and services online?
   a. It represents a small percentage of e-commerce.
   b. It represents a small and declining percentage of e-commerce.
   c. It represents a large but stable percentage of e-commerce.
   d. It represents the largest and most rapidly growing percentage of e-commerce.
9. The neighborhood pornographic movie theater
   a. has been experiencing a resurgence with a growing adult film industry.
   b. has all but disappeared due to the availability of sexually explicit materials available online and on cable television.
   c. has experienced a slow steady growth since 2000.
   d. is illegal in most states.
10. The Meese Commission, impaneled under President Reagan, found that exposure to non-violent pornography
   a. was harmful and prevented normal sexual development.
   b. was a leading cause of the increase in date rape.
   c. was the second leading cause of rape.
   d. was not harmful and did not lead to sexual aggression and violence.

Web Resources

National Task Force on Prostitution
www.bayswan.org/index.html

The Prostitutes' Education Network site, offering information about health, legislation, and other issues affecting prostitutes and sex workers. Provides many links to prostitution-related issues.

Blue Ribbon Campaign for Online Free Speech
www.eff.org/blueribbon.html

A site sponsored by the Electronic Frontier Foundation (EFF), a movement that opposes censorship on the Web. A section on the latest news from the government cites links for more information.

Sex, Censorship, and the Internet
www.eff.org/CAF/cafuiuc.html

The Electronic Frontier Foundation (EFF) is a non-profit, nonpartisan organization working to protect fundamental civil liberties and freedom of expression on Internet. This site is geared to college-related Internet freedom issues.

Sex Laws On-Line
www.geocities.com/CapitolHill/2269

This site is a gateway to current sex laws in the United States and in other countries.

References

Adult video, cable market surges. (1995). *Broadcasting & Cable, 125*(13) 47.

Ashe, D. (2009). Dani.cash Frequently Asked questions. http://www.dannicash.com/info/faq_unlogged.cfm

Attorney General's Commission on Pornography. (1986). *Report on pornography and obscenity.* Washington, DC: U.S. Department of Justice.

Bash, A. (1997, August 20). Age-based TV ratings slated as first planned. *USA Today On-line* [Online].

Board of Directors of the Society for the Scientific Study of Sex. (1987). SSSS responds to the U.S. Attorney General's Commission on Pornography. *Journal of Sex Research, 23*(2), 284–285.

Bradlee, N. C. (1997). The Bradlee files. *Newsweek, 126*(13), 82–88.

Brown, J. D. (2002). Mass media influences on sexuality. *Journal of Sex Research, 38*(4), 42–45.

Call for a crackdown on the 900 billing charade [editorial]. (1994). *Business Communications Review, 24*(5), 12.

Diamond, M., & Dannemiller, J. E. (1989). Pornography and community standards in Hawaii: Comparisons with other states. *Archives of Sexual Behavior, 18,* 6.

Edwards, M. (1996). The Net and the Web: Unlimited potential to communicate sexuality issues. *SIECUS Report, 25*(1), 2–4.

Elmer-Dewitti, P. (1995, July). "On a screen near you": Cyberporn. *Time, 146*(1).

Family Safe Media. (2009). Pornography Statistics. http://familysafemedia.com/pornography_ statistics.html#anchor1

Fisher, W. A., & Barak, A. (2002). Internet pornography: A psychosocial perspective on Internet sexuality. *Journal of Sex Research, 38*(4), 312–323.

Friedman, T. (2007). The World is Flat; Release 3.0. New York: Picador.

Gardetta, D. (1998, November). The LUST tycoons. *Los Angeles Magazine,* p. 141.

Guarding young Web-surfers: Don't count on special software to protect kids' privacy. (1997 September). *Consumer Reports, 62*(9), 17.

Heavy breathing: Phone sex. (1994). *Economist, 332*(7874), 71.

Hite, S. (1976). *The Hite report: A nationwide study on female sexuality.* New York: Macmillan.

Hunt, M. M. (1974). *Sexual behavior in the 1970's.* Chicago: Playboy.

Is your kid caught up in the Web? How to find the best parts and avoid the others. (1997, May). *Consumer Reports, 65*(5), 27–32.

Kaplan, J. (1995). The Triumph of Calvinism. (September 18), New York, 46–57.

Kent, R. E. (1907). Television ratings. *FCC-V-chip Homepage.* Available via e-mail: rekent@eecs. wsu.edu.

Lagnado, I. (1997). Is the PC party really over? *HFN: The Weekly Network for the Home Furnishing Network, 71*(3), 10.

Lewis, E. (2001, June 28). Sex education: Industry trends or event. *New Media Age,* pp. 47–56.

Masters, W. H., & Johnson, V. E. (1966). *Human sexual response.* Boston: Little, Brown.

McWilliams, P. (1998). *Ain't nobody's business if you do: The absurdity of consensual crimes in a free country.* Santa Monica, CA: Prelude.

Munro, K. (1997, April 8). Filtering utilities. *PC Magazine, 16*(7), 235–238.

Mustanski, B. S. (2002). Getting wired: Exploiting the Internet for the collection of valid sexuality data. *Journal of Sex Research, 38*(4), 292–301.

O'Kane, M. (1994, March 21). All in a night's work: Male escorts. *Guardian,* pp. 2–4.

Petersen, J. R. (1999). *The century of sex: Playboy's history of the sexual revolution 1990–1999.* New York: Grove.

Prostitutes' Education Network. (2003). Home page [Online]. Available: www.bayswan.org/index. html.

Richards, K. (1997). PCs on the Web: Researcher forecasts sales drive. *HFN: The Weekly Newspaper for the Home Furnishing Network, 71*(1), 79–81.

Rimm, M. (1995, June). Marketing pornography on the information superhighway. *Georgetown Law Journal, 83,* 1849–1934.

Roberts, D. (2000). Media and youth: Access, exposure, and privatization. *Journal of Adolescent Health, 27*(2), 814.

Schlosser, E. (1997, February 10). Pornography. *U.S. News & World Report,* pp. 43–50.

Seitz, P. (2003). Personal Computer Still Eludes A Fifth of U.S. Households. *Investor's Business Daily.* http://biz.yahoo.com/ibd/040109/tech_1. html

Shrage, L. (1996, Spring). Prostitution and the case for decriminalization. *Dissent.*

Silberg, L. (1996). Hot for your home PC. *HFN: The Weekly Newspaper for the Home Furnishing Network, 70*(48), 47–49.

Slade, J. (1986). Violence in the hard-core pornographic film: A historical survey. *Journal of Communication, 34*(3), 148–163.

Stern, S. E., & Handel, A. D. (2002). Sexuality and mass media: The historical context of psychology's reaction to sexuality on the Internet. *Journal of Sex Research, 38*(4), 283–291.

Topp, D. (1997). Virtual immorality [Online]. Available: walraven@iadfw.net and http:// web2.airmail.net/walraven/esquire.htm

U.S. Department of Labor. (2003). Cable and other pay television services [Online]. Bureau of Labor Statistics. Available: http://stats.bls.gov/ oco/cg/cgs017.htm

U.S. TV ratings system almost finalized. (1996, November 26). *Toronto Star.*

index